Innovative Teaching Strategies

in Nursing

and Related Health Professions

WY
18
F84
2017

Edited by

Martha J. Bradshaw, PhD, RN

Consultant
Professional Writing
Nursing Education
Dallas, Texas

Beth L. Hultquist, PhD, RN, CNE

Clinical Assistant Professor
Louise Herrington School of Nursing
Baylor University
Dallas, Texas

JONES & BARTLETT
LEARNING

World Headquarters
Jones & Bartlett Learning
5 Wall Street
Burlington, MA 01803
978-443-5000
info@jblearning.com
www.jblearning.com

Jones & Bartlett Learning books and products are available through most bookstores and online booksellers. To contact Jones & Bartlett Learning directly, call 800-832-0034, fax 978-443-8000, or visit our website, www.jblearning.com.

Substantial discounts on bulk quantities of Jones & Bartlett Learning publications are available to corporations, professional associations, and other qualified organizations. For details and specific discount information, contact the special sales department at Jones & Bartlett Learning via the above contact information or send an email to specialsales@jblearning.com.

The content, statements, views, and opinions herein are the sole expression of the respective authors and not that of Jones & Bartlett Learning, LLC. Reference herein to any specific commercial product, process, or service by trade name, trademark, manufacturer, or otherwise does not constitute or imply its endorsement or recommendation by Jones & Bartlett Learning, LLC and such reference shall not be used for advertising or product endorsement purposes. All trademarks displayed are the trademarks of the parties noted herein. *Innovative Teaching Strategies in Nursing and Related Health Professions, Seventh Edition* is an independent publication and has not been authorized, sponsored, or otherwise approved by the owners of the trademarks or service marks referenced in this product.

There may be images in this book that feature models; these models do not necessarily endorse, represent, or participate in the activities represented in the images. Any screenshots in this product are for educational and instructive purposes only. Any individuals and scenarios featured in the case studies throughout this product may be real or fictitious, but are used for instructional purposes only.

The authors, editor, and publisher have made every effort to provide accurate information. However, they are not responsible for errors, omissions, or for any outcomes related to the use of the contents of this book and take no responsibility for the use of the products and procedures described. Treatments and side effects described in this book may not be applicable to all people; likewise, some people may require a dose or experience a side effect that is not described herein. Drugs and medical devices are discussed that may have limited availability controlled by the Food and Drug Administration (FDA) for use only in a research study or clinical trial. Research, clinical practice, and government regulations often change the accepted standard in this field. When consideration is being given to use of any drug in the clinical setting, the healthcare provider or reader is responsible for determining FDA status of the drug, reading the package insert, and reviewing prescribing information for the most up-to-date recommendations on dose, precautions, and contraindications, and determining the appropriate usage for the product. This is especially important in the case of drugs that are new or seldom used.

Production Credits

VP, Executive Publisher: David D. Cella
Executive Editor: Amanda Martin
Associate Acquisitions Editor: Rebecca Stephenson
Editorial Assistant: Lauren Vaughn
Production Editor: Vanessa Richards
Senior Marketing Manager: Jennifer Scherzay
Product Fulfillment Manager: Wendy Kilborn
Composition: S4Carlisle Publishing Services

Cover Design: Scott Moden
Director of Rights & Media: Joanna Lundeen
Rights & Media Specialist: Wes DeShano
Media Development Editor: Troy Liston
Cover Image: © art_of_sun/Shutterstock
Printing and Binding: Edwards Brothers Malloy
Cover Printing: Edwards Brothers Malloy

Library of Congress Cataloging-in-Publication Data

Names: Bradshaw, Martha J., editor. | Hultquist, Beth L., editor.
Title: Innovative teaching strategies in nursing and related health
    professions / edited by Martha J. Bradshaw, Beth L. Hultquist.
Description: Seventh edition. | Burlington, Massachusetts: Jones & Bartlett
    Learning, [2017] | Includes bibliographical references and index.
Identifiers: LCCN 2016009603 | ISBN 9781284107074 (pbk.)
Subjects: | MESH: Education, Nursing—methods | Teaching—methods
Classification: LCC RT71 | NLM WY 18 | DDC 610.73071—dc23
LC record available at http://lccn.loc.gov/2016009603

6048

Printed in the United States of America
20 19 18 17 16   10 9 8 7 6 5 4 3 2 1

Contents

■ Section II: Educational Use of Technology   93

■ Section III: Teaching in Structured Settings   141

Foreword

There are only a few books in nursing education that have become classics, and *Innovative Teaching Strategies in Nursing*, now in its seventh edition, is one of them. In every edition of this book, the authors have added new content to keep health professions educators up to date with new teaching approaches based on evidence. This book will guide both novice and experienced educators in academic and clinical settings in selecting and using varied teaching methods.

Selecting teaching methods for a course is an important decision for educators. In choosing methods for teaching in the classroom, online environment, clinical setting, or laboratory, the teacher needs to consider—above all else—the specific learning outcomes to be achieved and the needs of the students. Although there are other factors that influence selection of teaching approaches, such as time for learning, resources, and student and teacher preferences, the learning outcomes and student needs must take priority. This book helps educators make good choices about teaching approaches that consider the learning outcomes, characteristics, and differences among students that can affect their learning, and the environment in which the learning takes place. To make those choices, one needs to understand learning processes and the potential impact of student characteristics on both learning and teaching, which are discussed in the first section of this book.

The use of technology in teaching has expanded at a rapid pace, and educators in the health professions need to understand how to integrate technology into their teaching. The goal is not to use the newest technology because it is available, but instead to assess if that technology will help students learn better and develop their skills and competencies more effectively. Many types of technology allow students to be actively involved in their own learning, and this is one of the reasons to read the chapters on multimedia, teaching in online environments, and using social media in this new edition of the book.

One of the goals of this book, and why I think it is a critical resource for both novice and experienced educators, is to describe varied teaching methods for use in the classroom, simulation and learning laboratories, and clinical settings. You will learn about many teaching strategies you can use when working with students face-to-face or online, or when teaching in other settings. The authors present evidence to support each teaching method and guidelines for implementing it with students.

Teaching is more than selecting and using various methods to guide learning. Health professions educators need to be continually evaluating whether students are learning and if changes are needed in teaching approaches. The book includes chapters to help readers understand the evaluation process, how to give good feedback to students, and other concepts of evaluation that are important when teaching in nursing and other health fields.

This book is intended to assist educators to select the best teaching methods and provide quality education across settings. With this reference, teachers in all types of health professions programs and those working with staff in clinical settings will have, under one cover, a resource to guide teaching. This is a "must read" book for all educators.

Marilyn H. Oermann, PhD, RN, ANEF, FAAN
Thelma M. Ingles Professor of Nursing
Director of Evaluation and Educational Research
Duke University School of Nursing
Durham, North Carolina

Preface

This edition of *Innovative Teaching Strategies in Nursing and Related Health Professions* continues the theme of interdisciplinary collaboration in health professions education. The need to capitalize on the contributions of numerous healthcare professionals is increasingly important in light of the current, complex healthcare system. Education has a knowledge base that crosses over disciplinary lines, and we need to understand that base in order to be effective in our work. The strategies presented are timely, are used by seasoned educators, and consider both the teachers and the learners. Strategies presented are for use in structured (classroom or online) settings, clinical practice lab settings, or patient care clinical practice settings (unstructured).

This text incorporates educational principles and techniques to encourage and advance learning for students in all higher education settings, at both the graduate and undergraduate levels. Learning is the focus, and educators can choose strategies that best address the learning needs of students in their professions. The diversity of learners continues to increase at all levels of higher education, so strategies for recognizing and working with a diverse student population are included throughout this book.

As technology continues to rapidly grow and evolve, it is not possible to present all methods and versions that are available; instead, new and different ways to utilize technology to enhance learning are presented. Educators need to remember that technology is a means, not an end, to enhance teaching effectiveness. It is the individual teacher who makes decisions, based upon best educational principles, about which strategy or form of technology to use in order to meet learning goals of both educators and students. The educational setting also may determine which technologies are most effective. Faculty certainly have input regarding the purchase and development of technologies in their settings when they are aware of how these technologies can be used to increase learning. Some students grasp the use of technology quickly and can benefit from the incorporation of technology in their learning, but other students are not as comfortable and may need additional faculty support to promote a positive outcome. Additionally, whereas technology may enhance immediate learning, educators need to continually assess retention of valuable information and skills.

Evaluation of learning is addressed in the chapters on concept mapping and the clinical pathway, and this edition contains a new chapter on how to give evaluation feedback. Other chapters provide information and strategies to use in relation to programmatic evaluation, as well as finding and evaluating resources for use in planning and teaching.

It is our intent that this book will be a useful resource for current and future educators in all health professions, so that they may become aware of and utilize strategies that encourage students to enhance and deepen their learning.

Martha J. Bradshaw
Beth L. Hultquist

The editors wish to acknowledge our wonderful chapter authors. These contributors have developed scholarly, timely, and helpful strategies that any health professions faculty can implement in their own classrooms. Throughout the process of preparing this edition, our chapter authors have been prompt, cooperative, and dedicated to producing excellent work. We hope our readers will see evidence of their caring and valuable contributions to educational practices.

I would like to personally thank my family for their continued support, especially my parents, Jim and Wanda Cantrell, for always believing in me. My students deserve a large portion of gratitude. Thank you for allowing me to be part of your path.

Beth L. Hultquist

Contributors

Stephanie S. Allen, MS, RN, CNS
Clinical Nurse Specialist
Children's Medical Center Dallas
Dallas, Texas

Catherine Bailey, CNE/PhD, MS, RN
College of Nursing
Texas Woman's University
Dallas, Texas

Martha J. Bradshaw, PhD, RN
Consultant
Professional Writing
Nursing Education
Dallas, Texas

LaDonna L. Christian, MSN, APRN-BC
Director of the Dotson Bridge and Mentoring Program
Simmons College
Boston, Massachusetts

Liliana Coman, BHSc(PT), MSc, MD
School of Rehabilitation Science
McMaster University
Hamilton, Ontario, Canada

Shelley F. Conroy, EdD, MS, RN, CNE
Louise Herrington School of Nursing
Baylor University
Dallas, Texas

Mariana D'Amico, EdD, OTR/L, BCP, FAOTA
Department of Occupational Therapy, OTD Program
Nova Southeastern University
Tampa, Florida

Brian M. French, RN, MS, BC
The Institute for Patient Care
Massachusetts General Hospital
Boston, Massachusetts

Shanti Freundlich, BA, MSLIS
Online and Educational Technology Librarian
MCPHS University
Boston, Massachusetts

Miriam Greenspan, RN, MS
Brigham and Women's Hospital
Boston, Massachusetts

Beth L. Hultquist, PhD, RN, CNE
Louise Herrington School of Nursing
Baylor University
Dallas, Texas

Lynn Jaffe, ScD, OTR/L, FAOTA
Florida Gulf Coast University
Fort Meyers, Florida

Kimberly Leighton, PhD, RN, ANEF
DeVry Medical International
Institute for Research & Clinical Strategy
Iselin, New Jersey

Arlene J. Lowenstein, PhD, RN
Simmons College
Boston, Massachusetts

Jennifer E. Mackey, MA, CCC-SLP
Department of Communication Sciences and Disorders
MGH Institute of Health Professions
Boston, Massachusetts

Hendrika Maltby, PhD, RN, FACN
College of Nursing and Health Sciences
University of Vermont
Burlington, Vermont

Gail Matthews-DeNatale, PhD
Emmanuel College
Boston, Massachusetts

Lesley Maxwell
Department of Communication Sciences and Disorders
MGH Institute of Health Professions
Boston, Massachusetts

Marjorie Nicholas, PhD
Department of Communication Sciences and Disorders
School of Health and Rehabilitation Sciences
MGH Institute of Health Professions
Boston, Massachusetts

Gregory G. Passmore, PhD, CNMT
Georgia Regents University
Augusta, Georgia

Lyn (Lynda) Pesta, RN, MSN
Louise Herrington School of Nursing
Baylor University
Dallas, Texas

Lyn (Llewellyn) S. Prater, RN, MSN, PhD
Louise Herrington School of Nursing
Baylor University
Dallas, Texas

Jenn Salfi, PhD, RN
Department of Nursing
Brock University
St. Catharines, Ontario, Canada

Patricia Solomon, PhD, PT
School of Rehabilitation Science
McMaster University
Hamilton, Ontario, Canada

Lori A. Spies, PhD, RN, NP-C
Louise Herrington School of Nursing
Baylor University
Dallas, Texas

Deborah Tapler, RN, CNE/BSN, MSN, PhD
College of Nursing
Texas Woman's University
Dallas, Texas

Karen H. Teeley, MS, RN, AHC-BC, CNE
Simmons College
Boston, Massachusetts

Cheryl A. Tucker, MSN, RN, CNE
Louise Herrington School of Nursing
Baylor University
Dallas, Texas

Barbara C. Woodring, EdD, RN, CPN
Dean and Professor, Retired
Byrdine F. Lewis School of Nursing
Georgia State University
Atlanta, Georgia

SECTION I

Introduction

Creating an effective learning environment is not an easy task in today's world, and it is even more complex in education programs for the health professions. Students entering the fields of health care are extremely diverse, both in age ranges and life experiences. Traditional undergraduates, entering college directly from high school, interact with a vast variety of nontraditional students returning to school after experiences in the workplace and/or having completed previous college degrees. Educators are challenged to recognize different learning needs and respect and utilize the knowledge and experiences that students bring to the learning settings. The teaching strategies and examples throughout this text may be adapted for use in a variety of situations, at undergraduate and graduate levels, taking into account the diversity of learning needs.

The chapters in Section I provide a foundation for understanding, selecting, and adapting specific teaching strategies to the educator's setting and student body. The contributors provide a theory base for learning and applied clinical reasoning, and also bring in various dimensions of effective learning that include creativity, humor, and exploration of varying, sometimes juxtaposed, viewpoints and ways of processing information.

CHAPTER 1

Effective Learning: What Teachers Need to Know

Martha J. Bradshaw
Beth L. Hultquist

Knowing is a process, not a product.

—Jerome Bruner (1966)[1]

What brings about effective learning in health professions students? Is it insight on the part of the student? A powerful clinical experience? Perhaps it is the dynamic, creative manner in which the nurse educator presents information or structures the learning experience. Effective learning likely is the culmination of all of these factors, in addition to others. In this chapter, dimensions of effective learning are explored as a foundation for use of the innovative teaching strategies presented in subsequent chapters. The monumental growth in the use of technology has definitely changed the teaching–learning environment. Learners also have changed regarding how they access and use information and their expectations regarding feedback. The field of health professions education is experiencing a difference in learners, yet how individuals learn is essentially unchanged.

■ Theories of Learning

We approach learning individually, based largely on cognitive style (awareness of and means of taking in relevant information) and preferred approaches to learning, or learning style. Some students are aware of their style and preference, some gain insight into these patterns as they become more sophisticated learners, and some students have never been guided to determine how they learn best.

Theoretical underpinnings classify learning as behavioristic or cognitive. Behavioristic learning was the earliest pattern identified through research.

---

[1]Bruner, J. S. (1966). *Toward a theory of instruction*. Cambridge, MA: The Belknap Press of Harvard University Press. Copyright © 1966 by the President and Fellows of Harvard College.

Psychologists such as Skinner and Thorndike described learning as a change in behavior and used stimulus response actions as an example. Subsequent theorists have described more complex forms of behaviorist learning. Bandura's (1977) theory of social learning describes human learning as coming from others through observation, imitation, and reinforcement. We learn from society, and we learn to be social. This type of learning is evident when we describe the need to socialize students to the health professions.

Robert Gagne (1968) formulated suggestions for sequencing of instruction, conditions by which learning takes place, and outcomes of learning, or categories in which human learning occurs. These learning categories are based on a hierarchical arrangement of learning theories, moving from simple to complex learning, and include intellectual and motor skills, verbal information, cognitive strategies, and attitudes. For example, within the category of intellectual skills are the following stages:

- *Discrimination learning*: Distinguishing differences, so as to respond appropriately
- *Concept learning*: Detecting similarities, so as to understand common characteristics
- *Rule learning*: Combination of two or more concepts, as a basis for action in new situations

Gagne's ideas seem to combine behaviorism and cognitive theories. Use of behaviorism in nursing education was especially popular in the 1970s and early 1980s through the use of concrete, measurable, specific behavioral objectives. Even though nursing education has moved away from the concrete methods of learning and evaluation, use of the hierarchical arrangement is seen in curriculum development and learning outcomes.

Cognitive theories address the perceptual aspect of learning. Cognitive learning results in the development of perceptions and insight—also called *gestalt*—that bring about a change in thought patterns (causing one to think, "Aha") and related actions. Jerome Bruner (1966) described cognitive learning as processes of conceptualization and categorization. He contended that intellectual development includes awareness of one's own thinking, the ability to recognize and deal with several alternatives and sequences, and the ability to prioritize. Bruner also saw the benefit of discovery learning to bring about insights. Ausubel's (1968) assimilation theory focuses on meaningful learning, in which the individual develops a more complex cognitive structure by associating new meanings with old ones that already exist within the learner's frame of reference. Ausubel's theory relies heavily on the acquisition of previous knowledge. These principles are useful for introducing the new student to the healthcare environment by relating information to what the student knows about health and illness. The same principles are fundamental to curriculum development, based upon transition from simple to complex situations. Having a good grasp of what is known is extremely helpful as learners move into new or unknown patient situations. This can be seen in the chapters on problem-based learning, clinical reasoning, and concept mapping.

Gardner's theory of multiple intelligences recognizes cognition as more than knowledge acquisition. Based on his definition of *intelligence* as "the ability to solve problems or fashion products that are valued in more than one setting" (Gardner & Hatch, 1990, p. 5), Gardner and Hatch have described the following seven forms of intelligence:

1. *Linguistic:* Related to written and spoken words and language, and use and meaning of language(s)
2. *Musical/rhythmic:* Based on sensitivity to rhythm and beat, recognition of tonal patterns and pitch, and appreciation of musical expression
3. *Logical/mathematical:* Related to inductive and deductive reasoning, abstractions, and discernment of numerical patterns
4. *Visual/spatial:* Ability to visualize an object or to create internal (mental) images, and thus able to transform or re-create the image
5. *Bodily kinesthetic.* The taking in and processing of knowledge through use of bodily sensations; learning is accomplished through physical movement or use of body language
6. *Interpersonal:* Emphasizes communication and interpersonal relationships, recognition of mood, temperament, and other behaviors
7. *Intrapersonal:* Related to inner thought processes, such as reflection and metacognition; includes spiritual awareness and self-knowledge (Gardner & Hatch, 1990)

Some educational programs use assessment tools based upon the work of Gardner and Hatch or similar assessments to guide incoming students on their approaches to learning and to better direct study skills. Faculty can benefit from this information as well and will find that student performance, as a group, is enhanced when a variety of teaching strategies are used. As an example, Slater, Lujan, and DiCarlo (2007) found that among first-year medical students, the females were more diverse in their sensory modalities and thus preferred multiple forms of information presentation.

Cognitive theories addressing learning stages appropriate for college students include Perry's (1970) model of intellectual and ethical development. This model recognizes the following four nonstatic stages in which students progress: (1) dualism (black versus white), (2) multiplicity (diversity and tolerance), (3) relativism (decision made by reasoned support), and (4) commitment to relativism (recognition of value set for decision making). Perry's ideas can be used to explain how critical thinking is developed over time.

A related behavior pattern that can be associated with success in professional education is categorized as executive functions (Lesaca, 2001). *Executive functions* are mental activities that are related to internal self-control and ability to employ goal-directed behavior. These functions then lead the individual to problem-solving ability and flexibility. Consequently, use of executive functions promotes better study skills and enhances the ability to apply content knowledge to purposeful, professional actions.

■ Approaches to Learning

Emerging from learning theories are descriptions of preferred styles or approaches to learning. Categorized as cognitive styles and learning styles, these approaches to learning are the ways individuals acquire knowledge, and are concerned more with form or process than content (Miller & Babcock, 1996). *Cognitive style* deals with information processing: the natural, unconscious internal process concerned with thinking and memory. It is the stable and enduring manner in which an individual organizes and handles information. The most common example of cognitive style is Witkin and colleagues' field-dependent–field-independent style (Witkin, Moore, Goodenough, & Cox, 1977). The field-dependent–field-independent style describes one's field of perception, or how one takes in information or data.

Although one style generally predominates, people possess the capacity for both styles. Field-dependent individuals are global, are open to external sources of information, are influenced by their surroundings, and therefore see the situation as a whole, rather than identifying and focusing on the separate aspects of it. Field-dependent people tend to be social, people oriented, and sensitive to social cues. Learners in which the field-dependent style predominates may be externally motivated and therefore take a spectator or passive role in the learning process, preferring to be taught rather than to actively participate. Field-independent individuals are less sensitive to the social environment than field-dependent individuals, and thus take on a more analytical approach to information. By identifying aspects of the situation separately, they are able to restructure information and develop their own system of classification. Field-independent learners enjoy concepts, challenges, and hypotheses and are task oriented (Miller & Babcock, 1996).

An aspect of learning style related to student behavior is response style. Kagan (1965) pioneered work, with school-age children, on the concepts of reflection and impulsiveness. These dimensions of cognitive response style describe personal tendencies regarding possibilities in solutions and choice selection. Individuals who have the impulsivity tendency prefer the quick, obvious answer, especially for highly uncertain problems, thus selecting the nearly correct answer as first choice. Reflective individuals identify and carefully consider alternatives before making a decision or choice. The implications for education in the health professions are apparent and will be discussed further. One problem that emerges with individuals who have a strong tendency in one of these dimensions is for the impulsive individual to act too quickly, based on an instant decision. Conversely, the reflective individual may be immobilized in decision making, which has obvious implications for outcomes.

Reflection, as associated with learning, was described as early as 1916 by John Dewey as being a process of inquiry (Miller & Babcock, 1996). To reflect on a situation, experience, or collection of information is to absorb, consider, weigh, speculate, contemplate, and deliberate. Such reflection serves either as a basis for reasoned action or to gain understanding or attach meaning to an experience. The most notable descriptions of reflection, especially as related to nursing, have been presented by Schön (1983). In his work, Schön related reflection to problem solving—and traditional means of teaching and learning result in structured problem solving where the ends are clear and fixed. In the reality of health care, such ends are not always so concrete or discernible.

Schön also believed that professionals in practice demonstrate a unique proficiency of thinking, and he has described the following three aspects of this thinking: (1) knowing-in-action (use of a personally constructed knowledge base), (2) reflection-in-action (conscious thinking about what one is doing, awareness of use of knowledge), and (3) reflection-on-action (a retrospective look at thoughts and actions, to conduct self-evaluation and make decisions for future events). Reflection results in synthesis. This outcome is evident when the individual carries over thoughts, feelings, and conclusions to other situations. Teaching includes reflection-in-action, in which the teacher spontaneously adapts to learner reactions. Thus, reflection is the foundation for growth through experience. Reflection, as a form of thinking and learning, can be cultivated. Educators improve their teaching when they reflect upon episodes of teaching that were successful as well as those that were failures (Pinsky, Monson, & Irby, 1998).

One of the best-known descriptions of learning styles is Kolb's, which emerged from Dewey's seminal theory on experiential learning (Kolb, 1984). Dewey pioneered educational thinking regarding the relationship between learning and experience. The relationship between the learning environment and personal factors such as motivation and goals can lead the learner through a stream of experiences that, once connected, bring about meaningful learning (Kelly & Young, 1996). Using these ideas, Kolb went on to describe learning as occurring in the following stages: concrete experiences, observation and reflection on the experience, conceptualization and generalization, then theoretical testing in new and more complex situations. Learning is cyclical, with new learning coming from new experiences. Consequently, learning occurs in a comprehensive means, beginning with performance (concrete experience) and ending with educational growth. Kolb further explained that individuals go about this learning along the following two basic dimensions: grasping experiences (prehension), with abstract–concrete poles; and transforming, with action–reflection poles (Kelly & Young, 1996). Applying his experiential learning theory to his dimensions, Kolb identified these four basic learning styles:

1. *Convergers:* Prefer abstract conceptualization and active experimentation. These individuals are detached and work better with objects than people. They are problem solvers and apply ideas in a practical manner.

2. *Divergers:* Prefer concrete experience and reflective observation. Individuals with this tendency are good at generating ideas and displaying emotionalism and interest in others. Divergers are imaginative and can see the big picture.

3. *Assimilators:* Prefer abstract conceptualization and reflective observation. Assimilators easily bring together diverse items into an integrated entity, sometimes overlooking practical aspects or input from others. Theoreticians likely are assimilators.

4. *Accommodators:* Prefer concrete experience and active experimentation. These individuals, while intuitive, are risk takers and engage in trial-and-error problem solving. Accommodators are willing to carry out plans, and they like and adapt to new circumstances (Miller & Babcock, 1996).

Gregorc's (1979) categorization of learning styles is similar to Kolb's, except that Gregorc believes that an individual's style is static, even in light of the changing educational setting. Thus, even after maturity and further learning, an individual still approaches learning in the same way. Gregorc uses the learning style categories of concrete sequential, concrete random, abstract sequential, and abstract random. In his research, Gregorc determined that individuals have preferences in one or two categories. In studying both first-year and fourth-year baccalaureate nursing students, Wells and Higgs (1990) discovered that these students have preferences in the concrete sequential and abstract random categories (total 81% of first-year students, 74% of fourth-year students).

■ Use of Learning Styles and Preferences

Theoretical foundations regarding learning and descriptive studies of cognitive and learning styles provide insight and understanding of self. It would be difficult to address research on all modes of learning in this one chapter. A summary application of information from the vast field of knowledge about learning theory and cognitive and learning styles has been developed by Svinicki (1994) as six operating principles, which are:

1. If information is to be learned, it must first be recognized.
2. During learning, learners act on information in ways that make it more meaningful.
3. Learners store information in long-term memory in an organized fashion related to their existing understanding of the world.
4. Learners continually check understanding, which results in refinement and revision of what is retained.
5. Transfer to new contexts is not automatic but results from exposure to multiple applications.
6. Learning is facilitated when learners are aware of their learning strategies and monitor their use. (p. 275)

To understand one's own learning styles helps to understand one's own thinking, to be aware of a fit between style and strategies for learning, and thus to select the most effective and efficient means to go about learning. Some students are aware of how they learn best and gravitate toward that strategy. Instructors see this process in students who choose to sit in the front row of the class, take many notes, and feel involved with the topic; or students who prefer online learning, choose not to come to class but instead read course material, watch Internet clips or videos, and acquire information as it pertains to a clinical assignment. Some students adhere to tradition-bound forms of learning, such as lecture and reading, yet do not maximize their learning. This result explains why these students benefit more from direct clinical experiences. Many students find learning to be more powerful when they experience something new or significant in a clinical environment, then explore information and reflect on the experience. Learning experiences can be adapted to the environment and are influenced by the environment in which they occur. Awareness and comprehension of one's style of learning enables one to tailor the learning environment for optimal outcomes. A simple test to guide the student in discovering his or her learning style(s) is presented in the teaching example at the end of this chapter.

Feedback from an observer, such as the instructor, can heighten awareness of personal styles. The knowledgeable educator also can guide the student in enhancing predominant styles or in beginning to cultivate additional dimensions of thinking and responding. For example, a student who is predominantly impulsive in decision making should be guided to explore outcomes of decisions and encouraged to increase reflection time as appropriate. Conversely, the student who is highly reflective may need to explore reasons that bring about hesitancy or prolonged deliberation and the outcomes of such behaviors.

■ Effective Teaching for Effective Learning

A knowledgeable and insightful educator is the key to effective learning in many situations. Consequently, the educator should call upon a knowledge base in learning and teaching as well as an extensive repertoire of useful strategies to reach learning goals. Faculty in health professions education are challenged to be directive in their teaching, addressing measurable learning outcomes that are directly linked to professional standards. This is juxtaposed with the importance of freeing the student from linear thinking and encouraging broader approaches to learning that are accomplished through dialogue, expression, and attribution of meaning. Instructors must determine best use of time, both for themselves and for students. So, difficult decisions must be made regarding what to leave in and what to omit from teaching episodes. In the health professions, faculty have to choose between teaching for practical judgment or for disciplinary knowledge. Specialized knowledge from within the discipline can clarify issues involved in practical situations, but it cannot determine judgment or a course of action (Sullivan & Rosin, 2008). This is where the role of the instructor, as a seasoned practitioner, is indispensable.

In their research to discover attributes of successful teachers at the rank of full professor, Rossetti and Fox (2009) developed these four categories for teaching success:

1. *Presence of the teacher:* Being there or available for the students, becoming acquainted with students, and cultivating mutual respect and trust
2. *Promotion of learning:* Interest in students' learning and finding meaning in their education
3. *Teachers as learners:* Staying current in the discipline and teaching strategies, and continually updating and refreshing courses
4. *Enthusiasm:* Conveying an interest in the subject and passion for the work

Regardless of setting, whether it be a traditional classroom, clinical care, synchronous or asynchronous electronic instruction, these principles of teaching success are applicable.

As students advance in their education, their established, comfortable ways of knowing, thinking, and reflection are challenged. This is especially true in the health professions, where students explore value systems that differ from their own and identify ethical dilemmas in practice or circumstances in which there is more than one right answer or no clear choice. In situations in which the research evidence diverges from existing paradigms that are known to students, and thus cause conflict in thinking, the instructor should be prepared to adapt and modify teaching to address this conflict (Fryer, 2008). Therefore, the instructor needs to be patently aware of his or her own teaching style and how to amend that style for the circumstances.

Regarding the teaching strategies presented in this text, each strategy will have different effects on the attainment of learning outcomes in each student, based on the attributes and use of the strategy, in addition to learning and cognitive styles and learning preferences. Here are some broad suggestions for applying information about learning in teaching situations. The specific strategies addressed in subsequent chapters provide detailed information to enable faculty to use each method in an optimal way.

Underlying assumptions regarding the nature of professional education are derived in part from principles of adult learning, as formulated by Knowles (1978). Key principles include assuming responsibility for one's own learning and recognition of meaning or usefulness of information to be learned. Students in health professions are career oriented and need to see practical value in their educational endeavors. As consumers, adult students need to believe that they are receiving the maximum benefit from learning experiences. Furthermore, taking charge of one's own learning is empowering. Students who gain a sense of self-responsibility can feel empowered in other areas of their lives, such as professional practice. Faculty, in turn, have the responsibility to cultivate empowerment and to affect learning outcomes.

The teaching–learning experience, whether it is in a classroom environment or online, should be fresh and challenging each time the class convenes. Faculty should endeavor to provide variety in the manner in which they teach, rather than the same, predictable, albeit comfortable method of telling rather than teaching. As providers of information, instructors need to remember that learning is best brought about by a combination of motivation and stimulation. The effective instructor should be the facilitator of learning in the students. In professional education, motivation is gained when the relationship to the well-being of the client is pointed out. The value of faculty experience is evident when the nurse-teacher shares from his or her own professional experiences and uses these anecdotes as examples of client outcomes. Nursing students and faculty agree that nontraditional strategies such as collaborative or cooperative learning, active involvement, and participation in the learning experience are desirable for effective learning. Students in professional education programs do respond positively to opportunities to choose or structure some of their learning experiences (Melrose, 2004). This approach should be used frequently by the teacher, not only to promote active learning but also to instill in students a sense of empowerment, which is an important attribute for the clinical setting. Technology-based learning activities direct the student to engage in independent learning, research, and use of visual cues, such as video, to enhance comprehension.

As can be seen from the information on learning styles, students are more likely to remember information with which they can agree or relate and if they can attach meaning to the item or information. Disagreement or disharmony should be explored in an objective fashion. Viewpoints can then be strengthened or altered. Questioning and discussion should be based on the diversity that exists among the students. An instructor who is able to establish a sense of trust and confidence with the students can promote the expression of different perspectives likely to be found in the group. Professional educators should support students who are at various levels of cognitive growth, looking upon students from a criterion framework rather than a normative one. Faculty should show that various viewpoints are welcome, legitimate, and worthy of discussion.

Effective educators guide students to see how their thought processes occur. They ask, "What do you know about ____?" or "How did you arrive at that answer/conclusion?" Teachers cultivate further development in the individual learners by demonstrating how to critique a theory, develop a rationale, or work through the steps of problem solving. These strategies will facilitate growth in students who are in an early cognitive stage such as dualism or will challenge more advanced students to a commitment to realism (Perry, 1970).

Delivery of information should be based on instructional theory in addition to content expertise. Using Ausubel's (1968) principles of advanced organizer, the teacher can develop inductive discovery by which students can build on previously acquired, simplistic knowledge to develop new or broader concepts. Effective learning experiences emerging from identified styles should be developed and used in both class and clinical settings. Information from Kolb's four dimensions serves as an excellent example. Students who are convergers readily become bored with straight lecture, especially with topics that are abstract in nature. These individuals work better by themselves, so they are less likely to participate well in group projects. Learners with the diverger style learn from case studies and will actively participate in discussion, but they may have difficulty detaching personal values from the issue. These students often are visionary group leaders. Individuals with the assimilator style manipulate ideas well, so they will participate well in discussion or write comprehensive papers; however, these students may be less practical and have difficulty with some of the realism of clinical practice. Accommodators usually enjoy case studies, new or unusual teaching strategies, skills labs, and tinkering with new equipment. These learners will be most responsive to a challenging, complex client. With the multitude of learning opportunities available through electronic resources and patient simulation, teachers can readily craft a learning experience that meets most learning styles and preferences.

Skiba, Connors, and Jeffries (2008) cite nursing education as the field considered by many to be a pioneer in the use of educational technology. Nursing, along with the other health professions, must face the challenges of incorporating core competencies, use of emerging technologies, and practice in informatics-intensive healthcare environments. However, one-way learning, such as web-based instruction, will not fully replace the competency-based instruction and verification that is needed in the applied disciplines of health care (Knapp, 2004).

In the clinical setting, the instructor may wish to provide introductory motivation through discovery learning. One way to accomplish this goal is to have each student observe or follow an individual in the clinical setting to gain exposure to the myriad tasks and responsibilities of a professional healthcare provider. Whereas students may have some rudimentary ideas of what healthcare providers do, they discover the depth and demands required in day-to-day work by observing actual practice. This strategy should broaden their perspectives and set the stage for meaningful learning, which includes increased retention of material and greater inquiry.

As students develop clinical written summaries about their clients, instructors should be flexible with the type of written work submitted. Traditionally, nursing students develop some form of a care plan based on the nursing process. The structured, linear method has taken criticism when regarded as the only way to look at clients. As a concrete, methodical strategy, the nursing process care plan is effective for students who are field independent and who can readily discern the data and related information needed for each step.

Additional methods of client summary or analysis should be introduced, and students should be encouraged to try each method. In doing so, students may broaden their ways of seeing clients and nursing problems, thus setting the stage for increased insight, analysis, and confidence. For example, use of the concept map is a way in which a student can envision the client or care situation in a holistic manner. Concept maps provide a fluidity that enhances the ability to determine relationships and make connections. Therefore, this strategy likely will be used positively by students who demonstrate Gardner's categories of visual/spatial or interpersonal intelligence. Learners who are field dependent also should do well with the concept map strategy because of their tendency to see the situation as a whole. Concept mapping should be effective for learners with all of Kolb's styles, but for different reasons and with different outcomes.

Guided reflection, especially reflection-on-action, helps the student bring closure to the clinical experience, as well as conduct self-evaluation and gain from the experience. Journal writing is one of the most effective means by which the student can capture thoughts and responses and preserve these ideas in writing for subsequent consideration. This strategy is particularly useful as a means by which students can identify and modify impulsive-reflective tendencies. Journal writing will have the best results with divergers and assimilators, and some students may benefit from open discussion about the experiences entered into their journals. Again, feedback from the faculty is crucial and should be as thoughtful as the entries provided by the student. Faculty who are reading these journals should guide the students in growth of insight and patterns of reflection.

Effective teachers in the health professions are those who possess content expertise, create an active learning environment, and use carefully selected teaching strategies (Wolf, Bender, Beitz, Wieland, & Vito, 2004). One of the greatest challenges for faculty is in developing a blend of strategies to bring about effective learning in all students. Part of the challenge is the fit between the faculty's styles and learning preferences and the styles and preferences of each of the learners. Faculty especially should be on guard against favoritism to students who possess the same attributes as the instructor. Conversely, the congruency between styles of the teacher and of the student may enhance a relationship that is especially meaningful and may evolve into professional mentoring.

■ Future Considerations

From this chapter, many ideas that are worthy of more detailed scrutiny emerge. The majority of research on cognitive styles, learning style, and learning preferences was conducted in the 1970s and 1980s. This was before the widespread accepted use of electronic technology. Use of technology in teaching and learning may be influenced by learning preferences, such as in visual and kinesthetic learners. Have some students learned to modify their preferences to become more comfortable with technology? Online education is widely accepted, and the role of the instructor is changing. The extent to which learners continue to value the presence of the instructor for spontaneous teaching is worthy of investigation. Currently, there is a shift in education toward student-centered, active learning for the development of critical thinking, coupled with generations of students who are used to immediate feedback and a variety of stimulation types. Educators must determine if selected strategies are useful for genuine learning or, if not used properly, merely providing entertainment.

■ Conclusion

Effective learning is more than merely the result of good teaching. It is enhanced by a learning environment that includes active interactions among faculty, students, and student peers. Effective learning is achieved through the use of creative strategies designed not to entertain but to inform and stimulate. The best ways faculty can bring about effective learning are by recognizing students as individuals, with unique, personal ways of knowing and learning; by creating learning situations that recognize diversity; and by providing empowering experiences in which students are challenged to think.

Teaching Example:
How Do I Learn Best?

This instrument typically takes 4 to 6 minutes to complete and can be self-scored. The style categories are visual, aural, read/write, and kinesthetic, which correspond with categories found in Gardner's multiple forms of intelligence. Students are directed to answer the brief questions, then are shown the learning modalities that best fit predominant styles.

How Do I Learn Best?
This test is to find out something about your preferred learning method. Research on left-brain/right-brain differences and on learning and personality differences suggests that each person has preferred ways to receive and communicate information.

(continues)

Choose the answer that best explains your preference and put the key letter in the box. If a single answer does not match your perception, please enter two or more choices in the box. Leave blank any question that does not apply. Once you have completed the test, find the totals for each of the letters (V, A, R, K) that correspond with a learning preference. Then look at the table of learning modalities (**Table 1-1**) to see which strategies best support your learning preference.

Table 1-1   Learning Modalities

	In Class	When Studying	For Exams
Visual	Underline Use different colors Use symbols, charts, arrangements on a page	Recall visual aspects of presentation Reconstruct images in different ways Redraw pages from memory Replace words with symbols and initials	Recall the pictures on the pages Draw, use diagrams where appropriate Practice turning visuals back into words
Aural	Attend lectures and listen Discuss topics with students Use a tape recorder Discuss overheads, pictures, and other visual aids Leave space in notes for later recall	May take poor notes because of preference for voices Expand notes by talking out ideas Explain new ideas to another student Read assignments out loud	Speak the answers/ tutorials Practice writing answers to an old exam Read questions to yourself or have someone read them to you
Reading/Writing	Use lists, headings Write out lists and definitions Use handouts and textbooks	Write out the words Reread notes silently Rewrite ideas in other words Use lecture notes/read	Practice with multiple-choice questions Write paragraphs, beginnings, endings Organize diagrams into statements
Kinesthetic: use all of the senses	May take notes poorly because topics do not seem relevant Go to lab, take field trips Use trial-and-error method Listen to real-life examples	Put examples in note summaries Talk about notes, especially with another kinesthetic person Use pictures and photos to illustrate	Write practice answers Role play the exam situation in one's head

Data from Gardner, H., & Hatch, T. (1990). *Multiple intelligences go to school: Educational implications of the theory of multiple intelligences* (Technical Report No. 4). New York, NY: Center for Technology in Education.

1. You are about to give directions to a person. She is staying in a hotel in town and wants to visit your house. She has a rental car. Would you:
   V) draw a map on paper?
   A) tell her the directions?
   R) write down the directions (without a map)?
   K) collect her from the hotel in your car?

2. You are staying in a hotel and have a rental car. You would like to visit a friend whose address/location you do not know. Would you like them to:
   V) draw you a map on paper?
   A) tell you the directions by phone?
   R) write down the directions (without a map)?
   K) collect you from the hotel in their car?

3. You have just received a copy of your itinerary for a world trip. This is of interest to a friend. Would you:
   A) ring her immediately and tell her about it?
   R) send her a copy of the printed itinerary?
   V) show her on a map of the world?

4. You are going to cook a dessert as a special treat for your family. Do you:
   K) cook something familiar without need for instructions?
   V) thumb through the cookbook looking for ideas from the pictures?
   R) refer to a specific cookbook where there is a good recipe?
   A) ask for advice from others?

5. A group of tourists have been assigned to you to find out about national parks. Would you:
   K) drive them to a national park?
   V) show them slides and photographs?
   R) give them a book on national parks?
   A) give them a talk on national parks?

6. You are about to purchase a new stereo. Other than price, what would most influence your decision?
   A) A friend talking about it
   R) Reading the details about it
   K) Listening to it
   V) It looks really upmarket

7. Recall a time in your life when you learned how to do something like playing a new board game. Try to avoid choosing a very physical skill, e.g. riding a bike. How did you learn best? By:
   V) visual clues—pictures, diagrams, charts?
   R) written instructions?
   A) listening to somebody explaining it?
   K) doing it?

(continues)

8. Which of these games do you prefer?
   V) Pictionary
   R) Scrabble
   K) Charades

9. You are about to learn to use a new program on a computer. Would you:
   K) ask a friend to show you?
   R) read the manual which comes with the program?
   A) telephone a friend and ask questions about it?

10. You are not sure whether a word should be spelled 'dependent' or 'dependant.'
    Do you:
    R) look it up in the dictionary?
    V) see the word in your mind and choose the best way it looks?
    A) sound it out in your mind?
    K) write both versions down?

11. Apart from price, what would most influence your decision to buy a particular textbook?
    K) Using a friend's copy
    A) A friend talking about it
    R) Skim reading of parts of it
    V) It looks OK

12. A new movie has arrived in town. What would most influence your decision to go (or not go)?
    A) Friends talked about it.
    R) You read a review about it.
    V) You saw a preview of it.

13. Do you prefer a lecturer/teacher who likes to use:
    R) handouts and/or a textbook?
    V) flow diagrams, charts, slides?
    K) field trips, labs, practical sessions?
    A) discussion, guest speakers?

Reproduced from Fleming, N. D., & Mills, C. (1992). Not another inventory, rather a catalyst for reflection. *To Improve the Academy*, 11, 137–155.

Discussion Questions

1. Reflect on the learning theorists mentioned in the chapter (Bandura, Skinner Thorndike, Gagne, Bruner, Ausubel, Gardner). Which theorist informs your own learning? Describe your own learning and how this theorist influences your classroom or clinical teaching.

2. Should the classroom teacher create learning activities or assignments tailored to all of the VARK learning styles as described in the Teaching Example?

3. Are traditional learning theories still relevant in today's technology-based educational system?

References

Ausubel, D. P. (1968). *Educational psychology: A cognitive view*. New York, NY: Holt, Rinehart & Winston.

Bandura, A. (1977). *Social learning theory*. Morristown, NJ: General Learning Press.

Bruner, J. (1966). *Toward a theory of instruction*. Cambridge, MA: The Belknap Press of Harvard University Press.

Fleming, N. D., & Mills, C. (1992). Not another inventory, rather a catalyst for reflection. *To Improve the Academy, 11,* 137–155.

Fryer, G. (2008). Teaching critical thinking in osteopathy: Integrating craft knowledge and evidence-informed approaches. *International Journal of Osteopathic Medicine, 11*(2), 56–61.

Gagne, R. M. (1968). Learning hierarchies. *Educational Psychologist, 6,* 1–9.

Gardner, H., & Hatch, T. (1990). *Multiple intelligences go to school: Educational implications of the theory of multiple intelligences* (Technical Report No. 4). New York, NY: Center for Technology in Education.

Gregorc, A. F. (1979). Learning/teaching styles: Their nature and effects. In National Association of Secondary School Principals (Ed.), *Student learning styles* (pp. 19–26). Reston, VA: National Association of Secondary School Principals.

Kagan, J. (1965). Reflection-impulsivity and reading ability in primary grade children. *Child Development, 36,* 609–628.

Kelly, E., & Young, A. (1996). Models of nursing education for the 21st century. In K. Stevens (Ed.), *Review of research in nursing education* (Vol. 7, pp. 1–39). New York, NY: National League for Nursing.

Knapp, B. (2004). Competency: An essential component of caring in nursing. *Nursing Administration Quarterly, 28,* 285–287.

Knowles, M. A. (1978). *The adult learner: A neglected species* (2nd ed.). Houston, TX: Gulf Publishing.

Kolb, D. A. (1984). *Experiential learning theory*. Englewood Cliffs, NJ: Prentice-Hall.

Lesaca, T. (2001). Executive functions in parents with ADHD. *Psychiatric Times, 18*(11), 4.

Melrose, S. (2004). What works? A personal account of clinical teaching strategies in nursing. *Education for Health, 17,* 236–239.

Miller, M. A., & Babcock, D. E. (1996). *Critical thinking applied to nursing*. St. Louis, MO: Mosby.

Perry, W. G. (1970). *Forms of intellectual and ethical development in the college years: A scheme*. New York, NY: Holt, Rinehart & Winston.

Pinsky, L. E., Monson, D., & Irby, D. M. (1998). How excellent teachers are made: Reflecting on success to improve teaching. *Advances in Health Sciences Education, 3,* 207–215.

Rossetti, J., & Fox, P. G. (2009). Factors related to successful teaching by outstanding professors: An interpretive study. *Journal of Nursing Education, 48*(1), 11–16.

Schön, D. A. (1983). *The reflective practitioner: How professionals think in action*. New York, NY: Basic Books.

Skiba, D. J., Connors, H. R., & Jeffries, P. R. (2008). Information technologies and the transformation of nursing education. *Nursing Outlook, 56*(5), 225–230.

Slater, J. A., Lujan, H. L., & DiCarlo, S. E. (2007). Does gender influence learning style preferences of first-year medical students? *Advances in Physiology Education, 31,* 336–342.

Sullivan, W. M., & Rosin, M. S. (2008). A life of the mind for practice: Bridging liberal and professional education. *Change, 40*(2), 44–47.

Svinicki, M. D. (1994). Practical implications of cognitive theories. In K. A. Feldman & M. B. Paulsen (Eds.), *Teaching and learning in the college classroom* (pp. 274–281). Needham Heights, MA: Ginn Press.

Wells, D., & Higgs, Z. R. (1990). Learning and learning preferences of first and fourth semester baccalaureate degree nursing students. *Journal of Nursing Education, 29,* 385–390.

Witkin, H. A., Moore, C. A., Goodenough, D. R., & Cox, P. W. (1977). Field-dependent and field-independent cognitive styles and their implications. *Review of Educational Research, 47,* 1–64.

Wolf, Z. R., Bender, P. J., Beitz, J. M., Wieland, D. M., & Vito, K. O. (2004). Strengths and weaknesses of faculty teaching performance reported by undergraduate and graduate nursing students: A descriptive study. *Journal of Professional Nursing, 20,* 118–128.

CHAPTER 2

Culture and Diversity in the Classroom

Arlene J. Lowenstein
LaDonna L. Christian

Today's classrooms are very different from those in the past. Immigration, both forced and voluntary, has shaped the face of the United States. Each new wave of immigrants adds to the mosaic that is the United States. A mosaic is made up of many pieces, each different in size and shape; some may be brightly colored and others pale, transparent, or with no color added. Each piece may not mean much by itself, but when put together, the pieces change, forming new designs and an overall effect very different from the mosaic's component pieces taken singly. The strength of the mosaic is the ability to capitalize on new and different ideas. Its weakness is the clash between cultures that feeds prejudice and discriminatory behaviors. Health professions educators and leaders have recognized this change, and cultural competence of practitioners is now being stressed in both education and service. By using the strengths and originality of diverse students, the final classroom product can be much stronger than the product of an assimilated, cookie-cutter culture.

A new emphasis on civil rights, feminism, sexuality, and morality issues in the late 1960s and 1970s brought about drastic changes in what had been considered accepted societal behavior. Those changes shaped the move toward increased diversity of both patients and the student body in our world today, and provided new and different opportunities and challenges from those of the past. Change continues as you read this, and classrooms in the future may look very different. Educators need to be flexible, aware of trends and patterns, and able to respond to continuing challenges. This chapter presents a brief glimpse of some of the diversity issues in the past and present day, and it discusses some of the issues and strategies involved in working with a diverse classroom population.

■ The Past

In the 1950s, healthcare professional education was almost nonexistent for African Americans (Blacks), other multicultural students, and persons with disabilities. Men went into medicine, while women became nurses. Other health professions may have had some of each gender, but women were often in the majority in nursing (Moffat, 2003). Educational facilities were often segregated culturally and religiously, not only in the South, which had a history of legal segregation at that time, but in the North as well (Carnegie, 1991, 2005). Catholic and Jewish hospitals often had their own schools of nursing, and there were religious and ethnic student quotas in many colleges and universities. This meant that most classes were homogenized, with a large majority of Caucasian (White) and Protestant students in all but the religion-sponsored or minority-established programs, and those were few and far between. Very few Hispanic, Asian, or Muslim students were admitted to the schools. For the multicultural students who were admitted, retention rates were often low (Carnegie, 1991).

Nursing education was founded in hospital diploma programs using the apprentice system of education. From the early days in the late 1800s through the 1950s, there were very few graduate nurses in hospitals. Most graduate nurses moved into private duty after graduation, with some going into public health and a few staying on primarily in managerial or teaching positions. Student nurses were the major providers of care for hospital patients. Very ill patients on the hospital wards were most often assigned a private-duty nurse to care for them, usually paid for by the patients and their families, although hospitals absorbed the cost in some instances.

In 1946, shortly after World War II, the Hill-Burton Act was passed in Congress and signed into law. It provided funds to hospitals for renovation, expansion, capital projects, and new hospital buildings. As hospitals expanded, more nurses and other healthcare professionals were needed. Another trend was the development of intensive care units in the mid-1950s, and skilled nurses were needed for those areas as well. The nursing students and nurses in the labor pool during those years were still primarily Caucasian and Protestant, with few minorities.

During that time, although it seems hard to believe in today's world, very few nursing schools admitted married students. Female students were dismissed from the program if they chose to get married; if the secret marriages that did occur were found out by school authorities, the students would be expelled, even if they were almost ready to graduate. In the few schools where married students were permitted, pregnant women were excluded, and pregnancy out of wedlock was an unforgivable sin for health professions education.

Nursing was viewed as a woman's profession, and few men were permitted in. Those men who were nurses had severe restrictions in clinical experiences such as obstetrics and gynecology, but they could be welcomed in psychiatric facilities because it was thought that they were stronger and could work better with distraught and violent patients. It was generally considered that students with disabilities would not be able to participate in providing all aspects of care, so they were not admitted to programs. No allowances were made. In Augusta, Georgia, from the early 1900s through the early 1960s, University Hospital had two schools of nursing, the Lamar school for Blacks and the Barrett school for Whites (Lowenstein, 1990, 1994). The two schools joined together in 1965, after the passage of civil rights legislation. The Barrett school accepted more nursing students and had a higher graduation rate than the Lamar school. One year, three Asian students applied and were admitted to the Barrett school, but only one graduated. In Augusta, as in most of the South, and often in the North (although no one talked about that), Black students were assigned to the units with Black patients, and White students to those with White patients. Supervisors, administrators, and teachers were almost always White.

The late 1960s and early 1970s brought revolutionary change, which has continued to expand since that time. The civil rights movement sparked a feminist movement, and those movements opened previously closed doors in education. Women had more opportunities to be admitted to healthcare professions that had theretofore been male dominated. A few men were admitted into programs that had only women students, although the numbers were still small and discrimination still prevalent, especially due to the belief that male nurses were homosexual. The sexual revolution of those years also brought a change in thinking about sexual orientation, although many attitudes of the past persist today, and discrimination still occurs. In nursing, the rules against marriage were dropped, and women could attend school while pregnant. Although the changes have been gradual, the face of the classroom is continuing its transformation.

During this period of time, the community college movement began, which provided more access to multicultural students, to those who could not afford private college tuition, and to students who needed educational facilities closer to their homes. This was a boon to older women, including women of color, and those with families, who could now attend less expensive schools that were closer to home. Part-time attendance was possible in some programs, and nursing students no longer needed to live at the hospitals. Graduates of associate degree programs in nursing were eligible for licensure as registered nurses and took less time to graduate than the typical 3-year diploma program students. Many hospital diploma schools began to close, although it was a prolonged fight. During those years, nursing leaders recognized the discrimination against women in college and university admissions. They were pleased that nursing education had moved out of the hospital program, but they were not satisfied. In an effort to raise the status of women in the profession, they began a move toward baccalaureate education for all nurses by 1984, which also speeded the demise of hospital programs. However, for many reasons, the baccalaureate goal was not achieved.

The physical therapy profession and its professional organization, the American Physical Therapy Association (APTA), were begun by women, but men were recognized in the profession by the 1920s. However, even with the feminist movements of the 1960s and 1970s, it took until the early 1990s for the APTA to feel it important enough to address women's issues and the inequities in the profession as they pertained to the disparities in the professional and economic status of women. The board of directors appointed the first Committee on Women in Physical Therapy, and in 1994 the Office of Women's Issues was created at APTA headquarters in Alexandria, Virginia. The Office of Minority Affairs also became an integral part of the APTA headquarters at this time, as the profession tried to recruit more minorities (Moffat, 2003). Those years also saw the beginning of affirmative action, and an increased number of multicultural students began to be admitted to colleges, although the numbers were still small. The end of the Vietnam War began an Asian migration to the United States, and we have seen other migrations since that time, creating increased Latino/Hispanic, Muslim, Indian, and Russian-Jewish populations in the United States, among others. Those migrations have meant more diverse students accepted into health professions programs. In 1990, the Americans with Disabilities Act (ADA) was passed by Congress and signed into law. It required educators to think differently about what could be done to provide access and retention for disabled persons who would be able to work in some, if not all, aspects of their chosen health profession and thereby provide a valuable service for the profession and its patients.

■ The Present

So where has this history led us in the classroom in today's world? The health professions classroom is more diverse than ever before. However, diversity no longer means ethnic background alone. The age range may be wide and gender ratios may have changed, although nursing still has a minority of male students. In medicine it worked the other way around, and more women have gone into that field than ever before. There is diversity in sexual orientation, although discrimination on this basis still exists.

There are diverse social and family issues in the classroom. Many divorced and single parents have gone back to school, but often have great responsibility in raising their children alone, which may interfere with the amount of time that can be allotted to school work (Grosz, 2005; Ogunsiji & Wilkes, 2005). In some places, disadvantaged students have come into the health professions classrooms as new economic relief programs are put into place (Wessling, 2000). Students, especially older ones, may have caretaker responsibilities for their parents or other relatives, including children with disabilities. Those in the "sandwich generation" may have caretaker responsibilities for both their parents and their children.

We also have wealthy students, for whom textbook purchases and other expenses are not a problem. However, need-based scholarship students and other students have real concerns about the financial issues affecting their ability to complete their programs. Tuition increases and the specter of repayment of student loans may create additional stress. Financially secure students may not have strictly financial concerns, but they may have other family and social problems that affect them and their classroom abilities.

The number of disabled students, with both physical and learning disabilities, has increased. Due to technological advances and better awareness, educational institutions are now able to provide more accommodations for students with disabilities. These may include policy modifications, equipment, and physical changes to increase handicap access. Students with disabilities often have concerns about how they are being perceived by others and worry other students and faculty are expecting them to fail. Research has shown creative problem solving and faculty support can be developed for students with disabilities, and health professions education programs can be enriched by their presence (Carroll, 2004).

Colleges and universities are being encouraged to promote diversity both in hiring faculty and in student recruitment and admissions, although success rates are still low (Silver, 2002; Barbee & Gibson, 2001). Even though affirmative action has been under fire, it is recognized there is still a need to make higher education more accessible for both minorities and students with disabilities. Although diversity in admissions and hiring may be strongly encouraged, retaining diverse students and faculty is often difficult. However, Splenser and his colleagues (Splenser, Canlas, Sanders, & Melzer, 2003), in a study of physical therapy educational programs, found when schools provided special retention efforts, they were effective in increasing the numbers of graduating multicultural students. They also found a positive correlation between increased applications from diverse students and the presence of multicultural faculty in a program.

Other researchers have found many multicultural students experience significant culture shock when entering the collegiate world, which may be very different from their previous life experiences. In schools or programs with low numbers of diverse students and faculty, the recruited multicultural students often feel excluded in an educational system where their values, knowledge, and practices are largely ignored. Because Blacks are frequently in the minority in such a classroom, feelings of isolation, alienation, and loneliness, as well as perceived racism, can cause academic difficulties. Inadequate academic preparation for the rigor of college, family conflicts, and lack of financial resources can contribute to failure. In many cases, support services are offered by institutions but might not be used (Kosowski, Grams, Taylor, & Wilson, 2001). Bain (2004) reported negative stereotypes are often internalized by multicultural students. The resulting educational disparities are evident in learning outcomes, which can apply to disabled persons as well (Bain, 2004). These feelings can be compounded by impersonal, and sometimes hostile, treatment from faculty, who are still predominately White. Multicultural faculty also face these feelings; in turn, this often leads to students dropping out of school and faculty leaving educational positions (Evans, 2004; Kosowski et al., 2001; Vasquez, 1990).

There are many causes for the lack of success of multicultural students in the classroom. Kirkland (1998) found a difference in psychological stress between Black and White nursing students. Blacks often felt more stress and perceived their environment differently. Because of the history of discrimination and their previous experiences with discrimination, Blacks may perceive discrimination even though White students, employers, or other employees in a healthcare setting do not feel that discrimination exists (Lowenstein & Glanville, 1995). Kosowski and colleagues (2001) noted the failure rate for Black students can be higher than for their White counterparts. These issues are not limited to Blacks, but often affect other multicultural students too, as well as White students from poorer economic strata. Evans (2004) found Hispanic/Latino and Native American nursing students struggled with similar feelings. Those in the study described the impact of perceived lack of options for multicultural students. Even before they entered the program, it was difficult for them to imagine themselves being successful in a healthcare profession. Language issues can be difficult to overcome. Lack of family support due to financial or cultural expectations and ignorance of academic demands was also identified as a barrier to success for some students, especially those who were the first in their families to attend college. Students who successfully confronted those barriers were helped by faculty who recognized these stressors, worked to respect students' intense obligation to family and community, and provided long-term, personal encouragement to continue in the program (Evans, 2004).

■ The Importance of Culture in Education

Language, ethnicity, religion, class, lifestyle, gender, and power shape culture. A person's cultural relevance is confirmed through values, beliefs, and traditions. Other cultural influences include ways of thinking and being. These characteristics are shared and identifiable in groups of people with a common geography, history, and communication system (Sieffert, 2006).

One of the main challenges of education is creating a learning environment that preserves cultural integrity for all students while enhancing their educational achievement (Phuntsog, 1999). Many educational institutions attempt to acknowledge cultures by offering a course in multicultural education, which is expected to address a breadth and depth of cultural diversity. Educators are expected to overcome years of deep-rooted societal beliefs, question or challenge cultural hegemony, and adopt transformational curricula of social justice. However, there is a need for educators to recognize culture is central to who we are. Attempts to dismiss it or mandate complete acculturation may have injurious effects on the ability of multicultural students to experience positive learning outcomes. Successful student-centered learning requires educators be prepared to adapt their curricula based on the cultural needs of the community in which they serve (Phuntsog, 1999). Teachers who have been successful with diverse students have set up situations where positive expectations are verbalized and integrated into the classroom. Letting multicultural students know there is respect for their abilities has been shown to lead to improvement in pass rates (Bain, 2004).

Researchers have confirmed the benefits of creating a learning environment that is relevant to, and reflective of, student realities, customs, and beliefs. Encouraging cultural and ethnic identity in the classroom diminishes negative experiences, increases self-confidence and self-esteem, and promotes resiliency in multicultural students (Kana'iaupuni, Ledward, & Jensen, 2010). Culturally inclusive pedagogical approaches are associated with the survival of ethnicity, tradition, and language. Culture is also vital to the functioning of social and family networks and support systems that may contribute to the sustainability of diverse ethnic groups in the classroom (Kana'iaupuni et al., 2010). However, a focus on individual groups and classrooms can obscure the role and responsibility of broader society in addressing educational inequity (Nasir & Hand, 2006). Hancock (2007) described the convergence of numerous aspects of social identity and memberships in marginalized multicultural communities as *intersectionality*. These inequities create a multiplicity of barriers and add important implications to our consideration of cultural differences in education (Hancock, 2007). Think about the term *minority*. This term is often used to describe multicultural and diverse students. What does that label mean to students? The connotation is they are out of the mainstream, not as good as the majority students, and often expected to fail. Bain noted even students who had a strong self-image could fall into the trap of feeling they needed to prove themselves, leading to increased anxiety, stress, and eventually failure (Bain, 2004).

Culture and Educational Theories

The definition of *culture* depends on whether the author's viewpoint is sociological or anthropological. In the sociological view, education socializes people into society's mainstream. Thus, education focuses on forming an organized social structure by bringing people together from multifarious backgrounds and Americanizing them (Sieffert, 2006). Early researchers in sociological education sought to explain racial deficits in learning and achievements as both biological and cultural. In the 1970s, educational sociologists began to argue that multicultural children were not deficient in their cognitive and social orientations, but rather were different from mainstream society in their learning styles. Sociologists then began to develop new conceptual models to better understand cultural differences and to explore ways to design pedagogical approaches and classroom environments to support culturally diverse children (Nasir & Hand, 2006).

Educational anthropologists define *culture* as a complex whole including knowledge, beliefs, morals, customs, and a social heritage that are transmitted and shared from one generation to another. The anthropological approach to education reduces ethnocentrism by instilling an appreciation for other cultures and contributes to the understanding of other human beings (Nasir & Hand, 2006). The anthropological theory of education takes into consideration the many aspects of culture and is concerned with cultural transmission. Cultural transmission involves both enculturation and acculturation, or the movement of cultural beliefs across traditional educational lines (Sieffert, 2006). Three major influences of the anthropological view contribute to our understanding of how culturally diverse students learn. First, there is the belief culturally diverse students are no less capable than members of the majority population; their variances in learning are attributed to language, culture, life experiences, and learning styles. Second, educational anthropology looks beyond exam scores and takes into account the entire schooling experience. Third, educational anthropologists view education as a process in which all participants contribute in shaping the outcomes (Jacob & Jordan, 1996, pp. 15–23).

Many theorists have attempted to rationalize the gaps in student performance. Most have focused on home, environment, communication styles, language, and cultural mismatch as the major problems with culture and learning (Jacob & Jordan, 1996). Oppositional theorists have cited societal inequities and experiences with discrimination as participatory causes explaining why many students of minority cultures have difficulty learning (Kana'iaupuni et al., 2010). Although both sociological and anthropological education theories have their advantages, current researchers have demonstrated that understanding the cultures of the populations we serve in our classroom makes a positive difference in learning outcomes. Anthropologists highlight the roles of communication styles, social interaction, and cultural norms, with a focus on ethnographic process-based descriptions of teaching and learning. The fundamental idea of educational anthropology is learning occurs as teachers negotiate complex social interactions that are often formed by a set of cultural differences in customs and resolutions (Nasir & Hand, 2006).

Pedagogy and Cultural Influences

All educational systems and institutions of learning are ingrained in a particular cultural worldview. The issue of culture has had a strong influence on pedagogy, and learning has not improved to date. Education is affected by culture, and the role of culture is germane to instructional design. Culture affects not only what students learn, but also how they learn. Cultural values and beliefs provide a basis for how a person interacts when learning and how a person perceives learning. Thus, culture and learning are intertwined and intricate. Pedagogy does not begin and end in the classroom. It should also reflect the practices of the community that it serves, locally, nationally, and internationally (Dale, 2009, pp. 27–37). Pedagogical strategies that include multicultural education, cultural competence, and cultural inclusivity must have an increased representation in curricula (Nasir & Hand, 2006). Because learning theories are not necessarily inclusive or compatible, educators must borrow from many different approaches (Vincent & Ross, 2001). Approaches to learning should be modified to include learning styles from different cultural backgrounds, because cultural diversity contributes to innovation and creativity within an educational environment (Sieffert, 2006).

Learning Styles and Cultural Implications

In most traditional classrooms, the pedagogical process functions according to mainstream assumptions about culture, which empowers some voices more than others. Some Asian Americans come from cultures where eye contact and active participation are not normal experiences and may be uncomfortable for them (Suinn, 2006). They also tend to remain silent out of consideration for others and do not interrupt other class members. This can manifest as minimal participation in class discussion, and they may sit back and not offer comments in class, even when they have a good understanding of the material and have information that would be helpful to the class, or when they need clarification and additional help with a concept (Fiume, 2005). Hawaiians and Native Americans are accustomed to helping one another instead of working at their desks independently. Both cultures feel strongly about this way of learning: collaboration is the norm. Participants may not want to stand out from the group because individual praise is discouraged. They believe that it spotlights a person and is culturally incongruous, whereas group praise is anthropologically acceptable (Swisher, 1991; Vogt, Jordan, & Tharp, 1987). Other researchers have indicated that students of African descent and Latinos are also more group oriented, cooperative, and less competitive than those of European descent. Traditionally, most educators see unassigned group work as cheating rather than collaborating or modeling (Griggs & Dunn, 1996). The cultural values of European Americans thrive on collaboration and discussion and getting their opinions heard. Class discussion is more acceptable because it is what they are used to and offers an opportunity to show off their knowledge base. They also tend to be more individualistic and often competitive

(Fiume, 2005). Of course, students raised in the American culture can also be shy or nonparticipating, especially in large classes, and small-group discussions can be helpful for them as well. In higher education, the phenomenon of group assessment, collaboration, and cooperative learning is becoming a positive trend.

Although we are making improvements toward developing new, innovative pedagogical assessment tools, group collaboration on exams is still viewed negatively and forbidden in many classrooms. Additionally, Pewewardy (2002) stated that many culturally diverse students are field dependent, where European-descent students are field independent. Field dependency or global processing is a learning style in which students are unable to perceive themselves as separate from their environment. These students are holistic learners, right-brain dominant, highly relational, visual/spatial, intuitive, integrative, and contextual. The field-dependent learner establishes meaning only in relation to the whole and prefers a loosely structured learning environment that includes group work and collaboration (Graybill, 1997). Field-independent learners tend to be linear or hierarchical, analytical, logical, and temporal. These learners often prefer classroom activity that requires competition and individual gain as well as impersonal work. Field-independent learners are able to divide and subdivide the whole into minute pieces. When classroom information is presented in an analytical and sequential manner, this places field-dependent learners at a disadvantage (Graybill, 1997).

Learning Styles and Pedagogical Strategies

Researchers have suggested no single instructional method will be effective in a culturally diverse classroom. Therefore, more attention must be given to helping educators develop a repertoire of instructional and assessment methods that include cultural differences and address various learning styles (Hurtado, 1996). Classroom teaching practices grounded in anthropological and constructivist education theory may be able to meet the challenges presented by culturally diverse classrooms. One of the primary beliefs of constructivist pedagogy is that knowledge comes about through the efforts of people interacting with each other and crossing various diverse social borders (Fuime, 2005). Phuntsog (1999) also acknowledged the need for culturally responsive teaching, which may require teachers to change the structure of classroom interactions and activities in order to meet the needs of students with different learning styles. Understanding the learning styles of our culturally diverse students can benefit not only educators, but also their students. When students understand how they learn, this empowers them to better manage their own learning. Educators benefit by developing curricula to include various classroom assessment tools to disseminate the information across the spectrum of learning styles (Vincent & Ross, 2001).

Teaching methods should be determined by distinct learning objectives adapted for variables such as goals to be attained and the learning styles of individual students. Some of the more well-known learning styles presented in the literature include Howard Gardner's seven distinct learning intelligences, Anthony Gregorc's learning styles models, Alice Kolb's four learning modes, Myers and Briggs's learning types preferences, and Carol Kanar's visual, auditory, and kinesthetic learning styles, which are related to physiological factors. Although most educators agree different learning styles do exist and have a substantial effect on the learning process, this wealth of available information can sometimes be confusing because there is no real consensus on acceptable criteria for practice (Vincent & Ross, 2001).

The diversity of cultures and learning styles in their classroom inspired Green and Stortz (2006) to search for a common culture that was accessible to everyone regardless of race, ethnicity, or culture. Their first goal was to understand the learning styles of their students. They were able to accomplish this by asking students about their own preferred modes of learning and their prior experiences. Second, they wanted to help the students better understand their own learning styles. Third, they wanted the students to learn to appreciate the diversity in the classroom and see it as a resource rather than an obstacle. According to Fuime (2005), active discussion is one instructional method that blends the many social borders that come together in culturally diverse classrooms. Other pedagogical practices that enhance learning include small-group work, debates on specific topics, case studies, dialogue, role play/simulation, and opportunities for open responses and language immersion (Fuime, 2005; Klein, 2008). It is important for the students' voices to be heard; an instructor can do this by relating their personal experiences to scholarship and by promoting these experiences as an essential pedagogical tool. When students feel comfortable contributing to discussion in the classroom, they are not only empowered, but also function as agents in construction of their own knowledge (Fuime, 2005). Classroom social interactions that cross age, gender, and cultural barriers, including cooperative learning, can help students make connections with other cultures and develop a community of learners. Student-taught classrooms require that each person act as an expert in an assigned subject. The students are then required to work collaboratively and teach one another. The use of this pedagogical tool will promote higher success for the entire class, rather than certain individuals (Ladson-Billings, 2008). Immediate assessment tools, called *feedback loops*, using free writing or specific questions, can help to evaluate whether the students are learning. The goal of culturally inclusive pedagogy is to combine cognitive and experiential learning strategies that allow exploration of individual learning styles and facilitate learning. Discovering their learning style will allow students to apply those strategies to actual interpersonal and cross-cultural situations, with an emphasis on personal growth and development (Reggy-Mamo, 2008). As educators, our role is to facilitate learning by setting a positive climate for learning. A better knowledge and understanding of learning styles allows the educator to teach in a multifarious fashion that both reaches the greatest number of students and challenges all students to grow as learners (Gilakjani, 2011).

■ Working with a Diverse Student Body

Diversity can have a positive impact on teaching and learning. When encouraged by faculty, recognition and understanding of differences and an introduction to other cultures can broaden viewpoints and stimulate discussion and ideas (Villaruel,

Canales, & Torres, 2001). However, it is important to point out that although this chapter covers some cultural traits, there is a wide range of cultural responses and traits within a single culture. Members of a racial or cultural group may or may not adhere to some of the traditions of their background culture and ethnic group, and they may not even identify as a member of that group. Gutierrez and Rogoff (2003) warned that relating learning styles to certain cultures may negate a person's individuality and result in stereotyping and defined limitations on how members of a certain culture can learn. Although it is important to understand the learning styles of individuals in different cultures, overgeneralizing can also be harmful (Morgan, 2009). Faculty members must remember that people are individuals who react differently and must be treated individually. A student who is a member of a particular cultural group cannot be expected to be a spokesperson for that group. There are too many variations within the groups themselves, and what is appropriate for one sect or subgroup within a group may not be acceptable to another sect in the group.

Discrimination is always a difficult issue, and faculty, staff, administrators, and patients are not immune from it. We all have our likes, dislikes, and moral beliefs. Because of their previous experiences, many multicultural students will see discrimination where others do not. This perception must be respected, and cannot be brushed off or dismissed, but sometimes it also must be faced, corrected, or worked with. The major thrust here should be concentration on providing appropriate learning opportunities and meeting learning objectives. Seeking ways to help students learn about each other can be a positive force in changing discriminatory attitudes. Many myths underlying prejudice and discrimination can be dismantled and dismissed when students who have led sheltered lives begin to know those who are different from them and understand that although there are cultural differences, there are also many similarities.

However, conflict between cultural groups does occur in the classroom. There can be other sources for conflict that have nothing to do with ethnicity, as well as conflicts that are based in ethnicity and values. In some instances, mediation may be helpful to define limits and focus the groups back on the learning tasks at hand. Separation may work for other groups, but this is usually a temporary situation until the strong feelings subside. Encouraging groups to learn about each other is a strategy that can be used to defuse potential conflict, but this strategy has to be carefully managed, and the instructor needs to observe group dynamics and be on the alert for peer-influenced negative ideas and peer pressure to adopt those ideas.

Baumgartner and Johnson-Bailey (2008) note that traditionally we, as teachers, work to avoid emotions in working with diversity, with negative emotions to be avoided and strong emotions to be kept under control. Engaged students oftentimes will display strong emotions. Baumgartner and Johnson-Bailey (2008) stress that while it is important not to get mired in emotions when discussing challenging issues, there is also an opportunity for a good teaching moment to explore.

> When a student expresses a strong emotion, it is a good time to take an intellectual breather and say, "Do you mind if we explore that?" . . . or "How about we step back

from this emotional terrain and deconstruct this premise." Take advantage of the energy learners bring to your classroom even when it means departing from the syllabus. These rare challenging teachable moments should be embraced as opportunities to knock down walls. (p. 52)

Developing a welcoming and supportive environment is essential, not only for multicultural students, but also for the other groups that are part of the diverse classroom, including single parents, disabled students, and those with age and gender disparities. Faculty availability and interest are critical elements in developing a positive environment. Instructors need to be aware of potential issues, know their students, and demonstrate interest in students and their success in the program. The importance of cultural and linguistic role models (e.g., community health professionals of color and/or those from minority-based professional organizations, including those who speak a similar language) cannot be overemphasized, because role modeling has a universal effect on overcoming obstacles and achieving academic success for students of color and English-as-a-second-language (ESL) students (Heller & Lichtenberg, 2003; Yoder, 1996). Mentoring has been successful, whether it comes from outside the school or from an advanced student of one's own ethnic or cultural origin, especially when there are no faculty members of color. Those same principles apply to gender-based multicultural students, who may also feel isolated or unwelcome in the profession.

When learning difficulties appear in any group of students, it is important to look for behavioral patterns that may be affecting their success or other stresses or anxieties that seem present. Some students need to be encouraged to be tested for learning disabilities. A diagnosis of a learning disorder, confirmed by testing, allows the student access to the resources required under ADA regulations. Faculty need to learn about student support services in their college. They need to know to whom and how to make referrals for students in areas such as financial aid, study skills, test-taking skills and tutorial assistance, mental and physical health services, and social services. It is extremely important for students to be supported and encouraged to take advantage of those services.

Age Range

Older students will have a sense of history during their lifetime that is very different from the 18-year-olds, and they have learned how to deal with many situations the 18-year-olds have not yet faced, which can be valuable when there are opportunities for sharing. However, depending on their success or frustration levels in working with those situations, older students can also hold an entrenched cynical or ingrained view that must be worked with and mediated at times. Older students may not value the young lifestyle and find younger students immature. Building on some of the strengths of the younger groups growing up in the technology age can be helpful to older students who are not comfortable with the technology.

Young students can be bored by the older students' experiences, tired of listening to them, or not relate those experiences to their own, or they can be interested in and learn from them. Younger students may relate to older students as parental figures—which can be good or bad—viewing them as caring or the extreme of dictatorial or authoritarian, which is often based in their prior experiences with older adults.

The most important task is getting students in different age groups to respect and learn from each other. Small-group work can create diverse working groups. Monitoring group work is important to identify conflict areas. However, when students in different age levels get to know each other better and have success in working together toward a common goal of meeting learning objectives, negative perceptions can change, and the students can be a positive support for each other.

Communication

Communication between minority cultural and ethnic groups and the majority group can be problematic. The learning goals and objectives have to be clearly understood by both students and the teacher in a diverse classroom. Communication is often an issue and at the same time is the key to understanding and acceptance of those goals. A diverse group of students may have their own individual goals and objectives based on their interests and learning experiences, and may or may not be willing to share them with the instructor. An instructor needs to be open to listen to and encourage ideas that may differ from the ones he or she planned for the class, and allow appropriate analytic, creative, and practical knowledge to be utilized. It may be easier for ESL students to read English than it is to understand English conversation, so written instructions or handouts may be helpful and allow students more time to clarify concepts. Instructors need to speak slowly and clearly in classroom presentations, and conversational pauses may have to be longer so students can be encouraged to speak up, but also to allow them to catch up with what is being said and with note taking.

Students and faculty may have a difference in perception, especially if English is not the primary language. Ideas may not translate well. One of the authors had the experience of presenting a lecture in Taiwan and working with a Taiwanese nurse who spoke English well and was responsible for translating comments to the audience into their native language. The author and translator met and went over the lecture notes. While the translator wrote her translations, things seemed to be going very well, until she asked the author, "What is custodial care?" The author immediately realized that she had assumed the translator understood everything that was being discussed—but that was not necessarily the case. The pair went over the speech again until the author was comfortable that the translator understood the concepts and would be able to translate them appropriately.

American ideals and values may be different from what some students are used to. One of the most important aspects in working with all students, but especially with multicultural and ESL students, is what the authors call "know your PVCs." This is not the cardiac term most of us are familiar with, but instead stands for *perception, validation,* and *clarification.* Each person perceives an event differently. An inquiry to see if there are any questions or areas they do not understand must have more depth than just asking if the students understand, and expecting and getting a *yes* answer. Students need to be encouraged to articulate what they think was said, and differences in understanding explored. Formal classroom assessment techniques can also be helpful in identifying problem areas (Angelo & Cross, 1994).

When an instructor feels that a student lacks understanding of the materials, it is important to question the *perception* with the student; *validate* that what was meant to be communicated is in reality what the student understood to be communicated; and, when there is a difference, *clarify*. Students who are not proficient in English may smile and seem to understand, but often they do not, and they may not want to ask for clarification or for statements to be repeated in front of the whole class. It is important for faculty to be aware of this possibility, and follow-through outside of the classroom environment may be necessary.

Accommodation

The passage of the Americans with Disabilities Act in 1990 has made a major difference in today's classroom. Instructors need to adjust to required accommodations. Think about the following: If a health professional is injured or comes down with a debilitating illness or has to use a wheelchair, can accommodations be made so he or she can continue working? In most cases employees can and will be accommodated in various jobs within the profession, even those employees who become deaf or legally blind. These jobs may not be those involving the usual clinical care, but they are still jobs a health professional must perform and are essential for quality care. Think about jobs that a disabled person could perform in your specialty—those that may be possible, despite the fact that some jobs will not be performed at all or as completely. Assistive devices can often be used to allow the employee to perform safely and appropriately in limited activities if he or she has the appropriate clinical knowledge required for the specific position. This being the case, why does the door to the profession have to be closed to these people, and applicants with disabilities turned away? Think about ways in which a disabled student could be prepared to work in those jobs within the profession, and the types of clinical experiences a disabled student can carry out that will provide appropriate experiences for a future job. The technology field is expanding rapidly, and assistive devices are improving and becoming more cost-effective and more available.

Faculty must become well aware of the disability regulations and student support services colleges have set up because of those regulations. Faculties need to develop awareness of the barriers and regulations that are present for disabled students and have to be addressed, and where resources can be found to help both faculty members and students. One issue that must be worked out in a positive manner is making sure these accommodations are fair to the nondisabled students. What does *fair* mean? Disabilities—in particular, learning disabilities or certain physical disabilities such as back problems—may not be visible to others. Rules of privacy may not allow faculty members to discuss a disabled student's condition, but they can encourage the student to discuss this issue with others and provide support as necessary.

For many years, teachers were authoritarians in the classrooms, with rigid standards and rules and regulations. Things are different today. Student demonstrations in the late 1960s and early 1970s began a students' rights movement that altered college cultures. But some questions have to be asked. How much compromise is possible, and how do we work within regulated issues? A very positive part of students' rights has been forcing faculties to look at what they were doing and assess whether they were working by ritual or providing real learning opportunities. Such faculties have learned to work successfully with students who, in the past, would not have had the opportunities available to them today.

Making accommodations is also an important concept for those with heavy personal responsibilities. Older students may be faced with family issues, such as caring for children and/or elderly parents. They and single parents may have responsibilities that interfere with their ability to meet deadlines or come to class. Rigid attendance policies are often more ritualistic than real: The focus should be on what is necessary for the learning experience. Sitting in a class does not guarantee that a student is attentive and learning. Teachers are well aware students daydream, have conversations with their classmates, and even fall asleep, and they will forget a good portion of what was presented, even though we as teachers believe every word we say is valuable. It may be more important for a student to attend a small seminar-type class, because the learning is more dependent on participation in discussion than it is when sitting in a large lecture session. The important, determining issue is what the goals and objectives are for the course, and whether there are other ways to meet them without perfect attendance. That may sound heretical, but there are other ways for conscientious and motivated students to meet learning objectives and set priorities. Use of the Internet, library services, and out-of-class assignments can afford some flexibility if needed. Attendance at clinical experiences may be more problematic because of the need for scheduling and faculty availability, but there are ways to design a program with a student that may afford some flexibility for specific instances. Again, it is important to keep the learning goal of the experience or class in mind and consider creative and flexible ways to work with students to plan for what they feel they can accomplish.

Financially challenged students may not be able to participate in some activities because they have to work in addition to their school responsibilities. They may have difficulty in buying books and special or technological equipment or participating in outside learning opportunities, such as conferences or lectures that have a fee attached. These students may not be able to spend hours in the library because of their work and family schedules, and finding study time may be difficult. Anxiety and worry over finances can seriously detract from their learning experience.

There is no easy solution to these issues, but again, student services can often be an ally. Student lives outside the classroom have to be respected, but the responsibility for learning is theirs, not yours. Students and faculty can work together to assess what is needed to achieve the objectives of the learning experiences and to facilitate their learning. Are there alternative ways of achieving those objectives that do not run up against the "Is it fair to others" question? It is important for instructors to meet with student services to find out just what they do and how they do it. Student services can help students set up workable schedules, tutorial services, and study and testing guidance. They can also counsel students on student life issues and refer students to outside resources when needed. Faculty should also be familiar with financial aid issues and regulations, which can be quite complicated because of differences in governmental and private sources, and be able to provide students with outside services for referrals when appropriate.

Academic Issues

Students with academic problems need to be identified early and encouraged to discuss the issue with faculty without the specter of punishment or embarrassment. It is important to discover patterns of negative behavior, discuss them directly with the students involved, and develop a plan the students and faculty agree to and believe can be implemented and carried out. Unfortunately, not all students can be helped, and some will drop out or fail the course, but others will be successful and benefit from the encouragement.

Students with learning disabilities and ESL students may have problems with timed tests. ESL students may need more time to read and digest test questions because they may be translating the questions into their primary language, and some words and phrases do not translate well. Students with learning disabilities are supported in the need for additional time by the ADA regulations, but that is not true for ESL students. To evaluate and accurately grade the level of knowledge, faculty can provide opportunities for various types of testing other than timed tests (take-home tests being one example). There may be a limit to this, however, when students need to improve in timed testing because of national licensing exams. Again, students with a learning disability may have additional time because the regulations support them, but ESL students can fail in timed tests, and those students may need practice and/ or tutorial assistance to become more proficient in testing so as to pass a licensing exam and enter the profession.

■ Conclusion

Although working with diverse students can be challenging, it can also be stimulating and exciting. As healthcare professionals, learning about new cultures and disabilities will be translated into increased cultural competence when working with patients.

Remember that although the responsibility for learning lies with the learner, feelings of anxiety and isolation can cause stress that negatively affects the learning process and may affect graduation rates and successful entrance into the profession. Family responsibilities can also interfere with a student's ability to carry out the required work. Faculty members need to learn to develop sensitivity to and awareness of issues that impact the learning process and work with students to meet the learning goals. They need to develop their knowledge of available services and resources that can be utilized by students. A culturally inclusive pedagogy also incorporates various learning styles, allowing the teacher to reach the greatest number of students. Flexibility, patience, and creativity are needed to develop a supportive environment that enhances learning. A major role of faculty is offering support, guidance, and referrals as appropriate and developing a community of students who view diversity as a strength that provides an opportunity to learn from each other as well as from their teachers. It is painful but necessary to understand this will not work for all students; however, it will be appreciated by and benefit many students. Our reward for the efforts expended is we can rightly celebrate and be proud of the successful students whom we have helped enter the profession and who are now providing a valuable service to their patients, communities, and profession.

Discussion Questions

1. Consider the difficult concept of death and dying in a culturally diverse health professions class. Which strategies will you, as the instructor, deploy to enrich this classroom discussion in your diverse classroom? Why did you choose these strategies?
2. Consider the cultural and educational theories as well as the learning styles and cultural implications discussed in this chapter. List three teaching modalities currently used in your classroom. What type of learner will benefit from these modalities, and which learners will be hindered? Reflect and describe strategies to enhance each learner's experience.
3. Consider a student with a learning disability in your classroom. How can you comply with ADA mandates and meet the learning needs of all your students?

References

Angelo, T. A., & Cross, K. P. (1994). *Classroom assessment techniques: A handbook for college teachers* (2nd ed.). San Francisco, CA: Jossey-Bass.

Bain, K. (2004). *What the best college teachers do*. Cambridge, MA: Harvard University Press.

Barbee, E., & Gibson, S. (2001). Our dismal progress: The recruitment of non-Whites into nursing [electronic version]. *Journal of Nursing Education, 40*, 243–244.

Baumgartner, L. M., & Johnson-Bailey, J. (2008). Fostering awareness of diversity and multiculturalism in adult and higher education. *New Directions for Adult & Continuing Education, 120*, 45–53.

Carnegie, M. E. (1991). *The path we tread: Blacks in nursing 1834–1990*. New York, NY: National League for Nursing.

Carnegie, M. E. (2005). Educational preparation of Black nurses: A historical perspective. *ABNF Journal, 16*(1), 6–7.

Carroll, S. M. (2004). Inclusion of people with physical disabilities in nursing education. *Journal of Nursing Education, 43*(5), 207–212.

Dale, R. (2009). *Education theories, cultures, and learning: A critical perspective*. New York, NY: Routledge, Taylor & Francis Group.

Evans, B. C. (2004). Application of the caring curriculum to education of Hispanic/Latino and American Indian nursing students. *Journal of Nursing Education, 43*(5), 219–228.

Fiume, P. (2005). Constructivist theory and border pedagogy foster diversity as a resource for learning. *Community College Enterprise, 11*(2), 51–64.

Gilakjani, A. P. (2011). Visual, auditory, kinesthetic learning styles and their impact on English language teaching. *Journal of Studies in Education, 2*(1), 104–112.

Graybill, S. W. (1997). Questions of race and culture: How they relate to the classroom for African American students. *Clearing House, 70*(6), 311–318.

Green, B., & Stortz, M. (2006). The syllabus as passport into a common culture of teaching and learning: Developing and assessing strategies for dealing with diversity. *Teaching Theology & Religion, 9*(4), 221–228.

Griggs, D., & Dunn, R. (1996). Hispanic-American students and learning style. *ERIC Digest*. Retrieved from ERIC database. (ED393607)

Grosz, R. C. (2005). The forgotten minority [Commentary]. *Internet Journal of Allied Health Sciences and Practice, 3*(3). Retrieved from http://ijahsp.nova.edu/articles/vol3num3/grosz_commentary.htm

Gutierrez, K. D., & Rogof, B. (2003). Cultural ways of learning: Individual traits or repertoires of practice. *Educational Researcher, 32*(5), 19–25.

Hancock, A. (2007). When multiplication doesn't equal quick addition: Examining intersectionally as a research paradigm. *Perspectives on Politics, 5*(1), 63–79.

Heller, B. R., & Lichtenberg, L. P. (2003). Addressing the shortage: Strategies for building the nursing workforce. *Nursing Leadership Forum, 8*(1), 34–39.

Hurtado, S. (1996). How diversity affects teaching and learning. *Educational Record, 77*(4), 27–29. Retrieved from http://www.diversityweb.org/research_and_trends/research_evaluation_impact/benefits_of_diversity/sylvia_hurtado.cfm

Jacob, E., & Jordan, C. (Eds.). (1996). *Minority education: Anthropological perspectives.* Norwood, NJ: Ablex Publishing.

Kana'iaupuni, S., Ledward, B., & Jensen, U. (2010). Culture based education and its relationship to student outcomes. *Kamehameha Schools Research and Evaluation.* Retrieved from http://www.ksbe.edu/_assets/spi/pdfs/CBE_relationship_to_student_outcomes.pdf

Kirkland, M. L. S. (1998). Stressors and coping strategies among successful female African American baccalaureate nursing students. *Journal of Nursing Education, 37*(1), 5–13.

Klein, A. M. (2008). Sensitivity to the learning needs of newcomers in foreign language settings. *Multicultural Education, 16*(2), 41–44. (ERIC document EJ832227) Retrieved from http://www.teqjournal.org/sample_issue/article_6.htm

Kosowski, M. M., Grams, K. M., Taylor, G. J., & Wilson, C. B. (2001). They took the time . . . they started to care: Stories of African-American nursing students in intercultural caring groups. *Advances in Nursing Science, 23*(3), 11–27.

Ladson-Billings, G. (2008). Toward a theory of culturally relevant pedagogy. *American Educational Research Journal, 32*(3), 465–491.

Lowenstein, A. (1990, March 28–April 1). Racial segregation and nursing education in Georgia: The Lamar experience. *Proceedings of the National Association for Equal Opportunity in Higher Education's (NAFEO's) 15th National Conference on Blacks in Higher Education,* Washington, DC.

Lowenstein, A. (1994, September). *Racial segregation and nursing education in Georgia: The Lamar experience.* Paper presented at the annual convention of the Transcultural Nursing Society, Atlanta, GA.

Lowenstein, A. J., & Glanville, C. (1995). Cultural diversity and conflict in the health care workplace. *Nursing Economics, 13*(4), 203–209, 247.

Moffat, M. (2003). The history of physical therapy practice in the United States. *Journal of Physical Therapy Education, 17*(3), 15–25.

Morgan, H. (2009). What every teacher needs to know to teach Native American students. *Multicultural Education, 16*(4), 10–12.

Nasir, S. N., & Hand, V. M. (2006). Exploring sociocultural perspectives on race, culture, and learning. *Review of Educational Research, 76*(4), 449–475.

Ogunsiji, O., & Wilkes, L. (2005). Managing family life while studying: Single mothers' lived experience of being students in a nursing program. *Contemporary Nurse, 18*(1–2), 108–123.

Pewewardy, C. (2002). Learning styles of American Indian/Alaska Native students: A review of the literature and implications for practice. *Journal of American Indian Education, 41*(3), 22–56.

Phuntsog, N. (1999). The magic of culturally responsive pedagogy: In search of the genie's lamp in multicultural education. *Teacher Education Quarterly, 26*(3). Retrieved from http://www.teqjournal.org/sample_issue/article_6.htm

Reggy-Mamo, M. (2008). An experiential approach to intercultural education. *Christian Higher Education, 7*(2), 110–122.

Sieffert, S. (2006). *Placing culture at the forefront.* Saskatoon, Canada: University of Saskachewan. Retrieved from http://www.usask.ca/education/coursework/802papers/seiffert/index.htm

Silver, J. H., Sr. (2002). Diversity issues. In R. Diamond (Ed.), *Field guide to academic leadership* (pp. 357–372). San Francisco, CA: Jossey-Bass.

Splenser, P. E., Canlas, H. L., Sanders, B., & Melzer, B. (2003). Minority recruitment and retention strategies in physical therapist education programs. *Journal of Physical Therapy Education, 17*(1), 18–26.

Suinn, R. M. (2006). Teaching culturally diverse students. In W. J. McKeachie & M. Svinicki (Eds.), *McKeachie's teaching tips* (12th ed., pp. 152–171). Boston, MA: Houghton Mifflin.

Swisher, K. (1991). American Indian/Native American learning styles: Research and practice. *ERIC Digest*. Retrieved from ERIC database. (ED335175)

Vasquez, J. (1990). Instructional responsibilities of college faculty to minority students. *Journal of Negro Education, 59*, 599–610.

Villaruel, A. M., Canales, M., & Torres, S. (2001). Educational mobility of Hispanic nurses. *Journal of Nursing Education, 40*(6), 245–251.

Vincent, A., & Ross, D. (2001). Learning styles awareness: A basis for developing teaching and learning strategies. *Journal of Research on Technology in Education, 33*(5), 1–10.

Vogt, L. A., Jordan, C., & Tharp, R. G. (1987). Explaining school failure, producing school success: Two cases. *Anthropology and Education Quarterly, 18*(4), 276–286.

Wessling, S. (2000, Fall). Coming home: Two unique programs are giving homeless and disadvantaged persons an opportunity to start again as nursing professionals. *Minority Nurse*, 32–35.

Yoder, M. (1996). Instructional responses to ethnically diverse nursing students. *Journal of Nursing Education, 35*, 315–321.

Recommended Reading

Byrne, M. (2001). Uncovering racial bias in nursing fundamentals textbooks. *Nursing and Health Care Perspectives, 22*, 299–303.

Dickerson, S., & Neary, M. (1999). Faculty experiences teaching Native Americans in a university setting. *Journal of Transcultural Nursing, 10*(1), 56–64.

Edward, J. (2000). Teaching strategies for foreign nurses. *Journal for Nurses in Staff Development, 16*(4), 171–173.

Griffiths, M., & Tagliareni, E. (1999). Challenging traditional assumptions about minority students in nursing education. *Nursing & Health Care Perspectives, 20*, 290–295.

Gurin, P., Dey, E. L., Hurtado, S., & Gurin, G. (2002). Diversity and higher education: Theory and impact on educational outcomes. *Harvard Educational Review, 72*(3), 330–366.

Maruyama, G., Moreno, J. F., Gudeman, R. H., & Marin, P. (2000). *Does diversity make a difference? Three research studies on diversity in college classrooms*. Washington, DC: American Association of University Professors. Retrieved from ERIC database. (ED444409)

Maville, J., & Huerta, C. (1997). Stress and social support among Hispanic student nurses: Implications for academic achievement. *Journal of Cultural Diversity, 4*(1), 18–25.

Miller, J. E., & Hollenshead, C. (2005). Gender, family, and flexibility—why they're important in the academic workplace. *Change, 37*(6), 58–62.

Taylor, V., & Rust, G. (1999). The needs of students from diverse cultures. *Academic Medicine, 74*, 302–304.

Weaver, H. (2001). Indigenous nurses and professional education: Friends or foe? *Journal of Nursing Education, 40*(6), 252–258.

Yurkovich, E. (2001). Working with American Indians toward educational success. *Journal of Nursing Education, 40*(6), 259–269.

Electronic Resources

U.S. Department of Justice. *ADA regulations and technical assistance materials*. Retrieved from http://www.usdoj.gov/crt/ada/publicat.htm

CHAPTER 3

The Teaching–Learning Experience from a Generational Perspective

Lyn Pesta

Cheryl A. Tucker

> Each generation sees farther than the generation that preceded it because it stands on the shoulders of that generation. You're going to have opportunities beyond anything that we've ever known.
>
> — *Ronald Reagan, 1981*

Much has been written in pedagogical and business literature about the learning differences among generations. Each generation is shaped in part by the cultural, technological, and political events that have transpired during the members' formative years. Therefore, each generation carries its own unique imprint from specific generational influences. Most of the college classrooms today are filled by generation X and Y (Xers and Yers) students, with the minority group being baby boomers. However, boomers have heavy influence on both of the younger generations as their parents and teachers.

Projection data for 2010–2020 from the U.S. Bureau of Labor Statistics (BLS) indicate that job growth is expected in all areas of healthcare occupations, and health care will generate more than 5.7 million new wage and salaried positions. There are currently 2,737,000 registered nurses in the United States. By 2020, the need is estimated to grow to 3,449,300 (BLS, 2012). Universities, colleges, and training centers that prepare people for health occupations may find several challenges in recruiting, admitting, and retaining a workforce prepared to meet the demand. Tension may arise between learners and educators of differing generations who may have conflicting expectations of each other.

■ Generational Perspectives of Faculty and Students

Several generations are bound together for the transference of essential knowledge, skills, and attitudes for the health professions. Faculty typically consist of three generations: the veterans/traditionalist/silent generation (veterans), who were born in the years between 1922 and 1945; the baby boom generation (boomers), who were born between 1946 and 1964; and generation X (Xers), who were born between 1965 and 1981. There is some overlap of years for each generation, depending on the source. Many healthcare programs, especially nursing, attract a wide group of students, including the traditional student who enters college after high school graduation, the slightly older student who has worked after high school or perhaps has a young family, and the seasoned individual who decides to pursue a healthcare career after raising a family or deciding to change professions. To help meet predicted needs for healthcare professions, recruitment efforts will remain focused on appealing to a younger demographic, fostering the idea throughout secondary educational settings that health care is an attractive career choice (Cohen et al., 2006). The majority of nursing students are either in generation Y, born between 1982 and 2001, or generation X. A minority of students today are boomers.

The Veterans

Cultural Setting

Most veterans experienced the effects of the Great Depression, where an estimated 25% to 30% of the U.S. population experienced unemployment or displacement. This ended when World War II broke out in 1941. Social programs such as Medicaid and Medicare were decades away. Credit cards had not arrived. Veterans are known for patriotism, loyalty, and duty. Many families were just beginning to be able to afford a family car, but the interstate highway system that linked remote areas of the nation had not been built. People listened to swing and the big band sounds of Tommy Dorsey and Glenn Miller on 78 rpm records. The whole family sat near the radio and listened to President Franklin Roosevelt's "fireside chats" or was spellbound by the *Shadow* series and other radio shows. Reel-to-reel tape recorders and televisions were new and extremely expensive. Any adult could correct a youngster, and such behavior was not considered extraordinary by a parent. The virtues of frugality, thriftiness, and self-restraint were necessary for survival.

Rapid advances in health care came about during and after World War II. However, polio and tuberculosis killed or crippled thousands of people during this era. Many died from infection or sepsis from simple traumas. The widespread availability of penicillin during the 1940s reduced infection death rates (Smith & Bradshaw, 2008).

Despite the United States being the "melting pot" of the world, cultural diversity was not the norm or routine part of life for veterans, especially in smaller cities, towns, or isolated rural communities. Most Americans lived in homogenous neighborhoods that were segregated by cultural practice, religious belief, race, or ethnicity. Family farms were still a way of life, and veterans were often isolated from outside influences. Life for the veterans was simpler, but they grew up in a formal and ordered society where manners and decorum were prized. They were taught not to question those in authority. Information from the outside world came from movie newsreels, *Life* magazine, newspapers, and postal delivery of handwritten letters. The digital age has made the world a smaller place, yet the veterans are not as accepting of cultural differences as are the younger generations.

Characteristics/Work Ethics/Learning Styles

Veterans are known to be disciplined, hardworking, patriotic, and loyal. Veterans are known to be team players. There is an almost universal belief within this generation in the motto, "All for one and one for all"—that is, the group good supersedes individual desires. Veterans believe that history has important lessons to be followed and used as bridges to the future. They have reached retirement age, but many work due to changes in retirement goals. Workplace stability and longevity in the work environment are prized by this cohort. Being raised in an environment that valued deference to established rules, veterans will usually follow the status quo. Veterans appreciate the wisdom of experienced leaders and elders, and they appreciate the mentor/mentee aspects of personal and professional relationships. Finally, veterans prefer a hierarchical structure in the workplace where lines of authority and responsibility are well defined. Veterans spent most of their lives without the convenience (or headaches) associated with personal computers, laptops, personal digital assistants (PDAs), instant messaging, e-mail, and Facebook. In fact, they often view technology suspiciously or as an intrusion. They put a higher value on face-to-face interaction, well-written notes, and telephone conversations (Outten, 2012).

The educational system in place during a veteran's upbringing placed a heavy emphasis on reading, writing, and arithmetic. Most learning acquisition occurred with an emphasis on process. Knowledge was obtained through sequential, step-by-step instruction and through memorization drills. Because of this, veterans may have a higher comfort level when these strategies are used in teaching. There are few veteran faculty, but their influences persist in traditional healthcare curricula, policies, and teaching strategies.

The Baby Boomers

Cultural Setting

Boomers are generally classified as being born between the years of 1946 and 1964. During this time, the middle class was growing along with the economy. Growth meant more resources to purchase goods. Automobiles, time-saving appliances, electronics, and store-bought clothing became the norm. The baby boomer generation learned that credit cards could provide more purchasing power and adopted a "buy now, pay later" mindset with respect to homes, cars, and big-ticket items (Johnson & Romanello, 2005). Advances in medicine and health care meant that people lived longer. Health insurance was an anticipated benefit when one worked for a company or corporation.

Boomers were born prior to digital technology. Because veterans and boomers needed to learn these digital technologies, often as a result of employer mandates, they are sometimes called *digital immigrants* (Prensky, 2001). Boomers needed to adapt and catch up to the rapid changes brought about by the introduction of the public Internet in the early 1990s and the ubiquitous presence of personal computing, e-mail, distance learning, cellular telephones, and rapid information access through powerful search engines. Boomers learned that some of their previously prized skills of penmanship and spelling were antiquated. Predigital education placed an emphasis on punctuation, writing, spelling, drills, rules, and memorization. Learners were taught in a highly structured, teacher-centered educational system that called for obedience to the rules. Computers were behemoths and, because of their large size, needed entire rooms to house them. The average person could neither afford nor use a personal computer. Simple arithmetic could not be done on calculators. Manual typewriters created important documents; correction fluid was considered a major time saver for correcting typed mistakes. Early television was not created as an educational tool but as entertainment that viewers watched on small, 9-inch screens in black and white with metal antennae. In the educational setting, challenging a teacher or parent was not usual or tolerated. Corporal punishment was not considered child abuse and was often used for a disobedient child.

Boomers used telephones to communicate when face-to-face encounters were not possible. Like learning a new language, they had to adjust to new technologies, such as e-mail and computer networks, as a necessity of work life and not a choice (Sherman, 2006). The boomers are not like the younger generations, who are fascinated with new technology and often view these inventions as time savers and vital connections to significant others (Oblinger, 2003). For the boomer, Friday nights meant attending a chaperoned dance at school. London's Twiggy was the epitome of fashion. Boomers relied on eight-track tapes or AM/FM radios for music. Now digital MP3 players provide a wide variety of music in an instant to almost every Xer and Yer. Boomers were enthralled with a variety of musical styles, the most influential being rock. The energetic sounds from a multitude of rock and roll bands emerged. The Woodstock music festival was a celebration of youth and freedom but with a downside of a culture laced with the idealization of illicit drugs, anger sparked by the Vietnam War, and the promotion of casual sex.

Other events of the day also influenced the boomer generation. Following World War II, the tension between Russia and the United States escalated the threat of nuclear war. Other major events that shaped the attitudes of the boomers were the draft, the Vietnam War, the Kent State massacre, the civil rights movement, the assassinations of Martin Luther King, Jr. and President John F. Kennedy, the feminist movement, and President Richard Nixon's Watergate scandal. Protests occurred in the street and on college campuses across the nation. Boomers are seen as idealists who want to right the wrongs of an unjust world (Gardner, Deloney, & Grando, 2007). The overall discontent of the era created an upheaval in the mores of society. Unlike their parents, many boomers came to mistrust authority figures and loudly questioned the wisdom of the institutions of organized religion, government, military, and marriage.

Characteristics/Work Ethics/Learning Styles

It is interesting that, as working adults, the boomers became known as the generation that put in long and hard hours—often at the expense of their families. Often referred to as the "me" generation, boomers sought individual accomplishment over the group good (Benedict, 2008). They often equate work with self-worth. In general, boomers crave positive acknowledgment for work performed and thrive on praise for their efforts. Boomers prefer a more casual style of dress than their predecessors and have an uneasy relationship with authority. The healthcare profession continues to have optimistic growth potential, and many baby boomers dispossessed from another industry, job, or profession may find changing to health care both an attractive and challenging alternative. Boomers are known to be committed, lifelong learners who tend to solve problems by action.

Generation X
Cultural Setting

There are differences among authors as to the exact years that define Xers. Some authors use the years between 1960 and 1977, while other ranges exist in the literature, such as 1965 to 1976 (Jones & Fox, 2009). The most agreed-upon years are in the range of 1965 to 1981. Regardless of the difference in defining age ranges, Xers comprise a much smaller group than the boomers who preceded them and the Yers who came after them. Culturally, this group was shaped by the important events of the time, including *Roe v. Wade* (1973), the U.S. Supreme Court decision that legalized abortion.

Xers were mostly raised by boomer parents. Demographic shifts meant that many generation X children were not raised near extended family or even by both parents. Many children were raised by single parents or parents who both worked. Xers grew up with the experiment of the Children's Workshop Network, known as *Sesame Street*. Some of these children participated in after-school programs manned by unrelated adults. The term *latchkey kid* was coined for the Xer child who was left alone after school hours while a parent or both parents remained at work. Left at home, often without adult supervision, they entertained themselves with television shows, computer games, and videos.

Xer children were exposed to a higher level of violence in movies, music, and in video games. During this time, various musical styles emerged. Music Television (MTV) first aired in 1981. Musical influences such as grunge, heavy metal, and rap entered the mainstream American culture during the typical Xer's formative years. These musical styles and videos contained graphic violence and obscene material that required close monitoring from busy parents. Xers grew up amidst both unprecedented economic prosperity and severe downturns in the economy. Middle-class children were exposed to more marketing commercialism for brand-name clothes, toiletries, and shoes than any other generation before them. Drugs such as ecstasy, heroin, and cocaine became prolific across the country. Major cities had increasing violence owing to gang warfare and violent initiation rites. Nationally, unwed teen pregnancy and divorce rates trended upward while marriage rates dropped (Boonstra, 2002; Stockmayer, 2004). The problems of acquired immune deficiency syndrome (AIDS) and homelessness were part of public discussions. Influential events included the Los Angeles riots of 1991, the *Challenger* space shuttle explosion, and the environmental disaster caused by the wreck of the *Exxon Valdez*. Overseas, the Tian'anmen Square protests of 1989, the unraveling of apartheid in South Africa, the Chernobyl nuclear accident, and the fall of communism helped shape this generation. Communication was instantaneous and brought to life in living color within moments after occurring. The Internet was introduced during this time. Xers became acclimated to learning on personal computers at school and during after-school hours.

Characteristics/Work Ethics/Learning Styles

Many conflicting characteristics are attributed to Xers. Generally they feel comfortable working alone and are considered independent. Due to their upbringing and isolation, it has been said that Xers have learned that they can only rely on themselves. They readily identify friends as extended family. As a learning group, Xers receive instant gratification related to technological advances and from obtaining information at the click of a button. They tend to see themselves as consumers of education, and tend to mistrust authority figures, which may include faculty. Xers become bored in meetings where there is much discussion prior to making decisions (Outten, 2012).

Leisure and time off to enjoy other interests are particularly critical to Xers. Unlike their parents who worked long hours, only to lose out on what their children consider to be the fun of living, Xers jealously guard their free time and view requests to work overtime as intrusions. Because of the higher value they place on personal time over the needs of their employers, they have been viewed as undependable. They highly value their individuality, but, as a group, widely adopted bizarre hair styles, tattoos, and body piercings as a sign of independence from the norm. This generation witnessed companies increasingly grow in international markets, thereby supplanting the local American worker for cheaper labor overseas. They realized that the years of loyalty their grandparents and parents gave in return for job security and a guaranteed pension no longer existed and, as a result, view government programs with skepticism and do not believe that social programs like Social Security will be available for them when they retire. Xers are described as cynical, ironic, clever, pragmatic, and resourceful (Johnson & Romanello, 2005). If there is a collective mantra that sums up the attitude of work versus leisure among Xers, it is "Work to live, not live to work."

Generation Y

Cultural Setting

Depending on the writer, there are many names and descriptions for generation Y. They are referred to as *nexters, generation N, millennials,* and *digital natives.* Collectively, Yers are usually placed as being born between 1981 and 2001. Despite variations in date, what is certain is that most Yers have never known a time before the age of digital technology. Culturally, Yers have been shaped by such events as the 1995 Oklahoma City bombing, the 1996 Summer Olympics bombing, the mass shootings at Columbine High School in 1999, and the terrorist attacks of September 11, 2001.

The War on Terror, with efforts in Iraq and Afghanistan, continues to affect the paradigm of this generation. Generation Yers show a taste for diverse music by rap, alternative, and socially conscious groups such as Coldplay, Yellow Card, and Green Day. Music and videos from Yers' favorite groups can accessed digitally in an instant while the audience is simultaneously performing other tasks (Taylor & Keeter, 2010).

The U.S. birth rate continued to decline in this era. Most children born in this generation were planned and wanted. As a benefit of caring and involved parents, most millennials are secure and value family relationships. Parents who become too involved in every aspect of their child's life are known as *helicopter parents* because of their hovering tendencies—they are ready to swoop down to supply any need or rescue their progeny from any threat (Pricer, 2008).

Characteristics/Work Ethics/Learning Styles

Yers are thought to be more sociable than Xers. While veterans and boomers are referred to as digital immigrants because they were not exposed to the digital world until adulthood, Xers and Yers are comfortable with new technologies and are considered as digital natives (Prensky, 2001). MP3 players, blogs, personal computers, Internet searches with Google or Yahoo, cell phones, instant messaging, text messaging, interactive gaming, video cameras, game technology such as Wii and PlayStation, wikis, Twitter, Flickr, YouTube, and Facebook/MySpace seem foreign to the digital immigrants. Digital natives, in contrast, were constantly exposed to the benefits of computer and digital technology and cannot remember a time before them. Many attributes have been assigned to Yers, including a high comfort level with computers and an insistence on being connected to family and friends technologically. There is no doubt that our world is becoming increasingly interconnected with wireless technology. Because Yers have never known a life without the presence of computers, cable, satellite radio, wireless connections, or cell phones, they are comfortable surfing the web, use digital music sources to download songs to MP3 players, and are usually experts in uploading or downloading videos through YouTube or other sources. Tweeting, texting, and using Facebook are activities that are as essential as breathing to the majority of the Yers (Hahn, 2011).

Parents of Yers have been known to involve their children in a multitude of activities—sports, music, private tutoring, and group activities. Therefore, Yers often have multiple and diverse talents. Generation Yers generally are considered more optimistic than Xers. They have lived structured, scheduled lives and generally are much closer to their parents and feel more comfortable in a structured environment than their earlier X counterparts. They are known to be enthusiastic learners but want to know that "what they are learning is connected to the bigger picture" (Sontag, 2009). Most millennials were encouraged early in life to express and voice their opinions (Piper, 2012). They are known to be deeply committed to causes of justice, environmentalism, and volunteerism for the greater good. Of all the generations before them, they are the most ethnically and racially diverse generation and not only readily accept those who are different, but also celebrate and prize diversity. They consider themselves to be global citizens (Johnson & Romanello, 2005).

The youngest generations have usually been exposed to a great deal of computer and digital technology in their formative years. Yers are comfortable in group settings yet feel isolated when unable to have instant access to friends through communication devices. They are more likely to treat technological innovations as integral to their lives, much like an appendage (Taylor & Keeter, 2010). It has been suggested that millennials may not have the verbal communication skills of their predecessors because they favor the use of digital communication media (Prensky, 2001).

There are similarities and differences among each of the generations. Although each generation is made up of individuals with unique characteristics, it is helpful to list some common characteristics that have been attributed to each generational cohort as outlined here. **Table 3-1** summarizes characteristics associated with each generation.

Table 3-1   Generational Characteristics

Veterans, 1922–1945	Boomers, 1946–1964	Xers, 1964–1981	Yers, 1982–2001
Attributes/Characteristics/Interpersonal Relationships/Communication Style			
• Unselfish; group oriented; loyal; patriotic; will delay gratification; responsible; accept line authority • Prizes the group welfare over individual needs; honors tradition; formal and proper • Prefers personal or written communication; not as comfortable with electronic style; prefers to communicate along established lines of authority	• Self-seeking behaviors; "me" generation • Inconsistent love-hate relationship with authority • Ambitious; challenge status quo; informal; casual; like fewer rules; idealistic • Early wave accused of sacrificing family for work obligations • Prefer face-to-face communication; adapt to technology as a necessity	• Confident; direct; assertive; fearless; adaptable; diverse; impatient; fun; informal; independent; pragmatic; outcome oriented • Challenge authority • Body piercings and tattoos are popular forms of expression; pessimistic tendencies • See friends as extensions of family • Hesitant to commit to marriage and long-term relationships • Prefer technology-enabled communication over face-to-face	• Instant access to desires; technology integrated into life • Assertive; ethnically diverse; optimistic; self-confident in most areas; embrace diversity; civic minded; consumer oriented; self-reliant; enthusiastic; easily bored; idealistic; patriotic; desire respect; optimistic; friendly; cooperative; open-minded; talented; less mature; interested in others; collegial • More respectful of rules and authority than Xers and boomers • Closer to parents than predecessors • Enjoy face-to-face communication; crave social connections via technology • Informal but schedule driven; being smart is cool; team players/collaborative

Table 3-1   Generational Characteristics (*continued*)

Veterans, 1922–1945	Boomers, 1946–1964	Xers, 1964–1981	Yers, 1982–2001
Learning/Work Styles			
• Dependable; follows established rules; prefers hierarchy • Educated in teacher-centered settings • Values mentorship with established leader or experienced person • Less likely to embrace newer technology than successors; more process oriented; seeks job security; very loyal to employer	• Prefers text over graphics; linear thinking; process oriented; step by step • Likes contact with faculty • Lifelong learning commitment; ties learning with life experiences; values rewards for work done; enjoys titles and accolades for achievements; willing to work long hours to get job done • Seeks secure retirement; loyal to employer • Technology reluctant • Does not enjoy games or being put on the spot	• Education began in student-centered settings; processes quickly; multitasks; enjoys fast pace; focused; parallel/mosaic thinking; nonlinear thinking; concrete thinking • Prefers to work alone; needs safe environment to participate; experiential; embraces technology • Little tolerance for extraneous information; dislikes assignments—does not view them as learning enhancements; discounts contact with faculty as important • Desires work and school flexibility; seeks instant results for efforts; self-directed; entrepreneurial • Values free time over work hours; little loyalty to employer; wants success and ambition on his or her own terms; may overestimate contributions to an organization; wants rapid advancement without expending long work hours	• Parallel/mosaic thinking; multitasks; expresses doubts about academic abilities; processes quickly; prefers graphics over text; likes to work in groups; curious; experiential; thrives on discovery; short attention spans; high incidences of ADD/ADHD diagnoses • Enjoys interactive learning and games with immediate response; demands 24/7 access to learning/faculty; learns best by trial and error; prefers more structure than Xers • Likes creatively presented learning materials; enjoys entertainment aspect of learning; no tolerance for delays in class beginning and endings • Has expressed concerns regarding academic abilities; enjoys mentoring relationships from experienced leaders; likes stories that are relevant to content; eager to learn new requirements for work/school • Prefers audio/visuals over reading; expresses higher reading comprehension than Xers

■ Generational Considerations for Educators

Changes in behavior, and thus learning, take place more readily when the student is fully engaged and can actively participate in the learning process. Faculty should plan teaching experiences carefully to achieve successful outcomes. With generational considerations in mind, an educator might ask the following questions:

- Which factors influence each generation involved in educational settings? What are the typical characteristics for each generation?
- How do my generational preferences and characteristics merge with or differ from those of the newer generations?
- What are the best teaching strategies to engage each generation of learners? How do generational differences affect communication?
- Could generational differences simply be maturity issues? How does technology affect the new learner?
- Who are digital natives and who are digital immigrants? Do digital natives think differently than other learners?
- Which strategies can engage the new generation of learners?

Educational Expectations of Teachers

Traditional teacher-centered learning has given way to a more student-centered approach (Brown, Kirkpatrick, Mangum, & Avery, 2008). Within nursing programs, there are decades of separation from the authoritarian, quasi-military chain-of-command programs that dominated training for most of the veterans and boomers. The hospital-based apprenticeship model of nursing education has long since moved into colleges and universities, where students spend much of their time in the classroom but less time with actual patients providing care—yet nursing curricula have not changed substantially (National League for Nursing [NLN], 2003). The challenges of a 21st-century acute care environment, with shortened lengths of stays while maintaining a high degree of safe, ethical, skillful, and efficient care, are emphasized. Increasingly, there are calls to reform nursing education into a model that espouses teaching in action (Benner, Sutphen, Leonard, & Day, 2010). A comprehensive study by the Institute of Medicine (IOM) recommended that nursing curricula be reexamined, updated, and adaptive enough to change with the changing needs of society and technological advances (IOM, 2011).

A well-prepared professional must be educated and equipped to manage the complexities of the system, or he or she will become overwhelmed by role performance demands. Faculty, armed with the knowledge and experience of the profession, challenge students through high ethical standards, self-discipline, professional development, and rigorous program curricula. Students who arrive late or do not attend class, communicate poorly, or appear to be inattentive in class are viewed with a certain amount of negativity. Students who text-message, shop online, do not keep appointments, talk in class, or use a disrespectful tone of voice are seen as uncivil by most boomer or veteran faculty. To maintain a positive rapport between faculty and students of different generations, the faculty member must clearly define behaviors that are acceptable in the classroom and clinical areas (Suplee, Lachman, Siebert, & Anselmi, 2008).

Educational Expectations of Students

Radical changes have occurred in primary, secondary, and postsecondary education for both parents and students in the past several decades. Advances in technology, the view that education is a commodity, developing maturity, tight schedules, previous life experiences, values, and cultural backgrounds have influenced learner attitudes. Education is no longer seen as a revered institution incapable of being criticized, but rather as a product—the result of a consumer-oriented culture. Whereas boomers appreciate a mentoring relationship with faculty, Xers believe they can teach themselves if given the right tools, while Yers view experienced faculty with admiration but not awe. Generation Y students, sheltered by doting parents, are said to be more grade conscious than their earlier counterparts. They are confident and not fearful of challenging faculty over a grade disagreement. They will quite readily voice dissent and demand their consumer rights. Younger students demand respect and to be listened to when their opinions are expressed. They prefer an egalitarian approach in the learning environment (Gardner et al., 2007). The newest generations want faculty who are not only experts in the field but also have recent relevant clinical practice in the subjects that are taught (Oblinger, 2003). Students in today's environment want clear connections and rationales as to why subject matter is to be learned. This coincides with adult learning theory and is not a foreign concept to experienced educators. Students today like personal attention and immediate constructive criticism for their performance. Above all, students seek a connection with faculty (Gardner et al., 2007). Younger generations seek 24/7 access to their instructors (American Association of State Colleges and Universities [AASCU], 2004). One study indicated that 64% of college students would be interested in communicating with faculty outside of the class schedule through postings created in blogs (Junco & Cole-Avent, 2008). Today, schools, colleges, and universities are striving to keep pace with these demands by putting the required technological infrastructures in place to support online access for students and faculty. Communication networks supported by colleges and universities enable communication methods to support the desire for increased learning activities or faculty support outside of the classroom.

Generation Yers anticipate support and nurturing from faculty (Gardner et al., 2007). Both the X and Y generations will adapt to a variety of teaching methods, with Xers being more comfortable with computer, online, and distance learning and self-paced modules. Experiential learning is preferred by both of these generations. Yers have a special penchant for hearing personal stories to illustrate points (e.g., analogies, humor, and wit) and seek an entertainment quality in teaching sessions. Despite their apparent addiction to new technologies, some studies indicate that nursing students actually prefer a well-designed and entertaining PowerPoint presentation with elements of multimedia embedded into the lecture material and a complete set of notes and slides over other methods (Paschal, 2003; Walker et al., 2007). Lecture and explanations are preferred for difficult content topics rather than group work. Undergraduate baccalaureate students younger than 25 years prefer to read about the subject first, followed by an expert's lecture, despite self-reports of reading comprehension difficulties (Walker et al., 2007). When attempting to learn a psychomotor skill, students in these cohorts favor demonstration over a lecture covering the material. Experiential learning fits easily within all three cognitive domains of nursing and is a valued methodology among all generations. Experiential learning is described as learning experiences (Kolb, 1984). Xers actually value doing over knowing, according to one author. Younger-generation learners have been reported to prefer to perform the skill first under the direction of the faculty and then independently, rather than hear a lecture on the material (Walker et al., 2007).

Barriers to the Teaching–Learning Experience

Education in a health professions program is challenging, especially for the incoming student. The sheer amount of reading and material can intimidate even the most scholarly student, yet it is clear that, to be successful in the program, one must be able to comprehend, analyze, and write well (Hawks et al., 2015). Typical Yers will have difficulty reading and studying for long periods of time (Gardner et al., 2007). Multitasking is second nature to the Yers, but sitting and reading for long periods of time is difficult. It is estimated that by the time students reach college, they will have spent 5,000 hours reading compared to 10,000 hours playing video games and 20,000 hours watching television (Prensky, 2001). There is no doubt that Yers have had more sensory input since childhood than earlier generations. Scientific evidence does show that environmental influences alter brain structures (Draganski et al., 2004; Sontag, 2009). It has also been suggested that the newer generations do learn differently from their predecessors because of the excessive amounts of visual stimulation they received throughout childhood.

Parallel/Mosaic Thinking Patterns

Mosaic thinking is a term coined by media theorist Marshall McLuhan (1978), who hypothesized that the electronic age sparked a revolutionary, or mosaic, way of processing information. Western civilization was formerly characterized by the dominance of reading and writing, which is now giving way to electronic media. Linear reasoning relies on a phonetic/alphabetical structure whose use is foundational to logical and sequential thought processes. Mosaic thinking is a consequence of visual symbols and images that are found in media today. According to McLuhan and others, this change in communication has radically altered the way information is processed and society functions. Similarly, parallel thinking is the ability to process information from a variety of sources simultaneously. These thinking/learning patterns have been ascribed especially to the newer generational cohorts who are comfortable in a fast-paced, technologically connected world.

Our newest cohorts connect with various digital technologies as they become available. Digital natives are said to gather information in parallel or a mosaic pattern. They process data quickly and have the ability to take in information simultaneously from various sources. Therefore, they do not always learn in a step-by-step sequential manner. Younger students have been exposed to endless hours of digitally enhanced games (Prensky, 2001). In gaming, trial-and-error methods meet with failure or reward. Quick motor reflexes for conquering spatial barriers and problem solving are rewarded and positively reinforced. A consequence of this is students' reduced tolerance for quiet reading, reflection, and listening. There is evidence that, because of changes in brain activity, technologically dependent students have a shorter attention span and poorer reading abilities than digital immigrants. As a result, boredom is not conducive to active learning.

Another downside to the reliance on instant feedback is the sometimes dubious accuracy of Internet sources. Easy distractibility due to the constant habit of multitasking is often observed in younger students. To engage today's learner, the experienced generations will need to understand their learners' preferred learning styles and adapt or enhance teaching strategies to help them connect with the material. The new generation prefers learning strategies that encourage exploration, discovery, and trial and error. Unfortunately, trial-and-error problem solving takes time and resources. It is not ideal in patient scenarios where the ultimate goal is to protect the patient's safety and comfort within limited time constraints.

Current nursing education may be outdated for digital natives as well as future generations of students. Curricula in health profession programs include a large demand for reading and sequencing. There is an emphasis on step-by-step processes to achieve learning outcomes. This method does not take into account new learners' propensity for a fast-paced, parallel, mosaic thinking pattern. Online access, virtual reality, simulation, and computer games could solve these needs. Because of this, many nursing leaders question whether current nursing curricula are preparing a viable workforce. The American Association of College Nurses and the NLN have published position papers calling for major changes to incorporate the technology of these younger generations (NLN, 2008). More schools are going online to adjust to the ever-increasing demand from students for increasing class schedule flexibility. It is estimated that online and distance nursing programs will continue to rise and remain a viable option for many. Despite the plethora of options for students today, recent studies indicate boomers and Yers prefer face-to-face communication over distance learning–type arrangements.

Strategies for Teaching Among the Generations

To best serve our successors, it will be necessary for faculty to understand our personal biases, learning styles, and preferred methods of teaching (Pardue & Morgan, 2008). The methods used to teach students are going through a radical upheaval because of changes in societal expectations, technological advances, and increased access to information. Adult learning theory rests on the accepted principle that learners will retain and retrieve information when meaning is associated with it. Another important principle of adult learning theory is the idea that adults want to learn what is applicable to them at the moment (Knowles, 1973). Knowledge of the technological advances in a digital age and methods to employ them in the classroom, lab, or clinical site will become increasingly important over time. To say that it would be a necessity to engage the students would be an understatement. Foreknowledge of general attributes of the digitally engaged student is useful for nurse educators who are products of a different generation. For any generation, faculty creativity, an open and honest dialogue, and availability will help create a positive environment for students to thrive.

From a learning perspective, Xers jealously guard their time; they prefer the bullet-point version of subjects. They want to know precisely what they need to know to pass to get good grades in the shortest way possible. They enjoy the presentation of specific information through e-mail, blogs, and instant messaging (Gibson, 2009). Xers have little tolerance for inefficiency and do not want their time wasted. They prefer brief learning episodes followed by group interaction and, because of their independence, will research information easily online (Gibson, 2009). They enjoy online courses because they provide more flexibility in scheduling. Xers are determined to complete tasks but see them only as a means to an end, not as learning for the sake of learning.

Yers learn best in an environment where there are multiple choices for obtaining the information, especially when the subject matter is difficult; choices include detailed notes, recordings of lectures, PowerPoint lectures, and videotapes of lectures that can be reviewed later. Yers value the joy of discovery more than their older counterparts. They are known to enjoy hearing the experiences of teachers whom they consider mentors. This trait may be especially heartening to the educator who has a rich history and experiences to share. Yers may need to be more directed by their educators than Xers (Gardner et al., 2007). Yers appreciate being asked for their opinions and relish opportunities to be part of a discussion. They are comfortable with technology and prefer peer collaboration, individual feedback, and interaction (Revell & McCurry, 2010). They demand respect from those who are in leadership roles. The Yer is more likely to be engaged when teaching strategies involve creative solutions (Gibson, 2009). The Yer prefers immediate feedback and instructors who are available beyond the classroom schedule.

The use of classroom clickers is a method to enhance classroom participation and may appeal to all generations within the classroom. They allow anonymous responses to classroom activities and provide immediate feedback to problems (Skiba & Barton, 2006). The risk for exposure is minimal; this aspect would appeal to a boomer student who chooses an incorrect response.

Technology and the role it plays in our lives will continue to expand, which may sometimes be intimidating and frustrating for the older generations but not so for the younger generations. In the workplace, the trend toward increasing reliance on electronic and digital equipment and electronic medical records underscores the fact that technology marches forward. It will be necessary to utilize the technology already in the workplace to prepare future health professionals. The Technology Informatics Guiding Education Reform (TIGER) initiative begun in 2007 is a national plan to move nursing practice and education into the digital age. Members and experts from nursing education, informational technology, practice areas, and government agencies are collaborating to meet a 10-year strategic plan. The TIGER vision is twofold. First, it aims to "allow informatics tools, principles, theories and practices to be used by nurses to make healthcare safer, effective, efficient, patient-centered, timely and equitable"; second, its goal is to "interweave enabling technologies transparently into nursing practice and education, making information technology the stethoscope for the 21st century" (TIGER, 2007, p. 6).

High-fidelity simulation (HFS) labs that use standardized patients and human-like computerized manikins to mimic real patient clinical situations are becoming more prevalent. This teaching methodology correlates with the preferences of the youngest generation to learn in an immersive and experiential approach that encourages important linkages between theory and practice. HFS fulfills the requirement to meet learning objectives, perform important skills, and develop clinical reasoning skills. Debriefing by faculty facilitators encourages students to analyze specific decisions and actions and reflect for future actions. Using a high-fidelity simulation lab requires dedication on the part of the program due to the added expense and time commitments (Garrett, MacPhee, & Jackson, 2010).

There are countless ways of involving and engaging students in experiential methods, with or without technological enhancements. Virtual clinical experiences and lab practice are becoming more affordable, reliable, and evidence based. They may be essential educator extensions as the shortage of qualified educators in the health professions continues. They blend well with the traditional methods to assist the learner in gaining psychomotor skills. The power of multisensory experiences embedded in curricular teaching strategies cannot be overestimated, because it increases the long-term memory retention and retrieval of the material for the learner. Increased networking with other faculty who are at distant universities, through electronic mailing lists or blogs, represents a viable way for faculty to increase their teaching method repertoires.

Computer-based video games have been part of entertainment and primary education for many years. Students are exposed to simulation experiences at increasingly younger ages. They become experts at manipulating objects in spatial environments repetitively throughout their childhoods. Applying trial-and-error methods in a safe environment allows the participant to practice necessary skills until perfection is achieved. Sources indicate that most younger students, especially digital natives, thrive on this type of learning. Older students may not embrace game playing as valuable, especially if they are not attuned to this particular modality. Fast-paced gaming may be threatening to an older student. There should be alternatives to this format if the class consists of multiple generations. Older students may need more time to practice or prefer a one-to-one, self-paced computer experience that focuses on decision making to enhance clinical reasoning skills. Simulation games have long been used for training purposes in aviation and the military. The learner plays out scenarios repetitively and receives immediate feedback for correct or incorrect responses. Virtual reality games for the purpose of skill acquisition are in the beginning stages in nursing education (Kilmon, Brown, Ghosh, & Mikitiuk, 2010).

As the technology becomes more sophisticated and realistic, it is not hard to imagine the possibilities for all areas of the healthcare professions. Learning and creative expression can also be taken into the virtual world of Second Life (Junco & Cole-Avent, 2008; Linden Research, Inc., 2009). Second Life is a virtual reality world where players interact locally or across the world. With the combination of enhanced video games, role play, simulation, and case studies comes a potential new learning methodology using this system. The educational goals might be collaborative skill development, communication, reasoning abilities, and/or practice of complex psychomotor skills. An exciting dimension to simulation learning has great potential in the healthcare professions. In 2005, Texas A&M University–Corpus Christi partnered with Breakaway Ltd., a gaming company, to launch a virtual reality simulation lab for training military and civilian emergency medical personnel in trauma care. This teaching modality immerses the learners in a high-fidelity, three-dimensional world that allows for multiple realistic patient scenarios to be played out in an emergency room setting. These experiential scenarios encourage critical thinking, psychomotor skill acquisition, and collaboration with other healthcare personnel—all in a low-risk, virtual environment (Breakaway, Ltd., 2012). Educators should anticipate that virtual simulations will be more widely used as they become increasingly available and reliable (Schmidt & Stewart, 2009). It should be noted that students are more receptive when experiential learning takes place in a low-stress environment.

There are many teaching strategies that can be employed to engage the younger generations of learners. Narrative pedagogy is a way of interpreting information from different perspectives; using a deconstruction (analytical) approach may work in classes that welcome and encourage student participation, analysis, and dialogue (Diekelmann, 2001). Concept maps use parallel/mosaic thinking to promote clinical reasoning (Burrell, 2014; Vacek, 2009). Reflection and critical thinking can be powerful and generationally relevant for promoting clinical thinking by experienced faculty. Students are guided in examining every angle through organized brainstorming techniques (Kenny, 2003). Another strategy that encourages clinical reasoning is engaging in Edward de Bono's six hats game (de Bono, 1999; Kenny, 2003). This encourages parallel thinking processes by looking at a problem from six different perspectives and discussing each of them.

Millennial students appear hardwired for action and engagement using web-based technology and resources. Educators identify lecture-based classes as transmitting low-level information that may actually reduce the ability to think critically. It is well known that learning is greater with an actively engaged learner than with a passive, bored one. In short, according to one expert in higher education, "class time is too valuable to spend time delivering content, which is, or can be, available elsewhere" (Taylor, 2010, p. 193).

■ Conclusion

Conflicts of younger generations with their elders have been documented for millennia. It may be debated whether the root causes of this conflict are student immaturity, undeveloped reasoning abilities, preferred learning styles, or alterations in brain structure.

Faculty reluctance to change or generational unawareness may also affect communication and learning. It will become increasingly requisite for healthcare curricula to change, modify, and adapt to strategies that coincide with technological advances and the societal expectations of new generations. Whatever the causes, these changes must be reckoned with. The timeless determinant for true educational success will most likely remain the connections from teacher to learner and from learner to teacher that transcend generational differences.

Discussion Questions

1. Discuss strategies you would use to meet the learning styles and educational expectations of a multigenerational classroom.
2. From a literature search, summarize the effectiveness of cutting-edge technology when utilized with multigenerational students.
3. You are planning group activities for your class. Each group has four students. Should each group have representatives from only one generation, or should each group contain all four generations?

References

American Association of State Colleges and Universities (AASCU). (2004). *The key to competitiveness: Understanding the next generation learner—A guide for college and university leaders.* Washington, DC: Author.

Benedict, S. I. (2008). How practitioners do and don't communicate: Part II. *Integrative Medicine, 7*(2), 54–59.

Benner, P., Sutphen, M., Leonard, V., & Day, L. (2010). *Educating nurses: A call for radical transformation.* San Francisco, CA: Jossey-Bass.

Boonstra, H. (2002). Teen pregnancy: Trends and lessons learned. *Guttmacher Report on Public Policy, 5*(1). Retrieved from http://www.guttmacher.org/pubs/tgr/05/1/gr050107.html

Breakaway, Ltd. (2012). Retrieved from http://www.breakawaygames.com/serious-games/solutions/healthcare/pulse

Brown, S., Kirkpatrick, M., Mangum, D., & Avery, J. (2008). A review of narrative pedagogy strategies to transform traditional nursing education. *Journal of Nursing Education, 47*(6), 283–286. http://dx.doi.org/10.3928/01484834-20080601-01

Bureau of Labor Statistics, U.S. Department of Labor (BLS). (2012). *Occupational outlook handbook, 2012–13 edition, registered nurses.* Retrieved from http://www.bls.gov/ooh/healthcare/registered-nurses.htm

Burrell, L. A. (2014). Integrating critical thinking strategies into nursing curricula. *Teaching and Learning in Nursing, 9*(2), 53. doi:10.1016/j.teln.2013.12.005

Cohen, R., Burns, K., Frank-Stromborg, M., Flanagan, J., Askins, D., & Ehrlich-Jones, L. (2006). Educational innovation: The Kids into Health Careers (KIHC) initiative: Innovative approaches to help solve the nursing shortage. *Journal of Nursing Education, 45*(5), 186–189.

de Bono, E. (1999). *Six thinking hats.* Boston, MA: Back Bay Books.

Diekelmann, N. (2001). Narrative pedagogy: Heideggerian hermeneutical analyses of lived experiences of students, teachers, and clinicians. *Advances in Nursing Science, 23*(3), 53–71.

Draganski, B., Gaser, C., Busch, V., Schuierer, G., Bogdahn, U., & May, A. (2004). Neuroplasticity: Changes in grey matter induced by training. *Nature, 427*(6972), 311–312. http://dx.doi.org/10.1038/427311a

Gardner, E. A., Deloney, L. A., & Grando, V. T. (2007). Nursing student descriptions that suggest changes for the classroom and reveal improvements needed in study skills and self-care. *Journal of Professional Nursing, 23*(2), 98–104. http://dx.doi.org/10.1016/j.profnurs.2006.07.006

Garrett, B., MacPhee, M., & Jackson, C. (2010). High-fidelity patient simulation: Considerations for effective learning. *Nursing Education Perspectives, 31*(5), 309–313.

Gibson, S. E. (2009). Enhancing intergenerational communication in the classroom: Recommendations for successful teacher–student relationships. *Nursing Education Perspectives, 30*(1), 37–39.

Hahn, J. A. (2011). Managing multiple generations: Scenarios from the workplace. *Nursing Forum, 46*(3), 119–127. doi:10.1111/j.1744-6198.2011.00223.x

Hawks, S. J., Turner, K. M., Derouin, A. L., Hueckel, R. M., Leonardelli, A. K., & Oermann, M. H. (2015, November 4). Writing across the curriculum: Strategies to improve the writing skills of nursing students. *Nursing Forum*. Advance online publication. http://dx.doi.org/10.1111/nuf.12151

Institute of Medicine (IOM). (2011). Committee on the Robert Wood Johnson Foundation initiative on the future of nursing. In *The future of nursing: Leading change, advancing health*. Washington, DC: National Academies Press. Retrieved from http://www.nap.edu/openbook.php?record_id=12956

Johnson, S. A., & Romanello, M. L. (2005). Generational diversity in teaching and learning approaches. *Nurse Educator, 30*(5), 212–216. http://dx.doi.org/10.1097/00006223-200509000-00009

Jones, S., & Fox, S. (2009, January). Generations online in 2009. *Pew Internet and American Life Project*. Retrieved from http://pewresearch.org/pubs/1093/generations-online

Junco, R., & Cole-Avent, G. A. (2008). An introduction to technologies commonly used by college students. *New Directions for Student Services, 124*, 3–17. http://dx.doi.org/10.1002/ss.292

Kenny, L. J. (2003). Using Edward de Bono's six hats game to aid critical thinking and reflection in palliative care. *International Journal of Palliative Nursing, 9*(3), 105–112.

Kilmon, C., Brown, L., Ghosh, S., & Mikitiuk, A. (2010). Immersive virtual reality simulations in nursing education. *Nursing Education Perspectives, 31*(5), 314–317.

Knowles, M. S. (1973). *The adult learner: A neglected species*. Houston, TX: Gulf Publishing.

Kolb, D. (1984). *Experiential learning: Experience as the source of learning and development*. Englewood Cliffs, NJ: Prentice-Hall.

Linden Research, Inc. (2009). *What is Second Life?* Retrieved from http://secondlife.com/whatis/?lang=en-US

McLuhan, M. (1978). The brain and the media: The Western hemisphere. *Journal of Communication, 28*(4), 54–60. doi:10.1111/j.1460-2466.1978.tb01656.x

National League for Nursing (NLN). (2003). *Innovation in nursing education: A call to reform*. New York, NY: Author.

National League for Nursing (NLN). (2008). *Preparing the next generation of nurses to practice in a technology-rich environment: An informatics agenda*. New York, NY: Author.

Oblinger, D. (2003, July/August). Boomers gen-Xers millenials: Understanding the new students. *EDUCAUSE Review*, 37–47. Retrieved from http://net.educause.edu/ir/library/pdf/erm0342.pdf

Outten, M. K. (2012). From veterans to nexters: Managing a multigenerational nursing workforce. *Nursing Management, 43*(4), 42–47. doi:10.1097/01.NUMA.0000413096.84832.a4

Pardue, K. T., & Morgan, P. (2008). Millennials considered: A new generation, new approaches, and implications for nursing education. *Nursing Education Perspectives, 29*(2), 75–79.

Paschal, J. (2003). *Understanding generation Y: Expectations of nursing education* (Unpublished thesis UMI No. 1414800). Waco, TX: Baylor University.

Piper, L. E. (2012). Generation Y in healthcare: Leadings millennial in an era of reform. *Frontiers of Health Services Management, 29*(1), 16–28.

Prensky, M. (2001, October). Digital natives, digital immigrants: Part II. Do they really think differently? *On the Horizon, 9*(5). Retrieved from http://www.marcprensky.com/writing

Pricer, W. (2008). *Helicopter parents, millennial students: An annotated bibliography*. Livonia, MI: Community College Enterprise. ERIC database (EJ837465). Retrieved from EBSCO.

Reagan, R. (1981, May 17). *Address at commencement exercises at the University of Notre Dame*. Retrieved from http://www.reagan.utexas.edu/archives/speeches/1981/517819.htm

Revell, S., & McCurry, M. (2010). Engaging millennial learners: Effectiveness of personal response system technology with nursing students in small and large classrooms. *Journal of Nursing Education, 49*(5), 272–275. http://dx.doi.org/10.3928/01484834-20091217-07

Roe v. Wade. (1973). 410 U.S. 113, 93 S. Ct. 705; 35 L. Ed. 2d 147.

Schmidt, B., & Stewart, S. (2009). Implementing the virtual reality learning environment: Second Life. *Nurse Educator, 34*(4), 152–155. http://dx.doi.org/10.1097/NNE.0b013e3181aabbe8

Sherman, R. (2006). Leading a multigenerational nursing workforce: Issues, challenges, and strategies. *Online Journal of Issues in Nursing, 11*(2). Doi:10.3912/OJIN.Vol11No02Man02

Skiba, D., & Barton, A. (2006). Adapting your teaching to accommodate the net generation of learners. *Online Journal of Issues in Nursing, 11*(2). Retrieved from CINAHL with full-text database.

Smith, D., & Bradshaw, B. S. (2008). Reduced variation in death rates after introduction of antimicrobial agents. *Population Research and Policy Review, 27*(3), 343–351. http://dx.doi.org/10.1007/s11113-007-9068-z

Sontag, M. (2009). A learning theory for 21st century students. *Journal of Online Education, 5*(4). Retrieved from http://www.eric.ed.gov/ERICWebPortal/detail?accno=EJ840530

Stockmayer, G. (2004, April). *Demographic rates and household change in the United States, 1900–2000.* Presentation at Population Association of America Annual Meeting, Boston, MA. Retrieved from http://www.demog.berkeley.edu/~gretchen/Stockmayer_Diss.pdf

Suplee, P., Lachman, V., Siebert, B., & Anselmi, K. (2008). Managing nursing student incivility in the classroom, clinical setting, and on-line. *Journal of Nursing Law, 12*(2), 68–77. http://dx.doi.org/10.1891/1073-7472.12.2.68

Taylor, M. (2010). Teaching generation next: A pedagogy for today's learners. In *A collection of papers on self-study and institutional improvement* (Vol. 3, pp. 192–196). Chicago, IL: Higher Learning Commission. Retrieved from http://www.taylorprograms.com/images/Teaching_Gen_NeXt.pdf

Taylor, P., & Keeter, S. (Eds.). (2010, February). Millennials: Confident. Connected. Open to change. In Millennials: A portrait of generation next. *Pew Research Foundation.* Retrieved from http://www.pewresearch.org/millennials

Technology Informatics Guiding Education Reform (TIGER). (2007). *Evidence and informatics transforming nursing: 3-year action steps toward a 10-year vision.* Retrieved from http://www.thetigerinitiative.org/docs/TIGERCollaborativeExecSummary_20090405.pdf

Vacek, J. (2009). Using a conceptual approach with concept mapping to promote critical thinking. *Journal of Nursing Education, 48*(1), 45–48. http://dx.doi.org/10.3928/01484834-20090101-11

Walker, J., Martin, T., Haynie, L., Norwood, A., White, J., & Grant, L. (2007). Preferences for teaching methods in a baccalaureate nursing program: How second-degree and traditional students differ. *Nursing Education Perspectives, 28*(5), 246–250.

CHAPTER 4

Strategies for Innovation

Arlene J. Lowenstein

The scope of change in health care has been enormous, and the rate at which change occurs continues to accelerate. Today's technology and therapeutics were inconceivable even a few decades ago. Over time, the growth of the health professions has been influenced by those new technologies and therapeutics, but there are many other influencing factors and forces as well, including, but not limited to:

- The appearance of new diseases, such as swine flu (H1N1), HIV/AIDS, Lyme disease, and Ebola and the rapid growth of new treatments, medications, and noninvasive surgeries.
- War and its consequences, which brought new techniques to care for burns and radiation, growth of the use of penicillin and other antibiotics, treatments for posttraumatic stress disorder, and growth of nursing and rehabilitation services in the military and veterans' systems.
- Sociocultural issues, including the civil rights movement, the feminist movement, the consumer revolution of the late 1960s and 1970s, and changing immigration and demographic patterns, which brought dramatic changes in maternity care ranging from shortened length of stay to sibling visitation and increased focus on care of the elderly and end-of-life care. Diversity has increased in healthcare education and practice, and more emphasis has been placed on culturally competent care.
- Religious issues, which brought ethical components of care and the development of parish nursing.
- Changing economics, as evidenced by the 2008 recession and political/legal issues, which brought us Medicare, Medicaid, managed care, and the Affordable Care Act passed by Congress in 2010.
- Changes in education brought nursing into academic settings and gave rise to nursing science and nursing research, thereby changing practice and creating new roles, such as advanced practice nursing and the newest credential, the doctor of nursing practice (DNP). Physical therapy embraced the doctor of physical therapy (DPT) as an entry-level degree, and other health professions have developed and evolved as well.

These forces are not isolated, but rather are part of the total environment in which we live and work. They are ever changing and interacting, challenging health professions educators to keep on top of the trends, technologies, and resources, while enabling self-directed student learning. Graduates who are self-directed learners understand and are responsive to healthcare system changes when they are in practice and out of the school setting, where there are no faculty members with whom to consult.

Healthcare educators straddle the fields of healthcare practice and education. They need to be knowledgeable about changes in practice and technology in both fields. What healthcare practitioners learn, as well as how they are taught, must keep pace with the changing milieu. The field of education has also changed over the years through many of the same forces that affected health care. Technology and therapeutics in health care can be compared to a new understanding of learning theories and teaching methods in education. The student entering a healthcare profession from high school today is most likely much more comfortable with the use of computers than the RN returning to school or an older student who has chosen a health profession as a second career. Online courses are now in the mainstream.

Health professions classrooms are also more culturally diverse than ever before. More men are entering the nursing profession, and more women are going to medical school. Younger students may have had very different cultural experiences in their secondary schools than did older students. Older students may be dealing with the added stress of parenthood and job responsibilities. Different cultures and experiences may produce different expectations of teaching and learning. Respecting learning-need differences and establishing an innovative climate in the classroom can help to prepare students for the changes they will face in practice. An educational climate that values different viewpoints and experiences among students encourages those students to create their own innovations. Those innovations will serve them well by enhancing positive interactions with the wide variety of persons for whom they will be caring and with whom they will be working.

Omachonu and Einspruch (2010) saw four areas of potential innovation in health care: product innovation, process innovation (which includes healthcare practices), marketing innovation, and organizational innovation. There are many new opportunities for innovation. Sources of information have multiplied. The Internet has laid at our doors the possibility of learning over long distances. The barrier of geography has been breached. Even nurses in rural communities have access to continued learning offered by highly qualified nurse educators. Innovative computer-based materials can provide technical training within the classroom—audio and video combining to offer a breadth of exposure previously available only through many hours at the bedside. Instant messaging is available, and we can listen to lectures over podcasts and locate reference material instantly through our personal cell phones. We can have two-way access between health settings and homes with the use of Skype, a software application that provides the ability to make voice calls, complete with pictures, over the Internet; and telemedicine, so a person many miles away can join you in your living room or in a health facility. The use of simulators has increased. This capability is becoming much more important as productivity pressures make clinical sites for student experience harder and harder to find.

How do we teach more and more information to our students without overwhelming them? And how do we maintain the underlying paradigm of care and compassion? How do we maintain the threads of patient-centered, holistic, and compassionate care within the complex scientific information our students must master? In this text, we hope to provide health professions educators with ideas and examples that have been used to allow students to master the facts and theory as well as the perspective of a caring professional. Implementing and adapting these methods will lead to further discovery of successful teaching strategies to keep pace with changes in the profession.

■ Examples of Innovation

Innovative teaching strategies can range from simple to complex. Innovations can be developed for an exercise within a course or for the method by which the entire course is taught. Teaching innovations can be developed for whole programs or even whole schools. They can be developed by one faculty member or by groups of faculty members. The prime objective is the teaching strategies selected must address what has to be learned in relation to the learning needs of students.

Think back to a favorite teacher or any strongly remembered event. Why does it stand out? What makes it unique among similar events? A major factor can be the realization that one object was completely different or out of its usually defined place, whereas the surrounding objects appeared normal. The teachers we remember often stood apart from our perception of others by only one or two details, but these details were out of the normal range. We remember the different much more than the normal, yet we can grasp only a small amount of the different and a large amount of the usual. The occasional nondigestible, completely different piece in the sea of the expected focuses our energies on analyzing not just the different piece, but also the other 99% rote material normally not given much attention and easily forgotten. Kirp, a professor of public policy, asked a former student, who had become a college professor, what she remembered about his teaching. He was astonished to hear that she remembered his baseball stories. She elaborated that the baseball anecdotes prodded her into thinking of him as more approachable and more human. Once she felt that way, she began to pay attention (Kirp, 1997).

Box 4-1 provides an example of using something different in a lesson: an analogy of pain management to the sinking of the *Titanic*. The objective is to allow students to discover what they know applies to other situations. Students will remember more if they can make the discovery.

Art, literature, storytelling, humor, and technology-assisted learning can all be used in innovative ways. Whitman and Rose (2003) had students choose media to express their nursing philosophy. This technique required students to think differently about what they were doing and what they believed. One student used a guitar and song to express his philosophy of healing. Another painted a brain within a heart, which symbolized her need to incorporate compassion as well as intellect into patient

---

Box 4-1   Analogy: Pain Management and the Sinking of the *Titanic*

The aftermath of bone surgery, such as ankle fusion, is very painful for patients. To create a more dynamic understanding of a patient's experience with pain and the need for appropriate pain relief measures, an analogy was used to discuss the issues involved. The choice of the *Titanic* disaster as an analogy actually came from a patient's description of the pain he felt in the postoperative period and his feeling that the nursing staff needed to pay more attention to pain relief. He felt there were times when he was totally immersed in the pain, and relief could have been started sooner and put him on a more even keel.

The *Titanic* was constructed with six watertight compartments that were expected to withstand a breach and keep the ship afloat. The compartments had very high walls but, unfortunately, those walls did not reach the ceilings. The design was appropriate for most possibilities, but not for the accident that actually happened. Students were told to think of the walls as the job of the pain medication and water as the pain. The wall of the pain medication isolates the water from the ship and the passengers' realization that they are surrounded by water. The pain is hidden. The danger lies in what happens if the water in the first compartment overflows its limit and then starts filling the second compartment. If up to three of these compartments fill with water (pain), it may not interfere with the ship's normal function; however, as the effect cascades into more of the compartments, the ship sinks at the bow until it's "all hands lost."

Patients initially don't understand that a sea of pain surrounds them. As the pain relief diminishes and they suddenly (perhaps by waking from sleep) find themselves immersed, a fear of this unexpected and uncomfortable situation is formed. This fear becomes a constant presence even after pain relief is restored, leading to anxiety and apprehension over the possibility of a repeat experience. In very painful procedures, this fear can result in clock-watching over the medication schedule as well as a compulsion to do anything to stay ahead of the pain curve. Appropriate pain relief measures, timing of administration, and other nursing measures can be discussed, continuing use of the analogy (such as the use of lifeboats in the pain relief cycle). Students can also be taught to develop and share their own analogies to improve learning retention.

---

care. A third wrote a poem to express her feelings and beliefs. This technique used sight, touch, and movement in addition to listening, which encouraged retention after class for both the creator of the piece and the viewer.

■ Developing Innovative Strategies

Innovation can occur at all levels of an educational organization. Support for innovation in education may begin at the top of the organization or be developed and implemented at program or individual class levels. Success is enhanced when administrators and faculty members work side by side to plan strategically and implement changes to improve the educational milieu (Woods, 1998).

Innovation at the school level was demonstrated by a group of business school educators. These educators chose to focus more on entrepreneurship and to move away from the traditional management study that prepared students to work in large organizations. This strategic innovation recognized the realities of the marketplace in a changing world. These schools set the pace for others to follow (They Create Winners, 1994). In working with social workers, Michael Chovanec (2008) recognized an educational need was not being met. While group processes may be in the curriculum for social workers, these practitioners often need to work with involuntary groups, such as court-ordered programs in domestic abuse and chemical dependency. A very different process is needed to work with people who do not want to be there but are forced to attend. Chovanec developed three innovative frameworks to teach social work students about this type of work. His article describes those frameworks as reactance theory for working with the reactions of those who do not want to be in the group, a stages-of-change model, and motivational interviewing, which encourages working with clients to improve their self-motivation. His model provides guidelines and exercises to model unpleasant experiences that students may be exposed to in their practice.

Nursing education has grown through innovation. Mildred Montag's introduction of the associate degree program in nursing, developed through research to meet an assessed need, changed the landscape of nursing education. The introduction of nurse practitioner programs also created a revolution in the profession. The physical therapy profession has endorsed the doctor of physical therapy (DPT) as the entry-level degree and strongly encouraged schools to provide transition programs for physical therapists currently in practice. The introduction of distance learning in all the health professions is the latest revolution and is growing rapidly, offering students different choices that are unfettered by the barrier of geography.

The Innovation Center for Medicare and Medicaid was established as a consequence of passage of the Affordable Care Act (CMS Innovation Center, 2013). Trossman (2012) noted that nursing was long governed by rules, regulations, and rigid schedules, but times are changing, and 21 nurses were among the 73 healthcare professionals who were selected as innovation advisors in December 2011 through the CMS Innovation Center.

Successful innovation does not come easily; it requires creativity, planning, and evaluation. **Box 4-2** describes a process for educators to work through to develop innovative teaching strategies. Just as health professions call for patient assessments, the educational process calls for learning and program assessments. *Assessment* of a course requires a look at both strengths and problems. How can the strengths be enhanced? What should be changed? Educators must focus on what the expected learning outcome ought to be, with awareness of learning theory and student learning styles and needs. Specific content requirements change often in health care, as new techniques, technologies, and research bring new knowledge needs. With the overwhelming amount of information available in today's healthcare world, it will not be possible to include everything students need. They will need to have appropriate resources to supplement classroom or clinical learning. The instructor must decide

---

Box 4-2   The Process of Innovation

Assessment

What is the content to be learned? What are the student learning needs? How are those needs being met? What is working and what is not?

Defining Options

How else can I look at this? Does the literature provide suggestions that would address the identified needs? Do students or other faculty members have suggestions that I could utilize?

Planning

1. Does this change require working with curriculum committees, collaborating with other faculty members, or individual instructor planning? How should this change be approached?
2. Will there be a need to work with technical specialists in the use of computer technology? Do I need additional technological knowledge to carry out this change?
3. How can I best use change theory in this planning? Who are the stakeholders who should be considered? How and where will I meet resistance? How will I develop support?
4. How will I plan to evaluate the effectiveness of this innovation?

Gaining Support for the Innovation

Which resources will be needed? How will they be acquired and funded? What level of administrative support is required and available? Which strategies will I use to gain additional support if needed?

Preparing Students for the Innovation

Do I need written student instructions? If so, are they clear? Have I provided a mechanism for troubleshooting problems, and do students know how to address problems?

Preparing Faculty Members for the Innovation

If other faculty members are involved, do they need additional education? How will that be carried out? Is everyone in agreement as to how the strategy will be run? Is rehearsal time needed?

Implementing the Innovation

How much flexibility is available if the intervention is not going well? Will follow-up be needed?

Evaluating the Outcome

How will I measure the learning outcome? How have students reacted to the strategy, and can they provide input for change or improvement? If other faculty members are involved, can a consensus be reached about the direction for needed change and/or support for continuation?

what and how much content will be needed—a decision that is often difficult. While addressing the content to be learned, it is also important to consider student learning needs. An understanding of the diversity in learning needs provides a foundation for the development of effective strategies.

To *define options*, the literature should be searched for research, suggestions, or techniques that address the identified needs. Asking students or other faculty members for suggestions can also be helpful. This is the place where creativity reigns. It is important to look at many different ways to address the learning objective before selecting one. Asking the question, "Is there another way to look at this?" can be fun and lead to additional options.

Once a strategy has been selected, *planning* is all-important. Understanding who the stakeholders are and what their investment is in the status quo or in change can be helpful in planning strategies to bring them on board. Many stakeholders, including students, do not like change and will resist new approaches. Using change theory can assist in demonstrating need and provide information that can make resisters more amenable to change. Some strategies will require curricular change, which is a complicated process and one that must be started early to avoid implementation delays. It is important to take enough time to develop support for the strategy. If this is a simple change within a course, then the instructor will need the support of students to participate effectively and not sabotage the effort. In more complex strategies, it may be important to bring in other faculty members or administrators.

Some strategies will require the help of technical specialists, who may be able to offer support and/or instruction for using the equipment. Time must be allotted for adequate instruction to enable faculty members and students to reach a comfort level. Most importantly, the technical staff must be available to help solve problems, which are bound to occur. Planning strategies for troubleshooting and providing access for problem solving—for both faculty members and students—must be thought out in advance of implementation.

Another phase of the planning process is planning for evaluation of the strategy. This is the time to decide what should be evaluated and how that evaluation should be done. This phase can range from how the strategy will be used in student grading to evaluating learning outcomes for the class as a whole, and should be developed to allow student and faculty input for future development. This can also be the time to develop an educational research project, if appropriate. Educational research and publication of results are extremely important, as they can assist all of us in understanding and applying an effective educational process.

Gaining support for the innovation is the next step. Some strategies require little or no resources to implement, whereas others require significant physical and/or financial resources. If resources are needed, then gaining support for acquisition of those resources is essential. Looking at alternative sources of funding is helpful. Grants can provide a good funding source, but require time and effort to secure and may last for only a limited time. Administrative support may be required, but administrators may also be an excellent resource to tap to discuss potential funding or acquisition of physical resources. Once the project has been developed, it is important to validate the support of stakeholders.

Class preparation is a given in education. ***Preparing students for the innovation*** is an important step. Student instructions have to be clear and specific. This is the time for motivating students to want to try this process, and for gaining their support. Students need to know how to address problems, especially when technology is involved. A learning curve may be required for some strategies. Students need to feel comfortable that they will not be punished for mistakes, but rather will benefit from those mistakes as part of the learning process. Evaluation methods or grading must be made clear.

Faculty members may also need preparation for the innovation. For some strategies, rehearsal time may be needed, or additional education may be required. Planning sufficient time for those activities will increase everyone's comfort level with the process. This is the time to be sure everyone agrees about how the strategy will be run. Use of *perception, validation,* and *clarification* (the author likes to use the mnemonic *PVCs* when teaching students about this) can be valuable here. Health professionals are familiar with cardiac premature ventricular contractions as PVCs, but using this term in a different context can help students relate to the term and remember it better. Too often, people interpret statements differently. Checking that everyone has the same perceptions (validating) and clarifying differences can provide unity in approach to students and reduce problems of students playing one instructor against another. Saying "Remember your PVCs" reminds us to think about this issue.

The best part of the process is ***implementing the innovation***, because it makes the innovation real for the innovator. It is hoped things will go well, but flexibility may be required if problems arise. Sometimes, unintended consequences, such as surfacing of emotional issues, can occur. Instructors should be alert to the need for follow-up or referral if problems arise.

Evaluating the outcome is the final step in the process. Remember learning can continue long after implementation of the strategy. It may be possible to measure short-term attainment of learning outcomes, but it may or may not be possible to explore long-term effects. For certain strategies that were developed to provide a foundation for other learning experiences, it may be possible to assess students at the end of their program. Students and faculty members should be able to provide input for future development and use of the strategy. A strong evaluation process provides an opportunity to participate in educational research. Even if a strategy is not suitable for research, it still may be appropriate for publication. Sharing teaching strategies presents the opportunity to improve the educational process. A catchword in health care today is *evidence-based practice*. We also need evidence-based practice in education.

■ Conclusion

Innovative teaching strategies must be based on both learning objectives and student learning needs. The wide diversity of student learning needs means that educators must recognize that although most students will benefit from the new approaches, some will not. This perspective can be disappointing, but it is realistic, and educators must take pride in what they have accomplished. Problems no one could foresee will occur despite adequate planning. These problems, although disturbing at the time, are often humorous memories later and can be addressed to improve future offerings.

Teaching Example:
Interdisciplinary Case Study Analysis

An example of an innovative strategy at the school level is the introduction of interdisciplinary case studies to health professions students. Healthcare providers interact daily with members of other disciplines. The mission statement of the health professions school, with programs in nursing, physical therapy, and communications sciences disorders, included the following:

> While health professionals must be prepared to provide expert care within their respective disciplines, they contribute to evaluating and improving health care delivery by working in close cooperation with professionals from other disciplines. Students educated in an interdisciplinary setting, one that integrates academic and clinical pursuits, will be well-equipped to function as members of the health care team. The involvement of active practitioners from different fields in program planning, student supervision, and teaching supports such an integrated program. (MGH Institute of Health Professions, 2000, p. 13)

Faculty members and administrators felt the need to strengthen the manner in which that portion of the mission statement was being addressed. Although students were exposed to a few multidisciplinary courses such as research and ethics, there was overall agreement that they needed more useful exposure to other disciplines within a clinical context. An interdisciplinary faculty task force was developed to explore possibilities. The academic dean staffed the task force and provided administrative support. After much discussion, the task force settled on a series of four required interdisciplinary clinical seminars as the preferred method.

The mechanics of developing and implementing the program were daunting, but the group was committed to the project. They enlisted other members of their departments to develop four case studies—one for each seminar. The subject of the case study would require care from each of the three disciplines: nursing, physical therapy, and speech pathology. Thought was given to the need for students to be involved with different age groups and various clinical settings. Teams of faculty members with expertise in each area developed the following cases:

- *Seminar case 1*: Pediatric patient with cerebral palsy who is starting school.
- *Seminar case 2*: Elderly patient with cerebral vascular accident and dysphagia in an acute care setting.
- *Seminar case 3*: Middle-aged adult with HIV and family issues in the community (end stages of illness).
- *Seminar case 4*: Young teen with traumatic brain injury in a rehabilitation center.

The intensive involvement of many faculty members in the development of the cases had some very beneficial effects. Interdisciplinary cooperation was necessary as the cases were developed. Faculty members were able to learn from each other and appreciate the role of the other disciplines. The faculty members who developed the cases were invested in the project and were able to support and commend it to other faculty members and to students in their classes, which reduced some resistance.

Each program was responsible for determining which students would be required to attend the seminars. The nursing program selected students who were in the spring semester of the second year of an entry-level master's program and were enrolled in the Primary Care I course. Nursing students in this program held a baccalaureate in any field prior to entry into the program. They had completed the first year and second fall semester in the generalist level

(continues)

of the nursing program. They were in the process of taking the RN licensing exam during this semester (they all passed). They were then in advanced-level course work that would lead to a master of science in nursing degree and eligibility to sit for certification as a nurse practitioner. Interdisciplinary seminar attendance was mandatory and counted as part of the clinical component in the Primary Care I course, so that students would not be required to add hours to the course. Compromise and negotiation were needed on the part of the course faculty to recognize and accept that the interdisciplinary seminar was a legitimate learning experience appropriate to the course.

Scheduling the seminars was a major problem. Coordinating three programs with students in different classes and in clinical sites was very difficult. The seminars were held in the late afternoon, and students in clinical placements were asked to leave their clinical sites early enough to return to the school. There is no easy solution to this problem. Each student was sent a letter outlining the purpose of the seminars and given the dates and times. The letter explained that attendance was mandatory and that the seminar would count as class hours.

Approximately 60 students were expected to attend the seminars. Four faculty members from each department were recruited to facilitate each seminar. In smaller departments, this meant that department faculty members participated in more than one seminar. The case discussions were designed so that students had an opportunity to participate in multidisciplinary groups, meet with their own specialty, and meet as a total group. The sessions were planned to last 2 hours each.

The role of the faculty members was to facilitate but not to lead the discussion among students. Faculty members were available to correct wrong information, but the focus was to have students take responsibility for explaining their discipline's role in working with the patient. Faculty members were not expected to be experts in the area under discussion or to introduce new material. The faculty role was explained to the students at the beginning of the session.

Previously prepared case materials presented assessment tools used by each discipline and questions to be addressed. The goals of the seminar were presented and clarified to all of the students before breaking students into groups. Students presented their assessments and plans for working with the patients, defining priorities of care. Faculty facilitators encouraged participation by all. Each small group took notes to be presented to the entire group for general discussion.

Evaluations of the seminars from both faculty members and students were excellent. The time selected for the seminars was problematic for many participants and seemed to be the major concern of students. Some students had various excuses for not being able to attend. Snow forced the cancellation of one session. All students attended a minimum of one seminar, but most attended the sessions as scheduled. Students remarked that the discussions were excellent and that they had gained new knowledge from each other as the different disciplinary approaches were presented. Faculty members also benefited from the discussions, and interdepartmental communications were enhanced. Some faculty members were uncomfortable at first with the expectation of their role and were concerned that they did not know enough about specific cases; however, most soon realized that the objectives of the session were valid for the level of their expertise and the expectation of facilitation rather than instruction. Overall, the project was deemed a strong success and was presented again, with minor changes.

The program has evolved, but the commitment to interdisciplinary education remains and has expanded. Students will have at least one interdisciplinary learning experience in each year. Each department is responsible for developing the experience for their students, and school-wide presentations will be carried out each semester.

Developing effective teaching strategies is challenging, and requires effort and persistence, but can also be exceedingly rewarding and fun. Sharing those strategies with others will benefit students and faculty alike. We hope you will take advantage of the strategies presented in this book and go on to develop, implement, and share your own innovative strategies.

Discussion Questions

Reflect on a classroom innovation: perhaps a change to concept-based teaching, or using active learning strategies in the classroom, or another innovative change. Using the process outlined in Box 4-2, answer the following questions:

1. Describe the assessment, defining options, and planning necessary for this innovation.
2. How will you gain support and prepare the students and faculty for the innovation?
3. Describe how the innovation will be implemented. What problems do you anticipate?
4. How will the innovation be evaluated?

References

Chovanec, M. (2008). Innovations applied to the classroom for involuntary groups: Implications for social work education. *Journal of Teaching in Social Work, 28*(1/2), 209–225.

CMS Innovation Center. (2013). *About the CMS Innovation Center.* Retrieved from http://innovation.cms .gov/About/index.html

Kirp, D. L. (1997). Those who can't: 27 ways of looking at a classroom. *Change, 29*(3), 10–19.

MGH Institute of Health Professions. (2000). Mission statement. *MGH Institute of Health Professions Self-Study, 13.*

Omachonu, V. K., & Einspruch, N. G. (2010). Innovation in healthcare delivery systems: A conceptual framework. *Innovation Journal, 15*(1), Article 2.

They Create Winners. (1994). *Success, 41*(7), 43–46.

Trossman, S. (2012, May/June). Nurses leading through innovation: Three nurses test strategies to improve care and reduce costs. *American Nurse,* pp. 1–7.

Whitman, B. L., & Rose, W. J. (2003). Using art to express a personal philosophy of nursing. *Nurse Educator, 28*(4), 166–169.

Woods, D. R. (1998). Getting support for your new approaches. *Journal of College Science Teaching, 27*(4), 285–286.

Recommended Reading

Butell, S. S., O'Donovan, P., & Taylor, J. D. (2004). Educational innovations: Instilling the value of reading literature through student-led book discussion groups. *Journal of Nursing Education, 43*(1), 40–44.

Jesse, D. E., & Blue, C. (2004). Mary Breckinridge meets Healthy People 2010: A teaching strategy for visioning and building healthy communities. *Journal of Midwifery & Women's Health, 49*(2), 126–131.

Nof, L., & Hill, C. (2005). On the cutting edge: A successful distance PhD degree program: A case study [Electronic version]. *Internet Journal of Allied Health Sciences and Practice, 3*(2). Retrieved from http:// ijahsp.nova.edu/articles/vol3num2/nof.htm

Travis, L., & Brennan, P. F. (1998). Information science for the future: An innovative nursing informatics curriculum. *Journal of Nursing Education, 37*(4), 162–168.

CHAPTER 5

Clinical Reasoning: Action-Focused Thinking

Cheryl A. Tucker
Martha J. Bradshaw

Instructors in the health professions, who also are practitioners in their fields, are compelled to assist students in developing their clinical reasoning skills as beginners in the health professions and as novice thinkers. Sound reasoning is essential in preserving the standards of the profession and promoting quality patient outcomes. Health professions literature has long addressed this process as *critical thinking*. However, the critical thinking model is limited in that it does not move learners to the level of thinking about their thinking. Recent literature is addressing this awareness and the need to move to a deeper level of thinking. This process is **clinical reasoning**. Within the various health professions, many terms and models exist. With the call to interdisciplinary education and collaborative patient care, healthcare professionals need a shared model of clinical reasoning. This chapter provides an overview of what clinical reasoning is and why it should be taught in a purposeful way, and it presents a model that can be implemented across the healthcare disciplines.

■ Clinical Reasoning Framework

In 2003, the Institute of Medicine (IOM) published its report *Health Professions Education: A Bridge to Quality,* which examined the need to transform health professions education. The IOM's vision for the education of health professionals is articulated in its core competencies, which assert, "All health professionals should be educated to deliver patient-centered care as members of an interdisciplinary team, emphasizing evidence-based practice, quality improvement approaches, and informatics" (IOM, 2003, p. 3). *The Future of Nursing: Leading Change, Advancing Health* (IOM, 2010) further addresses these core competencies and explores the necessity of transforming professional nursing education. The American Association of Colleges of Nurses (AACN) supports these core competencies as delineated in the *Essentials of Baccalaureate Education for Professional Nursing Practice,* which highlights such areas as "patient-centered care, interprofessional teams, evidence-based practice, quality improvement, patient safety, informatics, clinical reasoning/ critical thinking, genetics and genomics, cultural sensitivity, professionalism, practice across the lifespan, and end-of-life care" (AACN, 2008, p. 35).

Various professional organizations use *critical thinking, clinical judgment,* and *clinical reasoning* interchangeably. A definition of *clinical judgment* is "an interpretation or conclusion about a patient's needs, concerns, or health problems, and/or the decision to take action (or not), use or modify standard approaches, or improvise new ones as deemed appropriate by the patient's response" (Tanner, 2006, p. 204). *Clinical reasoning* is the ability of the health professions student to use critical thinking skills in the practice environment. It should include the "context and concerns of the patient and family" (Benner, Sutphen, Leonard, & Day, 2010, p. 85). Clinical imagination and reflection are also part of clinical reasoning (Benner et al., 2010). The thought is that critical thinking is a snapshot in time, whereas clinical reasoning can accommodate the changing nature of the clinical settings. Tanner (2006) acknowledges that *problem solving, critical thinking, decision making,* and *clinical judgment* are often used in the literature to mean the same thing.

In varying degrees, all students need guidance with transfer or application of knowledge to specific patient situations. This process, also called *knowledge translation*, is the means by which new knowledge is organized, given meaning or understood, and put in to action (Leahey & Svavarsdottir, 2009). As the teacher builds clinical reasoning abilities in the student, the individual student learns (or should learn) to recognize the meaning of knowledge (information) and then grasp how to use (apply) this knowledge. Transfer of knowledge is critical for success in the healthcare arena.

The IOM (2003) report *Health Professions Education: A Bridge to Quality* articulates the need for healthcare professionals to be amply prepared to address the healthcare needs of an ever-changing patient population. The IOM report calls for healthcare providers to collaborate on delivering individualized, yet comprehensive health care. This requires purposeful, thoughtful, analytical processing of information and deliberate communication of this process to other healthcare professionals. For this to happen, the educational process must be transformed into one that cultivates clinical reasoning.

What role does the health professions teacher play in the development of clinical reasoning in his or her students? Health professions teachers have been utilizing different tools in promoting clinical reasoning in their students. A few examples of various tools utilized in the thinking process include professional nursing's nursing process (assessment, nursing diagnosis, planning, implementation, and evaluation), medical education's SNAPPS (summarize, narrow, analyze, probe, plan, and select) (Nixon et al., 2014), and physical therapy's International Classification of Functioning, Disability and Health (ICF). These tools promote the student's thinking through various steps of the clinical reasoning process. When health professions students collaborate on patient care problems, the professionals must speak the same language as they develop their clinical reasoning skills. To develop those skills in an interdisciplinary manner, the students collectively should use a decision-making tree, based on the scientific method, as a clinical reasoning tool. Utilizing the clinical reasoning tool, students acknowledge the clinical problem and gather data; analyze the information, develop solutions or a plan, and make a decision; implement the decision(s); and evaluate the decision(s).

The scientific method of thinking, which uses problem definition, analysis, decision making, implementation, and evaluation, has long been used by healthcare providers. Every profession uses this method in some way, although each uses different nomenclature for the steps of the process. A proposed model for clinical reasoning (see **Table 5-1**) incorporates all of the analytical methods used by educators in the various health professions. The categories are similar in content, are sequential, and serve as a means for novices to understand their thinking as they move through the process.

Health care continues to grow more complex, and health professionals must be better prepared to utilize their clinical reasoning skills. Teaching clinical reasoning is difficult; it must be purposeful and can be both planned and spontaneous. In the IOM report (2010, p. 544) states, ". . . Faculty report spending most of their time supervising students in hands-on procedures, leaving little time focused on fostering the development of clinical reasoning skills" (McNelis & Ironside, 2009). It is essential that classroom and clinical experiences be interwoven with real-life clinical experiences. Health professions teachers assist the students to make connections between gaining and applying knowledge, so that students stitch a strong tapestry of clinical reasoning skills for the diverse and complex healthcare environment (Benner et al., 2010).

■ Types of Learners

Teaching of clinical reasoning to the student will vary in style and depth depending upon where the student is in the health professions program. Beginning students need a foundation based on the essential course work such as basic sciences, psychology, sociology, and the like. Furthermore, a fundamental condition for learning and practice in all health professions students is the ability to obtain and manipulate information from a variety of sources, organizing it in a meaningful way to bring about purposeful decision making. Students come to the learning environment with different learning styles and preferences. When faced with new knowledge, students gravitate to their dominant learning style and successfully assimilate new information when the teaching strategies utilized are in harmony with their preferred style. (Learning styles are discussed more thoroughly elsewhere in this text.)

Clinical practitioners also need the physical abilities to provide safe and competent care. To assist educators, the Americans with Disabilities Act (ADA) has defined core competencies, with the intent of clarifying minimal expectations for entry-level applicants (ADA, 1990). Each health profession then can develop specific criteria as appropriate for the benchmark of that profession. Examples of typical core competencies and the ways they are defined in nursing are displayed in **Table 5-2**.

Prerequisite courses and core competencies assist beginning health professions students as they progress to clinical courses where their thinking about patient problems is transformed into clinical reasoning. There also are essential attributes of learners that will contribute to the development of clinical reasoning. These attributes are:

- *Motivation:* A willing learner who desires to become a health professional
- *Attention to details:* Recognize and use vital information to promote safe patient outcomes

Table 5-1 A Clinical Reasoning Model for Healthcare Professions

Healthcare Professions	Scientific Method[a]	Nursing[a]	Medicine[b]	Physical Therapy[c]
Clinical reasoning model	Scientific process	Nursing process	SNAPPS	The physical therapy clinical reasoning and reflection tool (PT-CRT)
Recognition				
Identify the clinical situation and collect relevant data	Define the problem; gather information (data)	Assessment (data collection): History taking, physical assessment, results of diagnostic tests	Summarize briefly the history and findings	Initial data-gathering/interview
Appraisal				
Analyze findings and formulate conclusions	Analyze the information (data)	Nursing diagnostics: Consider assessment database and identify problems; choose nursing diagnosis	Narrow the differential to two or three relevant possibilities	Generate initial hypothesis
Formulate Actions				
Develop interdisciplinary strategies to resolve clinical situation	Develop solutions; make a decision	Planning: Determine desired outcomes; choose interventions to achieve those outcomes	Analyze the differential by comparing and contrasting the possibilities / Probe the preceptor by asking questions about uncertainties, difficulties, or alternative approaches	Examine/evaluate/plan of care
Implement Actions				
Accomplish strategies using interdisciplinary collaboration	Implement the decision	Implementation: Carry out the interventions	Plan management for the patient's medical issues	Interventions
Clinical Judgment				
Evaluate decisions and outcomes and revise strategies as needed	Evaluate the decision	Evaluation: Assess the result of the interventions; determine if outcomes have been achieved; revise the plan if outcomes are not being met; terminate interventions no longer needed	Select a case-related issue for self-directed learning	Reexamination/outcomes

[a]Data from deWit, S. C., & O'Neill, P. A. (2014). *Fundamental concepts and skills for nursing* (4th ed.). St. Louis, MO: W.B. Saunders.

[b]Data from Wolpaw, T., Papp, K. K., & Bordaage, G. (2009). Using SNAPPS to facilitate the expression of clinical reasoning and uncertainties: A randomized comparison group trial. *Academic Medicine, 84*, 517–524.

[c]Data from Atkinson, H. L., & Nixon-Cave, K. (2011). A tool for clinical reasoning and reflection using the International Classification of Functioning, Disability and Health (ICF) framework and patient management model. *Physical Therapy, 91*, 416–430.

Table 5-2   Example Core Performance Standards

Requirements	Standards	Examples
Critical Thinking	Critical thinking ability for effective clinical reasoning and clinical judgment consistent with level of education preparation	Identification of cause/effect relationships in clinical situations Use of scientific method in the development of patient care plans Evaluation of the effectiveness of nursing interventions
Professional Relationships	Interpersonal skills sufficient for professional interactions with a diverse population of individuals, families, and groups	Establishment of rapport with patients/clients and colleagues Capacity to engage in successful conflict resolution Peer accountability
Communication	Communication adeptness sufficient for verbal and written professional interactions	Explanation of treatment procedures, initiation of health teaching Documentation and interpretation of nursing actions and patient/client responses
Mobility	Physical abilities sufficient for movement from room to room and in small spaces	Movement about patient's room, work spaces, and treatment areas Administration of rescue procedures such as cardiopulmonary resuscitation
Motor Skills	Gross and fine motor abilities sufficient for providing safe, effective nursing care	Calibration and use of equipment Therapeutic positioning of patients
Hearing	Auditory ability sufficient for monitoring and assessing health needs	Ability to hear monitoring device alarm and other emergency signals Ability to discern auscultatory sounds and cries for help
Visual Ability	Visual ability sufficient for observation and assessment necessary in patient care	Ability to observe patient's condition and responses to treatments
Tactile Sense	Tactile ability sufficient for physical assessment	Ability to palpate in physical examinations and various therapeutic interventions

Reproduced from Sample Core Performance Standards table of the Americans with Disabilities Act, Implications for Nursing Education Web page, © Southern Regional Education Board. Used with permission.

- *Ability to formulate questions:* For the purposes of clarifying, acquiring, and processing information
- *Awareness of knowledge gaps:* Based upon known information, can identify what is not known and can identify resources for narrowing the knowledge gap
- *Awareness of own thinking:* Attention to own strategies for thinking through a problem and recognition of hindrances to effective problem solving
- *Ability to draw analogies:* Taking known information and applying it to new situations such as a challenging patient example

As learners gain more exposure in the clinical setting, they have more experiences and knowledge to draw on for their clinical reasoning. Individual students develop their own success strategies for developing clinical reasoning. Verbal learners, who process and absorb new knowledge through logic and sequence, are typically left-brain thinkers. These left-brain thinkers will learn clinical reasoning best through a linear process as exemplified by nursing process care plans. Students who have a learning tendency toward right-brain thinking processes absorb information visually, holistically, and often intuitively. Right-brain thinkers prefer a more global approach, such as the use of concept maps (Worden, Hinton, & Fischer, 2011).

■ Conditions for Learning
Effective Teaching for Clinical Reasoning

To cultivate clinical reasoning in the health professions student, the instructor should possess a comprehensive command of the subject and must facilitate thinking by the student rather than merely presenting information. Current practice knowledge is imperative and should include professional standards, guidelines, practice recommendations, and research evidence. The instructor's clinical practice background is beneficial in providing clinical scenarios that are realistic and promote retention of concepts that are useful in clinical practice. Furthermore, the instructor must possess the same attributes of the learner as listed in the previous section. Thus, the ideal teacher is one who can articulate and bring about clinical reasoning in his or her own self and in students.

A teaching style that incorporates Socratic questioning is ideal for developing clinical reasoning in the student. The questioning format stimulates clinical curiosity ("What would we expect in the patient when we see ____?"), and the process leads students to start thinking in the form of questions ("Why did this happen?"). The Socratic method also allows faculty and students to listen to each other's thinking processes and decision making (Oyler & Romanelli, 2014). When using Socratic questioning, the faculty member constructs questions purposefully to lead the student down a particular path of thinking. The process of moving through a scenario brings the student to outcomes the faculty wishes to reach. As the guide in this process, the faculty member redirects the student's thinking when needed, explores potential outcomes of the situation, challenges the student's clinical reasoning abilities by exploring options, and then discusses alternative actions. An example of this process appears in **Box 5-1**.

As can be seen in the example in Box 5-1, the student's clinical reasoning is not enhanced when the faculty member assumes control of the situation. Promoting clinical reasoning includes assessment, often through questioning, of the student's knowledge and potential knowledge gaps or misunderstandings. The instructor then can correct the student's thinking to bring about more accurate reasoning. Due to the nature of the clinical setting, the instructor, at times, may need to be more directive in the approach with the student. In another illustration, in the teaching example at the end of this chapter, it would be easier for the faculty

---

Box 5-1   Case Example: Guiding a Student in Clinical Reasoning

On a routine clinical day, it was time for the student to give his patient an insulin injection. The student and the instructor met in the medication room to review pertinent information prior to preparing the injection. The student had all the correct information and began to prepare the insulin injection. During the process of drawing up the medication, the student drew up the wrong dose of insulin—50 units of insulin instead of 5 units. The instructor remained calm and thought about how to point out the medication error to the student in such a way that the student could learn from the experience, accept constructive criticism, and not lose self-confidence.

The instructor gave the student the opportunity to recheck each step in the process, in hopes that the student would identify the medication error. Unfortunately, the student did not realize that he had prepared an incorrect dose. Using the Socratic method, the instructor began to ask the student questions concerning the medication in an effort to determine if a knowledge gap could be identified. If so, the instructor could provide additional direction and provide time for further review. Although the student knew the drug information, it became apparent that the student could not accurately read calibrations on a syringe. It was now time for the instructor to intervene. So, the instructor asked the student to identify where on the syringe the 5-unit mark was for the correct dose. The student pointed to the 50-unit mark. The instructor directed the student to the correct calibration on the syringe. The student immediately realized his mistake and corrected the medication dosage. The instructor discussed with the student the potential outcome if he had administered the wrong dosage. Working through the steps of the clinical reasoning model, this situation became an opportunity for the student to explore the potential negative consequences to the patient. He then administered the insulin injection correctly.

As a follow-up, the instructor referred the student to the clinical skills lab for remediation.

---

member to take action to correct the problem, but this does not promote the development of independent thinking and the student's clinical reasoning skills. Again, the role of faculty in developing clinical reasoning is to cultivate clinical reasoning in others.

Reflective practice serves as a basis for future action or as a guide in gaining understanding about an experience. Effective teachers can benefit from self-analysis through reflection prior to the teaching experience by asking such questions as "Where do I want them to demonstrate progress today?" "What are the clinical goals for the day?" "How can I promote clinical curiosity in my students?" "Is there anything about my teaching style that impedes the students?" Such self-reflection by teachers will lead to beneficial effects in students, in the form of development and enhancement of clinical reasoning.

Student Considerations That Promote Clinical Reasoning

An important condition that must be considered is that of student self-concept, which includes self-confidence. Learners who begin a program with limited self-concept or weak self-confidence lack the ability to trust their own judgment and feel good about their clinical decisions. Low self-confidence in a student often hinders initiation of care or projects to the patient and family a lack of competency. Thus, the patient may develop a lack of trust in the care provider, which jeopardizes the patient–care provider relationship. To guide the student in overcoming a lack of confidence, the instructor approaches the learning situation in progressive steps. A first step can be to identify a simplistic hurdle that can easily be overcome. An example is talking a student through improving a psychomotor skill such as sterile procedure. Often students need reassurance that they have the knowledge and skill to perform safely in the clinical environment. To assist the student in developing his confidence, the clinical instructor can talk through the steps with the student prior to entering the patient room. Also, the instructor can role play the patient situation with the student, anticipating questions the patient may have while care is being provided.

The goal of the educational program is to create a student who thinks like a health professional. In the skills practice lab, students prepare for clinical practicums, yet once in the patient care setting do not see themselves as the legitimate care providers. They do see themselves as students in an academic setting; therefore, the faculty member must elevate the student's concept of self as a health professional. Research by Etheridge (2007) addressed experiences students identified as beneficial in both their clinical nursing judgment and their role in making these judgments. Students stated that multiple clinical experiences helped them to increase self-confidence and learn responsibility for decisions and care outcomes. Also, students stated that having the opportunity to discuss clinical care experiences with their peers was helpful in validating decisions and gaining further insight. Active discussion assisted the students in learning to trust themselves and their thinking while developing collaborative care. Furthermore, students expressed personal growth through the support of the clinical instructor and through interactions with supportive professional staff. This evidence points to the value of the personal presence of the clinical teacher during student patient care experiences. The teaching example at the end of this chapter explains how the instructor guides the student through clinical reasoning to solve a clinical problem.

■ Potential Problems

For the student to develop clinical reasoning abilities, the student must be motivated to learn and apply information in the academic and clinical arenas. Preparation such as reading and completion of other assignments is fundamental for knowledge application, and is essential in both the classroom and clinical settings. In fact, college students often do not read prior to class, but wait to see what important content is covered in class, and then read that information (Starcher & Proffitt, 2011). However, the basis for clinical reasoning is core knowledge essential to the professional field. In the ideal learning environment, where Socratic questioning, active discussion, and case scenarios are used, it is assumed that at the time of class the student possesses preliminary information related to the topic of the day. Based on this assumption, learning outcomes are achieved and the student is equipped to use the information as a foundation for clinical decisions and actions. Without this fundamental information, the student will not be able to provide the appropriate level of care. Even though the faculty emphasizes the value of class preparation, the student may not appreciate this importance until after the first graded assignment. For those students who seek counseling after a failing grade, the instructor should explore time management and study strategies. If the student has been reading, the instructor can provide suggestions for more efficient reading. If the student has not been reading, the instructor can reiterate the benefit of reading and preparation.

In the clinical setting, the student who does not possess the fundamental information and skills will struggle with reasoned decisions necessary for safe and appropriate care. As can be seen in the example in Box 5-1, the unprepared student would not be able to move through the thought processes to arrive at the correct conclusions. A student who is unable to process the information and display clinical reasoning has the potential to jeopardize patient care and his or her own success in the clinical course. As the student gains more knowledge and skill and increases in confidence, she or he should increase in independence. If this is not occurring, the student will not employ clinical reasoning and the instructor will need to have a conference with the student to determine the obstacle(s) and develop a remediation plan.

Many students are successful in the didactic portions of their academic programs but are unable to demonstrate transfer of knowledge and concepts into the practice setting. Benner and colleagues (2010) indicate that this may be due to the type of teaching strategies employed. These strategies may be unidirectional, didactic, content-driven teacher-talk, with no opportunity for the students to manipulate and fully understand the information presented, much less apply it. Benner et al. further recommend that educators in health professions programs use strategies focused on the patient and care activities. Examples that can be found in this text include human patient simulation, case studies, and problem-based learning.

Educational programs must employ a continuous strategy that assesses a student's ability to transfer theoretical knowledge to the clinical practice. Part of this strategy should examine the learner's ability to overcome ethnocentrism and stereotypical thinking, because these limit the learner's ability to be open to clinical reasoning that is unbiased and patient centered. In a similar fashion, some students enter their professional program with a work-related background that influences their thinking. A typical example is a student who has been a paramedic and enters medical school. This student likely has preconceived notions about his or her chosen field of study and his or her personal abilities related to the practice. Likely this is a misdirected self-concept, in that the student sees himself or herself as competent and qualified to perform in the new clinical setting. The student may be competent in the previous field, yet not display clinical reasoning and skills appropriate in the new field. This can lead to overconfidence on the part of the student, which then leads to safety risks. It is the duty of the instructor to bring these erroneous notions to the student's attention and redirect his or her thinking.

Teaching Example:
Clinical Reasoning in Practice

It was the first day of clinical practice for first-semester nursing students. The students were prepared with care plans in nervous hands. A hundred thoughts raced through their heads. "Is my care plan good enough?" "Will my patient like me?" "I just have to get through this first day safely!" In preconference, the instructor discussed the student assignment for the day, which was to assist their patients with activities of daily living (including bathing, toileting, and nutritional needs), as well as assessment of vital signs. As a part of the assignment, the instructor went with the students to each patient's room to validate the students' assessment of the vital signs.

In one instance, as they entered the room, the instructor scanned the room and quickly noted two safety issues. First, the IV pump was blocking easy access to the bathroom for the patient. Second, the bedside table holding the patient's water, cell phone, and call light was across the room and out of the patient's reach. Furthermore, the head of the hospital bed was pressed up against the wall, preventing easy access to the sphygmomanometer (blood pressure cuff) attached to the wall above the headboard.

The instructor knew she needed to guide the student in recognizing and correcting these safety issues. The first step was for the instructor to ask the student to take a mental snapshot of everything in the room; the instructor patiently waited while the student complied. Then the instructor asked, "What is wrong with this picture?" The student accurately identified the two safety issues and rectified them immediately.

Then she proceeded with her assessment of the vital signs, which was her next priority. During this time, the instructor wondered how this particular student would reach the blood pressure cuff. It was challenging in this situation because this student had dwarfism and had abnormally short arms and legs for her age. The student successfully measured the patient's temperature, radial and apical pulse, and respirations. Then it was time to take the blood pressure. The student moved to reach the blood pressure cuff and was unable to reach the equipment. The student asked the instructor to please get the blood pressure cuff for her.

The instructor paused and thought about a correct response. The instructor recognized the unique teachable moment of this opportunity and acknowledged that the greatest benefit would be for the student to use clinical reasoning to solve the problem rather than seek assistance. The instructor said to the student, "As you move through your nursing career, you will have many challenges. You will need to solve this problem on your own without my assistance." The student received this response positively and proceeded to discuss a solution with the instructor. The student's first action was to find a step stool. Using the stool, the student still could not reach over the patient to retrieve the cuff. She then reasoned that she needed to move the bed. After having done so, she realized she could reach the cuff without the step stool. She then proceeded with the rest of her assessments and completed her clinical assignment.

In this actual scenario, the student approached the problem using a reliable fall-back method (step stool) that did not solve the problem in this new setting. Therefore, the student *recognized* that she needed to approach a challenge with a new way of thinking, which is the first step in clinical reasoning.

This student had success in this and subsequent clinical courses and graduated from the program.

■ Conclusion

Educators in the health professions are recognizing that successful patient outcomes call for more than critical thinking. Positive effects of patient care demand more than intellectual manipulation of content and critical analysis. The proficient healthcare provider fuses critical analysis with thoughtful, rational, and reflective deliberations. The healthcare professional faced with a clinical challenge must engage in clinical reasoning to process data from multiple sources, quickly synthesize the information to draw conclusions, and take action to bring about quality care. Teaching clinical reasoning calls for awareness of how students learn and think, and thus necessitates the use of a variety of teaching strategies. Effective teachers engage in self-reflection about their own teaching style, are willing to be flexible with students to accomplish learning on an individual basis, and are able to recognize and address barriers in the student that hinder clinical reasoning.

Discussion Questions

1. Discuss key strategies for application of the clinical reasoning model for the healthcare professional to your profession's designated decision-making tool.
2. Describe a personal clinical teaching experience that enhanced a student's clinical reasoning skills. Obtain feedback concerning your teaching experience with this student.
3. How would an instructor utilize the Socratic method in developing clinical reasoning skills in learners?

References

American Association of Colleges of Nursing (AACN). (2008). *The essentials of baccalaureate education for professional nursing practice.* Washington, DC: AACN. Retrieved from http://www.aacn.nche.edu/education/pdf/BaccEssentials08.pdf

Americans with Disabilities Act. (1990). Pub. L. No. 101-336, 42 U.S.C. § 12101.

Atkinson, H. L., & Nixon-Cave, K. (2011). A tool for clinical reasoning and reflection using the International Classification of Functioning, Disability and Health (ICF) framework and patient management model. *Physical Therapy, 91,* 416–430.

Benner, P., Sutphen, M., Leonard, V., & Day, L. (2010). *Educating nurses: A call for radical transformation.* Stanford, CA: Carnegie Foundation for the Advancement of Teaching.

deWit, S. C., & O'Neill, P. A. (2014). *Fundamental concepts and skills for nursing* (4th ed.). St. Louis, MO: W.B. Saunders.

Etheridge, S. (2007). Learning to think like a nurse: Stories from new nurse graduates. *Journal of Continuing Education in Nursing, 38*(1), 24–30.

Institute of Medicine (IOM). (2003). *Health professions education: A bridge to quality.* Washington, DC: National Academies Press.

Institute of Medicine (IOM). (2010). *The future of nursing: Leading change, advancing health.* Washington, DC: National Academies Press.

Leahey, M., & Svavarsdottir, E. K. (2009). Implementing family nursing: How do we translate knowledge into clinical practice? *Journal of Family Nursing, 15,* 445–560.

McNelis, A. M., & Ironside, P. M. (2009). National survey on clinical education in prelicensure nursing education programs. In N. Ard & T. M. Valiga (Eds.), *Clinical nursing education: Current reflections* (pp. 25–38). New York, NY: National League for Nursing.

Nixon, J., Wolpaw, T., Schwartz, A., Duffy, B., Menk, J., & Bordage, G. (2014). SNAPPS-plus: An educational prescription for students to facilitate formulating and answering clinical questions. *Academic Medicine, 89*(8), 1174–1179. doi:10.1097/ACM.0000000000000362

Oyler, D. R., & Romanelli, F. (2014). The fact of ignorance: Revisiting the Socratic method as a tool for teaching critical thinking. *American Journal of Pharmaceutical Education, 78*(7), 144.

Starcher, K., & Proffitt, D. (2011). Encouraging students to read: What professors are (and aren't) doing about it. *Journal of Teaching and Learning in Higher Education, 23,* 396–407.

Tanner, C. A. (2006). Thinking like a nurse: A research-based model of clinical judgment in nursing. *Journal of Nursing Education, 45*(6), 204–211.

Wolpaw, T., Papp, K. K., & Bordaage, G. (2009). Using SNAPPS to facilitate the expression of clinical reasoning and uncertainties: A randomized comparison group trial. *Academic Medicine, 84,* 517–524.

Worden, J. M., Hinton, C., & Fischer, K. W. (2011). What does the brain have to do with learning? *Phi Delta Kappan, 92*(8), 8–13.

CHAPTER 6

Finding the Information: Strategies for Conducting Searches

Shanti Freundlich

Educational approaches are constantly evolving and changing, as are student and educator expectations. The last decade has seen an elevation in our expectations regarding the availability and accessibility of information, and in the sophistication of the search tools at our disposal. Students and faculty now not only expect all information to be available immediately online (Brantley & Pickard, 2010), but also tend to work from the starting assumption that their search skills are sophisticated enough to easily find all the information they are looking for, on any given subject (Dahlstrom, 2012). Finding relevant, high-quality information that can be the basis of evidence-based nursing practice is not as simple as the quick and basic Google search most students enter college or graduate school comfortable performing. Search skills can be learned, and this chapter discusses strategies that will work regardless of search engine or interface design. These strategies are part of the mechanical skill set necessary for searching, as well as a larger critical thinking skill set concerning finding and evaluating the information students need throughout their nursing careers.

There is no one single correct search strategy, nor is there one single correct way to teach searching. Regardless of the professor's preferred teaching theory, or the student's learning style, the keys for developing searching proficiency and confidence are repetition and a clear search topic. The more often students search for and find academically or clinically relevant information, the less intimidating the resources and strategies become. The teaching of search strategies and appropriate resources should be closely followed by opportunities for students to test them out via assignments that require finding information (Duke, 2011). This type of assignment-based searching is also a good way for students to get familiar with articulating topic concepts. As students become proficient in using search strategies and navigating the various resource interfaces, they can then focus their attention on critically evaluating the information they find. Being able to find, identify, and use high-quality information is an integral part of lifelong information literacy, and speaks to a variety of teaching and learning core competencies (see **Box 6-1**).

Box 6-1   Relevant Teaching and Learning Core Competencies

Nurse educators who incorporate teaching of critical thinking about search strategies are working to meet the National League for Nursing Core Competencies of Nurse Educators: Facilitate Learning (C1), Use Assessment and Evaluation Strategies (C3), Function as a Change Agent and Leader (C5), and Function Within the Educational Environment (C8) (Massachusetts Department of Higher Education, 2010).

It also helps students meet the Association of College and Research Libraries (ACRL) *Framework for Information Literacy* for Higher Education (ACRL, 2015), specifically "research as inquiry," "scholarship as conversation," and "searching as strategic exploration."

■ Current Issues in Searching

According to the 2011 Pew Internet Health Topics survey, 80% of Internet users, or 59% of U.S. adults, look online for health information, and search engines have conditioned people, especially younger generations, to expect all information to be easy to find and free online (Fox, 2012). Even the delay of making a photocopy or entering an additional password can be the difference between reading or skipping an article (Sathe, Grady, & Giuse, 2002). Researchers at every level admit they would rather use a less relevant and less authoritative online journal article than a more relevant and more authoritative print article (Sathe et al., 2002). At the same time, another survey found teachers agreed that the amount of information available online can be discouraging or overwhelming to students (Purcell et al., 2012). Even more importantly for healthcare professionals, there are the serious accuracy concerns for more than half of health information–related web resources (Chung, Oden, Joyner, Sims, & Moon, 2012).

Unfortunately, while many students think they have "Google-fu" (the ability to find anything with a Google search), the ERIAL Project and other research have shown that instead they have a rather "stunted understanding of how to finely tune a search in order to hone in on usable sources" (Kolowich, 2011). Students' mental models seem to rely primarily on typing whole questions into any and all search boxes, not inquiring how the results are generated or arranged, trusting the first few search results, and rarely scrolling past the first page (Duke, 2011; Pan et al., 2007). They have limited experience using advanced search features and, quite understandably, sometimes compare academic databases to black holes. When teaching search strategies, one must acknowledge students' existing models and processes, encourage them to embrace the search frustrations and failures that they regularly experience (Bain, 2012) and comprehend the personal benefit of altering their search strategies, and give them time to try out the new strategies on a topic of their choice (see the example activity in **Box 6-2**).

■ Scaffolded Information Literacy Programs

An approach that is increasingly being adopted is direct collaboration between faculty members and their librarians to develop information literacy programs that focus on the critical thinking behind a search strategy, that teach the evaluation criteria necessary to make informed choices, and that tie directly into the course curriculum. These scaffolded programs rely on students receiving information literacy instruction

Box 6-2   Teaching with Google, Not Against It

Almost every resource has a scenario in which it is the best possible source to use. Instead of working against students' existing information-seeking habits, consider a classroom activity that draws on those habits and teaches students to place Google and Wikipedia within the larger information universe.

Start by having the students brainstorm what kinds of information they might need for a project, who might have authored it, and where it would be published. Next, have students do a side-by-side comparison of Google results and a Discovery Search (e.g., EBSCO Discovery Service or ProQuest Summon) as they work from their initial topic idea through the specific types of information they will need to complete an assignment. Instead of forbidding a resource or search platform, ask them to compare the types and quality of information they are finding. Prompt them to consider the advertising and personalization in Google, as well as their emotional reaction to familiar and unfamiliar resources. Encourage them to critically read the sources, and to understand the structure of a research article.

After an activity like this, most students will better understand when and how to use a combination of resources, and they will be more confident in screening their search results.

Box 6-3   Prompt Questions for Brainstorming a Topic

- What did you learn about in class this week that really caught your attention?
- What was the last news story you read?
- Is there something you can start from that you saw in clinic/with a patient?

repeatedly throughout their college experience. Learning objectives and skills are mapped to developmentally appropriate course requirements, so students are learning increasingly sophisticated ways to think about, find, and manipulate information as they progress through the program. Successful information literacy programs are built on close working relationships between librarians and faculty members, and scaffold the learning process so students have time to incorporate their new skills and knowledge into their existing mental models and demonstrate their newfound knowledge, skills, and abilities through course work. When developing a program, consider using the new ACRL *Framework for Information Literacy for Higher Education* (2015) as a basis for the learning outcomes.

Developing a Topic

The most basic skill for most students is that of choosing a topic of interest. **Box 6-3** lists some prompt questions that health professions educators could use to help them get started.

An instructor can also demonstrate how an article in a popular magazine or a song can lead to a research topic and keywords. For example, an article in *Mother Jones Magazine* on a program for homeless people in Utah could lead into a policy paper on funding "housing first" state policies. Or, hearing "Yuri Kochiyama" by the Blues Scholars might inspire a research project on her human rights activism.

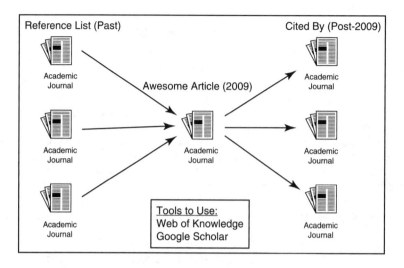

■ **Figure 6-1** Citation searching.
Courtesy of Shanti Freundlich.

A somewhat underappreciated but important part of the search process is translating a research topic into search terms (see **Figure 6-1**). Without clear research concepts to start from, search strategies will never yield fully satisfactory results because there is no clear goal for the search. The search process combines articulating an initial topic, expressing it in search terms, picking where to search, and refining the results to only the relevant results. Developing keyword search terms in many ways reverses the research question development process. That is, by necessity a research question is narrow and highly focused, whereas the combination of search terms necessary to find relevant literature must start deliberately broad: encompassing alternate and related terms to describe the topic. After all, the researcher is trying to find the universe of literature that surrounds the gap identified through the question. Once a student has an initial topic in mind (see **Box 6-4**), he or she can start translating it into keywords.

Box 6-4   Starting Research Projects with Broad, Long-Form Research Topics of Interest

"My topic is related to parent–nurse relationships and improved patient outcomes in the NICU."
"What are the best practices around interdisciplinary nursing and medical education?"
"We are hoping to improve communication between doctors and nurses in academic and clinical settings."
"Our interest is to find out more about the attitudes of both healthcare providers and patients toward screening for domestic violence."

Topics into Keywords

Without instructions or an explanation of how databases use keywords to produce search results, students will often try to type their whole question into a database's search box, and will not consider adding alternative terms to describe the topic. When their initial search fails to produce results, they become frustrated and revert to familiar Internet search engines. However, keywords can be explained simply and adopted quickly: they are the concepts that are core to your question. Any question complex enough to be a research question includes multiple core ideas, and a good search strategy tries to address all of them. Alternative terms for one idea are connected using OR between them, and different ideas are connected using AND (see **Box 6-5** and **Box 6-6**).

Most databases return articles that contain the literal word or phrase typed in, primarily based on the title, author, abstract, or subject headings; nevertheless, databases are becoming more flexible all the time. Turning a question into keywords can be a mental shift, but once students see the benefits to their search results, they often are open to adopting new habits (Bain, 2012).

Experienced researchers may recognize that "connecting terms" are Boolean operators, and that there is a third term: NOT. Similar to AND and OR, NOT defines the relationship between concepts. However, NOT is an exclusionary term, and removes concepts from the search, rather than broadening the concepts (OR) or narrowing the focus (AND). Students tend not to know enough about their topic at the beginning to say with certainty that a given concept is definitely of no interest to them and is not crucial to the topic at hand, so this exclusionary term may be more useful after they are already well into their iterative search. Assignment- and evidence-based projects will sometimes also ask for comparisons of topics, conditions, practices, and so on; thus, excluding a concept might remove relevant results.

Students are often reassured to hear their search strategies are not being compared to a "perfect" search: a good search is the one that returns the most relevant, accurate results. Search strategies and keywords are not precious or set in stone; rather, they are flexible tools to be changed or thrown away if the results are not good

---

Box 6-5   Concepts Connected to Each Other Using AND

Expressed as keywords, the examples from Box 6-4 could look like:

- parent–nurse relationships AND patient outcomes
- interdisciplinary nursing AND medical education AND communication AND clinical
- attitudes AND healthcare providers AND domestic violence

Box 6-6   Using the Same Example Search Topics

- Parent–nurse OR family-centered OR parent–professional AND patient outcomes
- Attitudes AND healthcare providers OR nurs* AND domestic violence OR intimate partner abuse OR spousal abuse

enough. For anxious searchers, it may also be reassuring to hear that most databases and search engines will save their search histories, so previous keyword choices can be recovered. There is no "correct" number of keywords, and there is no perfect combination of keywords for a topic. That said, usually a range of two to four concepts with a keyword for each one will suffice for most searches, although there are exceptions, including for systematic reviews.

The advantage of expressing concepts as keywords is students can express their ideas in their own words: there is no wrong keyword. However, this flexibility also means there are an almost unlimited number of ways to describe a topic, and it can be challenging to align one's keywords to the terms actually used in the literature. Although students might know exactly what concepts their keywords signify, it is quite possible that experts and researchers in the field describe their work in different or more technical/medical terms. Adding alternate or additional keywords or using subject terms can help bridge this conceptual gap (see Figure 6-1). Because a single concept can be described in many literal words, adding alternate keywords expands the potential search results for a concept. Keywords can also be methodologies, standardized instruments, population characteristics, or any other aspect of the literature that is significant for the research project.

Students sometimes assume that search boxes "understand" what they mean, rather than what they type, but most research-focused resources still depend on literal words and phrases, so providing multiple terms for a core idea lets the database do more work for you. Brainstorming alternate terms to describe a concept indicates the ability to think critically about a problem from multiple angles, a knowledge practice of the Searching as Strategic Exploration ACRL Frame (ACRL, 2015).

Finding Additional Keywords

Databases are built to assist with the mechanics of searching, so students are not required to think of every possible alternative term or search criterion on their own. In addition to the knowledge base they build through classroom and clinical learning, databases and other high-quality resources include tools to assist in this process, including the thesaurus and subject terms that students can use to find preferred and additional terms to use as keywords. Also, every found article is a gold mine for additional keywords: Their titles and abstracts are full of clues as to how leading voices in a field are describing the current research. Those terms can be added to, or even replace, initial keywords, and altering search terms based on the language used by researchers in the field will help bring back more results that are current, relevant, and of high quality. This stage of the process highlights that keywords are not precious or static; as soon as a better or additional keyword is identified, it should immediately be incorporated into the search (see the learning activity in **Box 6-7**).

Citation Searching

Mining article references is a long-standing method of enhancing a literature search and quickly gathering the significant, well-respected studies in a field. Students new to the research process often need to be encouraged to see articles as dynamic tools

---

Box 6-7   Searching for Search Terms Activity

It's impossible and unnecessary for students to know all potential keywords before they start a search. Once students are familiar with iterative searching and research terminology such as *systematic review*, that knowledge can be built upon.

Ask students to find a review article on a topic of their choice, locate and identify the methods section (the databases searched and the terms used), and then replicate the search as closely as possible.

This activity asks students to find information on their topic of choice; build confidence with search terms and database tools; and demonstrate that they can find, read, and evaluate a specific type of article. It's also an opportunity to grasp the scholarly conversation of the researchers and articles.

---

that are more than just the sum of their research content: They have references, methods, keywords, and more that students can use to shape their own processes. In addition to using an article's references, databases are also starting to offer links to "cited by" sources. That is, if an article was published in 2008, the "cited by" sources are the articles published since then using the initial article as a reference. Mining these sources is a way for students to stay within their search topic, but move forward into even more current research. It's also a visible, useful demonstration of how past, current, and potential sources are connected and influence each other (see Figure 6-1). This is a powerful search tool that can help students understand that past research informs future research, and how both of them inform practice.

Subject Headings

Searching primarily with keywords is still a fairly recent development, and the subject heading searches previously depended upon are still the backbone of how articles, journals, and books are organized: MeSH in Medline, CINAHL Headings, Library of Congress Headings, and so on. Simply put, subject headings are expertly applied tags that are pulled from a controlled list, and are used to connect like research to like research.

The advantage of a subject heading is that it is a term from a field of research (nursing, medicine, etc.), and it has a consistent, specific meaning that has been applied by an expert. That is, every article with "Family-Centered Care" as a subject heading will contain content on "Family-Centered Care," and a student can easily get to all the articles on "Family-Centered Care" through that subject heading. Most student search needs can be satisfied with a sophisticated keyword search in which subject headings are used as keywords. Searching only via subject headings is possible and is often a useful exercise for students who need to do an exhaustive literature search, integrative review, or systematic review (see **Box 6-8**). Understanding the theory of subject headings can reassure students that they are not attempted to pull structure out of chaos, and that databases are in fact highly organized repositories designed to facilitate their search process. Understanding the underlying structure of information may help students shift their mental models about searching for and finding information to include keywords, subject headings, citation mining, and connecting terms.

> ### Box 6-8   Keywords Versus Subject Terms
>
> Are your students still unclear about defining and using keywords versus subjects? Consider comparing them to platforms that students are familiar with from their own lives.
>
> Subject headings: When you tag a friend in a photo on Facebook; you're using subject headings—pulling from a controlled vocabulary of your friends.
> Keywords: When you use a hashtag on Twitter or Instagram; anyone can make one up, and it may or may not be the best way to describe the topic.

Database Limiters

Students are not solely dependent on the search box and keywords for narrowing down their results by relevance. Instead, there are an almost overwhelming number of limiting tools built into databases to do the work of narrowing down the results. There are limiters that can be used on any search for evidence-based literature, including date range, peer review, demographic options, methodology-based limiters, and a variety of others. None of them is required for a search, but they will do some of the work of narrowing down the literature. They help a researcher eliminate results that are not relevant to the topic at hand and would only confuse the issue rather than clarify it.

Searching Is Iterative

Anyone who has tried to search for research literature in an academic database has experienced the frustration of a failed search and the moment of panic wondering if perhaps there just isn't any literature on that topic. Experienced researchers know that a "no results found" message is really just a search engine's way of telling you to try the search again, but students need to be prepared by their teachers for their searches to fail. It is frustrating to labor through articulating a search strategy only to be told that there are no results matching your criteria. The truth is, except for very rare cases, there is *always* literature related to a research topic. The challenge, especially for students new to research, is to brainstorm additional search terms while still staying on topic; usually adding alternate terms gives a search engine enough flexibility to start returning results. For the students who are having difficulty reconceptualizing their topics into different terms, the subject heading and thesaurus functions built into most databases will give them hints and suggestions. For many initial student forays into the research literature, it is enough to simply broaden the keywords that represent the major concepts and remove keywords that represent minor concepts or demographic details. Suddenly seeing thousands of results can reassure students there are many potentially related articles, and the database has the tools to narrow down the list to the most relevant ones. The true challenge after a failed search is to figure out how to approach the same topic from a new direction, but still maintain the intended focus.

Where to Search

If approaching the topic with different keywords does not bring back more relevant and satisfactory results, the issue may be where students are conducting their searches. As we have established, students tend to expect that everything is available from one search box. However, academic libraries still subscribe to a multitude of databases because different content is available through each one, and the search results can only be as relevant as the content that the database search and draw from. Although many students are inclined to continue searching in resources with which they are already familiar, like JSTOR or Project MUSE, they will only be truly exploring the most relevant literature by also becoming familiar with Medline, PubMed, CINAHL, the Cochrane Library, and the Joanna Briggs Institute (JBI). Libraries will also usually list and describe additional databases related to any given topic on research guides and the library website.

■ Conclusion

With everything else that faculty are being asked to integrate into their curricula and classrooms—meaningful assessment, active learning activities, social media, the latest technology, all on top of the increasing amount of actual content and up-to-the-minute research—it can sound like one additional element too many to ask faculty to teach search strategies as well. Faculty can instead choose to view search strategies as a skill set that empowers students to take responsibility for their own learning, both immediately in the classroom and in their long-term practices; they can also draw on their librarian colleagues for teaching support. When students understand that research articles connect to practice guidelines and the everyday clinical choices they make, and they are able to confidently search for the latest evidence, they will be more empowered to take responsibility for their own learning. There is high-quality information available to support students throughout their learning process, but they need to develop confidence in their searching abilities, be willing to be flexible in their approach, and set high standards for the information they use. Teaching students to be empowered, confident searchers is the first step in training them to think critically about the information they choose to use in their academic work, their clinical practice, and their everyday lives. The next step beyond finding information is being able to evaluate it confidently, weighing its strengths and weaknesses before consciously deciding whether and/or how to use it as a foundation for evidence-based practice.

Discussion Questions

1. What are your assumptions about your students' experience and confidence with finding and using research literature? Do these assumptions align with students' questions and demonstrated abilities?
2. How could you incorporate information-seeking skills into assignments or conversations about where textbook information comes from?

References

Association of College and Research Libraries (ACRL). (2015). *Framework for information literacy for higher education*. Retrieved from http://www.ala.org/acrl/standards/ilframework

Bain, K. (2012, November). *What the best college teachers do—and how you can be among them*. Speech presented at the Colleges of the Fenway Teaching and Learning Collaborative Annual Fall Conference, Boston, MA.

Brantley, S., & Pickard, B. (2010). *The ERIAL project at UIC: Understanding how students search for information* [PDF document]. Retrieved from http://www.erialproject.org

Chung, M., Oden, R. P., Joyner, B. L., Sims, A., & Moon, R. (2012). Safe infant sleep recommendations on the Internet: Let's Google it. *Journal of Pediatrics, 161*(6), 1080–1084.e1. doi:10.1016/j.jpeds.2012.06.004

Dahlstrom, E. (foreword by C. Dziuban & J. D. Walker). (2012). *ECAR study of undergraduate students and information technology, 2012* [Research report]. Louisville, CO: EDUCAUSE Center for Applied Research. Retrieved from http://educause.edu/ecar

Duke, L. (2011). *Search skills of the 21st century student* [PDF document]. Retrieved from http://www.erialproject.org/wp-content/uploads/2011/04/ACRL-erial-results-presentation.pdf

Fox, S. (2012). Health topics. *Pew Internet & American Life Project.* Retrieved from http://www.pewinternet.org/Reports/2011/HealthTopics.aspx

Kolowich, S. (2011, August 22). What students don't know. *Inside Higher Ed.* Retrieved from http://www.insidehighered.com/news/2011/08/22/erial_study_of_student_research_habits_at_illinois_university_libraries_reveals_alarmingly_poor_information_literacy_and_skills

Massachusetts Department of Higher Education. (2010). *Nurse of the future: Nursing core competencies.* Retrieved from http://www.mass.edu/currentinit/documents/NursingCoreCompetencies.pdf

Pan, B., Hembrooke, H., Joachims, T., Lorigo, L., Gay, G., & Granka, L. (2007). In Google we trust: Users' decisions on rank, position, and relevance. *Journal of Computer-Mediated Communication, 12*(3), 801–823. doi:10.1111/j.1083-6101.2007.00351.x

Purcell, K., Raine, L., Heaps, A., Buchanan, J., Friedrich, L., Jacklin, A., . . . Zickuhr, K. (2012). How teens do research in the digital world. *Pew Internet & American Life Project.* Retrieved from http://pewinternet.org/Reports/2012/Student-Research.aspx

Sathe, N. A., Grady, J. L., & Giuse, N. B. (2002). Print versus electronic journals: A preliminary investigation into the effect of journal format on research processes. *Journal of the Medical Library Association, 90*(2), 235.

Recommended Reading

Bing, P., Hembrooke, H., Joachims, T., Lorigo, L., Gary, G., & Granka, L. (2007). In Google we trust: Users' decisions on rank, position, and relevance. *Journal of Computer-Mediated Communication, 12*(3), 801–823. doi:10.1111/j.1083-6101.2007.00351.x

Blanchett, H., Powis, C., & Webb, J. (2012). *A guide to teaching information literacy: 101 practical tips.* London, UK: Facet Publishing.

Booth, C. (2011). *Reflective teaching, effective learning: Instructional literacy for library educators.* Chicago, IL: American Library Association.

Carpenter, J., Wetheridge, L., Tanner, S., & Smith, N. (2012). *Researchers of tomorrow.* Retrieved from http://www.jisc.ac.uk/publications/reports/2012/researchers-of-tomorrow

Core competencies of nurse educators with task statements. (2005). Retrieved from http://www.nln.org/docs/default-source/default-document-library/core-competencies-of-nurse-educators-with-task-statements.pdf?sfvrsn=0

Gavin, C. (2008). *Teaching information literacy: A conceptual approach.* Lanham, MD: Scarecrow Press.

Gwyer, R., Stubbings, R., Walton, G., & International Federation of Library Associations and Institutions. (2012). *The road to information literacy: Librarians as facilitators of learning.* Berlin, Germany: De Gruyter Saur.

Kaplowitz, J. R. (2012). *Transforming information literacy instruction using learner-centered teaching.* New York, NY: Neal-Schuman.

Kvenild, C., & Calkins, K. (2011). *Embedded librarians: Moving beyond one-shot instruction.* Chicago, IL: Association of College and Research Libraries.

Palfrey, J., & Gasser, U. (2008). *Born digital: Understanding the first generation of digital natives.* New York, NY: Basic Books.

Walton, G., & Pope, A. (2011). *Information literacy: Infiltrating the agenda, challenging minds.* Oxford, UK: Chandos Publishing.

SECTION II

Educational Use of Technology

Educational technology continues to grow by leaps and bounds and has changed the complexion of the world of education. The technology can be as simple as communicating by e-mail or as complex as presenting full degree-granting programs by distance learning. Classroom teaching is utilizing more and more technology, from PowerPoint presentations and student- and faculty-made videos to blended learning, a combination of in-class and asynchronous discussions. Online courses are now using learning management systems (LMSs) that allow both synchronous and asynchronous technologies. Social media include blogs, wikis, Twitter, and YouTube. Libraries have become accessible to distance learners by use of technology, and full-text articles are now available online. The Internet has opened a new and extensive world of information not previously available, and both faculty and students need to learn not only how to take advantage of the wealth of information, but also how to use it discriminately. Students are increasingly involved in social technology, where they communicate with wide audiences. Teaching in a technological world requires faculty collaboration with academic information technology specialists, a specialty field in itself, to learn how to use the ever-changing systems, as well as to keep abreast of new resources as they become available and provide technological support for students.

The discussion in these chapters provides a look at different ways of utilizing available technologies and discusses strengths of the systems and problems that may occur. As technology has grown in the past few years, the technology discussion in this edition has increased as well. Chapter 7, on blended learning, explores the use of technological strategies in the classroom environment. Chapter 8, "Teaching in the Online Environment," details specific learning theories and strategies available for success in an online classroom. Social media are included in teaching strategies, as discussed in Chapter 9, "Social Media as a Context for Connected Learning." Distance learning techniques have moved into the classroom in blended or hybrid classes, and faculty need to learn to incorporate these strategies as a way to better achieve their learning objectives. Distance learning can be *asynchronous*, meaning that students can access the material and discussions at any time; or *synchronous*, meaning that students are online together regardless of their location.

Technology may be used to assist learning, but it does not replace the instructor. Teaching methods require adaptation to be effective in this new environment and should be evaluated for effectiveness. The amount of Internet information may be overwhelming, and it is critical for faculty and students to begin to cull the material to a reasonable amount, and validate its accuracy. The use of educational technologies may require extra time and effort from faculty, but can be very effective in enhancing learning and can be rewarding for students and faculty alike.

CHAPTER 7

Using Multimedia in the Blended Classroom

Karen H. Teeley
Arlene J. Lowenstein

To an experienced educator, who was also a digital immigrant, the first entry into online teaching was a challenge, but has now become a love affair.

—*Arlene J. Lowenstein*

■ Definition and Purposes

Garrison and Vaughan (2008) define *blended learning* as "a coherent design approach that openly assesses and integrates the strengths of face-to-face and online learning to address worthwhile educational goals" (p. x). They note that it is a thoughtful fusion of classroom teaching and online learning experiences. *Thoughtful* is the key word here, because the learning opportunities and experiences are crucial, and the course must be specifically designed to allow students to discover and work with those opportunities. Blended learning requires a restructuring of class contact hours with the goals of engaging students in the learning process and extending access to learning opportunities that may be found on the Internet (Garrison & Vaughan, 2008).

Online teaching can be *synchronous*, where students will be online at the same time (e.g., chat rooms, teleconferences, and online synchronous class sessions with programs such as Adobe Connect), or *asynchronous*, where students can access the course and post responses at any time, day or night, in different time zones. Blended learning, also known as *hybrid* or *mixed mode*, is a combination of online plus face-to-face (f2f) classroom sessions. Blended learning may utilize less face-to-face class time, but adds asynchronous learning time and could even include some synchronous class sessions, although that is not required. A blended course may be designed 50% onsite classroom and 50% online time, or 70% and 30%, or other percentages. The ratio will vary depending on the course and needed content. The method chosen and class design depend on the learning objectives and the technology available.

Understanding the Blended Course Environment

A learning management system (LMS) is used to allow students to access course information. Common systems include Blackboard, Moodle, and Sakai, among others. Depending on the school's procedures, students can log in with a user name and password at any time, beginning a few days before the first day of class. Access to class materials after the course ends is determined by school policies. The course syllabus and other posted classroom materials, including PowerPoint or other forms of presentation tools, videos, or other lecture materials, such as podcasts/audio lectures and interactive teaching modules, allow students to review materials and refresh their memories if they so choose. Announcements and communication methods, such as e-mailing the students, group discussion boards, blogs, Twitter, and wikis, may also be available. Use of social media is becoming more common in the classroom and can be used with blended learning as appropriate (McEwan, 2012; Moran, Seaman, & Tinit-Kane, 2011; Steer, 2012).

The instructor can post materials anytime during the course, so lecture materials may be posted before the class during which the lecture is given, to encourage preparation; or after the lecture has taken place, to allow the students to review for exams or assignments. However, a blended learning environment can enable the "flipping" of the classroom: where learners ingest the course materials for a lesson (readings, video lectures, podcasts) *outside* the classroom before a session (Berrett, 2012; Brunsell & Horejsi, 2011; Sams & Bergmann, 2013). That allows the valuable class time to be used for discussion of the material and active learning, rather than passive listening to a lecture.

Blended learning and other forms of web-based instruction require educators to adapt to the ever-growing list of technological opportunities. The challenge for the instructor is not just to master new and complicated technology, but instead to find more meaningful ways to engage the students. Expectations are higher with each succeeding generation as students are exposed to technology at earlier ages. Today's students have grown up with technology; they have been raised on the Internet, Google for information, have thrived in online communities, and are connected 24/7. John Sener addresses the "cyberization" of education as now being mainstream and unlikely to change in the future (Sener, 2012). Students expect educators to be adept with the current technology and its applications (Prensky, 2001).

Discussion Posts

Discussion posts may be assigned at varying times during the blended course, or weekly, again depending on class design. Students need clear instructions as to what is expected in the posts, the length of the post for assigned discussions, and what is expected for responses to classmates. A good discussion between students develops a learning community, where students learn from each other as well as from the instructor (and, especially when students are encouraged to use the literature to develop their discussions, the instructor can also learn from the students). One example is for the instructor to develop specific discussion questions based on course objectives, materials that have been presented online, and readings, but ask for more evidence than was given, such as finding a new reading on the question or a broader question. This type of question can help the student develop a higher level of critical thinking (Palloff & Pratt, 2005). Along with scholarly work, students can be asked to discuss appropriate experiences they have had or know about that illustrate some of the issues within the questions. Student responses to their classmates' threaded discussion postings and faculty comments help set up the learning community dialogue to the benefit of all.

Assignments

Papers and group and individual projects can be assigned along with specific assignments, such as searching for additional resources and websites to share through the postings. Assignments may be posted and graded online or turned in on class days, depending on teacher preference. Antiplagiarism software (e.g., TurnItIn and SafeAssign) may be used to help cut down on cheating and plagiarism. Quizzes and exams may be given online or in class.

■ Theoretical Foundations

In the 1990s, Badrul H. Khan (2007) was concerned with what it takes "to provide the best and most meaningful flexible learning environments for learners worldwide." His answer to this question was developed into a framework for online learning, and this model is used internationally. He understood that e-learning did not include just teaching, but required a combination of factors to be effective. His framework (**Figure 7-1**) consists of eight elements, the first being *institutional*, which discusses

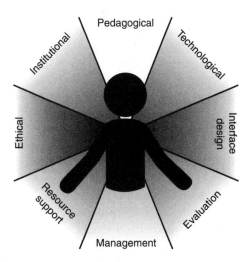

■ **Figure 7-1**   A framework for e-learning.

Reproduced from Khan, B. H. (2009). *E-learning framework.* Retrieved from http://www.badrulkhan.com

administrative elements and the need for administration understanding and support. *Pedagogical* refers to the learning goals and design, and the need for adaptation to the expansion of opportunities available through online learning. The *technological* section refers to the infrastructure available to produce effective online teaching, avoiding the frustration that can occur with poor technology, and this goes along with the *interface*, which discusses how the user gains access, through the technology, to those learning opportunities. *Evaluation* of both learners and content is critical to understand the problems and seek solutions to improve the learning. The *management* section refers to management of the learning environment, who is responsible, and how is it done; and the *resource support* refers to required resources other than the nontutorial components. The *ethical* portion is related to diversity issues and ethical concerns in e-learning.

Harvey Singh (2003) adapted Khan's framework to serve as a guide to planning, developing, delivering, managing, and evaluating blended learning programs. He noted that blended learning includes several forms of learning tools and mixes various event-based activities, including face-to-face and e-learning, which can include both synchronous and asynchronous learning activities along with self-paced learning.

Singh's (2003) studies found that blending provides various benefits over using any single learning delivery medium alone. He recognizes learning is not a one-time event, but rather a continuous process. The concepts in the Khan framework demonstrate the need for a broad base of support, as well as the instructional or pedagogical elements, to implement and carry out blended learning offerings. Singh has looked at each piece of Khan's framework in relation to how it can be developed to establish effective blended learning.

Ausbum (2004) explored instructional features most important to adult learners in blended classes. She found that most adults in her study valued course designs that contained options, personalization, self-direction, variety, and a learning community. They enjoyed and highly valued two-way communication with their classmates and instructor, and felt they benefited from frequent announcements and reminders from their instructors. However, she also found that in online instruction, as in more traditional environments, learners with different learning styles and characteristics do prefer and benefit from varied instructional features and goals, depending on their previous experiences or learning style. Their preferences were not all the same.

Means, Toyama, Murphy, and Baki (2013) carried out a meta-analysis of 45 studies contrasting fully or partially online (blended) with fully face-to-face instructional conditions. Most courses lasted more than 1 month. Results showed that on average, students in online learning conditions performed modestly better than those receiving all face-to-face instruction, but there was a significant advantage over face-to-face instruction for students in blended learning conditions. Active and self-paced learning established in blended learning can relate effectively to different learning styles and student preferences. Studies designed with blended learning tended to involve additional learning time, instructional resources, and course elements that encouraged interactions among learners (Means et al., 2013).

Faculty development is key to a successful blended program (Myers, Mixer, Wyatt, Paulus, & Lee, 2011). Faculty need to become comfortable with the technology and the movement between classroom and online. When attending a faculty development program about blended learning, faculty are required to shift their role from teacher to student. This shift can enrich their learning about teaching (Myers et al., 2011).

■ Types of Learners

Students enter the health professions in different stages in their lives. While some are traditional college students, most students have very busy lives with jobs and children and other family obligations. With the added expense of college tuition, it is a rare student who does not have to work in addition to attending school and fulfilling clinical placements. This changing profile of the learner suggests that most students fulfill the pedagogical description of the adult learner (Jairath & Stair, 2004). The more flexible and self-paced the course delivery is, the more likely it is the students will be able to fit it into their schedules and be successful.

Web-based courses using a learning management system such as Blackboard® or Moodle® require a comprehensive orientation to the format. Students must quickly become proficient in navigating the tools, troubleshooting common problems such as disabling pop-up blockers, and mastering e-mail and attachment functions. Most importantly, students need to know how to access help.

Students in higher education in the first decade of the 21st century fall into the generation called "millennials" (Howe & Strauss, 2000). These are students born between the years of 1982 and 2002. They are global, connected, and interactive. Although they grew up in a media age, they will undoubtedly have varying levels of proficiency, which will require access to support functions.

Marc Prensky (2001) differentiates *digital natives* from *digital immigrants*. He describes digital natives as the students today who are native speakers of the digital language of computers, video games, and the Internet; those who are not native to the digital language (most instructors) are said to be *digital immigrants*. Immigrants have to learn a new language and adapt to a new environment. "Digital natives are used to receiving information really fast. They like to parallel process and multi-task ... They function best when networked" (Prensky, 2001, p. 3). He suggests it is unlikely digital natives are going to learn the immigrant's language, so, in order to reach these students, immigrant instructors must learn to communicate in the language style of the student.

■ Conditions for Learning

Know Your Learners

It is important to understand who your learners are. What is the size of the class? Small classes should be treated differently than larger classes and will necessitate different teaching methodologies. What background do students have prior to entering this course? Have they taken courses that provide the background material for the current course? Can you assess, or can students tell you, what their preferred learning style is? Today's students may be very diverse. What are the forms of diversity in the class? Do you have students with specific learning disabilities? If so, how can they be supported in their learning activities? Cultural and ethnic diversities can enrich all students by fostering cultural understanding and learning, but monitoring may be necessary to avoid stereotyping and negative feelings and communications. Students with English as a second language may need assistance or specific programs to assist them in writing assignments. Some of these questions can be answered in the introduction to the course, either in class or online with an introductory exercise in which students introduce themselves to faculty and classmates.

Working with Technology

Faculty need to work with instructional technology to learn to work with the LMS and keep up to date with changing technology. It is critically important for you to have a good understanding of what the LMS offers and how to work with it *before* designing your course. It is very helpful to have a connection with the technology resources in your institution so you know whom to contact for support when technology glitches occur—but also to help you avoid those glitches. Success in online teaching requires close collaboration with those in the school's instructional technology department. Understand how to contact them, and make them your best friends if possible. It is very helpful to have a specific person to work with. Technology changes rapidly, with some older technological teaching strategies becoming outdated and new ones coming in. Technology personnel can help keep you up to date on new technological teaching strategies that have been developed, and can let you know if there are financial obligations for the use of some of those technologies.

Technologies such as wikis (excellent for group projects because students can access and edit a group paper, rather than using e-mail), blogs, voiceover Power Points, podcasts, and other technologies can be incorporated within the course, but too many different technologies can be overwhelming to students. It is critical to meet technology deadlines in preparing your classes, so the course template can be set up on time.

Check to see if there are faculty technology orientation programs or workshops that you can take advantage of. Encourage students to attend technology orientations and to contact the student technology support system with computer issues. Orientation to a course may include a scavenger hunt for students within the e-learning environment, which may allow students to download certain files, take practice quizzes, send an e-mail, and so on, and enter the results, information from the documents, or a special word from a mail message to guarantee they can successfully access all the e-learning tools required for the course.

■ Using the Method

Planning and Modifying

In online and blended learning courses, good planning is critical to a successful course. Planning out and posting the course prior to implementation makes teaching easier. Adjustments can be made as needed, but the course will be well organized and the instructor is freed up to focus on the discussions and other online activities, rather than taking time to prepare a weekly class. A schedule of in-class and online or out-of-class activities should be set up for each week. This allows the students to know what is required in class (readings or other assignments to bring to class) and what will be required out of class (such as discussion posts, podcasts, quizzes, or other online teaching methodologies).

Planning is also very important in developing a coherent course that stays within the expectations for a student workload that is necessary but not excessive for the topic. It is very important not to overload students with work for the course; when students feel the work is achievable, this perception can encourage student motivation in self-directed learning (Keller, 2008). The Simmons College Academic Technology Department presented a workshop for instructors interested in establishing a blended learning course, and participants were asked specific questions to think about as they worked on their course plans (see **Box 7-1**). Planning takes time and has to be carried out well before the classes begin. The online portion must be completely developed and posted prior to the beginning of the course (see **Box 7-2**). The last-minute preparation that may occur with traditional classroom lectures must be avoided, although modifications, such as adding additional information and resources or correcting information, can be made during the course with appropriate notification to students.

Box 7-1 Questions to Think About for Blended Course Design

1. What do you want students to know when they have finished taking your blended course?
2. As you think about learning objectives, which would be better achieved online and which would be best achieved face to face?
3. Blended teaching is not just a matter of transferring a portion of your traditional course to the web. Instead, it involves developing challenging and engaging online learning activities that complement your face-to-face activities. Which types of learning activities do you think you will be using for the online portion of your course?
4. Online asynchronous discussion is often an important part of blended courses. Which new learning opportunities will arise as a result of using asynchronous discussion? Which challenges do you anticipate in using online discussions? How would you address these?
5. Can synchronous online sessions be incorporated into the course? Is a synchronous program available, and what would the purpose of using it be? How much time can be allotted to those sessions? Would students have access to a synchronous online class from the technology and time perspectives?
6. How will the face-to-face and time-out-of-class components be integrated into a single course? In other words, how will the work done in each component feed back into and support the other component?
7. When working online, students frequently have problems scheduling their work and managing their time, as well as understanding the implications of the blended course module as related to learning. What do you plan to do to help your students address these issues?
8. How will you divide the percentage of time between the face-to-face portion and the online portion of your course? How will you schedule the percentage of time between the face-to-face and online portions of your course (e.g., one 2-hour face-to-face session followed by one 2-hour online session each week)?

(continues)

Box 7-1   Questions to Think About for Blended Course Design (*continued*)

9. How will you divide the course grading scheme between face-to-face and online activities? Which means will you use to assess student work in each of these two components?

10. Students sometimes have difficulty acclimating to the course website and to other instructional technologies you may be using for face-to-face and online activities. Which specific technologies will you use for the online and face-to-face portions of your course? Which proactive steps can you take to assist students to become familiar with your course's e-learning and those instructional technologies? If students need help with technology later in the course, how will you provide support?

11. There is a tendency for faculty to require students to do more work in a blended course than they normally would complete in a purely traditional course. What are you going to do to ensure that you have not created a course and a half? How will you evaluate the student workload as compared to that of a traditional class?

Courtesy of Blended Learning Institute, School for Health Studies. (2008). *Academic technology.* Boston, MA: Simmons College.

Box 7-2   Blended Learning Preparation

- Define course objectives
- Carry out a literature review of articles and websites
- Develop a detailed lesson plan for each class that includes each area of the f2f and online course environments, and note quizzes, exams, and other learning assessment strategies as appropriate
- Write discussion questions and assignments for each week of the course
- Prepare quizzes and exams
- Develop a grading rubric and clear expectations for discussions and other assignments
- Prepare the course syllabus to be posted on the Internet platform
- Prepare a welcome letter
- Post materials for student access prior to the first day of class (although access dates may be controlled)

Developing the Learning Community

It is important to develop a discussion learning community where students feel safe to talk to each other with little interference, except for guidance and nurturing from the instructor. Trust takes time to build, and the instructor needs to support students in this, so they do not keep quiet or hold back in the discussion because of fear of criticism. Students need to be given guidelines for discussion posts. For example, students should be instructed about *netiquette;* derogatory personal comments or attacks must be avoided. Instructor responses must demonstrate that mistakes are expected in a learning environment, and students need not be embarrassed, punished, or ashamed of those mistakes—because they will learn from them. Instructors can provide constructive critiques via e-mail to ensure privacy and avoid embarrassment for individual students as needed. Discussion boards can be more informal than required papers;

however, students using traditional Internet speak may need to define those abbreviations for new computer users, and the smiley face can be used to provide emotion :-).

Encouraging students to ask questions when unsure of the lecture material or e-learning environment is valuable; be sure they know not to hold back even if they may feel the question is a "silly" one. There are no silly questions! One student's question may also be in the mind of other students who were afraid to ask because they felt it was "dumb," or "they should have known" and did not want to receive criticism from the instructor and/or classmates or be embarrassed. It can be helpful to have a separate discussion board where students can ask the instructor questions, and the instructor's response is then available to all students. Depending on the technology available, it may be possible to allow a student to post a question anonymously. Personal questions or comments can be handled by e-mail.

Discussions should promote evidence-based practice, and encourage students to apply the research they are reading to their clinical environments. Asking students to apply the readings to case studies, to their clinical practices, and to their personal experiences promotes critical thinking and spurs interest by making the material come alive and become relevant, thereby enhancing the lecture material. While classroom discussions are limited in the numbers of students who can be active, online discussions involve everyone. In large classes, small discussion groups can be established, and it can be exciting to see the different impressions and experiences that students talk about among themselves.

Instructors need to stay in the background during the discussions, allowing the students to create a dialog among themselves—the "guide on the side," rather than the "sage on the stage" (Collison, Elbaum, Haavind, & Tinker, 2000). However, it is important that students recognize the instructor's contacts and presence in the online portion of the course. Instructors can correct or add information to the discussions when specific points require attention, but the discussion should to be student centered. Avoid a constant student-to-instructor and back again conversation and encourage students to discuss with each other instead. The student who provides a main post should be instructed to return to that thread and answer classmates' response posts, challenges, and questions. Students should also be instructed to avoid "cheerleading": a one-line post that says nothing more than "that was a good post" or "great post"; instead, they should say why it was a great post, but also constructively challenge and ask questions, and express their own experiences that relate to the thread under discussion. As you monitor the discussions, you will get to know your students well and learn from them as they learn from you.

Begin planning a blended course by defining course objectives (see Box 7-2). Meeting objectives is a prime responsibility in designing a course lesson plan. The next step is to carry out a literature review of articles and websites to be used for course readings, which can be assigned to students to supplement the textbook and used for post-assignment discussions. During the course, asking students to research and post appropriate articles and websites expands their learning opportunities.

Develop a detailed lesson plan for each class that includes each area of the f2f and online course environments, and note quizzes, exams, and other learning assessment strategies as appropriate (see **Box 7-3**). This is the "thoughtful" portion of

Box 7-3   Lesson Plan Template

Course Title: NUR 390 Theory and Research, Integration and Synthesis for Professional Nursing Practice
Course Developer: Arlene Lowenstein

Course Objectives

Upon completion of the course the student will:

1. Address the historical influences in health care, nursing research, and the nursing profession and their influences on the nursing profession today.
2. Explore the application of theories within the discipline of nursing and other disciplines and consider their use in practice and research.
3. Identify and explore the various research methods utilized to advance nursing science.
4. Recognize the responsibilities of the professional nurse to advance nursing through research critique and utilization.
5. Consider the role of the nurse in formulating research questions and contributing to conduct and dissemination of research findings.
6. Apply principles of evidence-based practice and research utilization as related to clinical practice issues.

Goals for Learning	As Evidenced By	Experiences	Online	Face-to-Face	Blend
(what graduates will know, understand, be able to do)	*(products of student work that correlate with the goal)*	*(course experiences that will generate this evidence)*	*(experiences most suited to online learning [OL])*	*(experiences most suited to f2f)*	*(integration/synergy between OL and f2f)*
Become aware of historical influences in the areas of health care, nursing research, and the nursing profession that have influenced the current-day nursing profession	Discussion posts relate readings that discuss historical issues to their nursing practice	View movie *Sentimental Nurses Need Not Apply* Lecture/discussion on historical issues—timeline		*Week 1* Viewing movie Classroom lecture/ discussion	
Explore the application of a theory from nursing and one other discipline and explain how they can be used in nursing practice and research	Following guidance from the instructor, select one nursing theorist and one theory from another discipline and search the literature for two to three articles and an appropriate website for each theory that include use in practice and research. Post the resources to the discussion board with a short explanation of key points and how they have been used.	Theory and theorist lecture will introduce students to basic areas to explore	Nursing theory podcast	*Part 2 of Week 1* Lecture introducing nursing theory and theories from other disciplines Classroom discussion	*Week 2 Online* Assignment to find website and articles for one nursing theorist and one additional theorist

104

Understand basic elements of quantitative and qualitative research design	Submit two 6- to 8-page papers, one critiquing a qualitative research article and one critiquing a quantitative research article; papers will follow guidelines that include analyzing the basic elements of the research design	Textbook readings Research examples	Discussion posts	*Week 3 Session 1* Quantitative research concepts *Week 3 Session 2* Qualitative research concepts Classroom discussion	*Prior to Week 3 Online* View "Reading a Research Article" PowerPoint and paper; select one research article and compare each section with the each section of the PowerPoint and paper Discussion posts in week 3 following the class session
Recognize the responsibilities of the professional nurse to advance nursing through research critique and utilization	Critiques of quantitative and qualitative research studies Select two articles and disseminate to the class	Textbook readings and lecture re critiquing	Exploring web and articles online	*Week 3 Concepts of Critiquing* Classroom discussion	Posting resources online *Week 4* Quantitative paper due *Week 5* Qualitative paper due
Consider the role of the nurse in formulating research questions and contributing to conduct and dissemination of research findings	Discussion posts show evidence of dissemination of research findings	Textbook readings Evidence-based practice examples	Online literature search	*Weeks 4 and 5* None	Discussion posts
Apply principles of evidence-based practice and research utilization as related to clinical practice issues	Presentation identifying evidence-based practice with references and recommendations for practice	Textbook examples and literature review Course wrap-up	Online literature search Develop PowerPoint presentation	Student presentations and discussion Course wrap-up and evaluation	None

Note: This 6-week course was taught in the summer for 12 undergraduate RN to BSN students. Because of the accelerated nature of the course, a discussion board was used each week.

the class, designing the course around the objectives and determining appropriate learning activities. Objectives and learning activities should be determined for each week of the course. It is important to develop a grading rubric and clear expectations for discussions and other assignments (**Table 7-1**). Writing discussion questions and assignments for each week of the course comes next. Discussion questions should relate to both the weekly class objectives and the overall course objectives. Students can also be asked to research articles or other materials and present them in the discussion board for that week, so the other students can see and develop a conversation about them. The next step is to prepare quizzes, exams, and guidelines for assignments. Exams may be offered in class or online. The instructional technologist should be able to help faculty with learning how to create, utilize, and post online quizzes.

Once the instructor has compiled the information and learning activities that will go into the course, it is time to prepare the course syllabus, which puts the lesson plan information into a document explaining what will be expected from students for the course; includes the grading rubric; and contains a schedule of the dates and time students are expected to be in class or posting on the discussion board, with deadlines for the posting process. Instructors can provide individual feedback by e-mail to students when needed instead of using the discussion board, but students need to know when they should or should not utilize e-mail rather than the discussion board. E-mail is usually used for personal or grading issues, to allow for and protect student privacy. It is helpful to prepare a welcoming letter clearly explaining your teaching methodology and expectations for student participation, and listing whom students should contact for technical issues and help. Materials for student access should be posted prior to the first day of class, although access dates may be controlled (see **Box 7-4**).

Course evaluations may be carried out in class on the last day of class, or online if the last class is a scheduled online class. As with quizzes and exams, evaluations can also be developed in an online format. Online capabilities also allow the instructor to keep statistics, such as how often students access the course online, to assist in course evaluation (Ginns & Ellis, 2009). A caution to be considered is that steps should be taken to see that course instructors do not have access to the evaluation posted online that includes identifying information from the student. Students need to be sure that their online posting is anonymous from their instructor, and this may be a technical issue to be resolved.

Potential Problems

Student Self-Direction

Successful students are self-disciplined in completing assignments and discussion posts on time. Patterns of late or missed discussions must be recognized and challenged using a positive and nonpunishment-oriented approach, especially early in the course as students are getting used to the process. Avoid criticizing students on the discussion board for everyone to see; instead, use e-mail or conferences to discuss

Table 7-1   Grading Rubric for Discussions

A Grade	B Grade	C Grade
Utilizes knowledge of adult learning theory in discussions and responses; meets objectives most of the time with minimal guidance and/or shows growth in learning from guidance and other student responses. Usually keeps up to date in responses.	Utilizes knowledge of adult learning theory in discussions and responses; meets objectives most of the time with consistent guidance. Responds late some of the time.	Content is usually satisfactory, but is late in responding much of the time.
Discussion submissions meet course objectives with minimal guidance and/or demonstrates growth in learning from guidance and other student responses. Usually keeps up to date in responses.	Discussion submissions meet course objectives in discussions and responses most of the time with consistent guidance. Responds late some of the time.	Content is usually minimally satisfactory but may lack thoroughness much of the time. Is often late in responding.

Box 7-4   Course Development Workflow Checklist

1. Outline the course into teaching modules
2. Identify online and face-to-face segments
3. Define learning objectives for each module
4. Outline module content
5. Define feedback and assessment strategies
6. Identify an integration link each week between online and classroom
7. Identify resources for content support
    a. Websites, books, articles
    b. Other
8. Determine teaching/learning activities to address course content and objectives
9. Determine assessment tasks
    a. Quizzes/tests
        i. Develop test questions based on objectives
        ii. Provide rationale for answers
    b. Discussion board questions/case studies
        i. Develop questions based on module objectives
        ii. Clearly define instructions for posting and responding, including length and deadlines (visual chart)
        iii. Provide rubric
        iv. Design method for weekly faculty communication with course coordinator
    c. Other written assignments
10. Develop grade plan based on the preceding assessment tasks
11. Communicate all of the preceding elements in the course syllabus
    a. Include time management expectation for students (e.g., 3 hours prep per hour class)
    b. Include help desk resources and academic technology support
12. Communicate all of the preceding to additional faculty in a faculty orientation/training session
    a. Develop faculty training materials

the problems individually with students. There will be some students who are exceptional in their postings, and others who will barely meet the minimum requirement. It is helpful to provide feedback to both types of students. It is important to remember that life can interfere with a student's ability to participate at times. Events such as illness, family celebrations, or a death of someone close have to be recognized and students supported as much as possible. Students need to understand that they must notify the instructor of such occurrences as soon as possible and make arrangements to make up missed work if possible.

Plagiarism

Plagiarism policies must be clearly spelled out. Many online platforms use or provide programs to examine papers for evidence of plagiarism. Instructors need to emphasize the importance of citing references.

■ Conclusion

Students entering the health professions in the 21st century are different learners than their instructors. Internet access to new information and the convergence of technology is a way of life and must be an integral part of the classroom if the goal is to be meaningful engagement and lifelong learning. Instructors need to learn to reach students in ways that encourage them to use the material and foster a love of learning. A successful student is one who knows learning will not end with graduation; rather, she or he will graduate with the necessary tools and skills to make lifelong contributions to the profession.

Comparison of Blended and F2F Courses

Blended Course Advantages

- Blended courses encourage active learning and student responsibility for their own learning. Increased student participation can increase retention of learning.
- Students learn from each other as well as the instructor, as experiences and resources are shared among them.
- Required onsite classroom time may be reduced, and students are able to work on their own time to avoid conflicts with family and work schedules.
- The online and in-class interactions allow faculty to get to know their students well, if not better than in the traditional classroom, through constant individual communications via the discussion board.

Blended Course Disadvantages

- Students require knowledge of working with computers. This can be more difficult for digital immigrants, usually older students, than for digital natives, younger students who have grown up with computers, although both groups may need strong support.
- Technical glitches can be frustrating and time-consuming.

■ Some students have difficulty with being self-directed and taking responsibility for their learning. This approach may be new to them if they have been used to lectures where all they had to do was sit in class. Change can be difficult. Patience, encouragement, and support may be needed until they become accustomed to the process.

I have also learned an inordinate amount of new information from students, which is a great benefit to me and has added to my reference and resource lists. I found that I was able to have students learn as much or more in a shorter period of time than in the traditional 12- or 14-week semester. The Teaching Example demonstrated that idea to me, as this was a 6-week session summer, whereas the usual fall semester was 14 weeks long. I found I was able to include all the information from the longer semester, and students were able to retain the material. However, adjusting to a new format definitely takes some getting used to, for both students and faculty. Faculty may need to experiment to see what teaching strategies work best at which time. All in all, I have found the rewards much greater than any problems that have surfaced, and so have my students.

Discussion Questions

1. Reflect on current students in higher education (use Chapter 3). Describe how blended learning strategies would engage this new generation of students.
2. Consider blended learning in relation to the nontraditional, older student. How can you, as the instructor, bridge the gap between blended learning strategies and a learner who may prefer more traditional teaching methods?
3. Read the comparison and teaching example. Discuss the points made, techniques suggested, and other information supplied based on the instructor's experience.

Teaching Example

The following example is from a nursing research course I taught for RN to BSN students. The course was held in the hospital in which the students were working. This was a summer course for 13 students, taught in a 6-week time frame rather than the traditional 12- to 14-week format used in the fall and spring courses. The traditional format for this four-credit summer course would have had two lecture sessions each week, but that would have been difficult for the students, who were all working as RNs, and for the hospital in which they were employed. Although I had taught fully online courses prior to this course, I had no experience with a blended format, but knew about that possibility. I decided to try that for this semester. I spoke with our academic technology department for advice, and was invited to a blended learning workshop for other faculty members who were interested in blended learning, and I was welcome to attend to begin to develop and plan the course. That workshop was extremely valuable to me as I looked at the differences between a strictly online course and a strictly classroom course and worked on the blended model of including both modalities. The course description and objectives were based on the traditional course description and objectives as follows.

(continues)

Course Description

The course is an upper-level course designed to assist the senior-level student in the continued integration and application of research and theory in nursing practice. Theoretical and historical perspectives will be discussed and integrated within the research process. A spirit of inquiry will also be fostered, as many clinical questions remain that require a nursing perspective for future study. Principles of nursing research, critique, and utilization in clinical practice will be highlighted, and students will be given the opportunity to develop a research-based project. Independent learning, self-direction, and understanding of group interaction in the teaching–learning process are also stressed. Intellectual integrity, creativity, and open communication are fostered in an environment of cooperative learning.

Course Objectives

Upon completion of the course the student will:

1. Address the historical influences in health care, nursing research, and the nursing profession and their influences on the nursing profession today.
2. Explore the application of theories within the discipline of nursing and other disciplines and consider their use in practice and research.
3. Identify and explore the various research methods utilized to advance nursing science.
4. Recognize the responsibilities of the professional nurse to advance nursing through research critique and utilization.
5. Consider the role of the nurse in formulating research questions and contributing to conduct and dissemination of research findings.
6. Apply principles of evidence-based practice and research utilization as related to clinical practice issues.

Based on the course objectives, developing the course lecture plan (see Box 7-3) was the first step, followed by the discussion board rubrics (see Table 7-1). The rubrics were developed on the basis of achieving the course objectives, and each rubric dealt with one or more of those objectives. However, in some instances I found the rubric to be too subjective, and may do some revision of it for future classes, but it serves as an example of the process. The course was implemented very successfully. Here are some of the undergraduate RN to BSN student comments to their classmates about the research hybrid course:

"Thanks to all my classmates, I think the term 'learning community' really summed up the experience very well. I do like the format and flexibility of online discussion. I think it allows a more considered participation than that of just classroom; often I will think about a discussion or response and have a question or comment later on. I think we did cover a really good amount of material in a relatively short time—and acquired some great skills to bring forward."

"First of all I want you all to know that I cannot believe how much I learned in this course. Although I felt at times to be in an ocean without a life jacket, you were all there to help. Thank you for letting me whine. I really appreciate all of the support you ladies have given."

"I liked the idea of online classes. This was my first one and I liked it."

"Hi Susi, thanks for another great post. I enjoy reading other people's interpretation of something I have read and getting their perception."

"Hi all, I just learned not to hit enter after the subject box or else it gets posted. And second thing I learned was if you save your thoughts as a draft, you have to remember to go back and actually post it."

References

Ausbum, L. J. (2004). Course design elements most valued by adult learners in blended online education environments: An American perspective. *Educational Media International, 42*(4), 327–337.

Berrett, D. (2012). How "flipping" the classroom can improve the traditional lecture. *Education Digest, 78*(1), 36–41.

Blended Learning Institute, School for Health Studies. (2008). *Academic technology*. Boston, MA: Simmons College.

Brunsell, E., & Horejsi, M. (2011). Flipping your classroom. *Science Teacher, 78*(2), 1.

Collison, G., Elbaum, B., Haavind, S., & Tinker, R. (2000). *Facilitating online learning: Effective strategies for moderators*. Madison, WI: Atwood Publishing.

Garrison, D. R., & Vaughan, N. D. (2008). *Blended learning in higher education: Framework, principles, and guidelines*. San Francisco, CA: Jossey-Bass.

Ginns, P., & Ellis, R. (2009). Evaluating the quality of e-learning at the degree level in the student experience of blended learning. *British Journal of Educational Technology, 40*(4), 652–663.

Howe, N., & Strauss, W. (2000). *Millennials rising: The next greatest generation*. New York, NY: Vintage Press.

Jairath, N., & Stair, N. (2004). A development and implementation framework for web-based nursing courses. *Nursing Education Perspectives, 25*(2), 67.

Keller, J. M. (2008). First principles of motivation to learn and e3-learning. *Distance Education, 29*(2), 175–185.

Khan, B. H. (2005). *Managing e-learning strategies: Design, delivery, implementation and evaluation*. Hershey, PA: Information Science Publishing.

Khan, B. H. (2007). *Flexible learning in an information society*. Englewood Cliffs, NJ: Idea Group.

Khan, B. H. (2009). *E-learning framework*. Retrieved from http://www.badrulkhan.com

McEwan, B. (2012). Managing boundaries in the Web 2.0 classroom. *New Directions for Teaching & Learning, 2012*(131), 15–28.

Means, B., Toyama, Y., Murphy, R., & Baki, M. (2013). The effectiveness of online and blended learning: A meta-analysis of the empirical literature. *Teachers College Record, 115*(3), 1–47.

Moran, M., Seaman, J., & Tinit-Kane, H. (2011). *Teaching, learning, and sharing: How today's higher education faculty use social media*. Babson Survey Research Group. Retrieved from ERIC database (ED 535130).

Myers, C. R., Mixer, S. J., Wyatt, T. H., Paulus, T. M., & Lee, D. S. (2011). Making the move to blended learning: Reflections on a faculty development program. *International Journal of Nursing Education Scholarship, 8*(1), Article 20.

Palloff, R. M., & Pratt, K. (2005). *Collaborating online: Learning together in community*. San Francisco, CA: Jossey Bass.

Prensky, M. (2001). Digital natives, digital immigrants. *On the Horizon, 9*(5), 1–6.

Sams, A., & Bergmann, J. (2013). Flip your students' learning. *Educational Leadership, 70*(6), 16–20.

Sener, J. (2012). *The seven futures of American education: Improving learning and teaching in a screen captured world*. North Charleston, SC: CreateSpace.

Singh, H. (2003). Building effective blended learning programs. *Educational Technology, 43*(6), 51–54.

Steer, D. (2012). Improve formal learning with social media. *T + D, 66*(12), 31–33.

CHAPTER 8

Teaching in the Online Environment

Karen H. Teeley

I will be sad when I won't have this class anymore. I am not sure I have ever said that before!!!

—*Student of Karen H. Teeley*

■ Introduction

Rapid changes in technology continue to open more doors to students seeking online educational opportunities. Recent advances in audio and video capabilities enable more live or synchronous—sometimes called "virtual" classroom options—where the teacher and the student are online at the same time and the teaching is "in person" with a real-time instructor presence. One of the biggest drawbacks of asynchronous learning—where the teacher and the student are *not* online at the same time—has been that the online class can be impersonal, often missing the connection with or online presence of the instructor (Mandernach, Gonzales, & Garrett, 2006).

This chapter looks at teaching online in general and specifically at teaching in a synchronous environment. Synchronous classrooms that utilize proven pedagogical strategies can be the best of both worlds: the best of online learning for convenience and accessibility of teaching tools plus the best of instructor-led learning.

From the instructor's perspective, this can be an ideal model for small classes. Often the instructor can interact with the students by audio, but ideally this is done by both audio and video. This model can be "flipped learning" at its best. The content is developed and posted online for the students to access asynchronously, and a "live" class time is regularly scheduled, much like a campus-based class, but held via the Internet. Because the students have already had access to the content, they come to class prepared and the live class time is spent reinforcing content through learning activities that are designed to produce the desired learning outcomes and provide students interaction with the instructor for real-time feedback and support.

■ Definitions and Purpose

Good online design is essential for student success. Clear learning outcomes, whether in the classroom, blended, or online, are dependent on a methodical and strategic design process based on evidence-based best practice. If faculty are not trained as instructional designers, they should work with experienced instructional designers to ensure meaningful content transformation to the online platform. Designing for on-line learning, if done correctly, can take anywhere from 6 months to a year, depending on the length of the course.

Content transformation for online learning does not mean recording lectures and posting them online, nor does it mean posting long PowerPoint lectures. Good online learning design means chunking the salient points from the identified con-tent and presenting the information in different ways, including learning activities, multimedia, audio and video, animations, and discussion boards, to name just a few style options. The content must be meaningful and associated with the learning outcomes.

The role of the faculty changes from the oft-quoted "sage on the stage" to being a "guide on the side." Faculty become facilitators and mentors, and the relationship with students changes to more of a partnership and less of an expert–novice dyad.

■ Theoretical Foundation

The creation of online learning environments has roots in our knowledge of adult learning. Components of adult learning are described by Malcolm Knowles (1990), who emphasizes adults are self-directed, that they are interested in topics that are relevant to their lives, and that they like to be actively involved in the learning process and have control over where and how they learn so they can learn at their own pace. Knowles's theory of andragogy makes the following assumptions about the design of learning:

1. Adults need to know why they need to learn something.
2. Adults need to learn experientially.
3. Adults approach learning as problem solving.
4. Adults learn best when the topic is of immediate value. (Knowles, 1990)

It is important for the instructor know the learners' needs and design learning activities that are relevant to those needs. The student should be actively involved in learning, with the instructor acting as a facilitator or guide. The instructor who rec-ognizes adults have different learning needs can tailor his or her instruction design to the characteristic ways adults prefer to learn.

Adult learning theory is important in online instructional design for several rea-sons: First, it is important to tailor the content specifically to the learner's level, or it will not be effective (Lee & Owens, 2000). Second, learner goals and objectives must utilize a variety of learning activities if adults are to be engaged in the learning (Fink, 2003). Lastly, by engaging in meaningful activity, students feel like they are making significant, sustainable contributions (Teeley, Lowe, Beal, & Knapp, 2006). Addition-ally, students need to connect with one another. Bornstein and Bruner (2014) point out that "development is intrinsically bound up with interactions" (p. 13); this research built upon Bruner's earlier work on reciprocity as the "deep human need to respond to others and to operate jointly with them towards an objective" (Bruner, 1966).

Problem-based learning (PBL) is based on interaction and meaningful learning. Learners work together in small teams to solve problems. Throughout this process, learners can "develop intellectual curiosity, confidence and engagement that will lead to lifelong learning" (Watson, 2004, p. 21). Interaction is a key theme and central to learning online. For collaborative acquisition of knowledge, one must build learning activities that require student interaction and encourage a sharing of ideas that will promote a deeper level of thought (Conrad & Donaldson, 2011, p. 5). Successful learning occurs when the online course design is centered on the learners and their interactions, and not on just a lecture-focused, instructor-centered approach.

The role of the instructor in an online class is to ensure a high degree of interactivity and participation (Kearsley, 2000). This means designing and conducting learning activities that result in engagement with the subject matter and with fellow students. Engaged learning does not just happen; it requires a conscious effort and purposeful design by the instructor. Well-planned learning activities that connect the students to the content and to each other will motivate learners to participate in knowledge building.

■ Types of Learners

Students who perform best in an online environment are students who are self-directed and are cognitively ready for participatory learning. Although most students in today's classroom are digital natives (Prensky, 2001), and they are often connected 24/7 to a device (and to each other), they may not all be suited for the self-directed, active learning environment of the online classroom. Some of today's students still claim to prefer a passive learning, predominantly lecture-based classroom. However, once exposed to a well-designed, active online classroom, they become engaged and ready to learn online.

It is important to set clear expectations from the outset so that students can assess their own readiness for online learning. Students in an online environment must be comfortable and skilled with technology.

Conditions for Learning

Online learning, along with the technology tools available, offers students active engagement, the opportunity to participate in groups, frequent interaction and feedback, and connections to real-world contexts (Roschelle, Pea, Hoadley, Gordin, & Means, 2000). Technology also expands what students can learn by providing them with access to an ever-expanding store of information. Researchers Roschelle et al. (2000) also emphasize that merely making computers available does not automatically lead to learning gains. They describe technology integration as only one element in "what must be a coordinated approach to improving curriculum, pedagogy, assessment, teacher development, and other aspects of school structure" (Roschelle et al., 2000, p. 78).

According to learning-science experts, the increasingly interactive nature of technology, exemplified by available interactive tools, creates new opportunities for students to learn by allowing them to do a task, receive feedback on it, and then build new knowledge. In *How People Learn: Brain, Mind, Experience, and School*, authors Bransford, Brown, and Cocking (1999, p. 207) explain that technology can be used to advance learning by:

- Bringing exciting curricula based on real-world problems into the classroom
- Providing scaffolds and tools to enhance learning, such as modeling programs and visualization tools
- Giving students and teachers more opportunities for feedback, reflection, and revision
- Building local and global communities that include teachers, administrators, students, parents, practicing scientists, and other interested people
- Expanding opportunities for teacher learning

Online learning, with its abundance and availability of technology tools, empowers students to take more control of their learning and makes the classroom student centered, rather than instructor or lecture centered. This creates both new opportunities and new challenges for the teacher and learner.

In his book *What the Best College Teachers Do* (2011), Bain emphasizes students are more likely to learn about what they are interested in. The challenge for the teacher is to create interesting and engaging learning experiences. Of course, this is true for campus-based instructor-led courses as well!

■ Synchronous Versus Asynchronous

Different teaching methodologies are utilized if the online class is designed to be asynchronous (when students log in at different times) rather than synchronous (when students are logged in at the same time as the instructor and a "live" class takes place).

Most online learning environments, including massive open online courses (MOOCs), are asynchronous. The main method of student–student and student–instructor interaction is on discussion boards. Discussion boards employ higher-order constructivist learning and contribute to the development of a learning community (Levine, 2007). When a discussion board is used, students post responses to the instructor's assignments and to each other. This strategy provides the maximum flexibility and convenience for online learning and is widely utilized.

The main benefit of asynchronous learning is that students and teachers do not have to be online at the same time. This makes access to the course materials much more convenient for learning on a variable schedule. In addition, students have time to prepare thoughtful discussion posts and responses, unlike in the classroom and the synchronous classroom, where the required discussion response is more immediate. Instructor presence is nevertheless an important consideration in asynchronous discussions; research shows the level of instructor presence preferred depends on the desired learning outcomes (Andresen, 2009). Mazzolini and Maddison (2003) found the instructor role of "sage, guide or ghost" depends on what the instructor wants to accomplish. Not enough instructor presence can leave the students feeling not connected, yet too much can interfere with student–student interaction. According to Palloff and Pratt (2003), the instructor should only intervene to keep the discussion on track or to take on a cheerleading role. The instructor should spend his or her time preparing carefully thought-out questions and topics that relate to the learning objectives (Andresen, 2009).

Although there is little research on the limits of asynchronous discussion forums (Andresen, 2009), several studies have emerged to show that problem-based learning can be difficult in an asynchronous format. Kortemeyer (2006) reported actual problem solving in physics was difficult, and Hong, Lai, and Holton (2003) reported similar results for a statistics class. Aside from practical scientific problem solving, however, asynchronous discussions are the mainstay of online learning.

With technology advancements in audio and video capabilities, there are more and more opportunities to bring instructors and students together in real time. This is often referred to as a synchronous class, a "live" class, or a "virtual" class. These can include chat rooms with just text, on up to video, teleconferencing, and even virtual environments such as Second Life (Skiba, 2009).

Synchronous classes usually take place by teleconferencing (phone only) or audio and video conferencing where students and instructors appear on web cameras. Synchronous environments are usually smaller classes (25 or less), more social, and have the potential to support learners in the development of learning communities (Hrastinski, 2008). Learners benefit from having the instructors be able to answer questions in real time, and instructors benefit from the smaller classes and more personal interactions with students. When cameras are present, body language adds to the richness (or not!) of the communication. Online synchronous classes allow students to connect and collaborate.

Synchronous classes present their own set of challenges. There are several things to watch for when considering synchronous classes:

1. Scheduling: Students and instructors must be able to come together at the same time.
2. Technology: Although technology is constantly improving, both students and instructors need to be technologically savvy. Technology interruptions must be expected, and solutions have to be in place for when interruptions do occur.
3. Personality and learning styles: Live classes favor extroverts. Some students do their best work alone and need time to carefully craft a response, rather than shout it out in the moment (Fuster, 2015).

■ Resources and Methods

Skilled Faculty

The most essential resource for a successful online course is the availability of experienced faculty to facilitate the online learning. Faculty must be trained in online teaching. Many colleges and universities require online teaching certification or, at the very least, for the faculty member to have taken an online class as a student before teaching online for the first time. Even skilled faculty teaching on a new platform should become totally familiar with the technology tools beforehand, and avail themselves of refresher sessions with faculty support if available. Platforms and tools vary widely across programs.

Technology

Students and faculty need access to Internet-enabled devices, web cams, and audio. Some audio is provided through the computer as VoIP (Voice over Internet Protocol) or through the telephone. Either way, for the best classroom experience, headsets with built-in microphones are recommended. Although laptops or desktop computers are preferred for teaching, many courses now are accessible for students through mobile devices and tablets.

Faculty must be proficient in the use of the online technology. This includes the tools available in the online platform that enhance learning. Some examples include the use of polls, whiteboards, and breakout rooms. Lecture-based classes online are just as boring as lecture-based classes in the physical campus classrooms. Faculty must learn to use the available tools, which are designed to engage students and enhance learning. The benefit of the online platforms is the tools are usually built into the software and do not require a different setup. Tools abound for creating engaging and meaningful online classroom learning activities.

Faculty Development

If the educational setting offers training for faculty, all faculty are advised to take advantage of it to learn the basics of online teaching, as well as to keep up with new and emerging educational technology. Nothing seems to diminish the important role of the faculty quicker than stumbling through the technology in front of savvy students.

■ Using the Method

There are numerous how-to texts and guides available for designing online courses; many of these resources are listed in the "Recommended Reading" section at the end of this chapter. This section looks specifically at developing the synchronous component, aimed at engaging the student during the live or virtual setting.

Planning

Just like any class, good execution requires a good plan. The synchronous session is the ultimate "flipped classroom," as the students have prepared the asynchronous materials (usually videos, texts, e-learning modules) on their own time and come to the live sessions prepared. With a smaller number of students, participants quickly realize that they are more accountable for the preparation work and consequently are more likely to come to class prepared. Of course this varies, but through peer pressure alone, students usually learn to come to class prepared, as they are likely to be called upon in the active and engaged live session. Additionally, faculty need to be well prepared for the live session. It is recommended to create a "Live Class Guide" that details the desired learning outcomes, the sequence of the learning activities,

Box 8-1   Synchronous Class Plan Workflow Checklist

1. Decide how much time will be allotted to the synchronous session.
2. Review the specific lesson objectives and determine the desired learning outcomes for the synchronous session.
3. Include the learning outcomes in your class plan.
4. Decide how the learning outcomes can be met with the (technology) tools available.
5. Design active learning exercises that meet the desired learning outcomes.
6. If possible, set up your synchronous classroom ahead of the class time, building in the activities using the available tools (e.g., set up poll questions, build breakout rooms, etc.).
7. Craft a detailed "Live Class Guide" so everyone can play a role in helping the class run smoothly.
8. Keep log-in and emergency numbers handy, just in case of a technology mishap.
9. Always have a Class Plan B!

and the time allotted to each (see **Box 8-1**). A clear plan will increase the probability of a smooth class flow.

Feedback and Assessment

Clearly articulating how and when the students will receive feedback, and how they will be assessed and graded, ensures success and prevents unwelcome feedback. Detailed participation rubrics are helpful to assure uniform grading criteria. In some programs, students take tests during their live sessions and are monitored while on camera. To ensure academic integrity during the online test, additional software can be employed, such as Proctortrack®, an automated remote proctoring product that verifies the student's identity.

Expectations

Setting student expectations in advance can help ensure a successful learning experience. The student's role, the faculty's role, and assignment expectations must be clear and easily accessed. Policies concerning student behavior (such as the use of social media and protection of intellectual property) must be specifically spelled out . . . otherwise, you may find your test answers posted on Facebook! The beginning of the course is an ideal time to set the expectations and start the class off on the right note. A welcoming and friendly setting will go a long way in soothing nervous students and sending a warm message. If it is helpful, post a list of Frequently Asked Questions and add to it as the course evolves.

Orientation

Student orientation to the live classroom environment should be just as thorough as the faculty's orientation, especially if this is a new way of learning. In addition to a program-sponsored orientation to the learning management system, the first live class should be spent going over course requirements, necessary technology skills, and live class behavior expectations. Additionally, it is important to set the stage for the formation of an engaged and collaborative learning community for successful live sessions for the remainder of the term.

■ Applied Example: Community Health Nursing—Converting to a Fully Online Class

Although this Community Health Nursing course had been previously developed by the instructor as a blended model (Bradshaw & Lowenstein, 2014, p. 291), there were new programmatic opportunities to reach larger audiences. A plan was developed to convert the undergraduate, senior-level community health class to an entirely online offering for a new RN to MSN program.

The nursing program was fortunate in having a technology partner, 2U®, which worked closely with the faculty to strategize the content transformation and filming production. It took a 7-month process of collaborative work between the production team from 2U and the faculty and instructional design team from the college to format and film the lecture content into small 10-minute chunks, include interactive features and discussions, and build out the course into the learning management system (LMS). The course as designed has a 3- to 5-year "shelf life," needing only minor semester updates; re-filming was reserved for major course revisions about every 5 years (depending on the content, of course).

The hallmark feature of each course is the weekly required synchronous live session. Students register for the live sessions as they would register for any class, but with a class capacity of no more than 15 students. Students receive training and guidance on technology needed, such as a web cam, a telephone headset, and a computer configured with the necessary plug-ins and downloads. Faculty also receive the same comprehensive training prior to their first class in this program. 2U provides extensive student and faculty support for technology issues that may arise and is available for live support whenever classes are running.

With the didactic content available to the student asynchronously, the faculty, called "section instructors," each manage a 15-student section and bring the students together for a live active learning session based on that week's learning objectives. The live session for Community Health meets weekly for 2 hours using Adobe Connect®. Adobe Connect offers numerous interactive tools that make the learning engaging and participatory. A valuable feature is the Breakout Room, which allows multiple small groups to work together simultaneously. In each Breakout Room, the students' audio and cameras connect only to each other and they can work together for a set period of time. At the end of the breakout session, the small groups rejoin the larger group and share their findings. The Breakout Rooms are a powerful learning feature that enables student-directed activities that are collaborative and engaging.

To illustrate a just a few examples from the community health class, **Table 8-1** shows the expected active learning outcome, the Adobe Connect tool used, and a description of the learning activity.

These classroom activities were easily adapted from the campus-based class design. The interactivity is actually much easier to administer online than on campus, as the tools are readily available. The Breakout Rooms replace small-group activities

Table 8-1   Examples of Outcome, Tool, and Learning Activity Coordination

Learning Outcome	Adobe Connect Tool	Learning Activity
Pool knowledge about resources available in the community	Breakout rooms	Students are grouped in breakout rooms by state or region to share local resources. Students benefit from sharing in small groups and then reporting their findings to the larger group.
Demonstrate knowledge from asynchronous readings	Polls	Students answer poll questions, set up by the instructor, designed to elicit baseline knowledge of weekly readings.
Demonstrate understanding or further clarification of presented content	Status icons	Students can use status icons to agree or disagree with the instructor, allowing the instructor to ascertain immediately whether a concept needs further explanation.
Generate new ideas	Whiteboard	Students use a whiteboard as they would a classroom whiteboard or flipchart to record ideas generated in a brainstorming session.
Capture stream-of-consciousness ideas as those ideas relate to the current topic	Chat	Students can use the chat feature (at the discretion of the faculty) to record ideas to share with their classmates.

without having to move chairs, and the polls replace the aggravation of classroom clickers. Status icons are easier and less intimidating than raising hands, and the digital whiteboards replace the cumbersome flipcharts. The chat tool replaces talking in the classroom or a backchannel. Like the campus classroom, the instructor can use discretion on how much or how little to allow background chat. A benefit to the online chat tool is that it can be saved and e-mailed for later perusal. Admittedly, there is an initial learning curve to master the technology tools within the Adobe Connect classroom—but once mastered, those tools offer endless possibilities for integrating active learning in the classroom.

Student feedback from the live sessions has been quite positive. Some comments include:

> *"This is such an interesting online classroom. I love the different pods with either surveys or notes; I really feel like you want us to be involved."*
> *"This layout is my favorite—lots of interaction between the students and the professor."*
> *"I really appreciate how this class is organized; it's engaging and interactive."*
> *"I will be sad when I won't have this class anymore. I am not sure I have ever said that before!!!"*
> *"This is such a fun class! I love seeing how the theories apply in real life."*

■ Conclusion

Students entering the health professions in the 21st century are more technologically savvy than previous generations, and are ready to take their learning online. New tools and learning research support rigorous and successful online learning. Student engagement through thoughtful use of available technologies contributes to a successful online experience for both students and teachers.

Discussion Questions

1. Reflect on your own learning styles. As an instructor, do you prefer to engage in synchronous or asynchronous teaching? How do you build a sense of community with each type of online learning?
2. Evaluate your current teaching. What concepts or activities could you transition to online learning? How can online teaching strategies improve your in-class teaching?

References

Andresen, M. A. (2009). Asynchronous discussion forums: Success factors, outcomes, assessments, and limitations. *Journal of Educational Technology & Society, 12*(1), 249–257.

Bain, K. (2011). *What the best college teachers do.* Cambridge, MA: Harvard University Press.

Bornstein, M. H., & Bruner, J. S. (2014). *Interaction in human development.* Hove, East Sussex, UK: Psychology Press.

Bradshaw, M., & Lowenstein, A. (2014). *Innovative teaching strategies in nursing and related health professions, 291.* Burlington, MA: Jones & Bartlett.

Bransford, J. D., Brown, A. L., & Cocking, R. R. (1999). *How people learn: Brain, mind, experience, and school.* Washington, DC: National Academy Press.

Bruner, J. S. (1966). *Toward a theory of instruction.* Cambridge, MA: Harvard University Press.

Conrad, R., & Donaldson, J. A. (2011). *Engaging the online learner: Activities and resources for creative instruction.* Hoboken, NJ: John Wiley & Sons.

Fink, L. D. (Ed.). (2003). *Creating significant learning experiences.* San Francisco, CA: Jossey-Bass.

Fuster, B. (2015, October 30). *Overcome 5 obstacles of live online classes.* Retrieved from http://www.usnews.com/education/online-learning-lessons/2015/10/30/overcome-5-obstacles-of-live-online-classes

Hong, K., Lai, K., & Holton, D. (2003). Students' satisfaction and perceived learning with a web-based course. *Educational Technology & Society, 6*(1), 116–124.

Hrastinski, S. (2008). Asynchronous and synchronous e-learning. *Educause Quarterly, 31*(4), 51–55.

Kearsley, G. (2000). *Explorations in learning & instruction: The theory in practice database.* George Washington University, Washington, DC. Retrieved from http://InstructionalDesign.org

Knowles, M. (1990). *The adult learner: A neglected species* (4th ed.). Houston, TX: Gulf Publishing.

Kortemeyer, G. (2006). An analysis of asynchronous online homework discussion in introductory physics courses. *American Journal of Physics, 74*(6), 526–536.

Lee, W. W., & Owens, D. L. (2000). *Multimedia-based instructional design.* San Francisco, CA: Jossey-Bass.

Levine, S. J. (2007). The online discussion board. *New Directions for Adult and Continuing Education, 2007*(113), 67–74.

Mandernach, B. J., Gonzales, R. M., & Garrett, A. L. (2006). An examination of online instructor presence via threaded discussion participation. *Journal of Online Learning and Teaching, 2*(4), 248.

Mazzolini, M., & Maddison, S. (2003). Sage, guide or ghost? The effect of instructor intervention on student participation in online discussion forums. *Computers & Education, 40*(3), 237–253.

Palloff, R. M., & Pratt, K. (2003). *The virtual student: A profile and guide to working with online learners.* Hoboken, NJ: John Wiley & Sons.

Prensky, M. (2001). Digital natives, digital immigrants. *On the Horizon, 9*(5), 1–6.

Roschelle, J. M., Pea, R., Hoadley, C., Gordin, D., & Means, B. (2000). Changing how and what children learn in school with computer-based technologies. *Future of Children, 10*(2), 76.

Skiba, D. J. (2009). Emerging technologies center nursing education 2.0: A second look at Second Life. *Nursing Education Perspectives, 30*(2), 129–131.

Teeley, K., Lowe, J., Beal, J., & Knapp, M. (2006). Incorporating quality improvement concepts and practice into a community health nursing course. *Journal of Nursing Education, 45*(2), 65–71.

Watson, G. (2004). Integrating problem-based learning and technology in education. In O. S. Tan (Ed.), *Enhancing thinking through problem-based learning approaches, 187–201*. Singapore: Thomson Learning.

Recommended Reading

Boettcher, J. V., & Conrad, R. (2010). *The online teaching survival guide: Simple and practical pedagogical tips.* Hoboken, NJ: John Wiley & Sons.

Brookfield, S. (1986). *Understanding and facilitating adult learning.* San Francisco, CA: Jossey-Bass.

Chickering, A. W., & Gamson, Z. F. (1991). Appendix A: Seven principles for good practice in undergraduate education. *New Directions for Teaching and Learning, 47.*

Clay, C. (2012). *Great webinars: Create interactive learning that is captivating, informative, and fun.* Hoboken, NJ: John Wiley & Sons.

Collison, G., Elbaum, B., Haavind, S., & Tinker, R. (2000). *Facilitating online learning: Effective strategies for moderators.* Madison, WI: Atwood.

Fink, L. D. (2005). *A self-directed guide to designing courses for significant learning.* Retrieved from http://www.ou.edu/idp/significant/Self-DirectedGuidetoCourseDesignAug%2005.doc

Matthews-Denatale, G., & Cotler, D. (2005). *Faculty as authors of online courses: Support and mentoring.* Retrieved from http://www.academiccommons.org/commons/essay/matthews-denatale-and-cotler

Novotny, J. M., & Davis, R. (Eds.). (2006). *Distance education in nursing.* New York, NY: Springer.

O'Neil, C. A., Fisher, C. A., & Newbold, S. K. (Eds.). (2004). *Developing an online course: Best practices for nurse educators.* New York, NY: Springer.

Palloff, R. M., & Pratt, K. (2001). *Lessons from the cyberspace classroom.* San Francisco, CA: Jossey-Bass.

Richardson, J. C., & Swan, K. (2003). *Examining social presence in online courses in relation to students' perceived learning and satisfaction.* Retrieved from http://hdl.handle.net/2142/18713

Tipton, S. (2015). Blended solutions. In Biech, E. (Ed.), *101 ways to make learning active beyond the classroom.* (pp. 99–107). Hoboken, NJ: John Wiley & Sons.

Vygotsky, L., Hanfmann, E., & Vakar, G. (2012). *Thought and language.* Cambridge, MA: MIT Press.

Wiske, M. S., & Breit, L. (2013). *Teaching for understanding with technology.* Hoboken, NJ: John Wiley & Sons.

CHAPTER 9

Social Media as a Context for Connected Learning

Gail Matthews-DeNatale

■ Introduction and Overview

It was only a few years ago that the now-shopworn term "21st-century learning" seemed fresh and exciting. With the turn of the century, we looked forward to the dawn of a new era in education with an optimism that seems naïve in hindsight. More recently, Harvard School of Management's Clayton Christensen has described higher education as an environment in peril. He posits that bigger, better, and more incremental improvement results in a behemoth that crumbles under its own weight (Christensen & Eyring, 2011, p. 13), and predicts many colleges and universities will succumb to that fate. In contrast, institutions that embrace disruptive change and fundamentally change their "DNA" by becoming more nimble and responsive will survive and thrive (2011, p. 25).

While technology features prominently in Christensen's work as an agent of disruption, it does not inevitably lead to positive change. For example, digital projection systems are no more revolutionary than the acetate overhead projectors that preceded them, and very few of us have achieved the paperless office that was forecasted with the advent of personal computers. Corporations often solicit Christensen's opinion on strategic directions for development, hoping to gain cutting-edge advantages through disruption instead of incremental change. Christensen demurs, saying he "doesn't have an opinion," but that his theory of disruptive change "has an opinion." If we understand the theory, we will be able to make prescient decisions about change within our own practice. As we incorporate the newest technologies into our teaching, how can we know if we are making a significant difference to improve learning instead of simply swapping in a digital teaching tool for its analog predecessor?

Past is prologue, even in the midst of disruption. Revisiting the history of technology in higher education can provide insight into the larger patterns and motivating factors at play—the DNA that Christensen says we need to change. If we understand the larger narrative arc associated with history, we will be better equipped to apply the theory of disruption and to make wise decisions about

---

The author wishes to thank Doug DeNatale for his review and contributions to this chapter.

what is worth disrupting in our teaching. This perspective helps us distinguish between superficial or even ineffective use of educational technology and learning designs that increase engagement and help students take learning to a deeper level.

Educators who have used technology for more than a decade will remember the early days when e-mail and listservs were considered cutting-edge technology. E-mail was useful for one-on-one communication, while listservs supported one-to-many discussion. The first iterations of these tools were clunky and unforgiving: Command-line interfaces made it difficult to correct even simple typos without having to start over. Over time, though, these technologies improved. Listservs still serve a purpose, and e-mail is central to our daily work in higher education.

In the early 1990s, the increasing popularity of the World Wide Web gave rise to learning management systems (LMSs). "Web Course in a Box," one of the first LMSs to be used widely in higher education, provided faculty and students with a suite of password-protected tools especially designed for learning contexts: a syllabus builder, threaded discussions, web-based quizzes, and a class roster that could include student-written biographies with photos. The invention of the LMS was important because it signaled a shift from technology as a discrete tool (i.e., software, hardware) to technology as an online *place* where learning could happen. The LMS provided us with a virtual classroom that could accommodate many modes of learning and the development of coherent learning communities: asynchronous and live, self-paced and group-based, text-based and audio/video. The first learning management systems were inexpensive or free to use, but commercial products such as WebCT and Blackboard soon followed, along with a series of mergers and acquisitions. Today only a few commercial LMS products dominate the field.

We have come a long way from the early days of blinking cursors and glowing iridescent green on tiny black screens, and our expectations have become increasingly sophisticated as well. Even though faculty and students assume their institutions will provide some form of LMS for coursework, many wish these online educational environments were more visually appealing and easier to use. In addition, LMS costs skyrocketed when a few major vendors acquired competitors and captured the market, reducing competition. Open source products such as Moodle are promising, but require in-house technical expertise and are often not robust enough for large-scale implementation. The LMS has gotten bigger, better, more sophisticated, and more expensive. Educational technology, the LMS in particular, has become the behemoth that Christensen's theory describes as ripe for disruption.

We find ourselves longing, simultaneously, for more *and* less: more flexibility to accommodate a wider range of learning preferences and scenarios, and less complexity to shorten the learning curve and lower barriers to entry. This is the near-recent context in which "Web 2.0" arrived on the scene in 2004–2005, bringing with it an explosion of social media tools that were visually engaging, elegantly designed, and easy to use. Unlike the LMS, a cumbersome Swiss Army knife of tools, these lightweight "apps" could be used separately or in conjunction with one another as mashups. They exemplified the best of the web because they were, in the words of David Weinberger, "small pieces loosely joined" (2003).

The rise of social media tools represented a radical departure because those tools did not try to be the best or most sophisticated. They embodied Web 2.0's "read-write" ethos, which made Internet multimedia authoring possible for the rest of us. Web 1.0 tools helped online authors connect things (hyperlinked documents, embedded images, and videos within documents). Web 2.0's social media tools helped people connect with people. These technologies felt, and continue to feel, like a breath of fresh air in the increasingly stodgy context of technology in higher education. They open up a host of possibilities for learning to engage all types of students in active and collaborative work.

First, social media have a strong visual component, making it possible for students to represent their developing understanding through a combination of text and images (and often audio/video). They help learners make their thinking visible to their peers and teachers (Ritchhart, Church, & Morrison, 2011). These multisensory artifacts of learning can also be used to assess progress and set goals for improvement, and can be revised to reflect the current state of understanding.

Second, these tools are designed to support networking among users, a process that can be leveraged to achieve social learning through social pedagogy. According to Holland and Judge, "By its very nature, and in the right hands, Web 2.0 technology has the capacity to transform existing pedagogic practices in higher education by creating a teaching and learning environment that supports participation, interactivity, communication and the development of learning communities where students can share and co-construct knowledge with each other and their instructors" (2013, p. 18).

Learning management systems are designed to support teacher-directed, course-centric learning. Students submit assignments and post messages, embedding their work within a course that disappears after the semester's close or graduation. Social media tools allow students to create work within personal accounts that can be networked, tagged, and commented upon, supporting a process of connected learning during which students pool originally produced media, compare differing perspectives, look for commonalities, analyze observations to discern meaning, and create an enduring record of learning. Learners both own and share their understanding.

By way of example, students enrolled in Michael Wesch's fall 2007 Cultural Anthropology course at Kansas State University (KSU) conducted primary research, created a polished 5-minute video about their findings, and posted the video, entitled "A Vision of Students Today," for public viewing on YouTube. This is not necessarily a novel assignment: students have been making "digital stories" for years. In 1994, Dana Atchley and Joe Lambert developed the first workshop on digital storytelling, and Lambert went on to found the Center for Digital Storytelling in 1998 (Lambert, n.d.). What is striking is that by September 2009, the video had been viewed more than 3,340,000 times, and as of March 2013 it had received 4,800,245 views (Wesch, 2007). In the words of social media, the video "went viral." The work of these students has extended beyond the duration of the class, beyond the KSU campus, and even after 5 years it continues to serve as a catalyst for intellectual discussion that spans continents. By March 2013, more than 9,676 people had used YouTube's commenting tool to post their thoughts about the video in the discussion area located directly below the piece.

Imagine the sense of accomplishment that Wesch's students must feel. No LMS-based assignment could claim this level of engagement and impact on society as a whole. According to George Siemens,

> Including technology and connection making as learning activities begins to move learning theories into a digital age. We can no longer personally experience and acquire learning that we need to act. We derive our competence from forming connections . . . (2004, para. 14)
>
> Personal knowledge is comprised of a network, which feeds into organizations and institutions, which in turn feed back into the network, and then continue to provide learning to individuals. This cycle of knowledge development (personal to network to organization) allows learners to remain current in their field through the connections they have formed. (2004, para. 27)

When used appropriately, with thoughtful guidance, social media can be a powerful conduit for helping students connect life and learning.

■ Theoretical Foundations

Given that technological options grow exponentially on a daily basis, how can educators avail themselves of emerging technologies without sacrificing precious learning time with their students? All too often, teachers who want to experiment with technology begin by selecting the tool and then determining its educational use. This strategy is both *inefficient*, because it forces educators to learn about all technologies regardless of their relevance to a particular learning scenario, and pedagogically *ineffective*, because it takes the focus off the most important drivers: learning goals, desired outcomes, and evidence of learning.

Ruben Puentedura's SAMR model for evaluating the impact of educational technology on learning focuses on transformational pedagogy (2012). SAMR is an acronym that stands for Substitution, Augmentation, Modification, and Redefinition (see **Figure 9-1**). For example, digital projectors serve as a *substitution* for overhead projectors and acetate pages. E-mail is an *augmentation* of written messages because it includes additional features such as the ability to attach files and distribute messages to hundreds of people simultaneously through the use of lists. Wikis *modify* the concept of authorship, turning what used to be a solitary, defined process into a crowd-sourced endeavor in which the formation of knowledge is distributed and infinite. Student-produced digital stories and multimodal online case studies *redefine* the communication of ideas because learners have an opportunity to integrate sounds, images, words, and video into a multisensory, multidimensional experience that conveys more than text alone.

Puentedura observes that new technologies can be used in place of previous tools (enhancement), or they can support a rethinking of how teaching and learning take place (transformation). Transformational pedagogy is not inherent to the tool; it is the intersection between innovative learning design and the new capabilities made possible by the technology. If we evaluate the use of social media from the perspective of SAMR, then sending classroom updates through Twitter is *augmented* use of the tool, whereas using Twitter as a platform for book discussions between

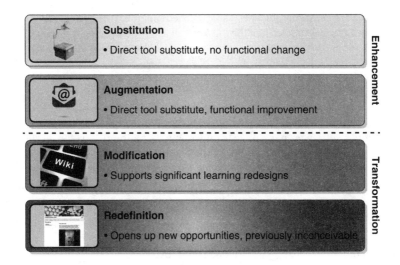

■ Figure 9-1   Reuben Puentedura's SAMR model.

Modified from Puentedura, R. (2014). *Learning, technology, and the SAMR model: Goals, processes, and practice.* Retrieved from http://www.hippasus.com/rrpweblog/archives/2014/06/29/Learning TechnologySAMRModel.pdf. Projector © chungking/Shutterstock, email icon © Artco/Shutterstock, Wiki key © Stuart Miles/Shutterstock.

students from different institutions is *transformational* (Matthews-DeNatale & Bullock, 2014).

Tanya Joosten's pathbreaking work *Social Media for Educators* (2012) encourages educators to focus on forms of engagement that enhance learning, such as building cooperation and feedback through dialogue. Social media evolves at a quick pace, and many of the technologies referenced in her book are not as popular as when it was written (e.g., Second Life), yet the strategies and best practices that she recommends are applicable to most forms of social media.

Lee Shulman, president emeritus of the Carnegie Foundation for the Advancement of Teaching, describes five dimensions that are central to effective teaching: vision, design, interactions, outcomes, and analysis (1998). A good course functions as a coherent whole: discrete assignments are engaging and often creative in design, yet the pieces are interconnected and create a synergistic learning experience. Likewise, good teaching is responsive to learners, differentiated to address a variety of capabilities, while also tailored to meet the needs of specific populations enrolled in the course. Georgetown University's Randy Bass describes this process of learning design as identifying "the problem":

> I realized I didn't know really if the better students in a course who demonstrated a real understanding of the material by the end of the semester were actually acquiring that understanding in my course, or were merely the percentage of students who entered the course with a high level of background and aptitude. Similarly, I realized

I didn't really know if the students who I watched "improve" from their early work to later work were really understanding the material and the paradigm from which I was operating, or merely learning to perform their knowledge in ways that had adapted to my expectations. (Bass, 1999, p. 4)

In response to these uncertainties, Bass and other proponents of the "scholarship of teaching and learning" advocate focusing on "the relationship between student prior understanding and their capacity to acquire new understanding" to investigate how students' "self-awareness of learning might help them develop a deeper understanding of certain disciplinary principles more quickly and meaningfully" (Bass, 1999, p. 6). With this approach, courses and assignments are developed in response to, and as an investigation of, students' learning needs and developing abilities.

In the article "Disrupting Ourselves: The Problem of Learning in Higher Education," Bass describes this approach to teaching and learning as a "porous" blurring of boundaries, a process that creates "not only promising changes in learning but also disruptive moments in teaching." He goes on to explain

By "disruptive moments," I'm not referring to students on Facebook in classrooms. I mean "disruption" in the way Clayton Christensen uses the term. Christensen coined the phrase *disruptive innovation* to refer to a process "by which a product or service takes root initially in simple applications at the bottom of a market and then relentlessly moves up market, eventually displacing established competitors." . . . I am asserting that one key source of disruption in higher education is coming not from the outside but from our own practices, from the growing body of experiential modes of learning, moving from margin to center, and proving to be critical and powerful in the overall quality and meaning of the undergraduate experience. (Bass, 2012, p. 24)

This problem-based approach helps faculty select emerging technologies that disrupt or transcend the confines of course-based learning in a way that is both meaningful and productive, realizing the full potential that technology holds for transforming higher education. The disruptive use of emerging technology in education is grounded in a vision for learning that:

- Is *responsive* to learner's intellectual and social needs;
- *Fosters connections* between the course at hand and students' life experiences (e.g., friends, family, regional, ethnic, and cultural affinity groups);
- *Creates a bridge* between the course and students' larger learning contexts (e.g., other courses, internships, service learning, and co-ops);
- *Taps into diverse preferences and perspectives,* allowing students to play to their strengths as they grapple with course concepts; and
- Helps students *achieve deeper conceptual understanding* and *develop core capabilities* in relationship to the course topic or discipline.

Expanded Approaches to Learning

Historically, higher education has best served students who learn best through reading, listening to lectures, taking notes, and doing sequential problem solving such as mathematical calculation. Educational theorists have developed a host of models designed to help teachers consider how to leverage the strengths and preferences found among learners in a heterogeneous classroom (Butler, 1986; Kolb, 1984; Felder & Soloman, n.d.). The four-part model put forth by Felder and Soloman is particularly useful in exploring the relevance of social media for higher education:

- *Reflective and Active*
  - Reflective involves learning by thinking.
  - Active involves learning by doing.
- *Sensing and Intuitive*
  - Sensing involves learning by facts and verifiable experience.
  - Intuitive involves learning through innovation and possibility-thinking.
- *Verbal and Visual*
  - Verbal involves learning through the written and spoken word.
  - Visual involves learning through images, diagrams, and timelines.
- *Sequential and Global*
  - Sequential involves drawing on details and facts to construct larger understanding.
  - Global involves starting with the "big picture" and then analyzing the whole to understand the sum of its parts.

Note that these pairs are continuums of learning preference, not dichotomies. All learners exhibit these eight capabilities in greater or lesser degrees. In addition, recent research indicates teaching to an individual's specific preference does not improve learning (Riener & Willingham, 2010). It is more effective to identify the most promising ways to learn a given topic or skill, design a learning experience that emphasizes the modality best aligned with the task, and also augment the plan with additional modalities to provide opportunities for differentiated engagement. For example, students need to engage in kinesthetic interaction (driving) if they want to learn how to drive a car. It would be absurd for a student to demand all driving lessons be taught through writing because she is a "verbal" learner. The most pedagogically effective method is to provide multiple opportunities for engagement through written materials, videos, live presentations, off-road simulations, and quizzes modeled on the DMV test, yet focus the majority of instruction on the kinesthetic experience of practice driving.

Social media are particularly adept at supporting differentiated instruction through active, intuitive, visual, and global learning. **Table 9-1** maps selected social media tools to Felder and Soloman's framework of learning preferences.

In recent years educators have increasingly focused on the role interpersonal interaction plays in learning, a concept that is often referred to as "social pedagogy." This concept is not new. According to Judha Hämäläinen, in 1889 theorist and philosopher Paul Natorp "claimed that all pedagogy should be social, that is, that in the philosophy of education the interaction of educational processes and society must be taken into consideration" (2003, p. 73). It stands to reason that social media are particularly good at supporting the social dimension of learning.

The online environment also has the potential to transform social pedagogy because it supports the development of intricate and geographically dispersed learning networks that are not possible in face-to-face settings. Echoing Oblinger, Bonnie Stewart observes, "Prior to the digital era, scholarly knowledge was traditionally organized

Table 9-1   Learning Preferences and Emerging Technologies

Preference	Social Media Example
Active (learning by doing)	Students pool labwork or field-gathered data into a wiki, authoring a collaborative analysis of their primary data.
Intuitive (innovation and possibility-thinking)	Students browse the TED Talks video site to identify thought leaders who can provide a "big-picture" analysis of a given topic (e.g., epidemiology students access a talk on pandemics given by Larry Brilliant).
Visual (images, diagrams, timelines)	Students identify stories of previous experiences that relate to a given topic, then create and share "digital stories" using VoiceThread (3- to 5-minute videos that combine images and words). Classmates use VoiceThread's annotation tool to comment on each other's stories.
Global (big-picture thinking)	Students use Bubbl.us to create mind maps that provide a holistic picture of a topic or concept, then use a blog or Twitter aggregator to compile an overview of all recent posts written about that topic.

around the premise that knowledge is scarce and its artifacts materially vulnerable" and the Internet "marks a shift from an era of knowledge scarcity to an era of knowledge abundance" (2015, para. 4). Stewart goes on to describe what she calls Networked Participatory Scholarship (NPS), an approach that "fosters extensive cross-disciplinary and public ties for scholars, and encourages scholars to be teacher-learners who engage and speak back in the midst of multiplicity and abundance" (2015, para. 51). When students are encouraged to access and create knowledge through online social networking, social media offers them the opportunity to experience the transformative richness of NPS firsthand. This is the power of connected learning.

Using the Method

When technology developers set out to create a new product, they begin by surveying the needs of their users. The next step is to develop a "spec," a specification document that describes all the things that the product will have to be able to do. In integrating emerging technologies into teaching, a similar process is useful. Begin with these questions:

1. What should my students know and understand by the end of the course (or assignment or module)?
2. What skills or capabilities, academic or disciplinary, are essential to achieving the goals for learning?
3. What is the "problem" (à la Randy Bass) that I am trying to solve—which of the goals for learning have been difficult for learners to achieve when I taught this course in the past?
4. What do I want for myself and for my students? For example, the teacher may want to obtain a clearer picture of students' thought processes, or she may want her students to connect course concepts to everyday life.
5. By the end of the learning sequence, what evidence will you and your students need to be confident that learning goals have been achieved? Along the way, what evidence would help you and your students identify trouble spots to address areas of concern and make adjustments as necessary?

6. What modes of learning are particularly relevant to the topic or learning goals? For example, epidemiology may lend itself to mapping clinical decision making to visual and other data analysis, and cultural competence or medical ethics to multimedia storytelling.

The answers to these questions provide a "spec" that can be used in seeking out emerging technologies that best align with the learning scenario. This preliminary work, often called "learning design," also saves time because the faculty member only needs to investigate technologies that will meet specific criteria for learning.

In evaluating emerging technologies, faculty need not be alone. Educause, the national organization dedicated to technology in higher education, publishes a series entitled 7 *Things You Should Know About* (Educause Learning Initiative, n.d.). Each brief focuses on a single technology or practice, describing what it is, how it works, and why it matters to teaching and learning. As of October 2015, there were 130 briefs in the series, with approximately 12 publications added to the collection each year. The Educause Learning Initiative, in collaboration with the New Media Consortium, also produces the *Horizon Report* (New Media Consortium, n.d.), an annual digest of technologies that are likely to have a significant impact on teaching and learning in the near future, along with examples of those technologies at use in higher education. An online self-paced workshop, 23 *Things* (n.d.), developed by the Public Library of Charlotte and Mecklenberg County as part of its "Learn 2.0" initiative, was also designed to provide a guided introduction to social media. Allan Carrington's regularly updated "Padagogy" wheel is a particularly useful tool for identifying educational uses for social media because he maps technologies to the SAMR framework (Carrington, 2015).

In addition, most colleges and universities have instructional designers who are current with recent developments in technology, eager to share their knowledge, and equipped to provide consultation on the use of technology for learning. These professionals are usually located within centers for teaching and learning, or centers for teaching and learning with technology. Whether consulting with an instructional designer or browsing 7 *Things* briefs, the result will be more satisfactory and efficient if the faculty member first uses "the method" to create a spec that identifies desired learning goals, processes, and outcomes.

Potential Problems

Despite social networking's capacity to increase student engagement, metacognition, and connected learning, educators have also found that these tools can be confusing, somewhat intimidating, and even scary. The associated terminology can sound like something penned by Lewis Carroll: *Twas pinterest and the slithy blogs did tweet and wiki in the wabe!*

Sometimes social media are *too* easy to use, with the consequence that embarrassing and inappropriate youthful dalliances are posted online for enduring public scrutiny. These horror stories might make some educators leery of incorporating social media into their work with students.

The accelerated pace of change is also dizzying: each week dozens of new resources arrive on the scene while others are either acquired or go out of business altogether. As soon as the public became accustomed to the term Web 2.0, technologists began speaking about a Web 3.0 featuring mobile technologies (e.g., GPS-enabled iPhones, iPads, Kindles, and Android devices) that are location-aware and context-tailored (e.g., tracking interests and setting to offer only pertinent resources and information). The use of version numbers (e.g., 2.0, 3.0, and beyond) quickly became as problematic as the hackneyed phrase "21st-century learning." Instead of focusing on the generation of a given technology and its specifics, perhaps we should focus our attention on the learning theories that, in the words of Christensen, "have an opinion" about the aspects of education that ought to be disrupted.

Emerging technologies are a grand adventure that can add a new dimension to learning, but there is a price for teaching "outside the box" of institution-supported learning management systems. Educational institutions are careful to make regular backups of courses in their LMSs; they cannot risk losing credit-bearing discussion posts or test results. In contrast, emerging technologies come with no guarantee of backups, security, or even ongoing existence. An assignment that previously worked well using a given technology may have to be adapted in response to new versions, acquisition by another company, or even the disappearance of a much-loved tool.

Unlike learning management systems, social media tools come unbundled and are rarely supported by technicians at the institutional level, therefore placing the onus for technical orientation and support on the teacher. Because the tools are selected *à la carte*, it is the educator's responsibility to weave technologies together into a coherent learning environment. Students can become frustrated when a course includes too many different technologies. When using an LMS, the student experiences it as *one* software application, even though the learning system can do many things. When using emerging technologies, students experience each one as a different tool: a different "place" to go to do course work, a different interface to learn, a different login, and a unique application that has its own technology troubleshooting challenges. One strategy is to use the LMS as a portal or door through which students can access all other tools used in the class. This can be accomplished by inserting links to all technologies on a course page or as needed within course modules. Another strategy is to integrate emerging technologies thoughtfully and sparingly: no more than two or three tools unless the course is about technology itself.

When taking the leap into emerging technologies, it is important to realize that this is uncharted territory. Students take their cue from their teachers, and these technologies require a pioneering spirit—so plan accordingly and encourage your students to take an adventurous approach as well.

■ Conclusion

Higher education is in a period of disruption, creating new opportunities for learning with social media that are visually rich, socially connected, and extend formal learning beyond the confines of school into everyday life. Emerging technologies provide educators with a rich palette of opportunities for enhancing learning, but technology should not lead the decision making. Newer, unbundled technologies are intuitive, particularly suited to learning that is active, social, global, and multimodal. Even though emerging technologies can breathe new life into coursework, enrich communication, increase student engagement, and promote social learning, these technologies often evolve, and therefore it is wise to have a contingency plan in place. Rather than selecting a tool and then deciding what to do with it in an assignment, those who want to incorporate emerging technologies into their teaching are cautioned to focus on pedagogy first—to identify the "problem of practice" or change that they wish to see in students' development—and then select tools that best meet these learning needs.

Teaching Example[1]

In 2011, Yale University launched an initiative to offer undergraduate core courses over the summer in two formats, with a face-to-face and fully online section of the same course running in parallel. As part of this initiative, Professor Ellen Lust worked with the author to develop the following exercise for a class entitled "Introduction to Middle East Politics."

On the first day of class, prior to any instruction or review of the syllabus, both the online and face-to-face students were asked to do the following exercise:

Where Is the Middle East?

This exercise is designed to be completed *before* you go through the syllabus, do Session One readings, and view the Session One videos—you are on your honor to not peek!!!

When you look at a map, the boundaries of nations and continents are clear. But regions such as the "Middle East" are open for interpretation. The regional boundaries that we draw can tell us a great deal about our underlying assumptions.

As we will discuss in more detail during the semester, one of the major goals of the course is to understand what factors unite the Middle East, what important distinctions exist across the region, and how this influences domestic and regional politics.

Before reading through the syllabus in detail, use ScribbleMaps to draw a map of the Middle East (see **Figure 9-2**). Session One's materials, located in the course website, include a ScribbleMaps "Quick Start Guide" that provides set-by-step directions for signing up for and using this online mapping tool. After you've completed your map, consider the following questions and capture your thoughts in writing.

1. What factors tie together the countries you identified as a region?
2. What are your reasons for excluding other, neighboring countries?
3. What important differences exist across countries that you, nevertheless, see as part of the Middle East?

When you have finished, post the link to your map and your responses online in the Session One dropbox. Your responses will serve as the basis for our discussion during the first session. Please note that we will view and refer to your maps during the discussion on Thursday, so it is very important for you to post your maps before the specified deadline.

In the face-to-face section of the class, students used the computer projector to navigate to their maps, discuss their decision-making process, and compare perspectives. In the online section, Ellen Lust held a "live classroom" synchronous webinar during which students used a similar process to share and discuss their maps.

---

[1] *The author would like to thank Ellen Lust for her contribution to this Teaching Example.*

(continues)

Teaching Example (*continued*)

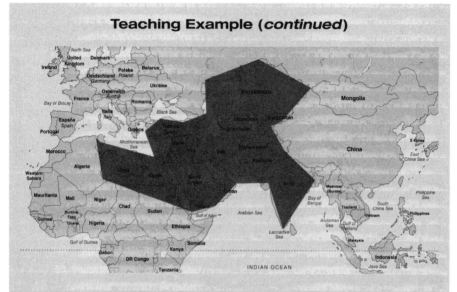

■ **Figure 9-2**   Rudimentary ScribbleMap created on the first day of class.
Data from Scribble Maps. (2016). Retrieved from http://www.scribblemaps.com.

In subsequent weeks, students granted advanced map access permission to each of their peers. This allowed them to use ScribbleMap's online commenting and tagging features to engage in dialogue within each other's maps, developing a differentiated yet shared understanding of the complexities of the region.

Each person's map continued to look different from the others, but every week students did a common set of exercises to refine and annotate their maps.

For example, during one week they posted markers on their maps to record the history of colonialism and independence in the countries they considered to be part of the "Middle East" region (see **Figure 9-3**). In other weeks they underwent a similar process to note the presence of Islam, fossil fuels, women's rights, and other dimensions that factor into the politics of the region. Sometimes students decided to change the boundaries of the Middle East in their maps in response to the rich patterns they identified during this annotation process; others kept the same construct but deepened their understanding of the decisions they had made. The map made their developing thinking visible to others, and also visible to themselves.

By the end of the course, each student had created an individualized, layered, and multimedia-rich map that represented his or her growth in understanding. By comparing the initial maps with those submitted for the culminating assignment, both the students and their teacher could see how far they had come.

As of this writing in 2013, Ellen Lust still uses ScribbleMaps in her teaching. When asked to reflect on the assignment and its pedagogical impact, she provided the following explanation:

The exercise serves two purposes. First, it provides a great discussion tool for the initial meetings of class. It engages students directly, as each makes active decisions about what countries are and aren't included in the region and, more importantly, why that's the case. These are easily put onto the screen for class discussion, and it's really the engagement

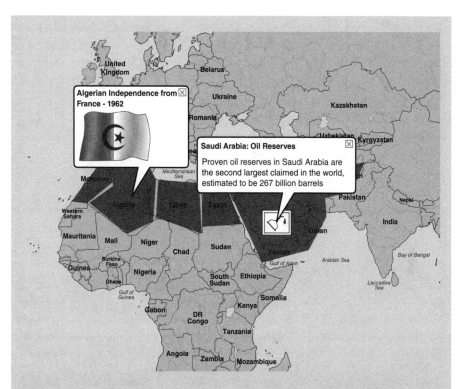

■ **Figure 9-3**   An illustration of an annotated ScribbleMap that includes embedded images and links to other websites.

Data from Scribble Maps. (2016). Retrieved from http://www.scribblemaps.com.

of students and a discussion about what "makes the Middle East" that I aim for at that first meeting (see **Figure 9-4**). Second, the map becomes a resource and sort of "diary" of the learning journey the students experience in the class. The students update the maps throughout the course, adding the dates of independence, colonial experience, resource wealth (especially oil), and other features into the map. At the end, they have an easy reference for many of the basic distinguishing features of the region, and also a way to look back at all that they have learned through the course.

Much of this could be done with a physical paper map, but the exercise would be much more cumbersome. Sharing the maps for discussion would be more difficult, and nearly impossible for distance learning. It's also more desirable than simply having a group discussion about boundaries based on a large classroom map (which is what I'd done previously), since this engages *all* of the students in making their own map, and not simply the more vocal students who are willing to describe boundaries. Updating the map is also technically feasible with a paper map, but often those maps get mangled over the course of a semester—a problem that doesn't exist with the electronic option.

In retrospect, Ellen Lust commented that the experience "really changed not just the course, but how I think about teaching" (personal communication).

(continues)

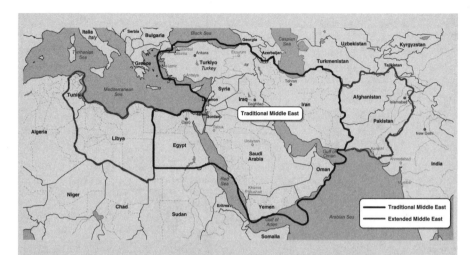

■ **Figure 9-4**   ScribbleMap conveys refined perspective on the region.

Data from Scribble Maps. (2016). Retrieved from http://www.scribblemaps.com.

Middle East ScribbleMaps created for the class in 2011 are still functional in 2013, despite the vagaries of social media. While the Middle East mapping assignment is designed for a course in political science, it is generalizable because it illustrates social media's capacity to engage students in the development of visible knowledge that persists for the duration of a course and long after the class has been completed. For example, within the field of nursing and health sciences, this exercise could be adapted for use in a community health windshield survey assignment, an epidemiological analysis, or any other experience in which health professionals need to be aware of, and sensitive to, their surrounding context.

Discussion Questions

1. In what ways do you use social media in your daily life? How do these experiences contribute to your informal and formal learning? What concerns do you have about integrating social media into your teaching? Conversely, what do you perceive to be opportunities?

2. What is your "problem of practice"? Identify a concept or skill that is particularly challenging for your students to learn. What makes it so difficult? What specific modality or modalities would provide your students with opportunities for working through those difficulties? What forms of social media are particularly good at engaging students in those modes of learning?

3. What forms of social media might support the "difficult" learning that you want your learners to attain? How will your lesson/course plan and use of technology address the development of complex skills and knowledge through social learning?

References

23 Things. (n.d.). *Self-paced online workshop developed by the Public Library of Charlotte and Mecklenberg County.* Retrieved from http://plcmcl2-things.blogspot.com

Bass, R. (1999). The scholarship of teaching: What's the problem? *Inventio: Creative Thinking about Learning and Teaching, 1*(1), 1–10.

Bass, R. (2012). Disrupting ourselves: The problem of learning in higher education. *The Educause Review Online.* Retrieved from http://www.educause.edu/ero/article/disrupting-ourselves-problem-learning-higher-education

Butler, K. (1986). *Learning and teaching style: In theory and practice.* Columbia, CT: Learners' Dimension.

Carrington, A. (2015). *The Padagogy wheel, V4.0.* Retrieved from http://www.designingoutcomes.net/PadWheelV4

Christensen, C., & Eyring, H. (2011). *The innovative university.* San Francisco, CA: Jossey-Bass.

Educause Learning Initiative. (n.d.). *7 things series.* Retrieved from http://www.educause.edu/ELI/ELIResources/7ThingsYouShouldKnowAbout/7495

Felder, R. M., & Soloman, B. A. (n.d.). *Learning styles and strategies.* Retrieved from http://www4.ncsu.edu/unity/lockers/users/f/felder/public/ILSdir/styles.htm

Hämäläinen, J. (2003). The concept of social pedagogy in the field of social work. *Journal of Social Work, 3*(1), 69–80.

Holland, C., & Judge, M. (2013). Future learning spaces: The potential and practice of Learning 2.0 in higher education. In B. Patrut, M. Patrut, & C.Cmeciu (Eds.), *Social media and the new academic environment* (pp. 1–25). Hershey, PA: IGI Global. Retrieved from http://www.igi-global.com/book/social-media-new-academic-environment/69841#table-of-contents

Joosten, T. (2012). *Social media for educators: Strategies and best practices.* Hoboken, NJ: John Wiley & Sons.

Kolb, D. A. (1984). *Experiential learning: Experience as the source of learning and development.* Englewood Cliffs, NJ: Prentice-Hall.

Lambert, J. (n.d.). *Digital storytelling: About: Press and history.* Berkeley, CA: Center for Digital Storytelling. Retrieved from http://www.storycenter.org/press

Matthews-DeNatale, G., & Bullock, B. (2014). *Twitter as a tool for engagement.* Poster presented at the College of Professional Studies Faculty Conference, Northeastern University, Boston, MA. Retrieved from http://www.slideshare.net/gmdenatale/twitter-as-a-tool-for-engagement

New Media Consortium. (n.d.). *The Horizon project.* Retrieved from http://www.nmc.org/horizon

Puentedura, R. (2012). *The SAMR model: Background and exemplars.* Retrieved from http://www.hippasus.com/rrpweblog/archives/2012/08/23/SAMR_BackgroundExemplars.pdf

Puentedura, R. (2014). *Learning, technology, and the SAMR model: Goals, processes, and practice.* Retrieved from http://www.hippasus.com/rrpweblog/archives/2014/06/29/LearningTechnologySAMRModel.pdf

Riener, C., & Willingham, D. (2010). The myth of learning styles. *Change: The Magazine of Higher Learning, 42*(5), 32–35.

Ritchhart, R., Church, M., & Morrison, K. (2011). *Making thinking visible: How to promote engagement, understanding, and independence for all learners.* San Francisco, CA: Jossey-Bass.

Scribble Maps. (2016). Retrieved from http://www.scribblemaps.com

Shulman, L. (1998). Course anatomy: The dissection & analysis of knowledge through teaching. In P. Hutchings (Ed.), *The course portfolio: How faculty can improve their teaching to advance practice and improve student learning* (pp. 5–12). Washington, DC: American Association of Higher Education.

Siemens, G. (2004). *Connectivism: A learning theory for the digital age.* Retrieved from http://www.elearnspace.org/Articles/connectivism.htm

Stewart, B. (2015). In abundance: Networked participatory practices as scholarship. *International Review of Research on Open and Distributed Learning, 16*(3). Retrieved from http://www.irrodl.org/index.php/irrodl/article/view/2158/3343

Weinberger, David. (2003). *Small pieces loosely joined.* Jackson, TN: Basic Books.

Wesch, M. (2007). *A vision of students today.* Retrieved from http://www.youtube.com/watch?v=dGCJ46vyR9o

Recommended Reading

Matthews-DeNatale, G. (2008). Digital story-making: Understanding the learner's perspective. Paper presented at Educause Learning Initiative Annual Conference, San Antonio, TX. Retrieved from http://www.educause.edu/Resources/DigitalStoryMakingUnderstandin/162538

Teaching in Structured Settings

This section focuses on teaching in structured (i.e., classroom) settings, which calls for focused planning and preparation on the part of the teacher. Concept-based topics that are applicable in a variety of teaching situations, regardless of the level of the learner, the topic, or the class size, are presented. Themes evident in each chapter include flexibility on the part of the teacher, a specific manner in which information is conveyed, and the importance of active student involvement and responsibility for one's own learning.

The principles introduced in the introductory section are used in the traditional classroom environments addressed in these chapters. Application of teaching and learning theories and use of planned activities enhance critical thinking in the learner and lead to clinical reasoning in practice settings. Educators can use creative innovations with time-honored strategies, such as lecture, to bring a fresh approach to teaching.

CHAPTER 10

Using Lecture in Active Classrooms

Barbara C. Woodring
Beth L. Hultquist

■ Setting the Stage

Take a good look at your home entertainment center (e.g., voice-activated digital TV with 156 channels, DVD, CD, electronic game board) with its 120-inch, touch-activated, 12-window screen accompanied by surround sound. It is in front of such centers that most adults and children spend 6–8 hours per day. Huntley (2009), an industrial chief learning officer, stated, "Education is no longer enough. Learners expect to be engaged and entertained more than ever . . . [Learners] are exposed to a variety of stimulating and on-demand media sources daily . . . learning modes need to be equally engaging" (p. 32). She identified a solution as *edutainment*, presenting knowledge in a way that engages and entertains.

Yet, with this concept of edutainment before us, we are reminded that the methodology that is the backbone for transmission of knowledge in most educational settings is the lecture. How, then, can educators satisfy the need for interactive variety and edutainment while implementing the most commonly utilized teaching method? The information in this chapter will assist in addressing this question.

The authors of other chapters in this text provide insight into creative and innovative teaching approaches that are currently used in higher education. The implementation and refinement of these strategies/methods during the last decade have often relegated lecture methodology to a lesser stature. Rather than revere what has previously been considered the educational gold standard, it became trendy to "lecture bash" (Woodring & Woodring, 2014)—that is, to describe colleagues who used lecture techniques as old-fashioned and out of step with educational trends. Many educators add the term *lecture* to their list of unspeakable, four-letter words. A Carnegie Foundation publication suggested that for the sake of being PC (pedagogically correct), the honorable tradition of lecturing has been relegated to an "Index of Forbidden Pedagogies" (Burgan, 2006, p. 31). In reality, a lecture is only a means to an end. Intrinsically, it is neither good nor bad; its success depends on why and how it is delivered.

The authors wish to thank Richard C. Woodring for his review and contributions to this chapter.

In practice, the lecture format is alive and well and remains one of the most frequently utilized teaching methods in the repertoire of postsecondary educators. When the objective is to communicate basic facts, introduce initial concepts, or convey passion about a topic, a well-prepared lecture is very useful (Cox & Rogers, 2005; Di Leonardi, 2007; Gleitman, 2006; Wolff, Wagner, Poznanski, Schiller, & Santen, 2015). In this chapter, readers will find a rationale for the long-term popularity of this teaching strategy and suggestions for becoming a better lecturer.

■ Definition and Purposes

The lecture is one method of presenting information to an audience. It should be a well-designed, instructor-led, interactive experience to engage students and support diverse styles of learning. Acceptance of this description indicates how far the educational process has come. Prior to the invention of the printing press, when only scholars had access to handwritten information sources, the lecture was the primary means of transmitting knowledge. Learners would gather around the master-teacher and take notes related to what was said. The lecture remained the common mode of disseminating information until printed resources and technological advancements became available and affordable.

It would appear that when students became able to purchase their own textbooks, and then their own technology (e.g., PC, laptop, tablet), methods of presenting information would have changed. Interestingly, though, change has occurred slowly. Today, with e-books and technology galore, the lecture remains a commonly used technique. We suggest there are two major reasons for this longevity: (1) most current educators learned via the lecture format, and it is well known that individuals teach as they were taught unless they make a specific effort to alter their approaches; and (2) the lecture is the safest and easiest teaching method, allowing the teacher the most control within the classroom setting. Some of the common advantages and disadvantages of using the lecture method are listed in **Tables 10-1** and **10-2**. Whatever rationale is used, positive outcomes can be achieved when both the lecture and the lecturer are well prepared.

■ Theoretical Rationale

Few lecturers take time to contemplate the theoretical basis of their practice, but the lack of a theoretical or organizational framework may be one reason that learners perceive some lectures to be disorganized and/or difficult to follow.

Foundational principles for a lecture presentation may be derived from a variety of philosophical and theoretical processes. Three common approaches flow from theories related to communication, cognitive learning, and pedagogical/andragogical approaches to teaching and learning. The theories supporting effective communications should be common knowledge to all healthcare providers; therefore, they are not discussed here. Healthcare educators should have an understanding of cognitive learning theory because it is the underpinning of developmental concepts found in most health-related courses. Pedagogical/andragogical approaches may not be as well understood and are addressed briefly.

Table 10-1   Advantages of Using Lectures as a Teaching Strategy

Advantages of a Lecture	Secondary Gain in Use of Lecture
Permits teacher maximum control of class.	Decreases teacher anxiety about entertaining unexpected questions (teacher sets the ground rules for when/if questions may be asked).
Creates minimal threats to students or teacher.	Lack of interaction or student participation may be desired and can be controlled by the teacher.
Clarifies and enlivens information that seems tedious in text.	Highlights enthusiasm/personality of teacher for topic.
Enables clarification of confusing/intricate points immediately.	May avoid frustration of time-delayed responses and clarification if teacher allows questions during the class time.
The teacher knows what has been presented.	Diminishes the "I never heard that before" comment by students.
Lecture material can become basis of publication.	Contributes to academic scholarship.
Students are provided with a common core of content.	May help students prepare for testing.
Accommodates larger numbers of listeners at one setting.	High priority in weak economy and/or teacher shortage.
May be time saving.	Teacher can present key points in much less time than it takes to elicit the same points from text or an extensive list of references.
Provides a venue to become known as an expert in a specific topic.	Contributes to the scholarship of teaching.
Encourages and allows deductive reasoning.	Can support principles of critical analysis if desired.
Enthusiasm of teacher motivates students to participate and learn more.	Reinforces professional role modeling.
Allows students addition of the newest information on a moment's notice.	Can support concepts of evidence-based practice with just-in-time data.
Permits auditory learners to receive succinct information quickly.	Encourages higher-level learning, not rote memorization.
Enables integration of pro and con aspects of topic.	Encourages critical thinking and analysis.

Over the past few decades, graduate education for many health professionals has emphasized disciplinary skills. Nursing and physical therapy, for instance, have focused on advanced practice skills, resulting in clinical nurse specialist (CNS), nurse practitioner (NP), and professional doctorate degree (DPT/DNP) designations. This change has resulted in limited numbers of newer faculty members who are prepared in the areas of curricular design and learning theory. *Pedagogy* is a portion of learning theory that loosely refers to educating the chronologically or experientially immature. In a pedagogical approach, someone external to the learner decides who, what, when, where, and how regarding the information to be taught; the learner becomes a passive recipient of knowledge. Historically, professional health-related content and practice have been

Table 10-2   Disadvantages of Using Lectures as a Teaching Strategy

Disadvantages of Lecture	Suggested Remedy
Teacher may attempt to cover too much material in abbreviated time frame.	Elicit questions at the conclusion of segments of time or content (e.g., every 15 minutes).
Less effective when not accompanied by another teaching strategy.	Include at least one audio and/or visual aid or interactive activity per hour.
Eighty percent of lecture information is forgotten 1 day later, and 80% of the remainder fades in 1 month.	Provide visual reinforcement or active learning (gaming).
Presumes that all students are auditory learners and learn at the same rate.	Add at least one handout, visual, or activity to support various learning styles.
Alone, the lecture is not suited to higher levels of thinking.	Intersperse scenarios or activities requiring problem-solving principles.
Not conducive to personalized instruction.	Call several students by name during each class. Encourage use of scheduled office hours for personal clarification and reviews.
Encourages passive learners.	Use clickers/automated response systems to encourage engagement of all class participants.
Provides little feedback to learners.	Encourage online/threaded discussion boards; use automated response clickers to allow immediate feedback.
Student attention wavers in 30 minutes or less.	Alter voice tone, classroom environment, teaching method (even turning off/on PowerPoint slides); change direction of students' attention.
Not appropriate for children below fourth-grade level.	Lectures for children must be brief and based on the children's cognitive abilities. This method is not fourth-grade reading level and/or attention span; if utilized, lecture must be accompanied by other learning activities.
Consistent use inhibits development of inductive reasoning.	Be flexible; incorporate creative teaching strategies described in previous chapters.
Poorly delivered lecture acts as a disincentive for learning.	Practice before you present! Be a positive professional role model.
Viewed by students as a complete learning experience wherein the lecturer presents all they need to know.	Encourage outside research, reviews, and readings, and set aside 5 minutes during each class to discuss them.
Effective learning seldom occurs in a lecture-only format.	Integrate use of lecture recitation, expository lecture, and/or provocative lecture techniques (described in this chapter).

taught from a framework based upon the medical model. Within the pedagogical context, the lecture strategy establishes the teacher as the one in command, the authority from whom answers come. This approach may provide a rationale for lecturing being viewed as traditional and out of step with innovation and creativity in the academy. Over the years, both the age and the experiential backgrounds of traditional college students have shifted, causing scholars to question the appropriateness of the previously used pedagogical methods. In response, educators such as Knowles (1970), Kidd (1973), and Cross (1986) introduced and refined the concept of andragogy. The principles previously utilized in teaching the young (pedagogy) were adapted and applied to mature learners (andragogy).

Those educators who ascribe to andragogical theory treat the learner as a mature individual who brings a variety of rich, valuable experiences to every learning situation. The who, what, when, and where of learning emanate from within the learner. Each model has value, and the needs of the learner should determine the singular or blended approach utilized. **Table 10-3** compares andragogy and pedagogy within the educational process.

Table 10-3   Comparison of Characteristics: Andragogy Versus Pedagogy

Characteristic	Pedagogy	Andragogy
Concept of learner	Dependent	Independent/autonomous
	Passive	Self-directed
	The learner needs someone outside self to make decisions about what, when, and how to learn	The learner wants to participate in decisions related to his or her own learning
Roles of learner's experiences	Narrow, focused interest	Wide range of experience, not just in nursing, that impacts life/learning
	Focuses on imitation	Focus on originality
	Past experiences are given little attention	The learner has broad interests and likes to share previous experiences with others
Readiness to learn	Determined by someone else (society, teachers)	Learners are usually in the educational process because they have chosen to be
	Focus on what is needed to survive and achieve	The learner wants to assist in setting the learning agenda
	The learner tends to respond impulsively	The learner tends to respond rationally
Orientation of teaching/learning	Needs clarity/specificity	Teachers are facilitators, providing resources and support for self-directed learners
	The learner looks to the teacher to identify what should be learned and to provide the information/process to learn	The learner likes challenging, independent assignments that are reality based
	The learner focuses on particulars concerned with the superficial aspects of learning (grades, due dates)	Evaluation is done jointly by the teacher, the learner, and/or peers
	Evaluation of learning is done by the teacher or society (grades, certificates)	The learner tolerates ambiguity

■ Types of Learners

The information included in Table 10-3 emphasizes that the teacher must know as much as possible about both the learners and the topic before deciding on a specific theoretical approach/model and/or selecting the teaching strategy. The concept of "know thy student" has always been important; however, now it is not only important, it is critical. Classrooms are filled with students born after 1990 who have been raised in the wireless, techno age and expect edutainment, even though the faculty may be uncomfortable communicating electronically or using social media. To bridge this generational communication gap, the teacher must understand and acknowledge many learners have a very short attention span, have an arsenal of electronic devices at their fingertips (including in the classroom), are used to multitasking (answering text messages and listening to e-tunes while reading about neuroanatomy), and are used to handling a rapid barrage of information. To address these different learning needs, the proficient teacher will accompany the lecture with adjuncts, such as electronic innovations like Second Life, video clips, electronic lecture retrieval (e.g., via MP3 players), lecture–discussion (addressed later in this chapter), realistic scenarios, questions/answers accompanied by automated audience response systems (the clicker) with real-time feedback (Caldwell, 2007), and other strategies presented in other chapters of this text.

A lecture can be used effectively with learners who represent a variety of developmental and cognitive levels. Adaptability is one of its most positive aspects. A teacher may, at a moment's notice, alter the teaching style, depth, sophistication, and level of the material being presented. These alterations can be made based on the needs, interests, and/or responses of the learners; new scientific revelations; or breaking news from the media. It is assumed the lecturer has a sufficient command of the subject matter, as well as the presence of mind and the flexibility, to alter the content and teaching plan; however, these assumptions may not be accurate with novice educators or when material is being presented for the first time.

Combining the lecture with pedagogical approaches can be especially useful in basic and beginning courses in a sequence, as well as in orientation to new clinical areas or agencies. Novice learners of any age tend to prefer the structure of pedagogy, rather than the more flexible andragogical approach; however, the more mature and secure teachers and learners become, the more they enjoy the flexibility and challenge of integrating andragogical concepts into the lecture format.

■ Types of Lectures

Lectures survive because, like most professional sports and the story line of *Gone with the Wind*, they continue to satisfy the need for dramatic spectacle and offer an arena in which psychological needs are met. A teacher may vary a lecture from a very formal presentation to a much more casual monologue. Although described more than a decade ago, Lowman's (1995) outline of three types of lectures is still accurate. He identified the formal, expository, and provocative formats as types most commonly used in higher education.

The *formal lecture* is sometimes referred to as an oral essay. In the formal setting, the lecturer delivers a well-organized, tightly constructed, highly polished presentation. The information provided primarily supports a specific point and usually is backed by theory and research. The presentation may be written and read to the audience, although recent data indicate most learners do not like having lecture materials read to them (Masie, 2006). Preparation of a formal lecture is time consuming; therefore, it is not used for every class period during a school term. It may, however, be appropriate to tie things together either at the beginning and/or end of a course or to address a specified topical area. One of the major problems with a formal lecture is that it ignores the interactive dimension and sometimes fails to motivate learners.

A variation on the formal lecture is *lecture recitation*. This process may be integrated into the formal lecture. The lecturer stops and asks a student to respond to a particular point or idea by reading/presenting prepared materials. An example of this approach is a formal lecture related to the pathophysiology of sickle cell anemia, followed by a student-presented case study about a patient experiencing the disorder.

The *expository lecture* is considered the most typical type of lecture. It is much less elaborate than the formal oral essay. Although the lecturer does most of the talking, questions from learners are entertained, or a critical thinking exercise may be introduced.

In the *provocative lecture*, the instructor still does most of the talking, but he or she provokes students' thoughts and challenges their knowledge and values with questions. This method is well suited for integration of video streaming or lecture capturing. Included in this category are lecture practice, lecture–discussion, punctuated lecture, and lecture–lab. *Lecture practice* utilizes props, illustrates the subject, and may include lectures with simulations, computer, or video integration. In *lecture–discussion*, the instructor speaks for 10–15 minutes and then stimulates student discussion around key points (the lecturer acts only as a facilitator to clarify and integrate student comments). In *punctuated lecture*, the presenter asks the students to write down their reflections on lecture points and submit them. In *lecture-lab*, the lecture is followed by students conducting experiments, interviews, observations, and other activities during the class period.

The introduction of automated audience response systems within the classroom has enhanced the possibilities for interactivity, especially in large classes (Caldwell, 2007). Similar to a game show, each student has a synchronized response unit—a clicker—similar to a TV remote control. This allows the students to reply to the lecturer's questions and allows the presenter to immediately verify the connections and involvement of students (Harper, 2009; Mayer et al., 2009).

Keep in mind that a lecture, in and of itself, is neither a good nor a bad/inappropriate approach to teaching. It may be deemed the best method when dealing with certain groups; however, like any strategy, it is most effective when not used as the singular, exclusive technique. Eble (1982), in *The Craft of Teaching*, suggested that the lecture should be thought of as a discourse—a talk or conversation—rather than an authoritative speech. As a discourse, the lecture can be viewed as a planned portion of the art or craft of teaching. As such, lecturing becomes a learnable skill that improves with practice.

Because the utilization of the lecture as a best practice in teaching has been called into question, numerous research studies have been undertaken. Amare (2006) studied the experiences of students in PowerPoint-enhanced versus non–PowerPoint-enhanced lectures. She found that, for 84 engineering, humanities, and education majors in a technical writing course, the performance scores were higher in the non-PowerPoint section. However, the students preferred the addition of PowerPoint slides. PowerPoint presentations, podcasts, and other technological enhancements were found to support the lecture by (1) bridging direct and constructionist teaching methods (Clark, 2008; Read, 2005), (2) supporting class attendance (Hove & Corcoran, 2008), and (3) reinforcing difficult concepts (Guertin, Bodek, Zappe, & Kim, 2007; Young, 2008). However, when Costa, van Rensburg, and Rushton (2007) compared group discussion to the lecture presentation method, the majority of medical student participants found the interactive, group discussion style more popular, the retention of knowledge better, and the scores on written tests higher. Generally, educational research findings support the notion lecture is still a valid, appropriate teaching strategy that is most effective when accompanied by other thought-provoking interludes (Wiebel, 2010). In "Sage on the Stage in the Digital Age," Chung (2005) presents a number of very salient points but concludes both graduate and undergraduate online education would suffer if the lecture component were absent.

■ Preparing Oneself to Lecture

Do not underestimate the time needed for preparation, regardless of how well versed you may be in the topic. When presenting an oral essay or formal lecture, preparation must begin well in advance of the presentation date. Planning, organization, and written preparation are essential and time consuming. Less formal forms of lecture may take less time, but their preparation should not be delayed by procrastination. If the lecture is one in a sequence (or within a course), the best time to add the finishing touches to the next lecture is at the completion of the preceding one. Significant ideas that should be reemphasized are still fresh in the presenter's mind, as are the questions raised (or that should have been raised) by the students. The lecturer can recall the presentation strategies that worked with a group of participants and those that did not. Changes that might have made the lecture more effective can be identified. Most lecturers, however, do not heed this advice, and lecture preparation is often relegated to a brief time immediately prior to the presentation.

Lectures are frequently used to deliver large amounts of information, typically to large groups of students. Unfortunately, the efficiency of this mode leads most educators to fail to use the lecture to stimulate thought, critical thinking, or problem solving. "It is important to model caring, judgment, and use of knowledge rather than simply overwhelming learners with facts and categories of facts" (Di Leonardi, 2007, p. 155).

The challenge then becomes involving the learner in what by definition is a one-way lecture format. Di Leonardi (2007) explored the characteristics of an effective lecture. She advocated for the use of questions during lecture to stimulate thought.

Multiple-choice questions, case-study questions, a 1-minute paper, or asking learners to write questions are all effective strategies. One of the authors of this chapter uses questions interspersed within a lecture format, pausing to allow students to think and reflect within the small group surrounding them. She then randomly picks a student name and asks for the answer. This strategy must be conveyed as a fun way to learn, and never become punitive. However, it also provides enough motivation for students to stay on task, listen to content being delivered, and work within small groups to attain answers. Another effective use of questions is at the end of any lecture vignette or lecture class. Clark (2013) details numerous methods of assessing learning in a class. Students feel valued when their questions are answered completely, and teachers can convey caring and civility by asking for and responding to learners' concerns. Handing out a 3 × 5 notecard at the beginning of class to each learner and making small talk is an effective way to make connections with each student, especially in a large class. The notecard can then be used for numerous strategies, such as reflecting on what students learned today, a think-pair-share activity, or for submission of questions at the end of the class regarding the day's material. The key to success is to gather all the "I do not understand" cards after class, review them, find themes, and address these questions in a follow-up e-mail. This strategy has been used effectively in many situations, from a beginner-level class where learners may be hesitant to raise questions in front of their peers, to a senior-level class when students may feel they are expected to know the content well and questions may be embarrassing.

A key concept in today's health professions education is active learning strategies (Di Leonardi, 2007; Waltz, Jenkins, & Han, 2014; Wolff et al., 2015). By and large, these strategies require students to prepare for the class by watching lecture vignettes, reading textbooks, and researching concepts before arriving for active learning in the classroom. In the case of a lecture, learner preparation is also essential. By providing students with an outline, questions to answer, and concepts to understand prior to arriving to class, the instructor allows lecture time to be used for exploration of more in-depth concepts and enhances the development of critical thinking as previously learned material is applied to several situations. The outline also allows effective note taking for the learner.

Any lecture must be planned and structured. Storytelling in lecture can be an effective method to create links between content and practice; however, lecturers must be intentional with the story and not use prior experiences as a way to fill time. Learners quickly become frustrated when time is used to explore topics irrelevant to the topic at hand (Di Leonardi, 2007). Likewise, technology can be a hindrance to learning if it is used ineffectively or technology issues arise that consume class time. Detailed planning is necessary to use technology to enhance learning.

Any lecture, whether given in an online class in the form of a video, voice-over PowerPoint, or live in a classroom, must be expertly planned and delivered. Di Leonardi (2007) encouraged teachers to improve their lecture techniques in order to engage students. Strategies for improvement include student and peer feedback, reflection on what is working in the classroom and what should be changed, and watching master lecturers at their craft.

■ Resources

The major resource needed to utilize the lecture techniques effectively is *you*, the well-prepared lecturer. Presenting an informative and interesting lecture is a craft and a learnable skill. Because the speaker is the crucial element for this strategy, some key points are identified in the following list to help polish your presentation skills, with additional suggestions summarized in **Table 10-4**. Remember, participants want to believe that you are smart, interesting, and a good speaker (Germano, 2003)!

- *Conveying enthusiasm is the key element in presenting an effective lecture.* Enthusiasm is contagious and is demonstrated by facial expressions, excitement in the voice, gestures, and body language. A lack of enthusiasm on the part of the speaker is interpreted by the listener as lack of self-confidence, lack of knowledge, disinterest in the learner, and/or disinterest in the topic. If you do not have an effusive personality, practice adding a smile and small hand gestures to each lecture. Once these movements are comfortable, add other interactive methods.

Table 10-4   Sample Lecture Plan

Time Allowed	Teacher	Learner	Supports
Introduction			
5 minutes	Personal introduction	Listen	*Visual No. 1:* Objectives
	Today's objectives	Take notes	*Handout:* Skeletal outline for note taking
	Overview of class process/ handouts	Ask for clarification	
Body			
15 minutes	Lecture Part I	Look	*Visuals No. 2, 3, 4*
		Listen	
		Take notes	
5 minutes	Q & A	Q & A	
10 minutes	Ask two questions related to the topic	Divide into pairs; discuss, then share responses with class	List common responses on board
10 minutes	Lecture Part II		*Visuals No. 5, 6, 7*
Conclusion			
5 minutes	State objectives achieved in the class		
	Ask three questions related to topic presented that day	Use clicker to respond	
	Ask two questions related to evaluation of the lecture	Use clicker to respond	

- *Know the content.* Even a written, formal lecture will not hide the insecurity of being unprepared or underprepared. Be certain you clearly explain key points in language understood by the audience; do not use jargon or attempt to impress with effusive speech.
- *Use notes.* The use of notes is generally the option of the speaker; however, to avoid the distress of losing your train of thought or incorrectly presenting complex information, the use of some type of handwritten or computer-based prompts is highly recommended. For ease of handling, record the notes on the computer or on pages/cards that are all the same size and sequentially numbered. If you are using PowerPoint slides to accompany the lecture, you may wish to operationalize the notation section and have your lecture notes or outline appear on the screen in front of you, with or without them being visible to the participants. The depth and content of lecture notes should fit the lecturer's comfort level. Use of anything from a skeletal outline to a full manuscript is acceptable. Notes should be prepared by leaving white space that is easy for your eye to follow.

  Major points should be highlighted so the eye can easily pick up a cue when scanning a page. Although the use of notes is perfectly acceptable, the verbatim reading of notes is *not* acceptable. Rehearse your presentation often enough to appear spontaneous and enthusiastic and to *complete it within the allotted time frame.*
- *Speak to an audience of 200 as if it were a single student.* Speak clearly and loudly enough to be heard in the back of the room. The use of a microphone may be necessary if you are presenting in a large room or auditorium. Always use the microphone if there is any doubt that your voice will not be heard in the last row. It is sometimes helpful to have a friend sit in the back and signal if your voice is not being heard during the presentation. A small clip-on microphone is preferable to a handheld or stationary microphone because it allows the speaker the flexibility to move away from the podium and frees the hands to handle notes and/or gesture. If a microphone is to be used, arrive in the assigned room early enough to try the equipment and to regulate microphone position and sound levels. If the lecture is being transmitted to multiple sites, as in distance/distributive education or video-conferencing settings, be certain to test the sound levels at all sites before beginning the lecture.
- *Make eye contact.* Select a participant at each corner of the room with whom you plan to make eye contact. Slowly scan the audience until you have seen each of the designated participants. Smile at familiar faces. If needed, review information related to the process of group dynamics. If the lecture is being transmitted to multiple sites, be certain to make eye contact via the monitors with participants in the distant sites. You may wish to make a concerted effort to look into each monitor or screen as you visually scan the lecture hall, and address participants at each site.

■ *Use creative movement.* Movements of the speaker's head and hands in gesturing should appear natural, not forced. Be careful when standing behind a podium; do not grip the sides tightly with your hands or lock your (shaky?) knees. This action produces a circulatory response that could cause the speaker to faint. Occasionally step away from the podium and toward the listeners. This conveys an attitude of warmth and acceptance. Avoid distracting mannerisms such as pacing, wringing your hands, clearing your throat, or jamming your hands into pockets and jingling pocket change/keys.

■ *Avoid barriers.* The use of a stage or podium places an automatic barrier between the speaker and the listeners. This gulf should be bridged early and often during the lecture. Suggestions for bridging the gulf include the following:

1. Use notecards rather than a manuscript because they are more portable and allow freedom to move away from the podium.

2. Step out from behind the podium, especially if you are short in stature; the audience does not wish to see a talking head.

3. Walk toward the listeners; this is interpreted as a sign of warmth and reaching out to the audience.

4. Address the right half of the audience, the left half of the audience, and then the audience at each distant site (each monitor or screen), but do not turn your back to either side of the audience or to the transmitting cameras.

5. Call on at least one participant in the audience and at each distant site by name.

6. Use hand gestures to accentuate words, but be careful not to overdo this action (this is especially important if the lecture is being transmitted to multiple sites because large or exaggerated hand gestures are more distracting when seen on a monitor than when viewed live).

7. If given the opportunity to be seated on a stage/platform, be aware of the eye level of the audience, especially if you are wearing a skirt/dress.

■ *Create a change of pace.* An astute lecturer constantly assesses the audience and interprets participants' signals. Facial cues indicate agreement/disagreement with what has been said and may express understanding/misunderstanding of content. Another signal is given when listeners begin having side conversations or squirm in their seats. These signals call for intervention, response, or a change of pace by the speaker. The change of pace can be as simple as turning off the computer/projector, shifting to a new slide, adding sound or animation to your visual, or changing the lighting—any of these actions will cause the listeners to refocus attention on the speaker or back on the visual. Shifting the focus from the speaker to a handout, using a humorous example, altering the tone or inflection of your voice, using automated interaction with feedback from participants, dividing into small groups for a brief discussion, or taking a "stand and stretch" break also can provide a needed change of pace. Keep this rule of thumb in mind: An individual's optimal attention span is roughly 1 minute per year of age up to the approximate age of 30 (e.g., a 5-year-old has a 5-minute attention span; a 25-year-old, 25 minutes), at which point it levels off. Therefore, plan a change of pace or break according to the average age of your audience. Bunce, Flens, and Neiles (2009) found that the attention of undergraduate chemistry students began to lapse within 30 seconds after the beginning of class but quickly returned, only to stray again within 9 minutes. These results cause one to question the necessity of more frequent breaks or changes of pace within class sessions and more specific research into the topic. At any rate, the adage "The mind can only absorb as much as the seat can endure" is a fairly valid and reasonable guideline. Know your audience.

- *Distribute a skeletal outline to help the learners identify key points.* Emphasize principles and concepts. Do not copy charts, graphs, and materials that are found in the learners' texts. Handout information should supplement the lecture. The lecture should not be a rehash of basic information from the learners' textbook. If handouts are used, they should be clear and contain a limited amount of information so the learner is not overwhelmed. Handouts printed on colored paper stand out and are more likely to be read than those printed on white paper. The reproduction or web posting of the PowerPoint slides or lecture notes is a hotly debated topic. Germano (2003) declares technology to be a tool, but notes tools are not friends and are often rivals. Stewart (2006) suggests that the distribution of full-text class notes or slides that contain a significant percentage of the lecture content truly discourages class attendance; however, students tend to request the maximum number of handouts related to the topic. The choice must be left to the individual lecturer.

Several timely publications that may be of assistance in keeping the lecture process fresh are *The Teaching Professor, Change, Masie's Learning Trends, The National Teaching & Learning Forum*, and the *Survival Skills for Scholars* series. In addition, websites maintained by most major universities offer guidance for teaching assistants and novice educators that are helpful.

■ Potential Issues

Factors That Contribute to a Successful Lecture

Nothing/no one is perfect. As with any method or technique, some problems exist when the lecture strategy is used. The key question to be answered is: "What makes lectures and lecturers successful or unsuccessful?" Over the past decade, Woodring has evaluated the response of nursing students to these questions, and each year responses have been consistent. The most frequently cited negative characteristics of lectures/lecturers focus on the person doing the presenting, *not* the method (Woodring & Woodring, 2014). In Tables 10-1 and 10-2, advantages and disadvantages of the lecture as a teaching method were outlined. Now we want to focus on the preparation and presentation of the faculty member as the implementer of the method. The teacher who consistently lectures without integrating other strategies into class time may be subjected to student-generated negative comments, such as "This class is so boring–all he does is lecture"; "It's awful–she reads to us right out of her book"; or "I can't learn to think critically if all she does is talk!" Based on comments such as these, lecturing is often identified as a poor teaching method, a last resort for instruction, when in fairness it is not the method (lecture) but the teacher who is generating the comments. Many lecturers, in fact, do not know how to impart information or stimulate interest effectively; consequently, their lectures are often poorly presented, badly organized, dull, and uninspiring (Gleitman, 2006) . . . all of which lead to boredom among those expecting edutainment.

To present an effective lecture, one must prepare oneself, plan ahead, organize the content, and integrate at least one additional teaching method (e.g., discussion, video stream, audience response system, small-group interaction, role play, or demonstrative props/simulation) into each lecture session. This approach will increase self-assurance (O'Malley & Fleming, 2012) and student interaction and should increase both student and teacher satisfaction. **Table 10-5** identifies attributes of lecturers that learners have perceived as negative and offers some suggestions for improvement.

Institutional Barriers That Lead to Negative Reactions to Lectures

There are certain physical, political, and situational barriers that exist within every institution—any or all of which may contribute to dissatisfaction with any instructional approach. The timing of a class offering is often a factor. Traditionally, teachers have disliked teaching, and students have disliked attending, classes offered at 7 AM or 9 PM. No one likes getting up early or staying in class that late! Classes taught immediately after meal times are considered sleepers because blood leaves the brain and moves to the gastrointestinal tract, making everyone sluggish. Classes taught late in the afternoon or early evenings are difficult because the students and teachers are tired. Try as one may, short of one-on-one teaching or total reliance on online/asynchronous education, the perfect time to hold a class will never be found. Speakers must make their presentations stimulating and motivating at any time of the day! Nevertheless, changes of pace, interactivity, occasional webcasting, and other technologic media that engage students can help offset undesirable time placement of classes.

Another institutional barrier to be considered is the number of students relative to the size of the classroom and the number of students in proportion to the number of faculty (student:faculty ratio). Lecturers are often placed in small, crowded classrooms with large numbers of students or large, cavernous classrooms with small numbers of students. Often, geographical relocation of desks/tables could ease the space configuration and provide a more positive learning atmosphere. Should the lecturer have the option, it is most ideal to be able to clearly see and make eye contact with each participant. This may be accomplished by arranging seating in semicircles around the lectern or angling tables/seats. If seating is fixed within the classroom, then it becomes the responsibility of the speaker to move away from the

Table 10-5 The Lecturer: Perceived Negative Factors and Suggestions for Improvement

Perceived Negative Factors	Suggestions for Improvement
Presentation disorganized or hard to follow	Spend time in practice and preparation.
Lack of outline or outline too detailed	Prepare and follow a brief outline for each lecture.
Presenter lacks professional appearance	Dress as a professional role model. If you are unsure what is acceptable for your role, consult a mentor or esteemed colleague.
Speaker lacks facial expression	Video one of your lectures; view the recording with a friend/colleague and establish goals for improvement.
Monotone voice or nervous/shaky voice	
Facial expression and/or voice lacks enthusiasm	Practice your lecture in front of a mirror until you know the main points by memory.
Reads lecture material; eyes do not meet those of listeners	Use only as many written notes as are absolutely essential; place cues in the margin for yourself. (Smile, walk, and relax!)
Remains behind podium to lecture (referred to as the talking head because that is all students see)	Avoid putting too much information in small print on slides and/or handouts.
Uses no visual aids or visuals of poor quality	Ask a librarian, media center, or learning center personnel for assistance in preparing visuals.
Too many PowerPoint slides	Use visuals to support, not replace, content.
Does not acknowledge that adult learners like to participate	Review techniques for keeping adult learners engaged.
	See references by Cross (1986), Kidd (1973), and Knowles (1970).
Inconsiderate of learners' needs	Schedule breaks and/or implement change-of-pace activities every 30–45 minutes.
Distracting habits of presenter: pacing, staring out windows, playing with objects (paper clips, rubber bands, change), using nonwords (*ah, um*) and repetitious phrases (*you know, like, well, uh*)	Use a video of your lecture to identify repetitive habits.
	Repositioning hands or holding notes may help the nervous-hands problem.
	Make a list of alternative words that could be substituted for the frequently repeated pet phrases.
	Nonwords are a verbalization that allows your speech to catch up to what your brain is thinking; becoming aware of the use of nonwords may or may not be all you need to eliminate them. When they occur, stop, take a deep breath, and then go on.

podium and make eye contact with as many learners as possible, as often as possible. Some of these logistical issues may be addressed as universities remodel or build new classroom facilities. The Masie Center's Classroom of the Future survey (Masie & Chen, 2011) found that despite the popularity of web-based and blended learning, classrooms are not going away. Eighty percent of the 654 respondents indicated plans for continued high usage of classrooms, plans for expanded classroom size, and plans for expanded classroom technologic capabilities (interactive whiteboards, video conferencing via webinar, audience response systems, cameras/microphones, and flexible furniture).

The large student:faculty ratio within classes will probably not decrease in postsecondary education in the near future. Large classes, especially at the freshman and sophomore levels, are very cost-effective. The bottom line will continue to impose restrictions exacerbated by the increase in distance and multisite class sessions and faculty shortages in many health-related professions. The disproportionate student:faculty ratio will require lecturers to implement the tips listed in this chapter, as well as utilize technological support, teaching assistants for smaller group interactions, and other creative strategies to enhance student learning for material presented in large lecture sections. The results of a study of undergraduate students (Long & Coldren, 2006) reinforced the need for the lecturer to make personal connections with students in large classes. There was a positive correlation between the students' perception of interpersonal connection with the faculty and student success in the class.

Helping the Student to Remember Tomorrow?

The problem of retaining information gained from a lecture should be acknowledged and addressed. Although those educators who enjoy using the lecture method hate to admit it, research conducted in the 1990s found that 80% of information gained by lecture alone cannot be recalled by students 1 day later, and that 80% of the remainder fades in a month. Because minimal research has been done to alter this perception, one must still heed the results. Educational data indicate that the more a learner's senses (taste, touch, smell, sight, and hearing) are involved in the learning activity, the longer the knowledge is retained. Therefore, if certain types of equipment are used to illustrate a point (touch, sight), a video clip is inserted into the midst of the lecture (sight, hearing), or any other active learning process (gaming, lab experiments, audience response activities) is introduced, the student's knowledge retention will increase.

In recent years, the use of *punctuated lectures* has also been viewed as a method to increase retention of information. The punctuated lecture requires students and teachers to go through five steps: (1) **listen** (to a portion of a lecture), (2) **stop**, (3) **reflect** (on what they were doing, thinking, and feeling during that portion of the lecture), (4) **write** (what they were doing, thinking, and feeling during that portion of the lecture), and (5) **give** (the written feedback to the lecturer) (Cross & Steadman, 1996). This approach provides the lecturer and the students with an opportunity to become engaged with the learning process, as well as to self-monitor their in-class behaviors. In addition, Brookfield (2006, pp. 100–101) suggests that students cannot read the lecturer's mind. Students cannot be expected to know what teachers expect, stand for, or wish them to value unless that information is explicitly and vigorously communicated to them. The reflective teacher, according to Brookfield, must continually work to build a case for learning, action, and practice rather than assume these values to be self-evident to the learner. Implementing these suggestions should enhance knowledge retention emanating from a lecture.

■ Evaluation

An evaluation of the lecture/lecturer must be completed in a timely manner. The most useful time to obtain this data is at the completion of an individual lecture. Obtaining this information need not be laborious. Ask the listeners to respond to a few specific questions and then allow them to provide additional comments, or pose the questions and allow automated clicker response before learners walk out the door. This type of feedback is especially helpful for the novice lecturer. The evaluation process should aim to provide constructive criticism and comments for improvement. One means of accomplishing this is to allow the students to make any comments they wish; however, a negative comment cannot be made without offering a suggestion for its resolution. When this evaluation technique is used routinely, the learners become accustomed to it. The process can be completed in 5 minutes or less, especially if automated response systems are used. Often, teachers are so interested in assessing whether the course objectives have been met that they forget to evaluate the means by which they were met. Lecturers will not improve without suggested change, and suggested change can best be obtained via the use of a planned evaluation tool/method completed by peers and/or class participants. The evaluation of a lecture or lecturer should not occur in isolation—it must be viewed as a portion of an overall evaluation and development plan—and should be conducted only when there are plans for growth, follow-up, and change. Rhem (2011) suggests that self-assessment and peer evaluation of even the most seasoned lecturer may result in improvement and professional reaffirmation. Be certain to provide feedback to your evaluators; let the class or colleagues know you have made a change in the way you are presenting some topic or how you have changed some assignment based on previous evaluative comments.

■ Conclusion

Presenting an effective lecture is more than a stand-and-deliver process. The lecturer must be knowledgeable, well spoken, organized, creative, and considerate of the learners' needs, abilities, learning styles, and cognitive/developmental level(s). The desired outcomes for the class and the individual objectives of the learners must be addressed. Each section should be planned and presented in an organized manner, never off the cuff. The prepared lecturer will be considerate, credible, and in control (not to be mistaken for rigid and controlling). Several factors enhance the presentation of a lecture, but none is more important than genuine enthusiasm. The lecture should not be considered a secondary teaching strategy. In many situations, it is the most appropriate methodology to be used. To elicit the best results, the lecture should be accompanied by at least one of the other effective strategies discussed in this text.

As we close this chapter on presenting a lecture, we suggest that attention should be paid to the words of the wise elder: Select your words carefully, be sure your words are sweet, because you never know when you will be called upon them to eat! Happy lecturing.

Discussion Questions

1. Reflect on Table 10-2. Pick three disadvantages and apply them to a topic you currently teach. How can you improve your lecture to mitigate the disadvantages?
2. What is the most effective method you use in teaching to capture and hold the attention of your students?

References

Amare, N. (2006). To slideware or not to slideware: Students' experiences with PowerPoint vs. lecture. *Journal of Technical Writing and Communication, 36*(3), 297–308.

Brookfield, S. (2006). *The skillful teacher* (2nd ed.). San Francisco, CA: Jossey-Bass.

Bunce, D., Flens, E., & Neiles, K. (2009). Teaching is more than lecturing and learning is more than memorizing. *Journal of Chemical Education, 86*(6), 674–680.

Burgan, M. (2006). In defense of lecturing. *Change: The Magazine of Higher Education, 38*(6), 30–34.

Caldwell, J. (2007). Clickers in the large classroom: Current research and best-practice tips. *CBE-Life Science Education, 6*(12), 9–20.

Chung, Q. B. (2005). Sage on the stage in the digital age: The role of online lecture in distance learning. *Electronic Journal of e-Learning, 3*(1), 1–14.

Clark, C. (2013). *Creating & sustaining civility in nursing education.* Indianapolis, IN: Sigma Theta Tau International.

Clark, J. (2008). PowerPoint and pedagogy: Maintaining student interest in university lectures. *College Teaching, 56*(1), 39–45.

Costa, M., van Rensburg, L., & Rushton, N. (2007). Does teaching style matter? A randomized trial of group discussion versus lectures in orthopaedic undergraduate teaching. *Medical Education, 41,* 214–217.

Cox, J., & Rogers, J. (2005). Enter: The (well-designed) lecture. *The Teaching Professor, 19*(5), 1–6.

Cross, K. P. (1986, September). A proposal to improve teaching. *AAHE Bulletin,* pp. 9–15.

Cross, K. P., & Steadman, M. H. (1996). *Classroom research: Implementing the scholarship of teaching.* San Francisco, CA: Jossey-Bass.

Di Leonardi, B. C. (2007). Tips for facilitating learning: The lecture deserves some respect. *The Journal of Continuing Education in Nursing, 38*(4), 154–161.

Eble, K. (1982). *The craft of teaching.* San Francisco, CA: Jossey-Bass.

Germano, W. (2003). The scholarly lecture: How to stand and deliver. *Chronicle of Higher Education, 50*(14), 14b.

Gleitman, H. (2006). Lecturing: Using a much maligned method of teaching. In *Teaching at Chicago: A handbook.* Chicago, IL: University of Chicago Center for Teaching and Learning. Retrieved from http://teaching.uchicago.edu/?/ctl-archive/course-design-tutorials/in-the-classroom/gleitman.html

Guertin, L., Bodek, M., Zappe, S., & Kim, H. (2007). Questioning the student use of and desire for lecture podcasts. *Journal of Online Learning and Teaching.* Retrieved from http://jolt.merlot.org/vol3no2/guertin.htm

Harper, B. (2009). I've never seen or heard it this way! Increasing student engagement through the use of technology-enhanced feedback. *Teaching Educational Psychology, 3*(2), 1–8.

Hove, M., & Corcoran, K. (2008). If you post it will they come? Lecture availability in introductory psychology. *Teaching Psychology, 35*(2), 91–95.

Huntley, J. (2009, June). Positioning the CLO. In B. Concevitch (Ed.), *The learning leaders fieldbook* (pp. 31–33). Saratoga Springs, NY: Masie Center. Retrieved from http://www.masie.com/fieldbook

Kidd, J. R. (1973). *How adults learn.* New York, NY: Association Press.

Knowles, M. (1970). *The modern practice of adult education: Andragogy versus pedagogy.* New York, NY: Association Press.

Long, E., & Coldren, J. (2006). Interpersonal influences in large lecture-based classes. *College Teaching, 54*(2), 237–243.

Lowman, J. (1995). *Mastering techniques of teaching* (2nd ed.). San Francisco, CA: Jossey-Bass.

Masie, E. (2006). *Learning trends*. Saratoga, NY: Masie Center. Retrieved from http://trends.masie.com

Masie, E., & Chen, J. (2011). *Classroom of the future & classroom of 2011 survey*. Retrieved from http://masie.com/classroom2011

Mayer, R., Stull, A., DeLeeuw, K., Almeroth, K., Bimber, B., Chun, D., . . . Zhang, H. (2009). Clickers in college classrooms: Fostering learning with questioning methods in large lecture class. *Contemporary Educational Psychology, 34*(1), 51–57.

O'Malley, D., & Fleming, S. (2012). Developing skills for teaching: Reflections on the lecture as a learning tool for the novice midwife educator. *Nurse Education in Practice, 12,* 253–257.

Read, B. (2005). Lectures on the go. *Chronicle of Higher Education, 52*(10), A39.

Rhem, J. (2011). Coaching and teaching. *National Teaching and Learning Forum, 21*(1), 8.

Stewart, E. (2006, February 6). *Class-conscious: Teachers want tech to enhance—not replace lectures. Deseret News (Utah)*. Retrieved from http://www.deseretnews.com/article/635181866/Class-conscious -Teachers-want-tech-to-enhance--not-replace--lectures.html

Waltz, C. F., Jenkins, L. S., & Han, N. (2014). The use and effectiveness of active learning methods in nursing and health professions education: A literature review. *Nursing Education Perspectives, 35*(6), 392–400).

Wiebel, G. (2010). Interactive lectures I. *History Tech*. Retrieved from http://historytech.wordpress .com/?s=interactive+lectures+I

Wolff, M., Wagner, M. J., Poznanski, S., Schiller, J., & Santen, S. (2015). Not another boring lecture: Engaging learners with active learning techniques. *The Journal of Emergency Medicine, 48*(1), 85–93.

Woodring, B., & Woodring, R. (2014). The lecture: Long-lasting, logical, and legitimate. In M. Bradshaw & A. Lowenstein (Eds.), *Innovative teaching strategies in nursing and related health professions* (6th ed., pp. 127–147). Sudbury, MA: Jones & Bartlett.

Young, J. (2008). The lectures are recorded, so why go to class? *Chronicle of Higher Education, 54*(36), A1, A12.

CHAPTER 11

Lighten Up Your Classroom

Mariana D'Amico
Lynn Jaffe

Humor is also a way of saying something serious.

—T. S. Eliot

He who laughs most, learns best.

—John Cleese (Priest, 2007)

■ Introduction

Most educators take learning very seriously, especially those in health care. They overlook the fact that humor is a lifeline to sanity and reality. Humor is not a primary teaching strategy, and it is quite difficult to measure the educational effect of humor in isolation from other teaching methods. However, the judicious use of humor can influence the cognitive and behavioral aspects of learning by engaging at least six of Gardner's seven forms of intelligence (as identified in Chapter 1). Research on humor has been a multidisciplinary endeavor, including a focus on use in classrooms and health care (Adamle, Chiang-Hanisko, Ludwick, Zeller, & Brown, 2007; Bennett, 2003; Chauvet & Hofmeyer, 2007; Garner, 2006; Mallett & A'Hern, 1996; Wrench & McCroskey, 2001; Ziegler, 1998). Well-placed humor can make the classroom environment a safe, comfortable, and effective arena for cognitive and professional growth (Halula, 2013; Jutras, 2009; Mayo, 2010; Nesi, 2012; Purzycki, 2010). Educators have used humor to alleviate classroom stress and facilitate knowledge acquisition and application for decades. Humor contributes to a positive affect and, to that end, humor has been used as a teaching tool for generations. Effectively using humor in the classroom requires knowledge, art, and skill, all of which may be learned (Chiarello, 2010; Garner, 2005, 2006; Hellman, 2007; Zeigler, 1998). This chapter highlights humor as an educator's tool and describes specific strategies for humor use in the classroom.

■ Definition and Purpose

Humor is a communication that induces amusement. Thus, it must be shared. It makes the learning environment a shared, pleasurable experience. In education, the most positive forms of humor are funny stories or comments, jokes, and professional humor. Sarcasm has been recorded as common in the classroom, but tends to be a negative form of humor. *Wit* is the cognitive process that elicits humor. *Mirth* is the emotional reaction to humor, joy, and pleasure. Laughter or smiling is a physical expression of humor. With all these elements, the formal study of humor in the classroom has been a challenge. A decade ago the literature on the use of humor in healthcare education was predominantly opinion pieces or reviews as opposed to actual evidence, although at least a dozen studies of humor were conducted in educational settings (Ziegler, 1998). Whether the evidence is as sound as it should be remains equivocal, but lately the majority of authors praise its contributions to the educational experience (Chauvet & Hofmeyer, 2007; Dormann & Biddle, 2006; Englert, 2010; Garner, 2005, 2006; Golchi & Jamali, 2011; Halula, 2013; Heitzmann, 2010; James, 2004; Makewa, Role, & Genga, 2011; Mayo, 2010; Nesi, 2012; Priest, 2007; Proctor, Maltby, & Linley, 2011; Southam & Schwartz, 2004; Symbaluk & Howell, 2010; Torok, McMorris, & Lin, 2004).

Humor has been studied and discussed from a variety of approaches—the physiologic, psychologic, emotional, and cognitive. Recent reviews have summarized these studies (Hart & Walton, 2010; Nesi, 2012; Purzycki, 2010; Southam & Schwartz, 2004; Torok et al., 2004) and confirmed that humor can promote health as well as learning through the physical benefits of reduced stress, increased productivity, and enhanced creativity. Humor has been deemed a primary vehicle for enhancing the learning environment through enlivening potentially dreary topics, keeping lectures engaging and enjoyable, and humanizing faculty in students' perceptions. The cultivation of the abilities to laugh at oneself and with others bridges many gaps between people and broadens the pathway from student to professional (Adamle et al., 2007; Chiarello, 2010; Field, 2009; Golchi & Jamali, 2011; Hart & Walton, 2010; James, Andershed, Gustavsson, & Ternestedt, 2012; Lei, Cohen, & Russler, 2010; Makewa et al., 2011; Nesi, 2012; Priest, 2007; Proctor et al., 2011). This broadening pathway of humor can level the ground for communication between professionals and patients or clients, and between students and educators (Bennett, 2003; Cleary, Horsfall, & DeCarlo, 2006; Halula, 2013).

The use of humor in the classroom can be productive, promoting comfortable, safe interactions between faculty and students. It has been shown to increase teacher credibility (Garner, 2006; Lei et al., 2010; Makewa et al., 2011; Symbaluk & Howell, 2010; Torok et al., 2004). The effective use of humor promotes creativity, learning, retention, and enculturation of professionals (Adamle et al., 2007; Chauvet & Hofmeyer, 2007; Chiarello, 2010; Dormann & Biddle, 2006; Flournoy, Turner, & Combs, 2001; Lei et al., 2010; Nesi, 2012; Purzycki, 2010; Southam & Schwartz, 2004). Counterproductive humor can cause fear and hostility, decrease self-esteem and motivation, and disrupt the community within classroom and work settings (Berk, 2009; Ciesielka, Conway, Penrose, & Risco, 2005; Laviosa, 2010; Shah & Inamullah, 2011).

Several studies (Chiarello, 2010; Golchi & Jamali, 2011; Makewa et al., 2011; Torok et al., 2004; White, 2001) compared perceptions regarding the use of humor between professors and students, whether students thought more favorably of professors who used humor, and what types of humor were preferred. Their findings had strong correlations between perceptions in the use of funny stories, funny comments, jokes, and professional humor. Students showed mixed support of humor in testing. The use of sarcasm and derogatory humor was not supported. Shibles's (1989) analysis of humor declares that ridicule and sarcasm are used as a superiority differentiation or as a defense mechanism and therefore do not qualify as types of humor. Berk (2009) articulated the need to avoid derogatory and cynical humor in clinical teaching and the workplace by healthcare providers. He advocated the importance of maintaining professionalism, as educators are models for the next generation of providers. Educators need to be cognizant of this because such a misuse of humor will be counterproductive in the classroom and the clinic. Students often found that positive humor facilitated attention, morale, and comprehension (Halula, 2013). Makewa et al. (2011) identified that affiliative humor and self-enhancing humor were most preferred by students. White's study identified agreement between professors and students regarding humor as a tool to relieve stress, create a healthy learning environment, gain attention, and motivate students. An item of greatest variation between faculty and student perceptions was in the use of humor to handle unpleasant situations—students believed it could be used, but faculty did not. Laviosa (2010) and Nesi (2012) identified the importance of cultural awareness of humor and humor context when using humor in the classroom, especially with a culturally diverse student body.

■ Theoretical Foundations

Humor is a complex phenomenon with a long and rich history. While no one has been able to establish when the first joke actually occurred, we know the Greek theater used both comedy and drama to entertain and enlighten. Many authors, such as Dickens and Swift, used satire to comment on society. Theoretical foundations of humor are multiple (Shibles, 1989). They have been categorized by discipline (biological, cognitive, physiological, linguistic, etc.) and construct (incongruity, superiority, affiliative, etc.) (Ziegler, 1998). Boyd (2004) proposes that humor and laughter relate to play theory, and thus create a sense of shared playfulness. He suggests that this sense of playfulness opens the participants to creative and critical thinking and action, while simultaneously alerting and disarming them in an environment of mutual trust and enjoyment. Effective use of humor may be a component of all learning theories. Humor and laughter contribute to all necessary principles of learning: enjoyment; creativity; interest; motivation; a relaxed, open, warm environment; a positive student–teacher relationship; and decreased tension and anxiety (Skinner, 2010). Being authentic is one of the most important qualities of an educator. Having a sense of humor is an aspect of authenticity (Hellman, 2007; Jackson, 2010; Lottes, 2008). Humor used constructively builds a positive self-image (Chauvet & Hofmeyer, 2007; Chiarello, 2010; Field, 2009; Garner, 2005, 2006; Golchi & Jamali, 2011; Hellman, 2007; Lei et al., 2010; Priest, 2007).

Cognitive and affective theories appear to be the most important for education, as they account for linguistic, intellectual, and emotional aspects of learning. Some humor theories state that laughter or amusement occurs as an intellectual reaction to something unexpected, illogical, or inappropriate in some way (Boyd, 2004; Mayo, 2010; Nesi, 2012; Purzycki, 2010; Shibles, 1989). Cognitive theory focuses on an understanding of language, knowledge, situation, and reasoning that addresses recognition of mistakes, incongruity, and wordplays. Research indicates that the recognition of incongruity begins in infancy (Boyd, 2004; Wild, Rodden, Grodd, & Ruch, 2003). Puns, irony, and satire require analysis and synthesis of words, knowledge, and context (Boyd, 2004; Wild et al., 2003). Without such understanding, students do not perceive the humor and may take affront or feel put down by the instructor. When students understand a concept well, they can make jokes or funny remarks about it, indicating their synthesis of the material. Cognition is shaped by culture, and humor has been defined as culturally appropriate incongruity (Boyd, 2004; Chauvet & Hofmeyer, 2007; Purzycki, 2010; Wrench & McCroskey, 2001).

According to Bloom, affect is an important domain of learning. Those theorists who subscribe to affective theory stress emotional components of humor. However, it seems inadequate to treat affect as separate from cognition, because emotion is largely constituted by thought (Shibles, 1989). There has been extensive discussion regarding the emotional and physiologic benefits of releasing psychic energy through laughter. Because of this, humor is an invaluable contribution to the educational process. Its use creates an affirmation of shared understanding and experience (Boyd, 2004). Research supports its use to reduce anxiety and stress, build confidence, improve productivity, reduce boredom, heighten interest, and encourage divergent thinking and the creation of new ideas (Chauvet & Hofmeyer, 2007; Chiarello, 2010; Dormann & Biddle, 2006; Field, 2009; Golchi & Jamali, 2011; Makewa et al., 2011; Mayo, 2010; Nesi, 2012; Purzycki, 2010; Ziegler, 1998).

The affective component of humor engages the limbic system, thereby enhancing both short- and long-term memory and increasing the learner's willingness to apply knowledge and skills (Flournoy et al., 2001; Southam & Schwartz, 2004). Some believe the best time to deliver serious points to students when teaching is right after they laugh (Field, 2009; Hogue, 2010; Makewa et al., 2011). The expression of feelings, such as empathy and anger, can be more constructive when approached in a witty manner (James et al., 2012; Makewa et al., 2011; Nesi, 2012). Both sides of the brain are actively engaged during laughter and the perception of humor (Southam & Schwartz, 2004). The right side of the brain involves reading and interpreting the visual, nonverbal information of humor, whereas the left side of the brain interprets the language nuances of humor. Novelty, imagination, and visualization help move information into long-term memory through the engagement of multiple brain cells firing simultaneously (Purzycki, 2010; Southam & Schwartz, 2004; Wild et al., 2003; Wrench & McCroskey, 2001). However, there is still much research to be done about the neuroscience related to humor and the perceptions about what is humorous (Purzycki, 2010; Wild et al., 2003).

■ Types of Learners

Humor is a type of playfulness that spans multiple ages and venues. Developmentally and intellectually appropriate humor can be employed with all levels of learners (Southam, 2005). Classroom humor relevant to course content is more appreciated by the adult learner than is random humor. It also is necessary to be aware of students' cultural backgrounds, because words and concepts may have different meanings and be misperceived, or worse, be taboo to discuss (Golchi & Jamali, 2011; Hogue, 2010; Jutras, 2009; Lei et al., 2010; Makewa et al., 2011; Mayo, 2010; Nesi, 2012).

Studies have provided mixed reviews about students' acceptance and appreciation of humor used by the teacher. Some studies have shown that gender impacts the acceptance and use of humor, as does the match between the educator's and students' sense of humor (Martin, Puhlik-Doris, Larsen, Gray, & Weir, 2003; Nesi, 2012). The associations found between intellectual ability and sense of humor suggest that educators need a firm check on the cognitive status of their students when employing wit, or they risk offending rather than amusing them (Boyd, 2004; LaFarge, 2004; Tallent, 2010; Wild et al., 2003). Gorham and Christophel (1990, as cited by Southam & Schwartz, 2004) found that learning outcomes of female students were not as influenced by teacher humor as were outcomes in male students, whose achievement was enhanced through the use of humor. Females, while not appreciably influenced by humor in that study, did prefer personal stories that illustrated pertinent points related to course content. Student reaction to humor has been differentially related to the gender of the educator as well, with female educators eliciting less overall appreciation of their efforts to be humorous (Golchi & Jamali, 2011; Nesi, 2012; White, 2001). Acceptance of humor in the classroom has been shown to be positively associated with a student's psychological health (Dziegielewski, Jacinto, Laudadio, & Legg-Rodriguez, 2003; Kuiper, Grimshaw, Leite, & Kirsh, 2004).

■ Conditions for Learning

Humor can be used judiciously throughout a class session or course and in all types of classroom situations: lecture, lab, fieldwork, and various course assignments. Mood can enhance or inhibit the reception of humor (Heitzmann, 2010; Wild et al., 2003), making it imperative to read the class members accurately and create a positive and pleasant classroom experience. Positive and constructive humor can be used to put the learner and the teacher at ease with the subject matter (Garner, 2005, 2006; Hellman, 2007; Lei et al., 2010; Makewa et al., 2011; Nesi, 2012; Purzycki, 2010). Humorous activities, or ice-breakers, that relate to the class session topic might begin a class. These activities can also be inserted at intervals to reaffirm the open, relaxed atmosphere that is most conducive to learning. Humor generated from course-content-related games can also create a fun learning environment and content retention (Glendon & Ulrich, 2005). Tension relievers before exams are usually helpful. As long as the humor remains embedded in the content, learners will internalize the new knowledge; otherwise, the flow of the lesson can be lost or misdirected (Weaver & Cotrell, 2001). Humor can be used to facilitate creativity and retention of material at any point in a lesson—from initial setup through final review (Chauvet & Hofmeyer, 2007; Garner, 2006; Hellman, 2007). Purzycki (2010) found that using minimally counterintuitive ideas increased recall and retention of new concepts. These ideas challenge the students' current cognitive knowledge template about a topic by presenting an exaggerated or unexpected parallel idea related to topic content or knowledge application.

Relationship between class size and classroom size may impact the effective use of humor. Berk (2002, as cited by Torok et al., 2004) noted that laughter is likely to be greater in larger, more crowded classes than in smaller classes in larger rooms. Laughter, like yawning, is contagious, so once a large group gets going it may take time to bring them back to focus. Dziegielewski and colleagues (2003) encourage the group leader (educator in this case) not to stop the laughter, but to let it stop of its own accord. They perceive that this laughter helps reduce anger and tension and may build cohesion and well-being—both of which are essential to productivity and learning.

Humor is a part of communication and not dependent on the natural comedic ability of an instructor. It is an attitude and permission for enjoyment of the educational process (Adamle et al., 2007; Chauvet & Hofmeyer, 2007; Golchi & Jamali, 2011; Joyner & Young, 2006; Makewa et al., 2011; Nesi, 2012; Weaver & Cotrell, 2001). It can be spontaneous or planned. Weaver and Cottrell recommend inserting humorous breaks every 15 minutes. Golchi and Jamali (2011) recommend delivering the most important content or concept for learning just after a good laugh, when the mind is relaxed and opened to new learning. Essential to creating open communication and allowing humor within the classroom is the teacher's nonverbal communication and voice tone, as these can convey openness or constrict enjoyment of learning. If the humor style of the teacher and that of the class do not mesh, then the use of humor in the learning process will not be effective (Golchi & Jamali, 2011; Makewa et al., 2011; Nesi, 2012). It is important to understand your audience—which in this case is the class—and to know one's own sense of humor and be willing to experiment with others (Garner, 2006; Hellman, 2007; Wild et al., 2003).

Humor is not necessarily universally appropriate. McMorris, Boothroyd, and Pietrangelo (1997) summarized studies that used humor in testing situations, with mixed results. Positive results depended on the type of humor used. Some studies found humor to reduce tension, but others found it to be distracting in a testing situation. Humor with a strong linguistic base may also disadvantage international students (Lei et al., 2010; Nesi, 2012). Likewise, as mentioned previously, any use of sarcasm was seen to be detrimental to learning (Berk, 2009; Garner, 2006; Hellman, 2007; Nesi, 2012; Shah & Inamullah, 2011; Torok et al., 2004).

Humor can be very useful in the enculturation of novices into one's profession, especially when dealing with the elements of embarrassing intimacy and reality shocks that may occur in healthcare provision (Adamle et al., 2007; Chiarello, 2010; Hart & Walton, 2010; James et al., 2012; Southam & Schwartz, 2004). A healthy sense of humor is related to being able to laugh at one's self and one's life without degrading oneself. Those who enter the health professions must be able to cope with adversity and be able to help others cope as well (Adamle et al., 2007; Hart & Walton, 2010; James et al., 2012). The development of a healthy sense of humor, beginning in preservice classes and continuing through professional in-services, benefits everyone.

■ Resources

As with any teaching strategy, the effective use of humor has to be learned and refined. Before using humor in teaching situations, educators may want to assess their own sense of humor using a humor profile such as the one developed by Richmond, Wrench, and Gorham (2001) (see **Appendix 11-1**). The score obtained on the humor profile reflects one's use of humor during communications. Completion of a humor profile is a preliminary step to learning one's current facility with humorous content.

Some ways to increase one's use of humor include exposing oneself to and collecting humorous experiences, such as reading comics, sitcoms, and joke books; visiting comedy clubs; and even looking for the humor around oneself. This may include viewing the world through exaggeration or broad, silly perspectives. Using exaggeration is a method to clarify concepts: the contrast assists understanding. Incongruity is another technique for promoting humor in the classroom, which Mayo's (2010) and Purzycki's (2010) studies found aided retention and recall of concepts and application. One such example is comparing a stripper and a corporate CEO regaining work skills (see the applied example in **Box 11-1**). Creating a top 10 list of teacher pet peeves or preferred learning behaviors can be a humorous way to share class performance expectations (Kher, Molstad, & Donahue, 1999). Using props in the classroom for role playing may also enhance the humor of a lesson (Joyner & Young, 2006;

Box 11-1   Applied Examples

At the beginning of a class, in this case a pediatrics class on toddler development, cartoons that related to the lecture topic were used as a starting point for discussion. The cartoons had been selected from the daily newspaper over a span of years, so there were many examples of toddler behaviors to choose from. Students who had their own children, or younger siblings, were able to immediately relate to the cartoon situations and discuss the behaviors depicted as well as other toddler behaviors and observations they had seen. Students without children and siblings participated in the discussion by asking questions of those with more experience. A lively discussion ensued. When presented with the accompanying reading material or tested on the material at a later date, students exhibited better retention and recall of the information and the discussion that occurred around the visual cue of the cartoon.

Another example of a humor-enhanced class discussion related to client-centered evaluation by using exaggerated comparison and contrast of a stripper's and a CEO's daily activity routines, expectations, and needs. Students started discussing their perceived stereotypes of these exaggerated individuals and, as new elements of typical activities of daily living were tossed out to the students to analyze for these individuals, another lively discussion occurred. When assessed for their understanding of activities of daily living evaluations, analyses, and syntheses for treatment plans, students exhibited a greater understanding of these processes related to individualized care with attention to details.

Polek, 2007; Priest, 2007). The cinema and YouTube are treasure troves of humorous situations just waiting to be tapped by the healthcare professional who is looking for examples of exaggeration, incongruity, or basic fun (Polek, 2007).

Articles about infusing humor into online courses have suggested a number of techniques to promote a positive learning environment in the virtual classroom that mirror applications of humor in the regular classroom. Primary among these techniques is the use of humor to project an authentic representation of the educator. The humor used, by necessity, is primarily linguistic, although cartoons are readily available (James, 2004; Nesi, 2012). Being humorous online requires extensive commitment, time, and effort, as it must be planned, personalized to the students, and monitored for receptivity (Boynton, as cited by James, 2004; Nesi, 2012). The following are a good start for the educator seeking humor:

1. Web resources (available as of publication; web addresses may change)
   Humor Matters Bibliography and Resources: http://www.humormatters.com/bibindex.htm
   Learning the art of using humor: http://www.humorproject.com/
2. Sources for cartoon humor (some resources are paid services)
   Cartoons from the *New Yorker* magazine: http://www.cartoonbank.com
   Single cartoons by Randy Glasbergen, often about business or family: http://www.glasbergen.com/
   Variety of popular newspaper cartoon serials: http://www.gocomics.com/explore/comics
3. Print resources
   Print versions of cartoons (*Far Side, For Better or Worse, Calvin and Hobbes, Zits,* etc.), local newspapers, bookstores
   Desk calendars such as "A Little Bit of Oy," "The Far Side," and "Charlie Brown"
   Cathcart, T., & Klein, D. (2007). *Plato and a Platypus Walk into a Bar: Understanding Philosophy Through Jokes*. New York, NY: Penguin Group.
   Cathcart, T., & Klein, D. (2009). *Heidegger and a Hippo Walk Through Those Pearly Gates: Using Philosophy (and Jokes!) to Explore, Life, Death, the After-life, and Everything in Between*. New York, NY: Penguin Group.
   Tibballs, G. (2000). *The Mammoth Book of Humor*. New York, NY: Carroll & Graf.
4. Check the humor section of any bookstore.

■ Using the Method

The use of humor can be learned and has a growing evidence base, yet remains highly individualized. The Humor Project, developed in 1977, is one workshop venue for learning how to use humor effectively. Humor is often a skill picked up and used by healthcare professionals when assessing health, recovery, and state of well-being of patients or residents in healthcare facilities (Hart & Walton, 2010; James et al., 2012; Proctor et al., 2011). Gender, culture, ethnicity, mood, and context affect the acceptance or rejection of this teaching strategy (Garner, 2005, 2006; Laviosa, 2010; Lei et al., 2010; Makewa et al., 2011; Nesi, 2012; Wild et al., 2003; Wimer & Beins,

2008; Ziegler, 1998). Nesi (2012) and Wanzer and Frymier (1999) found that witty, rather than funny, professors were considered interesting, entertaining, and motivating by adult learners. Robinson is often cited (Southam & Schwartz, 2004) as proposing four interrelated aspects to be considered in the area of education and humor: (1) enhancing the learning process itself through humor; (2) using humor to facilitate the process of socialization; (3) teaching the concept of humor as a communication and intervention tool; and (4) modeling the use of humor as a vehicle for facilitating the other three. Using humor in the classroom does not mean one must attempt to become a comedian. It involves assuming an attitude of authenticity and comfort within the classroom (Garner, 2005, 2006; Golchi & Jamali, 2011; Hellman, 2007; Jackson, 2010; Lottes, 2008; Makewa et al., 2011; Nesi, 2012; Polek, 2007; Purzycki, 2010). Chiarello (2010) conducted a qualitative study of a clinical supervisor's deliberate use of humor for eight nursing students. Seven of the eight students were responsive to the humor and identified the use of humor as beneficial to their learning and growth.

The ability to learn to use humor has been questioned by a few authors (Wrench & McCroskey, 2001). These authors distinguish sense of humor, a culturally taught trait, from the act of being humorous, which may be a genetic trait. However, most authors promote the idea that the use of humor not only can be learned, but also ought to be learned by educators to enhance the teaching–learning process (Adamle et al., 2007; Chauvet & Hofmeyer, 2007; Dormann & Biddle, 2006; Englert, 2010; Garner, 2006; Mayo, 2010; Nesi, 2012; Priest, 2007; Skinner, 2010; Symbaluk & Howell, 2010). Employing humorous methods is within every educator's reach and will enhance the educational experience for students.

Using humor in the learning process can take several forms. It is easy for most faculty to use spontaneous storytelling by relating their own experiences to enhance the learning process. Other faculty may need to collect jokes, cartoons, movie excerpts, and humorous exercises to insert into their regular teaching activities to enhance the learner's receptivity to information and participation during content presentations. **Box 11-2** collects some useful tips.

Box 11-2   Tips for Using Humor in the Classroom

1. Create a casual and safe atmosphere.
2. Smile; adopt a laugh-ready attitude.
3. Relax; use an open nonverbal posture; increase interpersonal contact through eye-to-eye and face-to-face contact.
4. Remove social inhibitions; establish a nonjudgmental forum for discussion.
5. Begin the class with a humorous example, cartoon, anecdote, or thought for the day.
6. Use personal stories, anecdotes, and current events related to class content.
7. Plan frequent breaks in content for application for humorous commercials or exaggerated examples; provide humorous materials.
8. Encourage give and take with students; laugh at yourself occasionally.

Data from Provine, R. R. (2000). *Laughter: A scientific investigation.* New York, NY: Viking Penguin; Weaver, R. L., & Cotrell, H. W. (2001). Ten specific techniques for developing humor in the classroom. *Education, 108*(2), 167–179.

Tamblyn (2003) highly recommends the frequent use of visuals such as cartoons, posters, and other images throughout an educational presentation to enhance the impact of the content. From a cognitive load perspective, the use of cartoons may enhance recall and retention due to the complementary effect of visual and verbal information processing, as long as the cartoon/text match is consistent with the course content and learning level of the student (Khalil, Paas, Johnson, & Payer, 2005; Makewa et al., 2011; Nesi, 2012). As has been mentioned, faculty must realize that what works for some people does not necessarily work for others (Boyd, 2004; Makewa et al., 2011; Mayo, 2010; Nesi, 2012; Tamblyn, 2003; Wild et al., 2003). Nesi (2012) found that some Asian cultures perceived humor used in the classroom as inappropriate.

Some specific techniques for including humor in a class situation include posting humorous situations on a bulletin board to teach interactive concepts (Flournoy et al., 2001). Using irony to contrast expected outcomes and actual occurrence enhances remembrance because of incongruity (Mayo, 2010; Nesi, 2012; Purzycki, 2010). Case studies with funny names related to topical content also enhance memory of the examples. (Example: Petunia Potter liked working in her garden. She needed some ergonomic changes to facilitate her participation in this avocation; how would you adapt this occupation for her?) Use of exaggerations and unusual professions increases awareness of people's needs in the healthcare arena. Personal stories about real-life experiences and challenges in one's role as a new professional, or unexpected circumstances (or embarrassing moments), can have teaching value. Sometimes when students are called on to do group presentations on a given topic, they will use humor (often in the form of mimicry or parody of the instructors) to engage their classmates and, possibly, to alleviate their own stress. Humor usage will be as variable as those using it, which can be quite diverse (Chauvet & Hofmeyer, 2007; Garner, 2006; Hellman, 2007; Makewa et al., 2011; Nesi, 2012; Priest, 2007).

A picture's meaning can express ten thousand words.

—Often misquoted Chinese proverb

■ Potential Problems

Not everyone gets a joke (Boyd, 2004; Wild et al., 2003). Some people are too serious. Some do not value humor in the educational process. Some find it too distracting to their learning. Using sarcasm, ridicule, and put-down humor can be counterproductive. Humor has the potential to be offensive, especially with ethnic, cultural, or gender issues. Incongruence between innate or cultural humor perceptions can be disruptive to the coordination of the learning environment. Besides potentially offending some members of a class, the use of deprecatory humor may affect students' perceptions of the faculty and undermine faculty effectiveness. Class clowns, who use humor for personal gain, also abuse the strategy and detract from the learning environment (Martin et al., 2003). It is essential for educators to remember that they are role models and exert power over students by their modeling (Berk, 2009; Shah & Inamullah, 2011), and thus should be cognizant of the type of humor used in communications (see **Box 11-3**).

**Box 11-3   Example of a Joke That May Be Appropriate for
a Class on Clinical Reasoning**

Sherlock Holmes and Dr. Watson went camping. After a good meal and an excellent bottle of wine, they lay down and went to sleep. A couple of hours later, Holmes woke up and nudged his faithful friend.

"Watson, Watson," he said. "Look up at the sky and tell me what you see?"
"I see millions and millions of stars," replied Watson.
"And what does that tell you?" inquired the master detective.

Watson thought for a moment, "Well, Holmes, astronomically, it tells me that there are millions of galaxies and potentially billions of planets. Astrologically, I observe that Saturn is in Leo. Horologically, I deduce that the time is approximately 2:25. Theologically, I can see that god is all powerful and that we are small and insignificant. Meteorologically, I believe we will have a glorious day tomorrow. What does it tell you, Holmes?"

"Watson, you imbecile! Some thief has stolen our tent!"

Reproduced from Tibballs, G. (2000). *The mammoth book of humor.* New York, NY: Carroll & Graf; joke 2470. Copyright © Dec 6, 2011 Geoff Tibballs. Reprinted by permission of Running Press, a member of the Perseus Books Group.

■ Conclusion

It has been said that Plato believed one could discover more about a person in an hour of play than in a year of conversation. The same could be said about the culture of a classroom, cohort, or department. Teaching–learning communities are built on engagement and communication among students and faculty. The development of respect and desire to learn can be facilitated with the thoughtful use of humor. All involved will find their creativity, enjoyment, and problem solving boosted by this cognitively stimulating and emotionally safe learning environment.

Discussion Questions

1. Discuss your level of agreement with the definition of humor in this chapter; give modifications and/or examples of when you have used or experienced humor in a classroom.
2. What types of humor might negatively affect classroom productivity?
3. Can the use of humor be learned, or must a person be naturally humorous?

References

Adamle, K., Chiang-Hanisko, L., Ludwick, R., Zeller, R, & Brown, R. (2007). Comparing teaching practices about humor among nursing faculty: An international collaborative study. *International Journal of Nursing Education, Scholarship, 4*(1), Article 2.

Bennett, H. J. (2003). Humor in medicine. *Southern Medical Journal, 96*(12), 1257–1261.

Berk, R. (2009). Derogatory and cynical humour in clinical teaching and the workplace: The need for professionalism. *Medical Education, 43,* 7–9. doi:10.1111/j.1365-2923.2008.03239

Boyd, B. (2004). Laughter and literature: A play theory of humor. *Philosophy and Literature, 28*(1), 1–22.

Chauvet, S., & Hofmeyer, A. (2007). Humor as a facilitative style in problem-based learning environments for nursing students. *Nurse Education Today, 27,* 286–292.

Chiarello, M. (2010). Humor as a teaching tool: Use in psychiatric undergraduate nursing. *Journal of Psychosocial Nursing, 48*(8), 34–41.

Ciesielka, D., Conway, A., Penrose, J., & Risco, K. (2005). Maximizing resources: The S.H.A.R.E. model of collaboration. *Nursing Education Perspectives, 26*(4), 224–226.

Cleary, M., Horsfall, J., & DeCarlo, P. (2006). Improving student learning in mental health settings: The views of clinical stakeholders. *Nurse Education in Practice, 6*, 141–148.

Dormann, C., & Biddle, R. (2006). Humour in game-based learning. *Learning, Media and Technology, 31*(4), 411–424.

Dziegielewski, S. F., Jacinto, G. A., Laudadio, A., & Legg-Rodriguez, L. (2003). Humor: An essential communication tool in therapy. *International Journal of Mental Health, 32*(3), 74–90.

Englert, L. (2010). Learning with laughter: Using humor in the classroom. *Nursing Education Perspectives, 33*(1), 48–49.

Field, A. (2009). Can humour make students love statistics? *The Psychologist, 22*(3), 210–213.

Flournoy, E., Turner, G., & Combs, D. (2001). Critical care: Read the writing on the wall. *Nursing, 31*(3), 8–10.

Garner, R. (2005). Humor, analogy, and metaphor: H.A.M. it up in teaching. *Radical Pedagogy, 6*(2). Retrieved from http://radicalpedagogy.icaap.org/content/issue6_2/garner.html

Garner, R. (2006). Humor in pedagogy: How ha-ha can lead to aha! *College Teaching, 54*(1), 177–180.

Glendon, K., & Ulrich, D. (2005). Syllabus selections: Innovative learning activities: Using games as a teaching strategy. *Journal of Nursing Education, 44*(7), 238–239.

Golchi, M., & Jamali, F. (2011). The effect of teacher's verbal humor on advanced EFL learners' classroom anxiety. *European Journal of Social Sciences, 26*(2), 185–192.

Halula, S. P. (2013). What role does humor in the higher education classroom play in student-perceived instructor effectiveness? *Dissertations (2009-)*, Paper 252. Retrieved from http://epublications.marquette.edu/dissertations_mu/252

Hart, R., & Walton, M. (2010). Magic as a therapeutic intervention to promote coping in hospitalized pediatric patients. *Pediatric Nursing, 36*(1), 11–17.

Heitzmann, R. (2010, May). *10 suggestions for enhancing lecturing.* Retrieved from http://www.eddigest.com

Hellman, S. V. (2007). Humor in the classroom: Stu's seven simple steps to success. *College Teaching, 55*(1), 37–39.

Hogue, B. (2010). I'm not making this up: Taking humor seriously in the creative nonfiction classroom. *Pedagogy: Critical Approaches to Teaching Literature, Language, Composition and Culture, 11*(1), 199–205.

Jackson, J. (2010). On ethnic sincerity. *Current Anthropology, 51*(2), S279–S287. doi:10.1086/653129

James, D. (2004). Commentary: A need for humor in online courses. *College Teaching, 52*(3), 93–94.

James, I., Andershed, B., Gustavsson, B., & Ternestedt, B. (2012). Knowledge constructions in nursing practice: Understanding and integrating different forms of knowledge. *Qualitative Health Research, 20*(11), 1500–1518. doi:10.1177/1049732310376042

Joyner, B., & Young, L. (2006). Teaching medical students using role play: Twelve tips for successful role plays. *Medical Teacher, 28*(3), 225–229.

Jutras, P. (2009, November/December). Could we use a good laugh? *Clavier Companion.*

Khalil, M. K., Paas, F., Johnson, T. E., & Payer, A. F. (2005). Interactive and dynamic visualizations in teaching and learning of anatomy: A cognitive load perspective. *Anatomical Record, 286B*, 8–14.

Kher, N., Molstad, S., & Donahue, R. (1999). Using humor in the college classroom to enhance teaching effectiveness in "dread courses." *College Student Journal, 33*, 400–404.

Kuiper, N. A., Grimshaw, M., Leite, C., & Kirsh, G. (2004). Humor is not always the best medicine: Specific components of sense of humor and psychological well-being. *Humor, 17*, 135–168.

LaFarge, B. (2004). Comedy's intention. *Philosophy and Literature, 28*(1), 118–136.

Laviosa, S. (2010). Deconstructing humour across languages and genres. *U.S.-China Foreign Language, 8*(7), 26–43.

Lei, S., Cohen, J., & Russler, K. (2010). Humor on learning in the college classroom: Evaluating benefits and drawbacks from instructors' perspectives. *Journal of Instructional Psychology, 37*(4), 326–331.

Lottes, N. (2008). FIRE UP: Tips for engaging student learning. *Journal of Nursing Education, 47*(7), 331–332.

Makewa, L., Role, E., & Genga, J. (2011). Teachers' use of humor in teaching and students' rating of their effectiveness. *International Journal of Education, 3*(2), 1–17.

Mallett, J., & A'Hern, R. (1996). Comparative distribution and use of humour within nurse-patient communication. *International Journal of Nursing Studies, 33*(5), 530–550.

Martin, R. A., Puhlik-Doris, P., Larsen, G., Gray, J., & Weir, K. (2003). Individual differences in uses of humor and their relation to psychological well-being: Development of the Humor Styles Questionnaire. *Journal of Research in Personality, 37,* 28–75.

Mayo, C. (2010). Incongruity and provisional safety: Thinking through humor. *Studies in Philosophy and Education, 29,* 509–521. doi:10.1007/s11217-010-9195-6

McMorris, R. F., Boothroyd, R. A., & Pietrangelo, D. J. (1997). Humor in educational testing: A review and discussion. *Applied Measurement in Education, 10*(3), 269–297.

Nesi, H. (2012). Laughter in university lectures. *Journal of English for Academic Purposes, 11,* 79–89. doi:10.1016/j.jeap.2011.12.003

Polek, C. (2007). The podium as a stage: A one woman act. *Nurse Educator, 32*(1), 8–10.

Priest, A. (2007). Learning through laughter. *Nursing BC, 39*(5), 8–11.

Proctor, C., Maltby, J., & Linley, P. A. (2011). Strengths use as a predictor of well being and health related quality of life. *Journal of Happiness Studies, 12,* 153–169. doi:10.1007/s10902-009-9181-2

Provine, R. R. (2000). *Laughter: A scientific investigation.* New York, NY: Viking Penguin.

Purzycki, B. G. (2010). Cognitive architecture, humor and counterintutiveness: Retention and recall of MCIs. *Journal of Cognition and Culture, 10*(1), 189–204. doi:10.1163/156853710X497239

Richmond, V. P., Wrench, J. S., & Gorham, J. (2001). *Communication, affect, and learning in the classroom.* Acton, MA: Tapestry Press.

Shah, J., & Inamullah, H. M. (2011). Social power of teacher. *European Journal of Social Sciences, 21*(4), 516–521.

Shibles, W. (1989). *Humor reference guide.* Retrieved from http://www.drbarbaramaier.at/shiblesw/humorbook/index.html

Skinner, M. E. (2010, October). All joking aside: Five reasons to use humor in the classroom. *The Education Digest,* 19–21.

Southam, M. (2005). Humor development: An important cognitive and social aid in the growing child. *Physical and Occupational Therapy in Pediatrics, 25*(1), 105–117. doi:0.1300/j006v25no1_07

Southam, M., & Schwartz, K. B. (2004). Laugh and learn: Humor as a teaching strategy in occupational therapy education. *Occupational Therapy in Health Care, 18,* 57–70.

Symbaluk, D., & Howell, A. (2010). Web-based student feedback: Comparing teaching-award and research-award recipients. *Assessment & Evaluation in Higher Education, 35*(1), 75–86.

Tallent, R. (2010, November/December). Education: What makes teaching worthwhile. *Quill, 12.*

Tamblyn, D. (2003). *Laugh and learn: 95 ways to use humor for more effective teaching and training.* New York, NY: American Management Association.

Tibballs, G. (2000). *The mammoth book of humor.* New York, NY: Carroll & Graf; joke 2470.

Torok, S. E., McMorris, R. F., & Lin, W-C. (2004). Is humor an appreciated teaching tool? Perceptions of professors' teaching styles and use of humor. *College Teaching, 52,* 14–20.

Wanzer, M. B., & Frymier, A. B. (1999). The relationship between student perceptions of instructor humor and students' reports of learning. *Communication Education, 48,* 48–62.

Weaver, R. L., & Cotrell, H. W. (2001). Ten specific techniques for developing humor in the classroom. *Education, 108*(2), 167–179.

White, G. W. (2001). Teachers' report of how they used humor with students' perceived use of such humor. *Education, 122*(2), 337–347.

Wild, B., Rodden, F., Grodd, W., & Ruch, W. (2003). Neural correlates of laughter and humour. *Brain, 126,* 2121–2138.

Wimer, D., & Beins, B. (2008). Expectations and perceived humor. *Humor, 21*(3), 347–363.

Wrench, J., & McCroskey, J. (2001). A temperamental understanding of humor communication and exhilaratability. *Communication Quarterly, 49,* 142–159.

Ziegler, J. B. (1998). Use of humour in medical teaching. *Medical Teacher, 20*(4), 341–348.

Richmond Humor Assessment Instrument

The Richmond Humor Assessment Instrument (RHAI) was designed to be a self-report measure of an individual's use of humor in communication. Unlike some other similar measures, this instrument does not focus on a particular kind of humor (e.g., storytelling). Alpha reliability estimates for this measure have been near 0.90.

■ Directions

The following statements apply to how people communicate humor when relating to others. Indicate the degree to which each of these statements applies to you by filling in the number of your response in the blank before each item:

5 = Strongly Agree; 4 = Agree; 3 = Undecided; 2 = Disagree; 1 = Strongly Disagree

_____1. I regularly communicate with others by joking with them.

_____2. People usually laugh when I make a humorous remark.

_____3. I am not funny or humorous.

_____4. I can be amusing or humorous without having to tell a joke.

_____5. Being humorous is a natural communication orientation for me.

_____6. I cannot relate an amusing idea well.

_____7. My friends would say that I am a humorous or funny person.

_____8. People don't seem to pay close attention when I am being funny.

_____9. Even funny ideas and stories seem dull when I tell them.

_____10. I can easily relate funny or humorous ideas to the class.

_____11. I would say that I am not a humorous person.

_____12. I cannot be funny, even when asked to do so.

_____13. I relate amusing stories, jokes, and funny things very well to others.

_____14. Of all the people I know, I am one of the least amusing or funny persons.

_____15. I use humor to communicate in a variety of situations.

_____16. On a regular basis, I do not communicate with others by being humorous or entertaining.

■ Scoring

To compute your scores, add your scores for each item as indicated here. Recode items 3, 6, 8, 9, 11, 12, 14, and 16 with the following format:

1 = 5

2 = 4

3 = 3

4 = 2

5 = 1

After you have recoded the previous questions, add all of the numbers together to get your composite RHAI score.

Score should be between 16 and 80. Scores of 60 and more indicate high degrees of humor usage; scores of 30 and less indicate low degrees of humor usage; scores between 30 and 60 indicate moderate degrees of humor usage.

Richmond, V. P., Wrench, J. S., & Gorham, J. (2001). *Communication, affect, and learning in the classroom.* Acton, MA: Tapestry Press; Wrench, J. S., & McCroskey, J. C. (2001). A temperamental understanding of humor communication and exhilaratability. *Communication Quarterly, 49,* 170–183.

CHAPTER 12

Problem-Based Learning

Liliana Coman
Patricia Solomon

Problem-based learning (PBL) is an educational process in which learning is centered on problems as opposed to discrete, subject-related courses. In small groups, students are presented with patient scenarios or problems, generate learning issues related to what they need to learn to understand the problem, engage in independent self-study, and return to their groups to apply their new knowledge to the patient problem. PBL is largely acknowledged as starting in the medical school at McMaster University in the mid-1960s in response to an educational environment that emphasized passive learning of large quantities of information that was quickly outdated and often appeared irrelevant. The emphasis in PBL is on learning all content in an integrative way through small-group, self-directed study of a problem with the assistance of a faculty instructor who is a facilitator of learning rather than an expert lecturer (Walton & Matthews, 1989). There is increasing support for the idea that PBL is effective because it encourages the activation of prior knowledge and provides the opportunity for elaborating on that knowledge in small-group settings (Hmelo-Silver, 2004; Schmidt, Rotgans, & Yew, 2011).

Shin and Kim (2013) conducted a meta-analysis of the available literature in order to synthesize the effects of PBL in nursing education. The authors found that PBL has positive effects on the outcome domains of satisfaction with training, clinical education, and skill course. Whereas PBL is theoretically more effective in structuring knowledge, the most agreed-upon advantage is that it is more enjoyable than traditional learning methods.

■ Background and Definitions

Since being introduced, PBL has been adopted by many health professional programs worldwide (Neville, 2009). The evolution of the scientific literature on PBL was described recently by Pinho, Mota, Conde, Alves, and Lopes (2015). Through a bibliometric analysis, the authors were able to show a strong, steady progression of scientific production on PBL since the end of the last century, with the United States, the United Kingdom, Canada, Australia, and The Netherlands having the highest number of publications since 1992.

Schmidt, van der Molen, Te Winkel, and Wijnen (2009) suggest that the literature includes at least three perspectives on PBL: PBL as a process of inquiry, as a learning-to-learn process, and as a constructivist approach to learning. Although many variants of PBL have been described, the following essential elements remain: (1) students are presented with a written problem or patient scenario in small groups; (2) there is a change in faculty role from imparter of information to facilitator of learning; (3) there is an emphasis on student responsibility and self-directed learning; and (4) a written problem is the stimulus for learning, with students engaging in a problem-solving process as they learn and discuss content related to the problem (Hmelo-Silver, 2004; Schmidt et al., 2011; Solomon, 1994).

Whereas PBL may be viewed as an educational methodology, it is most often associated with an overall curricular approach. PBL was originally viewed as an all-or-none phenomenon in which an educational program had to commit entirely to the curricular philosophy to attain the most benefits (Barrows & Tamblyn, 1980). Programs that had individual problem-based courses and more traditional courses running concurrently were thought to send mixed messages to the student and devalue the problem-based components (Walton & Matthews, 1989). Although there is still concern that isolated problem-based courses will not be successful (Albanese, 2000), there is greater acceptance of curricula that use mixed or partial PBL approaches. Fyrenius, Bergdahl, and Silén (2005) argue that lectures can be used as valuable tools for learning in a PBL curriculum.

There have been several attempts to define and classify PBL curricula. Barrows (1986) describes a taxonomy based largely on the problem design and role of the teacher. Charlin, Mann, and Hansen (1998) present an analytic framework to understand and compare PBL curricula that varies along 10 dimensions, such as the purpose of the problem and the nature of the task to be accomplished during study of the problem. Harden and Davis (1998) offer an 11-step continuum of PBL, with theoretical learning and an emphasis on traditional lectures and textbooks at one end, and task-based learning (essentially learning in clinical practice settings with real patients) at the other. As one moves along the continuum, there is greater emphasis on the problem, activation of prior knowledge, contextual learning, and discovery learning. Solomon, Binkley, and Stratford (1996) provide a simple distinction between a problem-based curriculum, which they describe as "fully integrated" (with few or no subject-related courses), and a transitional PBL curriculum, which uses traditional curricular elements early in the curriculum and incorporates increasingly larger components of PBL as the students progress through their program.

■ Theoretical Foundations

Some of the original theoretical premises for PBL have not found strong support within the literature. Contextual learning, with roots in the constructivist learning theory, was an appealing rationale for the superiority of PBL. The rationale was that by learning all content (including basic, clinical, and social sciences) within the context of a problem, a learner would be able to recall information better when he or she encountered a similar patient or problem within the clinical setting (Clifford & Wilson, 2000). However, there is weak empirical support for this theory, and it is likely too simplistic to integrate the complexities associated with PBL (Colliver, 2000).

The information processing theory, proposed by Miller in 1956, incorporates aspects of contextual learning theory and provides more comprehensive theoretical support for PBL, as it also considers activation of prior knowledge and elaboration of knowledge as core elements (Albanese, 2000; Schmidt et al., 2011). However, one theory may be insufficient support for PBL. Albanese (2000) outlines three others that are salient to PBL: cooperative learning theory, self-determination theory, and control theory.

Cooperative learning, based on Vygotsky's social development theory (McLeod, 2007), in which individuals are dependent on other group members to achieve their goals, is used extensively in small-group PBL. Learning occurs through mutual interaction and shared understanding (Dolmans, De Grave, Wolfhagen, & van der Vleuten, 2005). Additionally, accepting responsibility for learning as an individual and as a member of a group is thought to enhance intellectual development (Copp, 2002).

Self-determination theory identifies controlled, more maladaptive motivators of behavior and autonomous motivators that the learner finds more interesting and enjoyable (Williams, Saizow, & Ryan, 1999). *Controlled motivators*, which include external demands under which people act with a sense of pressure and anxiety, are more characteristic of traditional curricula. *Autonomous motivators*, which involve a sense of volition and choice, would be more characteristic of a PBL curriculum. Control theory states that all behavior is based on satisfying the five basic needs of freedom, power, love and belonging, fun, and survival and reproduction (Glaser, 1985). Instruction can fail if it does not meet these basic needs of the learner. PBL may be superior at meeting these needs. For example, fun, or enjoyment of learning, has been frequently associated with outcomes of PBL (Albanese & Mitchell, 1993).

Schmidt and colleagues (2011) summarized the evidence relevant to the mechanism by which PBL affects learning in terms of two hypotheses derived from cognitive psychology: the activation-elaboration hypothesis and the situational interest hypothesis. The authors conclude that elaboration in a small group (through self-explanation, discussion with peers, and practicing and responding to questions) facilitates the processing and adds to the long-term retention or memorability of the knowledge gained. The situational interest hypothesis stems from the literature on the psychology of curiosity and learning. The cognitively induced experience of knowledge deprivation (the gap between what one knows and what one wants to know) initiates information-seeking behavior intended to close the knowledge gap. As learning occurs, the situational interest decreases and knowledge equilibrium is achieved (Rotgans & Schmidt, 2011). It has been demonstrated that the presentation of the problem increased the level of situational interest significantly in the students in a PBL course, and this was maintained during the small-group discussion (Rotgans & Schmidt, 2011).

■ Types of Learners

PBL has been used extensively in many health professions programs. Health professions students at all levels can benefit from the use of PBL to simulate realistic clinical situations. It is important to note that students accustomed to more traditional ways of learning often experience stress and anxiety when adapting to this new student-centered style of learning (Solomon & Finch, 1998). Supports must be put in place to ease the students' transition to this type of learning.

■ Resources

PBL requires different resources to support its implementation. Unlike traditional programs in which one faculty member lectures to large numbers of students, learning occurs in small groups, necessitating additional faculty to support PBL. There also is a need for numerous small-group tutorial rooms and extensive library and other learning resources that enable self-directed learning. As elaborated upon next, there is an additional need for faculty who are well prepared to assume the role of facilitator.

■ Role of Faculty

The instructor's role in PBL is different from that in a conventional class or tutorial setting. In PBL, the role of the instructor is to activate and facilitate learning in the group by encouraging participation of all members and to monitor the depth and breadth of knowledge and intervene when the desired quality of learning is not achieved (Barrows & Tamblyn, 1980; Maudsley, 1999). The instructor also plays a key role in assisting students to become self-directed learners and guiding them to become metacognitively aware: learn to be conscious of what information they know, what information they need, and what strategies they should use to solve the problem. Students perceived stimulating active and self-directed learning as the most important tasks with regard to group functioning (Boelens, De Wever, Rosseel, Verstraete, & Derese, 2015).

There has been significant debate in the PBL literature as to whether teachers with subject-matter expertise or teachers with good facilitation skills are preferable. Content experts are thought to be more likely to play a directive role in the learning process, speak more often, and supply more direct answers to students' questions, which may have a negative effect on the collaborative learning (Silver & Wilkerson, 1991). By contrast, Eagle, Harasym, and Mandin (1992) and Davis, Nairn, Paine, Anderson, and Oh (1992) suggest that instructors with content expertise are better at posing questions at critical moments, which positively influences students' learning. Although some debate remains (Kaufman & Holmes, 1998), it is generally recognized that a combination of content and process expertise is preferable.

Dolmans, Wolfhagen, Scherpbier, and van der Vleuten (2001) provide an excellent summary of issues related to instructor expertise. Not surprisingly, they conclude that faculty instructors initiate activities with which they are most familiar. Hence, content experts use their expertise to direct learner performance, and non-content experts use their process facilitation skills to direct group dynamics. However, this relationship is not as simple as once believed. A teacher's performance is not likely to be stable, as it is influenced by contextual circumstances such as the quality of the written cases, the structure of the course, and students' prior knowledge. Thus, teacher expertise may compensate if the structure or content of the problem is low and/or the students have little prior knowledge of the case.

While the evidence suggests that there is not a simple distinction between expert and nonexpert teachers, the implications for faculty development are clear: Faculty require training to assume more facilitative roles. Hitchcock and Mylona (2000) note that there has been little systematic study on effective ways to train faculty to assume PBL roles, although many descriptions have appeared in the literature. They emphasize that although the most obvious training is in instructor facilitation skills, there are many other roles and skills that must be developed. They describe Irby's sequence of steps of skill development: (1) challenging assumptions and developing understanding of PBL, (2) experiencing and valuing the tutorial process, (3) acquiring general teaching skills, (4) developing content-specific instructor knowledge and skills, (5) acquiring advanced knowledge and skills, (6) developing leadership and scholarship skills, and (7) creating organizational vitality. Each of these steps is described at length in Hitchcock and Mylona's paper (2000).

It is clear that faculty members who possess a level of content expertise in the area under study are the preferred small-group facilitators. However, there is an equally important need for faculty who are well trained in PBL and the tutorial process. The skills needed to facilitate and evaluate the small-group process, to promote metacognitive skills such as self-monitoring of one's reasoning and decision-making skills, and to design curriculum and develop problems and other instructional materials to support self-directed learning are very different from the skills required in a traditional curriculum. These require long-term faculty development initiatives.

■ Using Problem-Based Learning Methods

There appears to be no one best way to implement PBL. Although some maintain that fully integrated PBL is preferable, this curricular design may not be feasible for many institutions. Diversity in curricular design and approach is to be expected because different institutional structures and philosophies and faculty knowledge and skill development will influence the extent to which PBL can be incorporated into the curriculum.

Typically the process is as follows: Students are presented with a written problem as a stimulus for learning. Problems are carefully designed to facilitate discussion related to specific learning objectives. In groups of six to eight, students read the problem (either aloud or to themselves) and brainstorm about what they need to learn to better understand the problem or hypothesize potential causes of the problem. During this initial process, students generate learning issues or questions for self-study. Learning issues can range from factual knowledge (e.g., which nerves innervate the upper extremity?), to more complex physiological questions (e.g., what is the process of inflammation?), to questions that include broader psychosocial issues (e.g., how would I apply a model of ethical decision making to this patient?), or questions that require evaluation of the literature and integration of evidence-based practice (e.g., what is the effectiveness of ultrasound in the treatment of lateral epicondylitis?). The process of developing a high-quality learning issue that is researchable may be quite time consuming for the learner who is new to PBL. Generation of the final list of learning issues that will be researched and discussed at the next learning session constitutes the end of the first stage of the PBL process. Students can choose to independently research all learning issues that have been generated for that session, or to divide up the learning issues among themselves for self-study. When students return for the next learning session, they discuss their findings and the implications for patient care. At the end of the session, students engage in a structured evaluation of the learning process and their performance. Each student provides a verbal self-evaluation of his or her performance that day, and both peers and faculty provide feedback.

During the learning session, the faculty instructor does not provide expert content information. Rather, his or her role is to establish the climate for learning, encourage problem solving, and promote debate and discussion within the group. The instructor also role-models effective self-evaluation and provision of feedback. Barrows (1988) describes the faculty teaching role as going through the following three stages: (1) *modeling* of the thinking process for the students by questioning and challenging them; (2) *coaching* by the faculty when the students are off track or confused, which occurs as the group becomes more comfortable with the process; and (3) *fading* the role of the teacher, which occurs as students progress further and develop into a well-functioning and effective learning group, leaving the group to work more independently. Barrows suggests that groups should meet for at least 8 weeks to allow for progression of these three stages.

The implementation of PBL in a curriculum is not an easy process, and erosions in a successfully implemented PBL program can occur (Hung, 2011). Azer, Mclean, Onishi, Tagawa, and Scherpbier (2013) published 12 tips as preventive measures that should assist in the maintenance of PBL programs.

■ Potential Problems

The costs associated with the number of faculty required to deliver education in small groups is a key concern and potential barrier to implementation (Albanese & Mitchell, 1993). Other costs related to space requirements for small-group rooms and development of self-directed learning resources may also pose barriers (Solomon, 1994). Without institutional support for curricular change, many program leaders may find it difficult to engage successfully in curriculum reform.

An additional barrier to the implementation of innovative problem-based curricula relates to the lack of rigorous long-term data that demonstrate significant differences between traditional and PBL curricula. Consequently, debate about the effects of this method on learning when compared to traditional methods continues (Colliver & Markwell, 2007; Schmidt et al., 2011). The lack of evidence reinforces the concerns of critics who ask, "Why bother?" Some argue that PBL is worth implementing even if the only benefit of PBL is its more personal, humane, and enjoyable approach. Federman (1999) noted advantages of PBL that are not amenable to measurement and relate more to the personal and interpersonal aspects of practice. Even the most ardent of critics would agree that these benefits are desirable in health professional education. Some of these include: (1) the person-to-person contact inherent in a small-group learning process; (2) the positive regard that is fostered by the respect afforded to the beginning student; (3) the focus on patients that promotes relevance of the curriculum from the early days; (4) increased opportunities to discuss moral and ethical issues and for the instructor to share his or her values; and (5) the positive effect on lectures because, with only a few lectures in the timetable, students are more committed to these lectures, which in turn has a stimulating effect on the faculty.

Recently, with the rise in popularity of online and web-based learning, there has been an interest in doing PBL online. Increased accessibility and opportunities for asynchronous learning are obvious advantages for distance and continuing education courses. In health professions educational programs, PBL online has inherent appeal because the number of facilitators required could be reduced, thus making it possible to implement in programs without sufficient resources to do face-to-face PBL. Although there have been a few descriptive articles (Bresnitz, 1996), few have examined the effectiveness of computer-based PBL. Some of the characteristics of PBL, such as using patient problems, sharing learning, promoting integration of knowledge, and self-directed learning, are relatively easy to transfer to online formats. Several authors (e.g., Donelly, 2009; Savin-Baden, 2007) consider PBL a pedagogical strategy that enables interaction, collaboration, discussion, and participation in online environments. In an e-learning context, PBL requires specific tools enabling group synchronization, document management, discussion, and task assignment to engage students in the group learning process. However, the advantage of flexibility, related to the ability to access the course in an asynchronous manner, may not be realized in intensive, integrated professional curricula in which the students' timetables are more restricted. Face-to-face PBL promotes the development of communication and verbal skills related to the ability to clearly articulate and present information, provide feedback to others, and develop and evaluate group skills. In an online PBL experience, the communication skills that are central to professional practice would clearly not be developed in the same way as they would in a small-group, face-to-face PBL experience.

■ Conclusion

PBL is an increasingly popular teaching and learning strategy within the health professions. The clinical relevance, small-group interactions, and active learning provided make PBL an appealing curricular alternative. Faculty training and expertise are essential for successful outcomes.

Discussion Questions

1. The healthcare problem is central to problem-based learning. What attributes would make a healthcare problem ideal for a class (successful for the student learning process)?
2. A cohort of learners in a program is divided into 10 tutorial small groups. How can the coherence of the curriculum be maintained while allowing students the flexibility of identifying their own learning objectives in the small groups?
3. What issues should be considered when designing assessment methods/tools in the PBL environment?

References

Albanese, M. (2000). Problem-based learning: Why curricula are likely to show little effect on knowledge and clinical skills. *Medical Education, 34*, 729–738.

Albanese, M. A., & Mitchell, S. (1993). Problem-based learning: A review of literature on its outcomes and implementation issues. *Academic Medicine, 68*, 52–81.

Azer, S. A., Mclean, M., Onishi, H., Tagawa, M., & Scherpbier, A. (2013). Cracks in problem-based learning: What is your action plan? *Medical Teacher, 35*, 806–814.

Barrows, H. S. (1986). A taxonomy of problem-based learning methods. *Medical Education, 20*, 481–486.

Barrows, H. S. (1988). *The tutorial process*. Springfield, IL: Southern Illinois University of Medicine.

Barrows, H. S., & Tamblyn, R. (1980). *Problem-based learning*. New York, NY: Springer.

Boelens, R., De Wever, B., Rosseel, Y., Verstraete, A. G., & Derese, A. (2015). What are the most important tasks of tutors during tutorials in hybrid problem-based learning curricula? *BMC Medical Education, 15*, 84–92.

Bresnitz, E. (1996). Computer-based learning in PBL. *Academic Medicine, 71*(5), 540.

Charlin, B., Mann, K., & Hansen, P. (1998). The many faces of problem-based learning: A framework for understanding and comparison. *Medical Teacher, 20*, 323–330.

Clifford, M., & Wilson, M. (2000). *Contextual teaching, professional learning, and student experiences: Lessons learned from implementation* (Educational Brief 2). Madison, WI: Center on Education and Work, University of Wisconsin–Madison.

Colliver, J. A. (2000). Effectiveness of problem-based learning: Research and theory. *Academic Medicine, 75*, 259–266.

Colliver, J. A., & Markwell, S. J. (2007). Research on problem-based learning: The need for critical analysis of methods and findings. *Medical Education, 41*, 533–535.

Copp, S. L. (2002). Using cooperative learning strategies to teach implications of the nurse practice act. *Nurse Educator, 27*(5), 236–241.

Davis, W. K., Nairn, R., Paine, M. E., Anderson, R. M., & Oh, M. S. (1992). Effects of expert and non-expert facilitators on the small-group process and on student performance. *Academic Medicine, 67*(7), 470–474.

Dolmans, D. H., De Grave, W., Wolfhagen, I. H., & van der Vleuten, C. P. (2005). Problem-based learning: Future challenges for educational practice and research. *Medical Education, 39*(7), 732–741.

Dolmans, D. H., Wolfhagen, I., Scherpbier, A., & van der Vleuten, C. (2001). Relationship of tutors' group-dynamics skills to their performance ratings in problem-based learning. *Academic Medicine, 76*, 473–476.

Donelly, R. (2009). Embedding interaction within a blend of learner centric pedagogy and technology. *World Journal on Educational Technology, 1*, 6–29.

Eagle, C. J., Harasym, P. H., & Mandin, H. (1992). Effects of tutors with case expertise on problem-based learning issues. *Academic Medicine, 67*(7), 465–469.

Federman, D. D. (1999). Little-heralded advantages of problem-based learning. *Academic Medicine, 74*, 93–94.

Fyrenius, A., Bergdahl, B., & Silén, C. (2005). Lectures in problem-based learning: Why, when and how? An example of interactive lecturing that simulates meaningful learning. *Medical Teacher, 27*, 61–65.

Glaser, R. (1985). *Control theory in the classroom*. New York, NY: Harper & Row.

Harden, R. M., & Davis, M. H. (1998). The continuum of problem-based learning. *Medical Teacher, 20*, 317–322.

Hitchcock, M. A., & Mylona, Z. (2000). Teaching faculty to conduct problem-based learning. *Teaching and Learning in Medicine, 12*, 52–57.

Hmelo-Silver, C. E. (2004). Problem-based learning: What and how do students learn? *Educational Psychology Review, 16*(3), 235–266.

Hung, W. (2011). Theory to reality: A few issues in implementing problem-based learning. *Educational Technology Resource and Development, 59*, 529–552. doi:10.1007/s11423-011-9198-1

Kaufman, D. M., & Holmes, D. B. (1998). The relationship of tutors' content expertise to interventions and perceptions in a PBL medical curriculum. *Medical Education, 32*, 255–261.

Maudsley, G. (1999). Roles and responsibilities of the problem-based tutor in the undergraduate medical curriculum. *British Medical Journal, 318*, 657–661.

McLeod, S. A. (2007). *Vygotsky: Social development theory*. Retrieved from http://www.simplypsychology.org/vygotsky.html

Neville, A. J. (2009). Problem-based learning and medical education forty years on: A review of its effects on knowledge and clinical performance. *Medical Principles and Practice, 18*, 1–9.

Pinho, L. A., Mota, F. B., Conde, M. V. F., Alves, A. A., & Lopes, R. (2015). Mapping knowledge produced on problem-based learning between 1945 and 2014: A bibliometric analysis. *Creative Education, 6*, 575–584. doi:10.4236/ce.2015.66057

Rotgans, J. I., & Schmidt, H. G. (2011). The role of teachers in facilitating situational interest in an active-learning classroom. *Teaching and Teacher Education, 27*(1), 37–42.

Savin-Baden, M. (2007). *A practical guide to problem-based learning online*. London, UK: Routledge.

Schmidt, H. G., Rotgans, J. I., & Yew, E. H. J. (2011). The process of problem-based learning: What works and why. *Medical Education, 45*, 792–806.

Schmidt, H. G., van der Molen, H. T., Te Winkel, W. W. R., & Wijnen, W. H. F. W. (2009). Constructivist, problem-based learning does work: A meta-analysis of curricular comparisons involving a single medical school. *Educational Psychologist, 44*(4), 227–249.

Shin, I., & Kim, J. (2013). The effect of problem-based learning in nursing education: A meta-analysis. *Advances in Health Science Education, 18*, 1103–1120.

Silver, M., & Wilkerson, L. A. (1991). Effects of tutors with subject expertise on the problem-based tutorial process. *Academic Medicine, 66*(5), 298–300.

Solomon, P. (1994). Problem-based learning: A direction for physical therapy education? *Physiotherapy Theory and Practice, 10*, 45–52.

Solomon, P., Binkley, J., & Stratford, P. (1996). A descriptive study of learning processes and outcomes in two problem-based curriculum designs. *Journal of Physical Therapy Education, 10*, 72–76.

Solomon, P., & Finch, E. (1998). A qualitative study identifying stressors associated with adapting to problem-based learning. *Teaching and Learning in Medicine, 10*, 58–64.

Walton, H., & Matthews, M. (1989). Essentials of problem-based learning. *Journal of Medical Education, 23*, 542–558.

Williams, G., Saizow, R., & Ryan, R. (1999). The importance of self-determination theory for medical education. *Academic Medicine, 74*, 992–999.

CHAPTER 13

Debate as a Teaching Strategy

Martha J. Bradshaw

The debate is a strategy long recognized as a means to address a topic on which there may be more than one viewpoint. Just as the value of a debate does not necessarily depend on the resolution of a topic or persuasive results, its value as a teaching strategy lies more in the process and presentation of the viewpoints.

■ Definition and Purposes

A traditional view of debate may be that of argument for the purpose of persuading the audience toward a clearly identified position. To *debate* an issue is to consider or discuss it from opposing positions or arguments (Berube & DeVinne, 1982). Political debates are used as opportunities for candidates to make their perspectives known on key issues. This form of structured argument has long been used in philosophy, theology, law, and the sciences (Tumposky, 2004). Martin, Moran, and Harrison (2009) point out that debate is beneficial in cultivating critical thinking about salient issues in any discipline, including athletic education. *Debate* has been defined as "a systematic contest of speakers in which two points of view of a proposition are advanced with proof"(Barnhart, 1966, p. 311). Koklanaris, MacKenzie, Fino, Arslan, and Seubert (2008) noted that debate is useful to promote active learning because "debating inherently involves a variety of positive features: the impetus for intense preparation, active participation, and a forum ideally suited to controversial topics" (p. 235). Based on these definitions, it is apparent that debate can be a useful teaching strategy.

Debate provides opportunities for students to analyze an issue or problem in depth and to reach an informed, unbiased conclusion or resolution. Debate encourages participants to identify quickly the essential nature of the issue as substantiated by evidence; to establish criteria for judging its successful resolution; and to weigh, compare, and contrast the merits of alternative strategies for resolution (Simonneaux, 2002). In addition, presentation of the debate allows students to practice oral communication skills, express professional opinions, and gain experience both in speaking to groups and in working in groups while preparing the debates.

■ Theoretical Rationale

Two important components of the professional role are the analysis of significant issues and the ability to communicate in efficient and effective ways. Professional communication is seen in many forms; scholarly publications, oral presentations, and electronic networking are a few examples. Similar to other skills, the development of effective communication skills must be fostered by faculty. The ability to communicate one's thoughts clearly and concisely evolves from the formulation of a perspective on a topic, analysis of that perspective and other views, and development of sound conclusions. Debate enables students to participate actively in a meaningful communication exercise.

The college environment is one that should develop the student's inquisitiveness and discriminating attitude (Vo & Morris, 2006). The debate is particularly helpful in causing a student to examine the position juxtaposed to a personally held view. Nyatanga and Howard (2015) point out that debate encourages healthy skepticism. One of the purposes of debate is to cause the learner to go beyond merely identifying an issue. Learners must actually analyze the issue: What are its key elements? What historical precedents have contributed to the issue? Who are the key proponents and opponents of the issue? What is the future of the issue? Students can learn how personal values or emotions influence thinking and responses to issues. Students also can identify what factors influence their thinking, such as the views of news analysts, popular literature, or peers (Simonneaux, 2002). Analysis on this level leads to powerful learning, calling for the use of reasoning and other forms of higher-order thinking. The learner first becomes more aware of his own thinking, then broadens and purposefully adapts his thinking (Tumposky, 2004). A study by Koklanaris et al. (2008) found that when the objective was learning about a controversial topic, resident physicians who prepared for and participated in a debate achieved higher test scores and retained information better than those who attended a lecture. They concluded that organizing a debate may be more effective than giving a lecture about a controversial topic.

■ Conditions for Learning

Debate is most useful as part of a course or seminar in professional and academic settings. Because of the nature of this strategy, it should be employed in a course that centers upon issues or topics that raise debatable questions. Questions employed in a debate should be those that can be addressed from more than one defensible perspective (Martin et al. 2009). Debate also is a means to validate and deepen content knowledge (Martens, 2007). This strategy can be used to facilitate students' ability to implement analytical skills, to systematically research and critique an issue, to arrive at salient points, and to demonstrate more professional development related to group processes (Candela, Michael, & Mitchell, 2003). Furthermore, debate provides students the opportunity to develop planned responses to an issue, rather than facing an awkward silence when asked to respond during a teacher-led class (Nyatanga & Howard, 2015).

The learning goals for the debate strategy include improving oral communication and research referencing skills, structuring and presenting an argument, and exercising analytical skills. The process for formulating and presenting the debate should facilitate these goals as much as possible; therefore, the faculty should provide as much freedom as possible for the students to reach these learning goals independently. Students should be given enough structure or direction to help them plan and organize their work, but they also should understand the responsibility they must take for researching debate positions, analyzing key issues, and practicing speaking skills. In the debate strategy described by Lowenstein and Bradshaw (1989), students were encouraged to take the viewpoint opposite the one they (personally) held. This approach promoted an understanding of existing oppositional perspectives and enhanced the ability to respond to opposing views (Lowenstein & Bradshaw, 1989).

Preparation for the debate should begin early in the course to provide adequate opportunity for library research and exploration of issues. Faculty facilitation is an essential part of the learning process. Conditions central to use of debate as an effective strategy include the following:

- Students need to be introduced to key issues in the course, and have to be able to identify controversial points suitable for debate.
- Students need to be familiar with one another in order to form working groups.
- Students need knowledge of existing resources to use in formulating debate. This includes increased familiarity with the faculty member(s) as a source of support and information.

■ Types of Learners

Debate can be used with all levels or types of learners, including undergraduate students, graduate students, and practitioners, because the learning goals of debate are suitable for all groups. Lowenstein and Bradshaw (1989) used debate with registered nurse students who were completing their BSN courses. Debate is a particularly successful strategy with this group because these students combine personal experience with actual patient or practice problems with the need to refine communication and analytical skills.

Swu-Jane and Crawford (2007) developed debate as a new component to an introductory core course for pharmacy students who were in their first professional year. Objectives were to facilitate the group process, improve critical thinking and communication skills, introduce controversial issues related to the U.S. healthcare system, enable students' ability to analyze and evaluate evidence, help develop skills in formulating written arguments, and encourage tolerance of diverse points of view. Thus, debate provides a true opportunity for professional growth in this type of student. By immersing themselves in the topic, students develop a better understanding of it than they would through other means of study.

By creating the need to objectively analyze an issue, debate becomes useful for a student who is strongly influenced by personal values or certain work experiences. An undergraduate who has not formed a worldview about sensitive ethical dilemmas, for example, can have the opportunity to examine the issues and how decisions are made. A practitioner who has been receiving negative influence in the work environment has the opportunity for objective analysis of the situation.

Debate is a strategy to be used when the instructor wishes to bring about active (rather than passive) learning, critical thinking, and creativity, and to introduce the learners to the role of conflict in professional endeavors. Direct confrontation—that is, face-to-face discussion—is particularly valuable in an educational environment in which students frequently converse in isolation through electronic means. Reliance upon technology hinders students from cultivating skills for professional, purposeful conversations. Furthermore, use of debate is an opportunity for a student to hone the ability to speak in front of a group, especially one that is not entirely supportive of the speaker's point of view.

■ Resources

Faculty members serve as an important resource by assuming the role of facilitator. Formal debate questions and positions can emerge from class discussion about important issues. Faculty members can assist students in formulating the debate question and can direct them to resources related to the issue. Clinical experiences and current issues in health care offer a wide range of debate topics. Faculty may wish to prepare the students early in the course by encouraging them to be alert to ethical dilemmas or patient care problems that are suitable for debate (Candela et al. 2003).

The library offers many resources for debate preparation. By using the professional literature to support the debate position, students are introduced to a wide range of journals, books, and other printed material. Electronic information systems can be extremely helpful to students as they identify debate issues and develop related positions. Database searches enable students to consider related topics and sources, outside of their own professional field, which may generate additional support for a position. The electronic media afford access to the most current information, which may be particularly helpful for students dealing with timely political topics. Electronic bulletin boards and other communication networks provide students an opportunity to interact with individuals outside their own institution who are involved with the issue.

The debate can be presented in any planned classroom setting. The environment should be such that the debate teams can be seen and heard by the audience. The debate process can be used in online courses as well (Swu-Jane & Crawford, 2007). Through a process of Informal Forum, students use critical thinking skills to research and retrieve information, then compile it in a manner by which they can make informed decisions or develop opinions on the issue under discussion (Huang, 2007). Just as with the traditional debate method, the Informal Forum is interactive among students, rather than being teacher directed. However, when conducted online, this approach does not provide the opportunity for face-to-face interaction and development of oral communication skills.

■ Using the Method

In the Lowenstein and Bradshaw method, faculty members define broad (topical) areas from the course outline and identify an advisor for each area. Students choose the general area in which they are interested and form groups of four or five members. At least one group is formed for each topical area, to guarantee that course objectives or topics are addressed. Depending on student interest and enrollment, a second group may be formed in certain areas. For example, two groups may choose to address the area of professional roles and responsibilities. Specific debate questions are formulated by the group in keeping with the objectives or broad topics of the course and personal interests of group members. Many of the topics are those currently being debated by our colleagues in all areas of health care: Patient care delivery systems, healthcare reform, genetic screening, and euthanasia are a few examples.

Each group should meet with the faculty advisor as needed to organize the debate presentation, gain insight into the points being presented, and receive assistance with resources. The instructor may assist the groups by refining their reasoning approaches. Martens (2007) identifies several types of reasoning as part of the argument:

Reasoning by:
Example
Analogy
Causal
Cost-benefit
Evidence

Students are guided to consider the perspectives of all individuals or interest groups (Simonneaux, 2002). For each debate group, two students select the affirmative position, two select the negative, and the fifth serves as moderator. In groups of four, the faculty advisor serves as moderator. Each group develops a reading list of significant articles related to the issue under debate. The list is circulated to the entire class at least 1 week prior to the debate. Students not involved in the presentation are expected to be prepared to discuss the issues under consideration.

The debate consists of opening remarks by a moderator, two affirmative and two negative presentations, rebuttal, and summary. Following the presentation, the floor is opened to the class for discussion. Questions and comments based on the presentations and readings are generated by the class. The debate moderator facilitates discussion and provides a final summary of the issues and discussion. In most situations, the burden of supporting the affirmative view is the more difficult position to hold (Law, 1998). With some issues, it may be appropriate to develop a resolution plan upon conclusion of the formal debate. This plan can incorporate some ideas from both positions, to encourage win-win negotiation. This process gives students experience in developing workable solutions to practice-related issues. Class members not participating in the debate are asked to evaluate each presenter based on a rating scale. Students evaluate the analysis of the issue, evidence presented, supporting resources, organization of the presentation, the argument presented, interaction

Date: _____   **Subject/Topic:** _____

Evaluate each speaker using the following scale:

Superior = 5; Excellent = 4; Good = 3; Fair = 2; Below standard =1

Team A		Team B
1 2 3 4 5	Bibliography (4 max)	1 2 3 4 5
	Overview of problem (Debater 1 or 2)	
1 2 3 4 5	Representing side of debate (Debater 1 or 2)	1 2 3 4 5
	Opening remarks	
Debater		Debater
1 2 3 4 5		1 2 3 4 5
	Resolution plan	
Debater		Debater
1 2 3 4 5		1 2 3 4 5
	Response to opposing team	
Debater		Debater
1 2 3 4 5		1 2 3 4 5

■ **Figure 13-1**   Grading tool: debate.

with the audience and opponents, and response to questions (**Figure 13-1**). An overall effectiveness score is given, and the evaluators indicate if their stand on the issue changed as a result of the debate. All faculty members participating in the seminar also evaluate the presenters. Debate grades are based on preparation, individual performance, and group efforts that were reflected in the effectiveness of the debate.

To reinforce the learning from the debate, students may be asked to write a formal paper on one of the professional issues discussed in the course. The paper can be evaluated on the presentation of the issue, arguments for both sides of the issue supported by literature, the student's position and rationale for selection of the position, application of ideas to practice, and use of references and format. Validation of learning through debate has been assessed by use of a pre- and posttest quiz (Koklanaris et al., 2008).

In the online format, Swu-Jane and Crawford (2007) developed a series of three debates over a 12-week term. Teams of four to five members were established and paired as pro (affirmative) or con (negative). Teams were encouraged to appoint a team leader to coordinate the work and communicate with an assigned teaching assistant. A forum was set up for discussion posts for the paired teams. Students were expected to post three arguments in an online forum that included two constructive arguments and one rebuttal and summary argument. Each group posted in one-week intervals, beginning with affirmative and followed by negative, then a second affirmative followed by negative; the final argument started with negative first and then positive. A word limit of 400 to 600 words (excluding references) was set to correspond to a speaker's time limit in an oral debate. Students were encouraged to read articles recommended by the instructors to provide an overview for both sides of the debate topic, and to search, use, and cite additional reference sources. An orientation to the debate process was accomplished by providing written materials to assist the students in understanding the expectations and flow. Three judges were appointed by the instructors to decide the winners of the debate.

■ Potential Problems

The debate strategy calls for significant student responsibility and preparation, for both debaters and the audience. Debaters are required to thoroughly research the issue and the position taken for the argument. From this preparation, they formulate a succinct and effective presentation. Debaters are expected to practice speaking skills and to prepare supporting materials for the oral presentation. The debate group provides an appropriate reading list for the other class members. Those students take the responsibility to read about the issue prior to the presentation, in order to understand the issue and participate effectively in discussion. Lack of preparation on the part of team members leads to inadequate presentation of the issue and superficial discussion. In contrast, students who are acquainted with the opposing team members may collaborate and develop a "planned" debate so as to maximize opportunity for a successful outcome. While this may be difficult to discover on the part of the instructor, it clearly is an example of academic dishonesty.

The debate causes students to clearly classify an issue as one that is right or wrong, or answered "yes" or "no." Many topics have no conclusions or answers, and thus may impose a false dualism (Tumposky, 2004). Students may have to defend a position to which they are not clearly committed. Students with strong moral beliefs about an issue may have difficulty defending a specified position or accepting the views of others. Faculty may have difficulty presenting a neutral position when moderating the debate and guiding discussion (Simonneaux, 2002). At some point during the presentations, it must be made very clear that there is no "right" or singular answer to most issues.

Nervousness about speaking in public can be a major concern. Some students have had little or no public speaking experience, or they may have had negative experiences that continue to generate anxiety. Tumposky (2004) asserts that female students may be more uncomfortable with the adversarial nature of this strategy than are their male peers. In addition, students of certain cultural groups may have difficulty with open debate as a way to learn. Students need encouragement and need to view the debate as an opportunity to speak to an open, receptive group in order to gain experience. What some students look upon with apprehension often results in being uplifting and beneficial. For example, one student was timid about speaking in groups and was extremely nervous before and during her debate presentation. Her nervousness was manifested in physical symptoms such as sweating, flushed face, tremulous voice, shaking hands, and rapid blinking. She received appropriate support from faculty and students, which encouraged her to work on this problem during the rest of her academic time. Three years later, she successfully defended her master's project in a dignified and professional manner. Her public speaking skills have now advanced to the point that she is able to address both groups and individuals effectively in her current employment as a clinical specialist.

The argumentative or confrontational nature of the debate may also create anxiety. In addition, debate or public speaking may be a new strategy on which students are graded, thus heightening anxiety. Faculty and students must continually emphasize that the debate is a learning experience. The excitement of defending a position, stressing key points, and deriving a workable solution should be presented as positive outcomes of the debate. Faculty members should stress that students will not be condemned or inappropriately criticized for taking unpopular viewpoints during the debate. Faculty members are prepared to handle strong emotional viewpoints and to help students understand that there is room for conflicting opinions in our society. In using debate as a teaching strategy, Candela et al. (2003) discovered that students liked the strategy and found it challenging, but did not see how they would use the skill or strategy in their professional careers. It is possible that, as novices, students are not aware of potential situations in which there will be a need to defend a position regarding health care. Students also need to be encouraged to see the benefit of the opportunity to practice speaking skills, research skills, and group work.

■ Conclusion

Debate is a strategy that promotes student interaction and involvement in course topics. There are many advantages to using this strategy. Debate expands the student's perspective on a given issue, creates doubt about the existence of one clear answer, and requires much thought and further evidence before a solution is derived. Debate also increases awareness of opposing viewpoints. As an interactive strategy, debate develops techniques of persuasion, serves as a means by which students confront a controversial issue, and promotes collaborative efforts and negotiation skills among peers. This strategy promotes independence and participation in the decision-making process, as well as enhancing writing and organizational skills. Debate allows for examination of broad issues that influence professional practice. Critical thinking is enhanced by the scrutiny of more than one position on the issue. Debate allows the student a wider forum than writing a paper does, and it may give a greater sense of accomplishment (DeYoung, 2003).

Selection of debate as a teaching strategy requires a strong commitment to preparation and guidance from faculty. Faculty members will have to deal with the emotions that can be elicited by the arguments. Faculty members will need to provide support for students who take minority or unpopular positions and for those who have limited public speaking skills. Following the debate, those students whose ideas are not accepted by the majority should be encouraged to recognize those parts of their work that were of value, even if others disagreed with their position. Those students whose ideas reflected the majority view should also recognize that public consensus can change quickly, and, as more information becomes available, opinions may be swayed. Finally, faculty members can help students to recognize that the debate is just a start to exploration of professional issues. Students will need to be encouraged to incorporate their newly learned and practiced skills into their professional practice.

Discussion Questions

1. What framework does the instructor need to create to keep the debate strategy from seeming confrontational and adversarial?
2. How can debate be used in a course that is fully online?
3. What are the advantages and disadvantages of having peers grade each other after a debate?

References

Barnhart, C. L. (Ed.). (1966). *The American college dictionary.* New York, NY: Random House.

Berube, M. S., & DeVinne, P. B. (Eds.). (1982). *The American heritage dictionary.* Boston, MA: Houghton Mifflin.

Candela, L., Michael, S. R., & Mitchell, S. (2003). Ethical debates: Enhancing critical thinking in nursing students. *Nurse Educator, 28,* 37–39.

DeYoung, S. (2003). *Teaching strategies for nurse educators.* Upper Saddle River, NJ: Prentice-Hall.

Huang, G. H. C. (2007). Informal forum: Fostering active learning in a teacher preparation program. *Education, 127*(1), 31–38.

Koklanaris, N., MacKenzie, A. P., Fino, M. E., Arslan, A. A., & Seubert, D. E. (2008). Debate preparation/participation: An active effective learning tool. *Teaching and Learning in Medicine, 20*(3), 235–238.

Law, C. F. (1998). Using argumentation to teach literature. *Exercise Exchange, 43,* 10–11.

Lowenstein, A. J., & Bradshaw, M. J. (1989). Seminar methods for RN to BSN students. *Nurse Educator, 14*(5), 27–31.

Martens, E. A. (2007). The instructional use of argument across the curriculum. *Middle School Journal, 38*(5), 4–13.

Martin, M., Moran, K. A., & Harrison, K. (2009). Utilizing debates in athletic training education. *Athletic Therapy Today, 14*(1), 31–34. Retrieved from http://ezproxy.baylor.edu/login?url=http://search.ebscohost.com/login.aspx?direct=true&db=c8h&AN=2010154594&site=ehost-live&scope=site

Nyatanga, L., & Howard, C. (2015). Using dialect debates to enhance innovative teaching of conceptual and historical issues in psychology. *History and Philosophy of Psychology, 16*(1), 27–35.

Simonneaux, L. (2002). Analysis of classroom debating strategies. *Journal of Biological Education, 37,* 9–12.

Swu-Jane, L., & Crawford, S. Y. (2007). An online debate series for first-year pharmacy students. *American Journal of Pharmaceutical Education, 71*(1), 1–8.

Tumposky, N. R. (2004). The debate debate. *Clearing House, 78,* 52–55.

Vo, H. X., & Morris, R. L. (2006). Debate as a tool in teaching economics: Rationale, technique, and some evidence. *Journal of Education for Business, 81*(6), 315–330.

CHAPTER 14

Games Are Multidimensional in Educational Situations

Lynn Jaffe

Games are central to human experience and an important way in which it is made meaningful.

—*Dormann & Biddle* (2006)[1]

In *Reality Is Broken,* Jane McGonigal (2011) expounds upon the failings of reality and how they might be repaired through games. It is appropriate to extend her arguments to education. Today's college students and adult learners are often bored and underserved with the simple lecture format, although they will cling to that format over having, in their impression, to "teach themselves" (Smith, 2008; Stanford University, n.d.). Current technology has fostered reduced attention spans and reinforced students' reliance on instant gratification, immediate feedback, innovation, and novelty to sustain interest in learning situations (Greenfield, 2009; Kanthan & Senger, 2011; Oblinger, 2006; Reiner & Siegel, 2008; Sauve, Renaud, Kaufman, & Marquis, 2007). Games can address these needs because they are experiential and can provide frequent feedback.

Games used for educational purposes, referred to as *serious games*, are a way to motivate, reinforce skills, and promote collaboration through their experiential format. There is extensive literature on game theory and gaming in multiple disciplines. Although the strength of the supporting evidence for the use of games in healthcare education is still equivocal (Aburahma & Mohamed, 2015; Alfarah, Schünemann, & Akl, 2010; Skiba, 2013), some randomized controlled trials are demonstrating significantly positive results in favor of game-based learning (Boeker, Andel, Vach, & Frankenschmidt, 2013). This chapter is an introduction to the use of games as a teaching/learning tool within the classroom or clinical setting. It also introduces the idea of "gamification" in education: the process of turning the entire learning experience into a multiplayer game (Sederstrom, 2014; Sheldon, 2012). Definitions, evidence regarding practice, and the types of

---

[1]Reproduced from Dormann, C., & Biddle, R. (2006). Humour in game-based learning. *Learning, Media and Technology, 31*(4), 411–424, reprinted by permission of the publisher (Taylor & Francis Ltd, http://www.tandfonline.com).

learning that fit most easily within the various game structures are described here, as are the limitations of game use within the educational or clinical environment.

■ Definition and Purpose

A *game* is an activity often classified as fun, governed by precise rules that involve varying degrees of strategy or chance, and one or more players who cooperate or compete (with self, the game, one another, or a computer) through the use of knowledge or skill in an attempt to reach a specified goal (Beylefeld & Struwig, 2007; Sauve et al., 2007). In addition, potentially the most salient feature of games is that they have a fairly immediate feedback system; this is necessary because modern students expect and desire immediate feedback on the accuracy of the knowledge they are acquiring (Johnson & Romanello, 2005; McGonigal, 2011; Nevin et al., 2014). Educational or serious games are believed to provide learning benefits that last beyond the game itself for all participants, and evidence to that effect forms the basis of this chapter. There are three major categories within the genre: games, simulations, and simulation games.

Game is a generic term that includes board, card, digital, and skilled activities. Many simple educational games use popular formats, such as bingo, *Jeopardy!*, *Trivial Pursuit*, *Monopoly*, and *Who Wants to Be a Millionaire?*, that provide familiar frameworks for inserting content and creating learning activities. These "frame" games typically involve a set of rules for player moves and termination criteria so that winners may be determined. The frameworks are easily adaptable to a wide variety of content and instructional objectives, usually in the lower cognitive domain areas. These games have been described in the literature, and examples are listed in the "Recommended Reading" section at the end of this chapter. Also see the websites listed in the "Resources" section for templates of popular game shows for educational use.

Simulations, in this context, are role-playing games and are discussed in other chapters. *Simulation games* are contrived reality-based conflicts that must be resolved within the constraints of the game rules; these have been shown to enhance competency development among health professionals (Graham & Richardson, 2008; Kanthan & Senger, 2011; Sauve et al., 2007). They have the potential to attain new heights of efficacy in digital game formats where they can be used to enhance other aspects of the educational experience more than mere review of content. Within authentic contexts, students have the opportunity to get immersed in the game and call on past knowledge and experience to solve problems, make decisions, and examine attitudes, affect, and empathy (Alfarah et al., 2010; Chen, Kiersma, Yehle, & Plake, 2015; Gleason, 2015; Skiba, 2008).

Debriefing is an important aspect of the learning process that occurs after the game. It is a discussion focusing on the concepts, generalizations, and applications of the topics covered within the game (Aburahma & Mohamed, 2015; Gee, 2008; Graham & Richardson, 2008). This process assists learners in recognizing the learning that has occurred within the fun experience of the game and contributes to the learners' ability to use self-reflection, especially for the modern learner (Allery, 2004; Johnson & Romanello, 2005). Effective debriefing requires a good deal of skill and experience from the facilitator and should be allotted as much time as was spent actually playing the game (Blakely, Skirton, Cooper, Allum, & Nelmes, 2010).

■ Theoretical Foundations

The use of games for educational purposes is a very old idea. The earliest recorded use was of war games 3,000 years ago in China; games were also used for such purposes in the 18th century in Europe and this century by the U.S. military. Game use was brought to the business community by former-military officers to provide training in problem solving and decision making. It was considered a bridge between academic instruction and on-the-job training. In the 1950s and 1960s, as the theoretical focus of learning shifted from the instructor to the student, experience-based learning became prominent, and games were used to meet this goal. In health-related areas, psychologists and nurses made numerous contributions to the literature on game use in both academic and clinical education, although the research is still inconclusive in judging the effectiveness of game use, primarily due to small sample sizes, poor operational definitions, and other design flaws (Akl et al., 2010; Alfarah et al., 2010; Beylefeld & Struwig, 2007; Blakely, Skirton, Cooper, Allum, & Nelmes, 2009; Bochennek, Wittekindt, Zimmermann, & Klingebiel, 2007; Royse & Newton, 2007; Shiroma, Massa, & Alarcon, 2011).

Game use falls under the theoretical umbrellas of active learning strategies and cooperative learning described previously in this text, and under the concept of *flow* coined by Csikszentmihalyi, which refers to a psychological state achieved when learning and enjoyment coincide (Beylefeld & Struwig, 2007). The focus is on actual engagement with both the educational material and classmates, engendering positive attitudes that promote deep processing of the learning experience. Learning through games can be intense, absorbing, and motivating (Dormann & Biddle, 2006; Kanthan & Senger, 2011).

■ Types of Learners

Games are being used throughout the educational continuum, from preschool through graduate education. They can be used for students who like to compete and for those who prefer to cooperate. For learners with achievement needs, games motivate through competitiveness (Nevin et al., 2014). Games may also be motivating for those with strong affiliation needs, such as millennial learners, because games can require team play and cooperation for completion. The element of luck within an educational game gives all students, not just the studious ones, a chance at winning and thereby keeps engagement higher. Educators must appreciate the different maturational stages students pass through. Adult learners have a particular need to engage meaningfully with content and apply it through a variety of methods, which can be accomplished through the interactive, immediate, and diverse formats of gaming.

Games can be structured to require a degree of flexibility on the part of the student to adapt to changing circumstances, especially when addressing the development of interdisciplinary awareness, problem solving, cultural sensitivity, and empathy with clients (Graham & Richardson, 2008; Jarrell, Alpers, Brown, & Wotring, 2008). Finally, particularly with the use of digital simulation games, some degree of computer/technology comfort is required on the part of both the students and the faculty/trainer. Most millennial and postmillennial students arrive on campus equipped and eager to use web-based technologies (Lynch-Sauer et al., 2011); some faculty need to increase their comfort level with this method.

■ Conditions for Learning

Games can be used to address all levels of cognitive objectives, from reinforcing the learning of basic facts, through developing application and analysis skills, and culminating in promoting synthesis and evaluation. They do this through the promotion of initiative, creative thought, and affective components within a safe forum for listening to others. Games are credited with supplementing rote memorization, providing useful organization of material, encouraging application of ideas, and providing comic relief from the otherwise anxiety-provoking task of preparing for exams.

Games are inherently student-centered and interactive, generating enthusiasm, excitement, and enjoyment. It has been found that students often prefer multiple methods, or styles, of learning (Lujan & DiCarlo, 2006; Wright, 2012). When new occupational therapy students are asked what their preferred learning style is, the predominant answer is usually hands-on/experiential (M. D'Amico, personal communication, September 12, 2012). An experiential learning method, such as gaming, creates an environment that requires a participant to be involved in a personally meaningful activity using multiple styles of learning, such as visual, auditory, and kinesthetic styles. Fostering a match between teaching strategies and student needs is one of the key factors in effective education. In addition, learning has greater impact when it has an element of emotional arousal, takes place within a safe environment, and has a period of debriefing to provide a cognitive map for understanding the experience (Allery, 2004; Medina, 2008).

Board or card games tend to be most appropriate for skill-based knowledge and practice in the cognitive domain, such as memorizing or concept matching (Bochennek et al., 2007; Van Eck, 2006). *Jeopardy!* and *Trivial Pursuit* are quite popular in many disciplines for reviewing course information in such subjects as abnormal psychology and research methods, because of the quick mobilization of facts or labels required. In health care, both would lend themselves to reviews in human development, clinical conditions, or other primary knowledge topics. These games are used to review facts, reinforce or test knowledge and understanding, and foster application (Patel, 2008). The games can be adapted in multiple ways: through the content and through the external attributes of the game itself, such as time limits and the degree of luck built into the format. Crossword puzzles, word searches, and bingo-style games have been used in nursing in-service training to review required materials as well as increase staff attendance and compliance. Games can also be created for the psychomotor domain; speed of manipulation, safety in transfers, and knowledge of intervention techniques could all be addressed through a game format that would reward an individual or a team.

Simulation games, referred to as *adventure games* when in digital format, are adapted to teaching problem solving, hypothesis testing, and the affective domain outcomes. Problem solving is best taught through practice and reflection. Within the format of the simulation game, especially in a computer or video game format, there is more opportunity for such repetition and practice than is available during limited classroom or clinical practice time (Reiner & Siegel, 2008). Video games also may offer consistent assessment of clinical reasoning skills in case-study situations of home or clinic visits (Duque, Fung, Mallet, Posel, & Fleiszer, 2008). The potential is there for multiple users in these virtual environments, and professional exploration may be accomplished through digital simulation games. Serious game design works best when communication is built in through blogs, wikis, and other Internet technologies (Derryberry, 2007). The time/effort involved in creating such environments becomes less feasible when faculty members are faced with overloaded clinical placements (Skiba, 2008).

A recent academic development is to structure an entire class as a game, referred to as *gamification* (Lee & Hammer, 2011; Sederstrom, 2014; Sheldon, 2012). The concept employs elements of games, such as experience points for accomplishments as opposed to grades, levels that students rise through as they gain the experience points, and assignments that are structured as quests or challenges, to promote engagement in learning. One gamification approach is to have assignments that can be repeated until competence is achieved (challenges). These challenges are created for the student's current skill level and increase in difficulty as the student's skill level advances. Another approach is to have group-based activities (quests) that foster teamwork and critical thinking. The gamification approach sparks motivation and emotional engagement through the choices offered to students—choices to engage in select activities or not, and to plot one's own path through the course material (Lee & Hammer, 2011; Sheldon, 2012). The take-away message is to provide feedback often and keep the stakes low while initial learning is taking place, so that the repetition needed to actually master the material can be a positive emotional experience, rather than a punishment. A game format is not required to accomplish this, but a game format can keep the focus on active, engaged learning that is within the learner's control rather than assignments being seen as an obstacle a professor is throwing in the path of perfect grades.

■ Resources

Creating games for the classroom usually takes time, imagination, and desire. The rewards can be great, although in this productivity-driven age, the tradeoffs must be considered. As has been described, the quickest resources are based on those games that are currently available in toy stores or on television. Using the frames of these games requires loading in course material, and thereafter it is easy to introduce such games to the students because of their familiarity with the format.

As of the publication date of this text, the following websites offered templates for such games:

> PowerPoint games at http://people.uncw.edu/ertzbergerj/msgames.htm or
>   http://powerpointgames.wikispaces.com/PowerPoint+Game+Templates
> Crossword puzzles or word games at http://www.crossword-puzzles.co.uk
> Eclipse crosswords at http://www.eclipsecrossword.com

A more challenging approach than using the aforementioned sites is developing the entire game from one's own imagination, although if the educator engages small groups from a class to create the game using some of the guiding principles in the next section, this may become more feasible (Patel, 2008). Dr. Martha Rosenthal has had great success in having her students create games from class topics as an assessment assignment within her classes; she describes the need to think about the material, opportunity to be creative, increased interest, and fun as some of the benefits (M. Rosenthal, personal communication, September 21, 2015).

Digital game developers have been creating structures that may be available as frameworks for cognitive and affective domain objectives. These frameworks range from addressing the lower/moderate end of knowledge/awareness, as in a WebQuest (http://www.webquest.org/index.php) search for specific information, through to the high-end evaluating/internalizing found in the Pod Game (ZaidLearn), where one is making judgments and decisions under a time constraint. The challenge for the educator is in finding and then using such formats, because of the technological knowledge required on top of the content application (Van Eck, 2006). Currently there are only a few such games that are directly applicable to health care. An international group has developed a small series of games to teach research and statistics that it offers for free to anyone wanting access (http://www.chermug.eu/index.html).

For those who like the recommendation that it is better to use teaching practices that are game-like rather than to try to develop whole games that may actually detract from the educational intent because of the novelty or the development time involved (Begg, 2008), a key resource for gamification is a blog with many linked resources found at http://top5onlinecolleges.org/gamification.

The "Recommended Reading" section at the end of this chapter has a variety of articles and websites describing gaming used in classroom education and in-service training. Some articles specifically target a greater use of technology, such as computer or web-based games. The references that describe active learning and cooperative learning are excellent background information for the new academician and are available online.

■ Using the Method: Basic How-To

Many authors have described the methodology behind using games in the classroom, and their advice is summarized in **Table 14-1**. To begin, games rarely succeed as add-ons; they must be integrated into the overall educational strategy (Nicholson, 2011; Ridley, 2004). A game pulled out of nowhere, just to be novel, will have no effect on outcome measures. In essence, when developing a game, the educator must determine the content area, statement of the problem, and objectives of the game. After this, he or she must determine the game format, number of players, time frame, and rules. If using a frame game, the generic rules already exist and can be adapted for the topic within health care. The next decisions have to set up the roles players assume and the scenarios in which play occurs. These can be simple adaptations for frame games, or more complex if setting up a game that is a simulation of a clinic.

Table 14-1   Process for Game Development

Step	Element	Probes
1	Specific objectives for game	Does the game parallel and/or facilitate the course objectives?
2	Fit within the curriculum and the environment	Are the concepts relevant? Is this for review or to move understanding forward? Is there adequate functional space for implementation? If digital, are there enough computers (or smartphones) and technical support?
2a	Employs conflict	This could be a time limit, competition between teams, or competition with the manager, depending on the objectives. Does it provide a just-right challenge? Can the student alter the level of challenge?
2b	Rules of play and criteria for closure are easily communicated	Are all the rules known up front, or are they learned over time? If there are dead ends or eliminations, what happens next?
2c	It is fun	If not, stop right here and rework or discard
2d	Provides immediate feedback to participants	Do students know how they are doing at all times? Is uncertainty part of the game? Does the feedback assist the student in modifying beliefs or performance in order to improve?
2e	Meets the needs of students	Does the game help organize the course material? Is it a reliable measure of their comprehension, or will it mislead them? Does the game encourage the players to "laugh with" as opposed to "laugh at" one another? Is it inclusive in nature?
3	Field-test to eliminate bugs	Did it go as planned, or are revisions needed?
4	Mechanism (such as pretesting and posttesting) that allows measurement of learning	Other than student satisfaction, check to see if actual learning occurs.
5	Share it with colleagues	Publish or post—there are many educational game websites.

The scoring system and physical elements of a frame game tend to remain consistent with the original game; for simulation games, they often have to be created outright. The designer chooses the media used, whether they are common materials or specially constructed components, based on available time and resources. The game must be tested on a small sample initially, critiqued, and possibly revised. Finally, it is beneficial to the community of healthcare educators if the game is then disseminated (Blakely et al., 2009; Nicholson, 2011).

Overarching elements that must be considered when using instructional games include the layout and amount of space in the classroom or availability of technology, to ensure equal opportunity to play. Time to be spent during the game, with enough time for the debriefing, must be planned. Also essential in planning are the method by which the students will become aware of the rules of the game and rewards for results, including whether the rewards are intrinsic or extrinsic. Remember that for best effect, the game must be integrated into the instructional strategy of the course and directly related to the subject. It must be challenging enough and not feel like work.

■ Potential Problems

Effective use of games in the classroom can be undermined in the ways most strategies fail: poor planning, lack of attention, and lack of follow-up. One example of inappropriate game use stemming from each of these obstacles was the use of a simulation game to evaluate treatment skills. There was a specific scoring sheet to test students on the use of a computer program for cognitive rehabilitation. The students were *therapists* with faculty *clients*. This experience was intended to provide feedback on the student's knowledge of the computer program, as well as to provide valuable lessons on therapist–client interaction and use of the environment (e.g., paying attention to the physical environment even though students were intervening for a cognitive task). The main drawbacks to this experience were neglecting to emphasize the game nature of the simulation to reduce trepidation, and having faculty be the clients, which increased anxiety. More planning would have improved the introduction of the activity. More pre-planning may have provided the impetus to revise the format so that there could have been *peer* clients. Knowledge about the use of educational games is essential to create a relaxed and appreciated learning experience.

Other potential pitfalls of game use require the instructor to be aware of:

- *Timing.* Monitor play, termination, and transition to the next learning activities. Fun activities can take on a life of their own. Simulations (especially) and games reduce control of the timing of the class period; the instructor must be comfortable with that reduced control or it will not work. While spontaneity and flexibility are admirable, there is also a need for planned sequences of activities and firm timekeeping.

- *Competition.* Motivation may be limited to those who win; losing may produce a failure experience that decreases self-esteem. Be conscious of all class members and monitor the degree of competition and cooperation required to achieve educational goals. Be ready to change out key players or use teams to encourage more extensive participation.

- *Initial high costs of developing and running a game.* It is quite time consuming to create or flesh out even a frame game. In some instances the task involves no more than developing more test questions/answers (as in *Jeopardy!* or *Trivial Pursuit* games), but that is often easier said than done. The outcome of a recent study found that educators did not have the time to develop appropriate games, and that class sizes made using games even more intimidating (Blakely et al., 2010). In the case of simulation games, a lot of thought is necessary to create an adequate situation and produce a complete cast of characters with goals and belief systems.

- *Unmet needs of participants.* Not all students' learning needs will be met within a simulation or game; therefore, instructors should not depend on these strategies as solo teaching approaches.

- *Closure.* Facilitate appropriate debriefing by allowing adequate time for this phase of the learning experience and being an active listener.

Teaching Examples:
Descriptions of Strategy in Use

The format of *Jeopardy!* lends itself to review of lots of material. One example is pre-exam reviews in an undergraduate mental health class for occupational therapy students, with categories covering such areas as theories, *Diagnostic and Statistical Manual of Mental Disorders, Fifth Edition* (*DSM-5*), defense mechanisms, leadership techniques, and pharmaceuticals. The class was divided into three teams. The regular jeopardy and double jeopardy rounds were employed, although final jeopardy was not. Each team had a person designated as the beeper, and the beepers could collaborate within the team to come up with the question that matched the answer on the overhead projector. Most of the class engaged in the spirit of the game. During the process there was time for discussion and clarification of the topic areas. Errors were made on the exam itself, despite the review, so the game did not lead to the degree of achievement expected. However, it was not formally evaluated or compared with other methods. The participation and apparent enjoyment of that review class were clear, though. (For an example using *Jeopardy!* in nursing education, see Boctor, 2013). A modification of *Jeopardy!* for large groups is to use a multiple-choice format for the potential question and have everyone (or the representative of a small team) write their name on a small piece of paper and drop it into a letter-identified bucket. The winner of the round is selected from the bucket corresponding with the correct answer. That person gets a "prize" and chooses the next category.

An example of a simulation game used in a class on life span development employed the use of percentage dice rolls that each pair of students used to create families and newborns who would function throughout the semester to demonstrate typical human development from birth through adolescence. Each newborn had characteristics (e.g., motor skill, cognitive level, appearance, longevity, social environment, financial environment) that would be based on a limited number of dice rolls. The higher the dice roll, the better the performance or status of the attribute to which it was assigned. The students' first objective was to determine which combination of attributes would lead to the best life outcomes for their children. Was it more important to be very smart or to be very attractive? Could you be successful in life with poor motor skills? After these decisions, there were journaling assignments regarding the development of the children and lots of negotiation between the partners regarding a series of developmental issues, culminating in special dice rolls in adolescence that determined whether the adolescent engaged in smoking and/or sexual activity, was involved in violence, and so on. Student feedback on this experiential assignment was mostly positive, although some did report that it was quite time-consuming. The expected degree of learning regarding human development was demonstrated in the journals. However, the greater learning experience was attitudinal change based on the discussions between partners of differing backgrounds and how they managed to cope with some of the unexpected events of these simulated lives.

■ Conclusion

Games are a suitable supplement for a variety of academic and clinical situations. They are a method of helping students recognize how much they know or how much they still need to study. Different types have been described, as has the appropriate usage within the wide variety of instructional objectives and content in healthcare curricula. The choices and time management required may seem daunting, but educators have found they enjoyed the respite from standard classroom practice while developing and implementing an educational game. It is well worth the effort.

Discussion Questions

1. What aspect of your teaching content lends itself most readily to adaptation into a frame game?
2. Given your teaching environment/context, what are the pros and cons of developing a game within your course?
3. What are your thoughts on use of student-developed games related to class content as part of your assessment of their learning?

References

Aburahma, M. H., & Mohamed, H. M. (2015). Educational games as a teaching tool in pharmacy curriculum. *American Journal of Pharmaceutical Education, 79*(4), 1–9.

Akl, E. A., Pretorius, R. W., Sackett, K., Erdley, W. S., Bhoopathi, P. S., Alfarah, Z., & Schünemann, H. J. (2010). The effect of educational games on medical students' learning outcomes: A systematic review (BEME Guide No. 14). *Medical Teacher, 32*, 16–27.

Alfarah, Z., Schünemann, H. J., & Akl, E. A. (2010). Educational games in geriatric medicine education: A systematic review. *Biomed Central Geriatrics, 10*, 19. Retrieved from http://www.biomedcentral.com/1471-2318/10/19

Allery, L. A. (2004). Educational games and structured experiences [Commentary]. *Medical Teacher, 26*(6), 504–505.

Begg, M. (2008). Leveraging game-informed healthcare education. *Medical Teacher, 30*, 155–158.

Beylefeld, A. A., & Struwig, M. C. (2007). A gaming approach to learning medical microbiology: Students' experiences of flow. *Medical Teacher, 29*, 933–940.

Blakely, G., Skirton, H., Cooper, S., Allum, P., & Nelmes, P. (2009). Educational gaming in the health sciences: Systematic review. *Journal of Advanced Nursing, 65*(2), 259–269.

Blakely, G., Skirton, H., Cooper, S., Allum, P., & Nelmes, P. (2010). Use of educational games in the health professions: A mixed-methods study of educators' perspectives in the UK. *Nursing and Health Sciences, 12*, 27–32.

Bochennek, K., Wittekindt, B., Zimmermann, S., & Klingebiel, T. (2007). More than mere games: A review of card and board games for medical education. *Medical Teacher, 29*, 941–948.

Boctor, L. (2013). Active-learning strategies: The use of a game to reinforce learning in nursing education: A case study. *Nurse Education in Practice, 13*, 96–100.

Boeker, M., Andel, P., Vach, W., & Frankenschmidt, A. (2013). Game-based e-learning is more effective than a conventional instructional method: A randomized controlled trial with third-year medical students. *PLOS ONE, 8*(12), 1–10. Retrieved from http://journals.plos.org/plosone/article?id=10.1371/journal.pone.0082328

Chen, A. M. H., Kiersma, M. E., Yehle, K. S., & Plake, K. S. (2015). Impact of an aging simulation game on pharmacy students' empathy for older adults. *American Journal of Pharmaceutical Education, 79*(5), 1–10.

Derryberry, A. (2007). *Serious games: Online games for learning* [White paper]. Retrieved from http://www.adobe.com/resources/elearning/pdfs/serious_games_wp.pdf

Dormann, C., & Biddle, R. (2006). Humour in game-based learning. *Learning, Media and Technology, 31*(4), 411–424.

Duque, G., Fung, S., Mallet, L., Posel, N., & Fleiszer, D. (2008). Learning while having fun: The use of video gaming to teach geriatric house calls to medical students. *Journal of the American Geriatric Society, 56*, 1328–1332.

Gee, J. P. (2008). Learning and games. In K. Salen (Ed.), *The ecology of games: Connecting youth, games, and learning* (pp. 21–40). Cambridge, MA: MIT Press.

Gleason, A. W. (2015). RELM: Developing a serious game to teach evidence-based medicine in an academic health sciences setting. *Medical Reference Services Quarterly, 34*(1), 17–28.

Graham, I., & Richardson, E. (2008). Experiential gaming to facilitate cultural awareness: Its implication for developing emotional caring in nursing. *Learning in Health and Social Care, 7*, 37–45.

Greenfield, P. M. (2009). Technology and informal education: What is taught, what is learned. *Science, 323,* 69–71.

Jarrell, K., Alpers, R., Brown, G., & Wotring, R. (2008). Using BaFa' BaFa' in evaluating cultural competence of nursing students. *Teaching and Learning in Nursing, 3,* 141–142.

Johnson, S. A., & Romanello, M. L. (2005). Generational diversity: Teaching and learning approaches. *Nurse Educator, 30*(5), 212–216.

Kanthan, R., & Senger, J-L. (2011). The impact of specially designed digital games-based learning in undergraduate pathology and medical education. *Archives of Pathology & Laboratory Medicine, 135,* 135–142.

Lee, J. J., & Hammer, J. (2011). Gamification in education: What, how, why bother? *Academic Exchange Quarterly, 15*(2), 1–5.

Lujan, H. L., & DiCarlo, S. E. (2006). First-year medical students prefer multiple learning styles. *Advances in Physiology Education, 30,* 13–16.

Lynch-Sauer, J., VandenBosch, T. M., Kron, F., Gjerde, C. L., Arato, N., Sen, A., & Fetters, M. D. (2011). Nursing students' attitudes toward video games and related new media technologies. *Journal of Nursing Education, 50*(9), 513–523.

McGonigal, J. (2011). *Reality is broken: Why games make us better and how they can change the world.* New York, NY: Penguin Books.

Medina, J. (2008). *Brain rules.* Seattle, WA: Pear Press.

Nevin, C. R., Westfall, A. O., Rodriguez, J. M., Dempsey, D. M., Cherrington, A., Roy, B., . . .Willig, J. H. (2014). Gamification as a tool for enhancing graduate medical education. *Postgraduate Medical Journal, 90,* 685–693. doi:10.1136/postgradmedj-2013-132486

Nicholson, S. (2011, September–October). Making gameplay matter: Designing modern educational tabletop games. *Knowledge Quest, 40*(1), 60–65. Retrieved from http://eric.ed.gov/?id=EJ964283

Oblinger, D. (2006). Games and learning. *EDUCAUSE Quarterly, 29*(3), 5–7.

Patel, J. (2008). Using game format in small group classes for pharmacotherapeutics case studies. *American Journal of Pharmaceutical Education, 72*(1), 1–5.

Reiner, B., & Siegel, E. (2008). The potential for gaming techniques in radiology education and practice. *Journal of the American College of Radiology, 5,* 110–114.

Ridley, R. T. (2004). Classroom games are COOL: Collaborative opportunities of learning. *Nurse Educator, 29*(2), 47–48.

Royse, M. A., & Newton, S. E. (2007). How gaming is used as an innovative strategy for nursing education. *Nursing Education Perspectives, 28*(5), 263–267.

Sauve, L., Renaud, L., Kaufman, D., & Marquis, J. (2007). Distinguishing between games and simulations: A systematic review. *Educational Technology & Society, 10*(3), 247–256.

Sederstrom, J. (2014, June 9). Develop a gamification game plan. *Managed Healthcare Executive.* Retrieved from http://managedhealthcareexecutive.modernmedicine.com/managed-healthcare-executive/content/tags/consumer-engagement/develop-gamification-game-plan

Sheldon, L. (2012). *The multiplayer classroom: Designing coursework as a game.* Boston, MA: Course Technology/Cengage Learning.

Shiroma, P. R., Massa, A. A., & Alarcon, R. D. (2011). Using game format to teach psychopharmacology to medical students. *Medical Teacher, 33,* 156–160.

Skiba, D. J. (2008). Nursing education 2.0: Games as pedagogical platforms. *Nursing Education Perspectives, 29*(3), 174–175.

Skiba, D. J. (2013). Emerging technology: On the horizon: The year of the MOOCs. *Nursing Education Perspectives, 34*(2), 136–137.

Smith, G. (2008). First day questions for the learner-centered classroom. *National Teaching & Learning Forum, 17*(5), 1–4.

Stanford University. (n.d.). *Is the lecture dead? The large lecture course in the humanities today.* Retrieved from https://teachingcommons.stanford.edu/events/lecture-dead-large-lecture-course-humanities-today

Van Eck, R. (2006). Digital game-based learning: It's not just the digital natives who are restless. *EDUCAUSE Review, 41*(2), 16–30.

Wright, K. (2012). Student nurses' perceptions of how they learn drug calculation skills. *Nurse Education Today, 32,* 721–726.

Recommended Reading

Cowen, K. J., & Tesh, A. S. (2002). Effects of gaming on nursing students' knowledge of pediatric cardiovascular dysfunction. *Journal of Nursing Education, 41*(11), 507–509.

Dologite, K. A., Willner, K. C., Klepeiss, D. J., York, S. A., & Cericola, L. M. (2003). Sharpen customer service skills with PCRAFT Pursuit©. *Journal for Nurses in Staff Development, 19*(1), 47–51.

Dunn, J. (2012). *The 100-second guide to gamification in education.* Retrieved from http://edudemic.com/2012/09/the-100-second-guide-to-gamification-in-education/

Flanagan, N., & McCausland, L. (2007). Teaching around the cycle: Strategies for teaching theory to undergraduate nursing students. *Nursing Education Perspectives, 28,* 310–314.

Gifford, K. E. (2001). Using instructional games: A teaching strategy for increasing student participation and retention. *Occupational Therapy in Health Care, 15,* 13–21.

Horsley, T. L. (2010). Education theory and classroom games: Increasing knowledge and fun in the classroom. *Journal of Nursing Education, 49*(6), 363–364.

Johnston, B., Boyle, L., MacArthur, E., & Manion, B. F. (2013). The role of technology and digital gaming in nurse education. *Nursing Standard, 27*(28), 35–38.

Jones, A. G., Jasperson, J., & Gusa, D. (2000). Cranial nerve wheel of competencies. *Journal of Continuing Education in Nursing, 31*(4), 152–154.

Masters, K. (2005). Development and use of an educator-developed community assessment board game. *Nurse Educator, 30*(5), 189–190.

Morton, P. G., & Tarvin, L. (2001). The pain game: Pain assessment, management, and related JCAHO standards. *Journal of Continuing Education in Nursing, 32*(5), 223–227.

Pearce-Smith, N. (2007). Teaching tip: Using the "Who Wants to Be a Millionaire?" game to teach searching skills. *Evidence-Based Nursing, 10,* 72.

Persky, A. M., Stegall-Zanation, J., & Dupuis, R. E. (2007). Students' perceptions of the incorporation of games into classroom instruction for basic and clinical pharmacokinetics. *American Journal of Pharmaceutical Education, 71*(2), 1–9.

Smith-Stoner, M. (2005, September/October). Innovative use of the Internet and intranets to provide education by adding games. *CIN: Computers, Informatics, Nursing,* 237–241.

Stringer, E. C. (1997). Word games as a cost-effective and innovative inservice method. *Journal of Nursing Staff Development, 13*(3), 155–160.

Ward, A. K., & O'Brien, H. L. (2005). A gaming adventure. *Journal for Nurses in Staff Development, 21*(1), 37–41.

CHAPTER 15

Role Play

Arlene J. Lowenstein

■ Definition and Purposes

Role play is a dramatic technique that encourages participants to improvise behaviors illustrating expected actions of persons involved in defined situations. A scenario is outlined, and character roles are assigned. The scenario can be scripted and rehearsed, but it is usually unscripted, relying on spontaneous interplay among characters to provide material about reactions and behaviors for students to analyze following the presentation. Those class members not assigned character roles participate as observers in the audience and provide feedback to contribute to the overall analysis. Role playing allows students to engage their imaginations to explore scenarios that target potential issues and stimulate team building. For the exercise to be productive, all the students must be committed to participating and feel comfortable and safe in the environment (Sasha, 2011). Role-play exercises are an ideal way for the participants to practice skills and experience ethical or culturally sensitive situations. To be most effective in developing practical skills, these learning experiences should be applicable to the actual context in which they will be used (Lane, Hood, & Rollnick, 2008).

Part of the category of simulation, role play allows participants to explore why people behave as they do. Participants can test communication skills, behaviors, and decisions in an environment that allows experimentation without risk. The scenario and behaviors of the actors are analyzed and discussed to provide opportunity to clarify feelings, increase observational skills, provide rationale for potential behaviors, improve communication skills, and anticipate reactions to decisions. New behaviors and communication techniques can be suggested and tried in response to the analysis.

Role play is used to enable students to practice interacting with others in certain roles and to afford them an opportunity to experience other people's reactions to actions they have taken. The scenario may be outlined to provide a background for the problem and the constraints that may apply. Defining the important characteristics of the major players establishes role expectations and provides a framework for behaviors and actions to be elicited.

The author wishes to thank Maureen Harris for her review and contributions to this chapter.

The postplay discussion provides opportunity for analysis and new strategy formation. Repeating a role play after the debriefing session provides the students with the opportunity for a second chance or do-over, thereby giving them confidence in handling tough situations (Silberman, 2006). Although it is a dramatic technique, the focus is on the actions of the characters and not on acting ability. An actor plays to the audience; the role player plays to the characters in the scenario. The audience also has a role: that of observing the interplay among characters and analyzing the dynamics occurring. The instructor's role is facilitator rather than director. The impetus for the analysis and discussion belongs with the learners. The instructor's role is passive—clarifying and gently guiding.

The role play, regardless of its length, develops communicative competence. Throughout this creative process, the student group must work together to exchange information and polish the presentation as they both speak and listen. The peer feedback offered by the audience will be valuable in assessing how well the players adopted cultural roles and expressed opinions (Qing, 2011).

Clinical simulations often incorporate role play. Although the simulation computer and mannequin provide the physiological issues in the scenario, students or faculty members may play the human roles, such as the doctor or family members. The computer operator may also provide a voice for the patient, to which the healthcare provider needs to relate, and this technique allows for better assessment of a patient's response to issues such as anxiety or pain. The use of role play creates the opportunity to provide care to the simulated patient in a realistic environment and requires reactions to complexity in the situation. Smith-Stoner used high-fidelity simulation together with role play to provide a scenario in which a student nurse, who was caring for a simulated patient who died during the scenario, needed to interact with the family member who was in the room. The exercise allowed the students in the class to explore their attitudes toward death and caring for dying patients (Smith-Stoner, 2009).

The use of the simulated patient has been effective to provide the practice and rehearsal necessary to increase competence in motivational interviewing, which is a method that works on influencing individuals to consider changing their behavior. Lane and colleagues (2008) found experienced practitioners engaging in role-play scenarios achieved the same level of competence in motivational interviewing whether they practiced with a peer or a simulated patient.

Role play can also be used in online courses. Although there may be no person-to-person drama, a scenario can be set up, parts assigned, and the conversation carried out via a chat room or discussion board. Riddle (2009) noted online educational role plays engage students in the learning and can be an improvement over didactic teaching strategies alone. Online role-play systems afford students the opportunity of acting and doing instead of only reading and listening.

Role play is a particularly effective means for developing decision-making and problem-solving skills (Hess & Giligannon, 1985). Imholz (2008) studied clinical research on the psychodrama practice of role play, looking at the therapeutic activity as both cognitive and emotional outcomes of the role play as change agent and also as a process that contributes to personal growth. Through role play, the learner can identify the systematic steps in the process of making judgments and decisions. The problem-solving process—identification of the problem, data collection, evaluation of possible outcomes, exploration of alternatives, and arrival at a decision to be implemented—can be analyzed in the context of the role-play situation. The scenario can include reactions to the implementation of the decision as well as the evaluation and reformulation process (Alden, 1999; Domazzo & Hanson, 1997). Role play has also been used to increase student cultural awareness, aiding in the development of cultural competence in patient care (Shearer & Davidhizar, 2003).

Role play can be utilized to develop competence in overall communications as well as to increase students' intercultural awareness. Collaborative role plays, which are performed in groups, can be beneficial as the students create the entire story complete with the cast of characters and dialogue. This can be a long-term process where one or more cultural considerations are raised during each role-play scenario and the interpersonal communication skills of the group develop. Eventually, the group rehearses the scenario and performs it for the audience, followed by a peer feedback session (Qing, 2011).

Role play provides immediate feedback to learners regarding their success in using interpersonal skills as well as decision-making and problem-solving skills. At the same time, role play offers learners an opportunity to become actively involved in the learning experience in a nonthreatening environment. Role play is not limited to use in the classroom. Corless and colleagues (2004) successfully used role play as a student assignment that required the adoption of the persona of a person with HIV who was required to take a number of medications over a specific period of time. Students carried out the role play in their homes, taking placebos in place of medication over a specific time frame. Their experiences in following the HIV regimen were then discussed in class, leading to an awareness of the difficulties patients faced in following the regimen. Role play is also being used as a teaching strategy in online courses (Mar, Chabal, Anderson, & Vore, 2003).

Giving feedback to the role-play performers, also called the *debriefing*, is a reflective process. Feedback is provided by peers, teacher, and a self-assessment. A feedback session is held at the conclusion of the role-play exercise to engage all the students in reflective discussion. The teacher's observations and opinions are highly regarded, but the entire audience needs to provide productive comments. The class as a whole or small groups offer their reactions and feedback to the role-play exercise. Prior to the feedback session, the teacher should instruct the students to offer positive and then constructive comments and to be specific. The teacher may assign specific students in the audience to attend to a player or group of players, a particular nuance (e.g., nonverbal behavior), and/or specific open-ended or closed-ended questions. The teacher seeks feedback from the players and the audience. What went well? What did not go well? What could be done to improve each player's performance? The teacher may offer observations or seek audience observations with a comparison to a benchmark/ideal script. Each role player is required to self-assess his or her performance and feelings about the experience (Silberman, 2006). Videotaping the role-play exercise can be an effective debriefing technique if used to review specific points in the recording. The teacher should attempt to draw the problem solving and decision making from the students to facilitate long-term carryover and learning (Silberman, 2006).

Verbal and nonverbal communication must be considered. Students may experiment with various facial expressions; pace, volume, and tone of voice; body language and physical gestures; and use of humor or drama. Role play has the potential to create an active atmosphere within the classroom that mobilizes the entire audience with enthusiasm (Qing, 2011).

■ Theoretical Rationale

Role play developed in response to the need to effect attitudinal changes in psychotherapy and counseling (Shaffer & Galinsky, 1974). Psychodrama, a forerunner of role play, was developed by Moreno as a psychotherapy technique. Moreno brought psychodrama to the United States in 1925 and continued to develop it during the 1940s and 1950s (Moreno, 1946). In psychodrama, players may be required to recite specific lines or answer specific questions and may represent themselves, whereas in role play, players are encouraged to express their thoughts and feelings spontaneously, as if they were the persons whose roles they are playing (Sharon & Sharon, 1976).

Psychodrama provided a foundation for further development of role play as an educational technique. Corsini (1957) and other psychotherapists and group dynamicists began using role play to assist patients to clarify people's behavior toward each other. Further development led to the use of role play in sensitivity training, a technique that became popular in the 1970s. Human relations and sensitivity training events share a common educational strategy. The learners in the group are encouraged to become involved in examining their thought patterns, perceptions, feelings, and inadequacies. The training events are also designed to encourage each learner, with the support of fellow learners, to invent and experiment with different patterns of functioning (Gordon, 1970). Role play can be used to meet those educational objectives; it is often used in human relations and sensitivity training, but has many other uses as well. DeNeve and Hepner (1997), in a study comparing role play to traditional lectures, found that (1) students believed the use of role play was stimulating and valuable in comparison to the traditional lecture method, (2) their learning increased, and (3) they remembered what they had learned.

In a study that looked at nursing students who role played with theater students and those who role played with other nursing students, Reams and Bashford (2011) noted that the students who played with the theater students gained confidence in their approach to patients and interdisciplinary colleagues by practicing repeatedly within a safe environment. However, when nursing students role played with a nursing student peer, they were inadvertently assisted by the peer. This assistance interfered with the nursing students' gaining confidence in their approach to patients, and it may be something for the instructor to watch out for.

■ Conditions

Role playing is a versatile technique that can be used in a wide variety of situations. One set of learning objectives might be role play dealing with the practice of skills and techniques, whereas a different group of objectives would use role play to deal with changes in understanding, feelings, and attitudes. Van Ments (1983) points out role play is conducted differently for these two sets of learning objectives. The role play used for the practice of skills may be planned with the emphasis on outcome and overcoming problems. The second type of objective may best be met with an emphasis on the problems and relationships. This method explores why certain behaviors are exhibited and requires expertise from the instructor in dealing with emotions and human behavior. The teacher is responsible for helping the students to avoid the negative effects that could come from the exploration of their feelings and behaviors. In any scenario, there is potential for conflict. The students may struggle to control their feelings so as to clearly relay their message without emotion. To resolve disagreements, confusions, and obstacles, students will need to understand the motives behind their actions. The teacher helps the players stay focused on achieving the objectives (Sasha, 2011).

Role play is a useful tool for developing communication skills. The role players assume personalities and act according to their understanding of their characters. The scenarios help prepare participants for future situations by allowing them to experience different perspectives. These lessons may be retained for long periods of time (Sasha, 2011).

Laughter can play a role in group communication and group dynamics even when the situation is not humorous. Laughter can be a tool, used intentionally and strategically, to direct communication and affect group dynamics (Keyton & Beck, 2010). Keep in mind that a role play is an exercise, not a reality, so it should not be taken too seriously. Humor should be encouraged, as it can be effective in defusing tension or hostility provoked during the role-play exercise, thus fostering positive attitudes (Bartle, 2007).

Role-play exercises can be designed with more than one student playing a role, to decrease the stress placed on an individual student. Two to four students can play one role, thereby allowing the shy students to feel more comfortable about actively participating in front of the audience. This technique also allows students to work as a team to create the dialogue, whether rehearsed or improvised. This collaboration is valuable training for what is required in practical healthcare situations where a team of doctors, nurses, therapists, nutritionists, and social workers provide patient care. Also, students in the audience have the opportunity to tap a role player on the shoulder and replace him or her as the character in the scenario so as to contribute something they feel is worthwhile. Likewise, a role player can tap an audience member on the shoulder and take that person's place as an audience member; thus, all students are potential role players. This exercise may be set up in two rows facing each other, in a half circle, or in a full circle, which has been referred to as a *fishbowl*.

■ Planning and Modifying

Teachers who are new to the technique need to plan before class, but they should monitor the needs of the group as the experience progresses and be able to modify those plans if necessary. The situation developed should be familiar enough that learners can understand the roles and their potential responses, but it should not have a direct relationship to students' own personal problems (McKeachie, 2002). It can also be effective to use two or more presentations of the same situation with different students in the roles if the objective is to point out different responses or solutions to a given problem. When this method is used, the instructor may choose to keep those students involved in the second presentation away from viewing the first presentation, to avoid biasing their reactions. The same role-play scenario can be used throughout the semester to allow students to react to changing events within the same scenario (Rabinowitz, 1997).

Role-play strategy qualifies as an adult-learning approach because it presents a real-life situation and tries to stimulate the involvement of the student. It has special value because it uses peer evaluation and involves active participation. However, it must be carefully guided to be sure participants have an understanding of the objectives and to ensure that feedback received from other players is congruent with outcomes that would exist in the real world (Mann & Corsun, 2002).

■ Types of Learners

Role play is appropriate for both undergraduate and graduate students. It is especially effective in staff development programs because of its association with reality. It is used effectively to reach effective outcomes. Role play can be simple or complex, depending on the learning objectives. Regardless of the simplicity of the play itself, it is important to allow adequate time for planning, preparation of the students for the experience, and postplay discussion and analysis. The actual role play may be as brief as 5 minutes, although 10–20 minutes is more common. Van Ments (1983) suggests that the technique be broken into the following three sections: briefing, running, and debriefing. Equal amounts of time may be spent in each session on simple objectives, or a ratio of 1:2:3, with most time spent on the debriefing or analysis for more complex learning objectives.

■ Resources

Role play can be used in most settings, although tiered lecture rooms may inhibit the ability of the players to relate to each other and to the observing students. In that setting, the theatricality of the technique is likely to be emphasized over the needed behavioral focus (Van Ments, 1983). Special equipment or props may be simple or not used at all, again depending on the objectives. An instructor may choose to use video- or audio taping. This can be especially helpful to review portions of the action during the debriefing and analysis section. Reviewing tapes may also be helpful for participating students who, because of their roles, were not in the room to hear and see some of the interactions that occurred in other role plays. A checklist of specific observations may be helpful to the students when developing their debriefing skills, tone of voice, eye contact, response to constructive criticism, and other aspects of communication.

Outside resources are not usually needed for most role-play situations, although additional instructors, trained observers, or specific experts may appropriately be used to meet certain objectives. The technique is best for small groups of students so that those not involved in the character parts can be actively involved in observing and discussing the action in the debriefing or analyzing portion. Van Ments (1983) found role play increasingly unsatisfactory as a technique in groups with more than 25 students, although there may be exceptions, depending on objectives and strategies for involving the audience. Creative role-play methods to accommodate more than 25 students are discussed in the next section.

■ Using the Method

When designing role-playing exercises, start with the script, which consists of the roles to be played via improvisation, prescription, or rehearsal followed by the drama or situation. Improvisation, which promotes spontaneity, is often difficult and intimidating for some students. The teacher has the option of assigning the roles and instructing the students in how to behave. Although this approach is less intimidating to the students, it may be more challenging for the students to identify with their assigned characters. Some role plays involve a detailed description of the situation, but the students have creative license regarding how to handle it. Student improvisations are risky, and the teacher's intended objectives may not be met (Silberman, 2006).

The situation may or may not be dramatic and may be a replay of a past situation or of a hypothetical event. Students may be most comfortable replaying a situation they have previously experienced. This can be performed informally as a conversation or with a rehearsed script. Realistic situations can provide valuable learning opportunities for all the students (Silberman, 2006). Next, consider the staging options, which include informal conversation between the teacher and a student that develops into a class discussion; formal setup with a pair or a trio in front of the group; simultaneous pairs acting out a scenario, which reduces anxiety as all the students are participating at the same time; rotational role play in front of the class, where the students tap in and out of the exercise; or one role played by three or four individuals simultaneously as a team (Silberman, 2006). These various models utilize more players, thereby accommodating groups of more than 25 students.

Planning is crucial to effective use of role play as a learning technique. It may be helpful to test the exercise before running it in the class situation to allow the instructor to anticipate potential problems and evaluate if the learning objectives can be met. Discussing critical elements of the role play with colleagues can be useful if full-scale testing is not feasible. A small amount of time spent going through the plans with someone else may prevent a critical element from going wrong and disrupting the exercise (Van Ments, 1983).

Selecting a scenario and deciding on character roles is an important part of planning. McKeachie (2002) cautions that situations involving morals or subjects of high emotional significance, such as sexual taboos, are apt to be traumatic to some students. He found the most interesting situations, and those revealing the greatest differences in responses, are those involving some choice or conflict of motives. Student input into planning can also be effective.

To implement the role play, the scenario and characters must be described briefly but with enough information to elicit responses that will meet the learning objectives. This planning is extremely important for obtaining good results. Spontaneity should be encouraged, so it is preferable to avoid a script, other than bare outlines of the action. Although spontaneity is valued in character dialogue, students need to have a clear understanding of their characters and those characters' basic attitudes and/or thought patterns. In some instances, spontaneity in the character description area could compromise the objectives and results, but if students understand the expected character, they can still be spontaneous within the character parameters. Allowing students in the character roles to have a few minutes to warm up and relate to the roles they will be playing is often helpful. Observing students absolutely must be briefed on their role. Enough time must be allotted for discussion and analysis of the action. The debriefing following the role play also allows for evaluation of the success in meeting the learning objectives.

In addition to the development of learning objectives and planning, the instructor is responsible for setting the stage for the role play, monitoring the action, and leading the analysis. Students need a clear understanding of the objectives, the scenario, the characters they are to play, the importance of the role of the observers, and the analysis as a vital part of the process. On occasion, the instructor may take a character role, but usually character roles are given to students.

When planning a role-play session, the instructor needs to be concerned with the amount of time students may be excluded from the room while waiting for their turn to participate. This issue is especially important when two or more presentations of the same situation are to be used, or when the role play has characters who should not be exposed to the dialogue that occurs before they appear in their roles. In some instances, it may be appropriate to have students switch roles during the role play to provide them with an opportunity to see and feel different reactions to similar situations, thereby experiencing a new perspective. For example, to achieve the learning objective of how to conduct a group, students may benefit by playing a group member and then switching to the leader, or vice versa, during the exercise.

Students must practice their listening skills during role-play exercises. Individuals must quiet their own thoughts when the characters are speaking. It is constructive for the students to prepare their thoughts before speaking, but listening is equally important. Players may jot down thoughts that pop into their minds on a notepad to ensure that they remain focused on other people's responses (Sasha, 2011).

The instructor needs to encourage students to respond to interactions in the role play in a spontaneous, natural manner, avoiding melodrama and inappropriate laughing or silliness. Effective use of role play focuses on student participation and interaction. The instructor, as facilitator, channels the discussion to meet the learning objectives but avoids monopolizing the play or discussion. The instructor must also be able to monitor and control the depth of emotional responses to the situation or interplay as needed, terminating the play when the objective has been met or the emotional climate calls for intervention.

Students need to understand the importance of playing the character roles in ways in which they believe those characters would act in a real-life situation (Mann & Corsun, 2002). Students in the observer role must be strongly encouraged to present their observations and contribute to the discussion and analysis. Students can also take part in the development of role-play scenarios, identifying the learning objectives, issues and problems they feel should be explored, as well as scenarios that may provide that exploration.

Graduate schools are catering to the full-time-worker market by offering online courses, provided either asynchronously, without attendance on campus required; or synchronously, where there is a designated login time for class. Given that today's health care is team oriented and interdisciplinary with each member required to speak, whether it is to ask questions or defend his or her position, in immediate time frames, the synchronous online course may be favored. Using real problem scenarios is an authentic learning approach that is effective in stimulating communication. Culley and Polyakova-Norwood (2012) had students work in teams to discuss and reflect upon their experiences and practice professional behaviors in a safe environment. Synchronous online role play was effective in fostering collaborative communication, which significantly improved their learning experience. Synchronous online role play requires coordination of all students' schedules and mastery of communication technology (e.g., web cams and microphones to create a virtual meeting room) to be successful. Some students preferred to participate anonymously and thus were reluctant to engage in synchronous online role play (Culley & Polyakova-Norwood, 2012).

Role play in the online environment uses the same basic principles, but with some differences, since the characters will not be visible to each other or to the audience (Mar et al., 2003). A synchronous environment, where all parties are online at the same time, will allow for a written dialogue flow between parties, with more similarity to an actual conversation (Phillips, 2005). An asynchronous environment, where parties log on at different times, will take longer to carry out the scenario and may not have as much spontaneity, but can be equally effective (Lebaron & Miller, 2005). As in all cases of role play, the design of an online role play will depend on the learning objectives.

■ Potential Problems

Van Ments (1983) refers to the hidden agenda and stereotyping that may occur as roles are presented, often reflecting the expectations and values of the students or the teacher. This stereotyping may lead to unanticipated learning that reinforces prejudices and preconceptions. Instructors need to be aware of this possibility and avoid writing in stereotypes. They should describe only functions, powers, and constraints of the role described. Roles should be rotated to avoid overidentification of one student with a specific role. In the debriefing session, the students are invited to question and challenge assumptions. Students may not always make a distinction between an actor and a role. Criticism of the student playing the role must be avoided, while allowing for critique of the behavior of the role character. The instructor must be aware of the emotional tones involved in the role play and channel the emotions into activities that will lead to successful attainment of the learning objectives.

Planning and learning objectives should determine the course of the role play. Students may take the role play in an unexpected direction, possibly because they have a need to explore another issue or problem. If it is not appropriate to revise the learning objectives to accommodate student needs, then the play can be terminated. In that case, the postplay discussion can be used to assist students in recognizing why the technique was not effective. Students should advise how to improve the role play or develop a different teaching strategy. Repeating a scenario with the same or different characters can sometimes afford a more in-depth examination and add to the experience.

The instructor and students need to be aware this is not a professional drama. Some students, because of stage fright, shyness, or other reasons, do not like participating (Middleton, 2005; Turner, 2005). Although at times it may be appropriate to change actors if the role play does not seem to be going well, it is important not to blame the students. In most cases, the teaching strategy requires changing, rather than the actors.

The environment must be arranged so all the role players can see and hear each other and the audience can see and hear all the players' verbal and nonverbal communication. Tone of voice and eye contact can affect how a verbal message is received. Some students multitask while participating in class. At times some students use social media site(s) while also attending classroom presentations. Such incidents of divided attention displayed by the audience during a role-play experience may be counterproductive to their ability to actively participate in the analysis portion of the exercise. Videotaping a role-play exercise may be highly effective in providing a replay of specific sections of the exercise during the debriefing; however, the role players may feel self-conscious being videotaped, thereby inhibiting their performance (Silberman, 2006). If these issues are understood and addressed, role play can be an effective and creative strategy to provide active student participation to meet specific learning objectives.

Teaching Examples:
Group Dynamics—Conflict Resolution and Role-Play Scenarios: Fishbowl

These role-play scenarios are a hands-on approach to engage learners in the process of identifying a conflict early in its development, negotiating and implementing its resolution, and using interpersonal skills to foster a positive working relationship and successful outcome. When conflict arises, work to be part of the solution, not part of the problem.

The fishbowl format enables multiple students to be actively involved in the role-play activity while giving the players the comfort of playing the same role as several other classmates. The participants' comments build on each other while the audience observes and analyzes the role play as it evolves.

The content regarding identifying conflicts, strategies for negotiating, reducing, and resolving conflict(s) by successfully utilizing an effective interpersonal approach is presented after the role play is completed. The instructor may attempt to facilitate the objectives during the role-play exercise.

Objectives

1. To use role playing to practice communication skills when in situations where conflict arises, so as to learn by doing.
2. To clearly identify a problem situation related to group dynamics.
3. To accurately state the problem identified in a nonemotional manner conducive to negotiation.
4. To establish a mechanism to clearly state a problem situation that has been identified.
5. To develop a process to deal with group situations involving a variety of personalities, to foster relationship-building opportunities.
6. To effectively employ interpersonal skills when utilizing strategies for reducing conflict(s).
7. To efficiently implement steps to resolve problems to facilitate collaborative dynamics for students working in groups.
8. To establish boundaries within which a group should work to achieve an effective work product in a timely manner.

Role Play Fishbowl Instructions

The instructor divides the class into four groups with 10–12 students in each group, as follows:

Group 1: Sally Slacker
Group 2: The four other students in Sally's group
Group 3: Carol Controller
Group 4: The four other students in Carol's group

Each group meets for 10 minutes to discuss its assigned role in the scenario. The students determine what the character they are assigned to play would say to explain or justify the character's behavior. Also, they must devise a plan of how to approach the situation in a manner to successfully resolve the conflict.

Each group chooses four students to enter the fishbowl.

Setting: Classroom

Setting up the Fishbowl

Two sets of four chairs are set up facing each other in the front of the classroom. See **Figure 15-1** for classroom setup.

Fishbowl Rules

The groups of students not sitting in the fishbowl act as the audience. Students can tap in and tap out of the fishbowl. Any audience member can tap in to verbalize something he or she feels needs to be said. When a student taps in, one of the students sitting in the fishbowl returns to the audience. Students in the fishbowl can tap out by picking a member of their group in the audience to take their place.

Group 1 and Group 2 Scenario

Sally Slacker

You are working in a group of 5 on a project that is due at the end of a 12-week semester. Your group divides up the work evenly and sets deadlines for the work to be completed in increments. At each deadline, the group meets and reevaluates the progress of the project. Assignments are modified and the group produces the final project in phases. Sally does not complete her aspect of the assigned project on time and is not able to take on additional work during the group reevaluation

(continues)

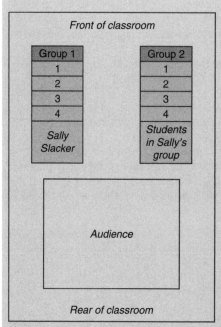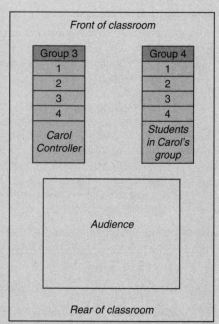

■ **Figure 15-1**   Classroom setup for fishbowl.

sessions. During the final meeting, Sally reports that she will complete her section and submit it to the group editor 24 hours before the final due date. When this 24-hour deadline arrives, there is silence from Sally. Twelve hours later, Sally has still not responded to queries from the group editor. The group needs to decide how to approach Sally Slacker to obtain her section of the project so they can submit the project on time for the best possible grade. They schedule a meeting for 1:00 PM.

In the dialogue that follows, the characters are represented by letters and numbers as follows:

SS = Sally Slacker
SSG1 = Sally Slacker group member No. 1
SSG2 = Sally Slacker group member No. 2
SSG3 = Sally Slacker group member No. 3
SSG4 = Sally Slacker group member No. 4
SSG4R = Audience replacement for SSG4
SSG2R = Audience replacement for SSG2
A = Audience
I = Instructor

Role-Play Dialogue
SSG1:   Sally, we have called this meeting to discuss the section of the project you were assigned. I need to add your section into the document and submit the project by 5:00 PM
today. Is your section ready to turn in?
SS: Well, there really isn't a problem; I am doing it and it will be finished by the time it is due.

SSG2:   The project is due by 5:00 PM today!

SSG3:   We all finished our sections 2 days ago!

SSG4:   I finished my section last week. I need a good grade on this project and you are not taking this seriously!

SS: Well, I work better under pressure. I never finish a project a week early. I feel like you are all ganging up on me.

SSG4:   Maybe it is better if SSG1 speaks for the group so you won't feel like we are ganging up on you.

SSG1:   Sally, we respect that you work best under a deadline, but we are concerned that you have not turned in anything for the past 12 weeks and now the project is due in 4 hours and we still have nothing to add for your section. Are you okay?

SS: You are all so organized and I know I haven't been able to keep up with the project. This has been a really tough semester for me. I couldn't afford my rent so I moved home, which is a 4-hour commute, round trip. I feel so disorganized. I never seem to have everything I need with me to work on my section.

SSG1:   I wish you had told us so we could have been supportive.

I: As a group, how could you have handled this situation differently?

SSG4R (A new group member taps in and replaces SSG4):   This meeting/ conversation should have been initiated early in the semester during the group reevaluation sessions when it was clear that SS was not completing her aspect of the assigned project on time and was not able to take on additional work.

SSG2R (SSG2 taps out and is replaced with one of Group 2's audience members):   How do we, as a group, complete the project today? Do we discuss our problem with the course instructor? Do we request an extension?

I: Let's open this discussion up to the audience.

Debriefing of Sally Slacker Role Play

Overall, good strategies for reducing conflict were employed, especially when SSG1 acted as the spokesperson for the group. These strategies include the following:

> Listen.
> State the problem clearly.
> Be respectful.
> Consider other perspectives.
> Be open to compromise.

Although there was a problem, the group did not address it until hours before the project was due. When the group confronted SS, several members exhibited elevated emotions and anxiety levels, as they were concerned about completing the project on time to get a good grade.

Negotiation strategies were successfully employed by SSG1. These strategies included the following:

> Call a meeting.
> State the rationale for the meeting.
> Give specific examples that illustrate the problem. State why it is a problem.
> Confirm the facts.
> Listen to the other side.

(continues)

This role play focused on the negotiation of the problem, whereas the active audience discussion focused on problem resolution, including the following:

Make suggestions for a solution.
Confirm feasibility of solution(s) and consider other solutions. Achieve consensus regarding solution(s).
Offer help to make the changes.
Share responsibility for managing the outcome.

In discussing the interpersonal approach, it was noted that SSG1 effectively used *I/we* (versus *you*) when presenting the problem and focused on SS's behavior, not on her as a person.

Group 3 and Group 4 Scenario

Carol Controller

You are working in a group of 5, on a project that is due at the end of a 12-week semester. Your group divides up the work evenly and sets deadlines for the work to be completed in increments. At each deadline the group meets and reevaluates the progress of the project. Assignments are modified and the group produces the final project in phases.

Carol is the self-appointed leader of this group. Carol assigns each group member a section, and during the reevaluation meetings she determines the modifications needed. Carol Controller is out of control; she shoots down any ideas that the group members propose and is making all the decisions regarding the direction of the project. The group needs to approach Carol so that all ideas are heard and considered. In the dialogue that follows, the characters are represented according to the following key:

CC = Carol Controller
CCG1 = Carol Controller group member No. 1
CCG2 = Carol Controller group member No. 2
CCG3 = Carol Controller group member No. 3
CCG4 = Carol Controller group member No. 4
CCG4R = Audience replacement for CCG4
CCG2R = Audience replacement for CCG2
A = Audience
I = Instructor

Role-Play Dialogue

CCG1: Carol, we like the way you have organized the workload and moved the project along. However, we are feeling like our project is not a true reflection of our work. We would like to have a more democratic process for determining which aspects of the project make the final edit.

CC: I have always been a good leader. I am well organized and know what needs to be done to get assignments done on time.

CCG2: We appreciate that you are organized and good at moving things along and getting things done. But, we would like to work together to fine-tune the final draft, choose the color schemes, and even choose the font that we feel make our project unique to our style as a group.

CC: We do work together. I always ask for input before I make changes.

CCG1: When I used a background color of green, you changed it to pink without even discussing it with me.

CC: I have taken courses with this teacher before, so I know what the teacher wants. I know pink is her favorite color, so we need to use pink.

CCG3:   We have also taken courses with this teacher before, so we also know what she wants. There is more than one style, and variety is not a bad thing. The goal is to produce a product that represents the whole group. We all need to participate.

CCG3:   When we discuss the direction of the project, you don't seem to listen to us. No matter what we come up with, you shoot us down without even considering that our ideas were worth pursuing.

CCG3:   And when you take my paper and change it so it is in your writing style, it makes me feel like you don't value my input and contribution. You should not change my words simply because you think your style is better.

CC: Why are you all being so sensitive? You should be happy that I am willing to carry this group.

CCG2:   I see no point in putting hours into a product when Carol is going to edit all our work out and use only her ideas. Maybe we should be okay with Carol doing it all as long as we get a good grade.

SSG2R (A taps in and replaces SSG2): Let me just jump in here and say (to CC) that when you shoot down our ideas and edit out our words, it makes us feel like you do not value our contribution.

CCG4R (CCG4 taps out and is replaced with one of Group 4's audience members):   Perhaps we should vote to pick someone else be the leader of the project and someone different to be the final editor.

CC: Well, I see no reason to change the way we are doing things, but if you don't care about getting a good grade, then I guess I don't have any say in this.

I: How can the group help CC reflect on the role of each group member so she can embrace the group's decision to restructure the way the project is being managed? Let's open this discussion up to the audience.

Debriefing of Carol Controller Role Play

Overall, good strategies for reducing conflict were employed by the group. These strategies included the following:

Listen.
State the problem clearly.
Be respectful.
Consider other perspectives.
Be open to compromise.

CC, however, was resistant to seeing her role as a collaborative team player. CC's responses were indicative of poor self-awareness, which ultimately leaves the impression that her motivation to make changes is poor.

All the students want to get a good grade, and this group appreciates the importance making their project unique to their style as a group. CC is confident that she knows the teacher's preferences better than anyone else, and even the color scheme is of utmost importance for her to dictate.

Negotiation strategies were successfully employed by most of the group members despite CC's inability to relinquish her control over any aspect of the project. The strategies included the following:

Call a meeting.
State the rationale for the meeting.
Give specific examples that illustrate the problem. State why it is a problem.
Confirm the facts.
Listen to the other side.

(continues)

This role play focused on the negotiation of the problem, followed by the discussion related to problem resolution, including:

Make suggestions for a solution.
Confirm feasibility of solution(s) and consider other solutions. Achieve consensus regarding solution(s).
Offer help to make the changes.
Share responsibility for managing the outcome.

The group suggested changes in the management of the project and voted on the solution to employ. CC was not fully committed to changing the current structure of the project, so implementing the solutions chosen by the group may become an issue.

In regard to the interpersonal approach, it was noted that the group effectively used *I/we* (versus *you*) when presenting the problem and focused on CC's behavior, not on her as a person. However, CC appeared to take the message personally and denied all ownership of the conflict.

Discussion Questions

1. Reflect on a topic in your course that could be taught using role play. Describe the roles you would use, and how the role play would be implemented in your own course.

2. Consider a role play in communication between healthcare professionals. What potential problems would you need to be aware of, and how would you resolve these issues? What are the differences in role playing this scenario between undergraduate students and graduate?

References

Alden, D. (1999). Experience with scripted role play in environmental economics. *Journal of Economic Education, 20*(2), 127–132.

Bartle, P. (2007). *Role playing and simulation games: A training technique.* Retrieved from http://cec.vcn.bc.ca/cmp/modules/tm-rply.htm

Corless, I., Gallagher, D., Borans, R., Crary, E., Dolan, S. E., & Kressy, S. (2004). Understanding patient adherence. In A. J. Lowenstein & M. J. Bradshaw (Eds.), *Fuszard's innovative teaching strategies in nursing* (3rd ed., pp. 128–132). Sudbury, MA: Jones & Bartlett.

Corsini, R. J. (1957). *Methods of group psychotherapy.* New York, NY: McGraw-Hill.

Culley, J. M., & Polyakova-Norwood, V. (2012, January/February). Synchronous online role play for enhancing community, collaboration, and oral presentation proficiency. *Nursing Education Perspectives, 33*(1), 51–54.

DeNeve, K. M., & Hepner, M. J. (1997). Role play simulations: The assessment of an active learning technique and comparisons with traditional lectures. *Innovative Higher Education, 21*, 231–246.

Domazzo, R., & Hanson, P. (1997). Community health problems, apparent vs. hidden: A classroom exercise to demonstrate prioritization of community health problems for programs. *Journal of Health Education, 258*, 383–385.

Gordon, G. K. (1970). Human relations: Sensitivity training. In R. M. Smith, G. F. Aker, & J. R. Kidd (Eds.), *Handbook of adult education* (pp. 427–440). New York, NY: Macmillan.

Hess, C. M., & Gilgannon, N. (1985, April). *Gaming: A curriculum technique for elementary counselors.* Paper presented at the Annual Convention of the American Association for Counseling and Development, Los Angeles, CA. (ERIC document no. 267327).

Imholz, S. (2008). The therapeutic stage encounters the virtual world. *Thinking Skills and Creativity, 3*(1), 47–52.

Keyton, J., & Beck, S. (2010). Examining laughter functionality in jury deliberations. *Small Group Research, 41*(4), 386–407.

Lane, C., Hood, K., & Rollnick, S. (2008). Teaching motivational interviewing: Using role play is as effective as using simulated patients. *Medical Education, 42,* 637–644.

Lebaron, J., & Miller, D. (2005). The potential of jigsaw role playing to promote the social construction of knowledge in an online graduate education course. *Teachers College Record, 107*(8), 1652–1674.

Mann, S., & Corsun, D. L. (2002). Charting the experiential territory: Clarifying definitions and uses of computer simulation, games and role play. *Journal of Management Development, 21*(9–10), 732–745.

Mar, C. M., Chabal, C., Anderson, R. A., & Vore, A. E. (2003). An interactive computer tutorial to teach pain assessment. *Journal of Health Psychology, 8*(1), 161–173.

McKeachie, W. J. (2002). *McKeachie's teaching tips: Strategies, research, and theory for college and university teachers* (11th ed.). Boston, MA: Houghton Mifflin.

Middleton, J. (2005). Role play is not everyone's scene. *Nursing Standard, 19*(24), 31.

Moreno, J. L. (1946). *Psychodrama* (Vol. 1). Boston, MA: Beacon.

Phillips, J. M. (2005). Syllabus selections: Innovative learning activities: Chat role play as an online learning strategy. *Journal of Nursing Education, 44*(1), 43.

Qing, X. (2011). Role play: An effective approach to developing overall communicative competence. *Cross-Cultural Communication, 7*(4), 36–39.

Rabinowitz, F. E. (1997). Teaching counseling through a semester-long role play. *Counselor Education and Supervision, 36,* 216–223.

Reams, S., & Bashford, C. (2011, Summer). Interdisciplinary role play: Nursing and theater students advance skills in communication. *Delta Kappa Gamma Bulletin, 77*(4), 42–48.

Riddle, M. D. (2009). The campaign: A case study in identity construction through performance authors. *Association for Learning Technology Journal, 17*(1), 63–72.

Sasha, I. (2011, May 3). *Role play ideas for effective communication.* Retrieved from http://www.livestrong .com/article/87296-role-play-ideas-effective-communication

Shaffer, J. B. P., & Galinsky, M. D. (1974). *Models of group therapy and sensitivity training.* Englewood Cliffs, NJ: Prentice-Hall.

Sharon, S., & Sharon, Y. (1976). *Small group teaching.* Englewood Cliffs, NJ: Educational Technology Publications.

Shearer, R., & Davidhizar, R. (2003). Educational innovations: Using role play to develop cultural competence. *Journal of Nursing Education, 42*(6), 273–276.

Silberman, M. (2006). *Active training: A textbook of techniques, designs, case examples, and tips.* Malden, MA: John Wiley & Sons.

Smith-Stoner, M. (2009). Using high-fidelity simulation to educate nursing students about end-of-life care. *Nursing Education Perspectives, 30*(2), 115–120.

Turner, T. (2005). Stage fright. *Nursing Standard, 19*(22), 22–23.

Van Ments, M. (1983). *The effective use of role play: A handbook for teachers and trainers.* London, UK: Kogan Page.

Recommended Reading

Ashmore, R., & Banks, D. (2004). Student nurses' use of their interpersonal skills within clinical role plays. *Nurse Education Today, 24*(1), 20–29.

Chester, M., & Fox, R. (1996). *Role playing methods in the classroom.* Chicago, IL: Science Research Associates.

Goldenberg, D., Andrusyszyn, M., & Iwasiw, C. (2005). The effect of classroom simulation on nursing students' self-efficacy related to health teaching. *Journal of Nursing Education, 44*(7), 310–314.

Greenberg, E., & Miller, P. (1991). The player and professor: Theatrical techniques in teaching. *Journal of Management Education, 15*(4), 428–446.

Griggs, K. (2005). A role play for revising style and applying management theories. *Business Communication Quarterly, 68*(1), 60–65.

Kane, M. (2003). Teaching direct practice techniques for work with elders with Alzheimer's disease: A simulated group experience. *Educational Gerontology, 29,* 777–794.

Loprinzi, C. L., Johnson, M. E., & Steer, G. (2003). Doc, how much time do I have? *Journal of Clinical Oncology, 21*(9 suppl.), 5S–7S.

Northcott, N. (2002). Role play: Proceed with caution! *Nursing Education in Practice, 2*(2), 87–91.

SECTION IV

Teaching in Guided Practice Settings

The teaching-learning strategies in this section are intended to encourage new ways of thinking and cultivating innovative approaches for applying patient care concepts. Learning is most effective when students assume a participatory role, occasionally counter to roles previously held. By challenging their thought processes in structured practice settings, students realize how they can independently, safely, and successfully approach and solve problems. As the facilitator, the teacher can individualize the learning situation and modify the level of challenge to meet learner needs.

Clinical experiences have long been the mainstay of health professions education. Students need guided practice opportunities in which to develop skills in patient care, interdisciplinary communications, and clinical reasoning. These practice opportunities also can incorporate use of various forms of technology. The chapters on high-fidelity patient simulation provide foundational information and detail a prescribed amount of control of the learning experience. Furthermore, creation of challenging or unique opportunities through all forms of simulation extends learning opportunities that are not always available in patient care settings.

CHAPTER 16

The Nursing Skills Laboratory: Application of Theory, Teaching, and Technology

Deborah Tapler

Creating an effective skills laboratory can energize students and facilitate the transition from practice of required skills to delivery of direct care to clients. The skills laboratory, using multiple modes of teaching and learning, provides an atmosphere for students to acquire new skill knowledge and implement those new skills. With emerging restrictions on clinical placement of health professions-related students, the increasing number of enrolled nursing students, and the shortage of nursing faculty, the skills lab can be used as an effective learning environment without the presence of clients (Curl, Smith, Chisholm, Hamilton, & McGee, 2007; McNett, 2012). Nursing programs are debating proposals that would allow students to spend much more clinical time in practice labs instead of in actual hospital units. With unlimited hours of operation, the lab can provide needed opportunities to practice procedures, evaluate learning outcomes, and reinforce clinical reasoning objectives. As technology increases in complexity, through the use of advanced human patient simulators, the skills laboratory can now provide almost true-to-life clinical situations.

■ Definitions and Purposes

Acquisition of new knowledge and skills is an important component of the educational curriculum for healthcare professionals. Nurses must be able to perform procedures such as wound care, intravenous therapy, and endotracheal suctioning. Through the use of a skills laboratory, these and other integral patient care skills are learned and practiced before implementation on patients. The instructor educating students about skills uses several sources for instruction.

The roles and responsibilities of the skills lab have changed with time and advances in learning technology. The skills lab takes on various labels based on its broad offering of services or purposes (Childs, 2002). Schools of nursing across the country suggest the following names: clinical skills laboratory, clinical resource center, learning resource center, clinical competencies learning laboratory, or, simply, nursing laboratory. Current laboratory facilities offer assessment labs, bed labs, static mannequins, simulation, training devices such as intravenous insertion simulators, video libraries, and computer services. Some universities support patient clinics associated with the skills lab for student experiences with actual patients. The skills lab offers a continuum of services depending on the school's interests, specific curriculum needs, and financial capability.

Theory-based practice guides the educator when preparing to teach new skills. Theory has a direct link to practice. Educational theories relate the instructor to students through the development of effective learning strategies appropriate for selected students. Theory also influences practice through theory-driven research that impacts patient care. For example, germ theory dictates the procedure of successful handwashing, which is a skill that every student must master to prevent infection. When learning in the skills lab, the student must progress beyond the how of a procedure to the more complex level of thinking to ask "why."

Evidence-based practice must also be used in the skills laboratory. Evidence-based practice is a systematic approach to problem solving that can be applied to patient care delivery as well as education (Pravikoff, Tanner, & Pierce, 2005). Teaching skills that are based on valid research provides students with state-of-the-art information for safe implementation of skills in actual clinical experiences. It is imperative to educate students about the process of accessing research evidence as part of a lifelong learning goal. Inviting students to participate in the evidence-based process is an important teaching opportunity to allow students to discover best practices regarding content reviewed in the skills lab. For example, students are assigned a particular topic, such as blood pressure monitoring or safe medication administration, to seek reputable best-practice standards regarding the psychomotor skill. Elements of procedures and relevancy of skills change as knowledge and technology grow. The skills laboratory must reflect the most current information when educating nurses for the future.

The skills lab is well suited for the development of clinical reasoning abilities in students representing all levels of the curriculum. From beginning students to students who are nearing graduation, specific planned activities in the skills lab can provide opportunities to learn, expand, and evaluate each student's ability to use clinical reasoning when delivering simulated patient care. Given a dynamic patient scenario in the lab, a faculty member may observe the student's ease of decision making and prioritization based on a set of simple to complex patient data. This type of evaluation, whether formative or summative in nature, is very effective when creating individualized goals to enhance student progress or success. In the lab, it is important that any teaching strategy be implemented with the purpose of promoting the progression of advancing levels of thinking (Billings & Halstead, 2011).

The purpose of this chapter is to explore the roles, diverse uses, and effectiveness of a skills laboratory. Based on current theory, valuable teaching modalities, and advanced technology, the skills laboratory can be an effective tool of education for a wide range of health-related disciplines.

■ Theoretical Rationale

Knowles's theory of adult learning has shaped the way that educators present information to adult learners (Knowles, 1989). Adults approach a learning situation differently than do children. With life experiences to color the acquisition of new knowledge and skills, adults thrive in a learning environment that is open to creativity, values personal knowledge, and is relevant to immediate learning goals. Adult learners desire to make individual choices and decisions. Education in the skills laboratory is hands-on and relevant to direct patient care. Students are allowed and encouraged to self-evaluate their competence prior to clinical placement (Clarke, Davies, & McNee, 2002). They develop self-confidence as they learn psychomotor skills without fear of failure. After the students attend traditional learning presentations, such as lectures, the adult learners are motivated to learn those things in the skills lab that they know will be necessary to accomplish course objectives. Practice in the skills lab allows the students to cope effectively with future patient interactions. The skills lab can also provide academic assistance when a student has difficulty integrating knowledge regarding a psychomotor skill.

Benner's theory of skill acquisition plays an important part in the nursing education curriculum (Benner, 2001). Benner proposed a model for the nursing profession based on the Dreyfus model, explaining that nurses function at various levels of skill, from novice to expert. The novice level is characterized by a lack of experience of the situations in which the person is involved and is expected to perform. The beginning nursing student functions at the novice level. The nursing curriculum gives students entry to nursing situations and allows them to gain the experience through skills development. The skills lab acts as an instrument to transfer knowledge and skills to novice nursing students so that they may progress to increasingly more complex levels of understanding. The skills lab can be used to teach about situations in terms of "objective attributes" such as intake and output, blood pressure, and temperature (Benner, 2001, p. 20). These features of the task world of nursing have to be learned before the prospective nurse has actual situational experiences with patients. The behavior of the novice is rule-governed and very limited and inflexible. Faculty members impart rules to guide performance before the information makes sense to students. Practice and rehearsal of new behaviors allow the students to gain confidence in their abilities despite little understanding of the contextual meanings of recently learned nursing concepts. Thus, the skills lab plays an important role in the learning process of new students who have no contextual cues. As the nursing student progresses through the nursing curriculum to graduation, the role of the skills lab can evolve and change to meet the expectations for learning dictated by the faculty and content objectives. According to Benner, students may progress from novice to advanced beginner, and then to the competent, proficient, and expert levels of nursing ability over the course of a career.

■ Selecting Learning Experiences

The skills laboratory can be used effectively throughout the curriculum. According to Infante (1985), the purpose of a skills laboratory is to offer students the appearance of reality in an artificial environment where the setting is controlled and offers practical application. The students are encouraged to achieve a predefined level of skill competence (Clarke et al., 2002). As skills move from simple (such as bathing) to complex (such as suctioning), the skills lab can be a learning experience that advances levels of knowledge and abilities.

Faculty involved in undergraduate curricula should identify skills associated with each level of progression to ensure that all necessary content is reflected in the educational goals of the laboratory. In addition, identified skills should be appropriate to the skill level of the student. Typically, nursing education has utilized the skills lab to provide psychomotor skill acquisition at the beginning of the curriculum. However, with technologies used in the lab, such as computer-based interactive case studies and human patient simulators, new modalities have provided unlimited opportunities for knowledge as well as skill development. Clinical reasoning scenarios are appropriate and can be facilitated by skills lab experiences. Human patient simulation offered in the skills laboratory has positively impacted the level of clinical reasoning development in undergraduate students (Lapkin, Levett-Jones, Bellchambers, & Fernandez, 2010). The use of simulation appears to improve knowledge acquisition, but may also enhance the decision-making process necessary to provide effective and competent patient care. With the high-stress, low-risk teaching situation of simulation, students have the opportunity to demonstrate clinical judgment abilities that are commensurate with the expected outcome of a course. Some professional disciplines, such as pharmacy, have reported the enhancement of clinical reasoning, problem-solving skills, and teamwork when implementing human patient simulation for students (Vyas, Ottis, & Caligiuri, 2011).

Faculty members using the skills lab should strive to teach a diversity of skills to students. Even though the skills lab environment typically lends itself to the training of psychomotor skills, other cognitive and affective domain skills can be developed there as well. According to Tarnow and Butcher (2005), the learning lab can be used to facilitate the development of caring actions by students that are key to the practice of the art of nursing. By observing role modeling of caring behaviors by faculty with lab mannequins, students can gain an appreciation of the elements of a therapeutic relationship and begin to demonstrate empathetic interactions. Students learn therapeutic communication and interpersonal skills through staged interactions with mannequins. For example, students can approach a mannequin and practice greeting the patient, introducing themselves, and explaining procedures to be performed as if it were a real patient encounter. Despite the fact that labs are most often used for the practice of psychomotor skills, a personal approach to the mannequin is encouraged so that students may gain confidence and become more comfortable with patient exchanges in the clinical environment. Collaboration is instilled when students work in groups to deliver patient care through participation in simulation. Faculty-developed case studies used in the lab should be structured with a communication component, such as telephoning the physician to clarify an order or suggesting strategies to interact with a distressed family member.

Learning situations can be enhanced by the contained setting of the skills laboratory. With close supervision and responsive interactions between students and faculty, the students learn in an environment of collaboration and inquiry. Questions about new procedures or concepts can be answered and discussed promptly without the constraints of a fast-paced patient care area. Faculty members act as facilitators and have opportunities to present information regarding advances in evidence-based practice. Students feel confident about trying new skills in a low-risk situation without fear of harming patients. Mistakes are excellent sources of learning and do not have to result in penalizing consequences. However, if the skills laboratory is used for mastery performance evaluation of student abilities, the results can be recorded as a component of a course grade or used for remedial identification. Students who have weaknesses in psychomotor or clinical reasoning skills can use the environment of the skills laboratory for tutoring assistance from faculty. Through one-on-one interaction, the weak student can practice and receive immediate feedback from a qualified evaluator to gain knowledge and confidence.

■ Types of Learners

Undergraduate nursing students possess various learning styles. The skills laboratory can provide a rich learning experience for all types of learners. Whether the student learner is self-directed or takes a dependent approach, the faculty can individualize instruction based on each student's abilities and learning style. (Cognitive styles, learning styles, and learning preferences were discussed previously in this text.) Kolb's theory of experiential learning proposes cycles of learning along a continuum from concrete experience to abstract conceptualization of knowledge (Dobbin, 2001). Nursing students possess a concrete, active-pattern learning style characterized by the need for dynamic involvement when learning new concepts and skills (Schroeder, 2004). According to Dobbin (2001), "learners also can have a preference for reflective observation (watching to learn) or active experimentation (learning by doing)" (p. 5). For example, tactile exploration by touching and manipulating syringes and needles is essential for the concrete learner. Lecturing has only limited ability to educate in regard to psychomotor skill acquisition. As the student learns new skills in the lab, questions arise and what-ifs are posed to enhance the learning experience. The use of return demonstration strengthens mastery and confidence.

Faculty must ensure that instruction in the skills laboratory is directed to students with a wide range of learning styles. Students may possess any one or a combination of the following learning styles: visual (spatial), aural (auditory-musical), verbal (linguistic), physical (kinesthetic), logical (mathematical), social (interpersonal), or solitary (intrapersonal) (Schroeder, 2004). Through the use of simulators, audiovisual software, graphs and diagrams, charts, pictures, demonstrations, practice, discussion, or even music, the skills laboratory can address the needs of all students when acquiring new nursing knowledge. The key to effective teaching in the lab is dependent on the faculty's use of a varied and innovative approach to education.

Generational differences among students are addressed by the variety of teaching strategies that are offered by faculty in the skills lab. Whether a generation Xer, millennial, or baby boomer, each student approaches the learning environment with different characteristics and learning needs (Billings & Halstead, 2011). The skills lab offers an array of options to capture the attention of students in today's society. For example, the millennial student prefers to work with a team and be socially involved. (Generational perspectives were discussed previously in this text.)

According to Godson, Wilson, and Goodman (2007), third-year students working with first-year students in a nursing program proved very effective. The third-year students were asked to teach a psychomotor skill related to patient care to the first-year students. The first-year students then practiced the skill that they had learned from their fellow nursing students. The mentors' support helped to comfort and ease the beginning nursing students' anxiety regarding learning a new skill. Each group described benefits of working together as a team.

■ Conditions for Learning and Resources

Opportunities to learn skills in the clinical environment continue to dwindle due to fewer clinical placements available in healthcare institutions. With often fierce competition among educational programs for optimal student assignments in hospital and community resources, the skills lab takes on increased importance for all clinical courses in the curriculum. Skills, which were once discussed and practiced briefly in the lab and then performed on clients, may no longer be practiced in the clinical area due to patient availability, acuity level of patients in clinical agencies, and legal ramifications (McNett, 2012). Practice in the skills lab may be the only opportunity for learning many basic as well as complex skills needed after graduation. Therefore, skills taught in each course must be identified and additional time and supplies allotted for practice in the lab. Skills will not only be taught in isolation with low-fidelity simulators such as static mannequins, but can also become a part of scenarios with high-fidelity human patient simulators. These scenarios offer students opportunities to interact with simulators presenting specific problems, and the skills learned are carried out as interventions become necessary, rather than in isolation. Thus, scenarios based on learning objectives for each course throughout the curriculum, and embedded with increasingly complex skills, become an important avenue for assisting the student to progress from novice to higher levels of ability and clinical reasoning. As a student's professional knowledge increases in complexity with each course, clinical reasoning proficiency must also be increased through practice in the skills lab and refined through activities delivering direct patient care in the clinical area. Skills performed within scenarios also allow the adult learner to apply knowledge and psychomotor ability to immediate learning goals.

According to Gonzol and Newby (2013), clinical reasoning is important when asking students to practice psychomotor skills. They suggest that students must understand the scientific rationale or purpose of performing each step of a procedure or skill, not just the mechanical performance of accomplishing a set of actions. For example, a student should know the reason why air is injected into a vial before a medication is drawn out with a needle and syringe. This knowledge contributes to the student's ability to think through clinical challenges when faced with diverse variables and complex situations. The authors used Webber's IRUEPIC (Identify, Relate, Understand, Explain, Predict, Influence, Control) reasoning model, which offers steps that build progressively when trying to understand the reasoning behind actions. The model was applied when teaching psychomotor skills and revealed a statistically significant difference in student outcomes when compared to a nursing process-based skills checklist. The reasoning model asked the students to be aware of and react to more contextual patient care elements, including speaking to the patient about the procedure and possible complications.

Skills labs must take on a new look that mimics the hospital environment, as simulators become patients and assist the student in the suspension of disbelief while practicing necessary skills. This environment includes not only sights, but also the sounds that are inherent in a busy clinical area. Labs must include the equipment, technology, and resources that are currently found in the clinical environment. Labs must be designed to provide rooms/bays that are essentially self-contained hospital units where scenarios can be carried out. Although the rooms may be used for a variety of scenarios, different rooms may have to be designed and equipped for areas such as obstetrics, emergency care, acute care, home care, pediatrics, and intensive care units, in addition to ancillary units. As the hospital environment changes and innovations such as telenursing and eICUs become commonplace, skills labs will require design elements that provide multiple-screen workstations connected to multiple simulators.

The skills laboratory includes not only typical equipment, such as intravenous pumps, but also technology devices and the ability to access the Internet. Through the use of available computers or laptops in the lab, students can engage in self-directed learning during lab activities, by finding answers to questions or searching for information about skills independently and when needed to enhance learning (Tracey, DiStefano, Morris-Hackett, & Steefel, 2013). Students should have access to best-practice guidelines and evidence-based resources that will be needed to assist them with problem solving and clinical reasoning as they work through scenarios. Informatics should be accessible, as students must learn to work with databases and documentation software.

■ Using the Method

Teaching within the new skills lab combines the best of the traditional methods of instruction with the new technological advances. Regardless of the complexity of the skill, acquisition begins with didactic instruction and practice in the lab on low-fidelity mannequins. Additionally, students may be provided with kits of equipment and supplies to continue practicing skills at home. These include such things as mock wounds for dressing changes and Styrofoam wig heads with tracheostomy tubes for practicing tracheostomy care. As mentioned previously, performance of skills at this time is rule-governed and inflexible. These skills can then be embedded within a scenario that presents the appropriate complexity of care based on the course objectives. Three to five students can work through the scenario on a high-fidelity human patient simulator, identifying indicators for various skills, perhaps obtaining orders for the skill, collecting supplies needed, performing the skills, observing the effects, and documenting and reporting the procedure and effects. Although only one student actually performs any one skill, other students actively participate in the skill through discussion and support. The importance of the skill takes on a new meaning as it becomes a part of patient care for an illness and a patient with specific needs and responses. Communication and professionalism are fostered with other team members, such as healthcare providers, and among other members of the student's peer group. Debriefing following completion of the scenario should be considered integral to the process. Discussions with the faculty as facilitators can assist the students in applying theory to practice, correcting mistakes, answering questions, identifying learning needs, and making connections to the real world.

The use of appropriate scenarios and all levels of human patient simulators and mannequins is invaluable for teaching skills in a safe environment where patient cooperation is not needed, where repetition is essential, and especially where skills could potentially cause harm to the patient. Clinical reasoning and problem solving, obtaining appropriate supplies, manipulating equipment, looking up resources, performing procedures accurately and safely, and communicating verbally and in writing are all activities that require considerable amounts of practice by the novice learner. In the fast-paced clinical environment, time is of the essence, and students are often expected to perform beyond the level of novice learner. Students can move beyond the novice level with the use of credible scenarios and simulated patients in the realistic, transferable environment of the skills lab.

Skills labs may include evaluation of specific skills as a part of outcome measurements at the end of the semester. Students are often evaluated while performing a specific skill or skills as the faculty observe and record their performance. Return demonstration to determine mastery of specified skills is an effective method to determine the safety of transition to patient care in the clinical setting. One type of summative evaluation is called objective structured clinical examination (OSCE) (McWilliam & Botwinski, 2010; Oranye, Ahmad, Ahmad, & Bakar, 2012). OSCE is a practical test that is used to determine proficiency in one or more skills. This evaluation strategy has been used in the clinical field to evaluate both undergraduate and graduate student competence in all areas of the health-related fields. OSCE offers an effective teaching option for faculty to evaluate students at multiple stations using standardized patients. For example, a student may proceed through a series of skills stations to perform a particular skill, such as bandaging or interviewing, while being observed by a faculty member guided by a rubric of required actions to successfully complete the skill in a predetermined time frame. If students perform poorly when evaluated, immediate remedial action can be taken to correct deficiencies before exposure to patients. Patient safety must be the overriding consideration when documenting student abilities. For example, if during a lab checkoff a student draws up 10 mL of a medication instead of the required 3-mL dose, the faculty can reeducate the student immediately, validate that accurate knowledge is mastered, and avert a potential patient injury in subsequent clinical encounters.

Simulated patients also are used in effectively evaluating skills. The required skills are developed in a short scenario. Three to five students care for the patient using a mannequin and perform the skills as the intervention becomes necessary in the scenario. Students should be aware of the criteria and expected behaviors, having previously practiced all the skills to be evaluated. At the beginning of the scenario, students can draw from a hat for the skills they are to perform during the scenario. As the scenario progresses, students care for the patient together, except when a specific skill is needed. Peers then become observers as the student who was assigned a skill performs according to the criteria outlined and is evaluated by the instructor. Peer observers become active learners as they mentally rehearse and evaluate the skills as they are being performed. Once the skill has been completed, the scenario resumes until another skill is needed. The process is repeated throughout the scenario until all students have demonstrated their selected skills. Verbal and/or written feedback can be given to the students individually by the instructor following the scenario. Students may also give their peers feedback about their performance. This same strategy can be utilized for standardized or real human patients or actors as opposed to static mannequins. A standardized patient actor is paid by the institution to act like a patient with a specific disease state or case scenario as prescribed by the faculty. According to McWilliam and Botwinski (2010, 2012), the use of faculty to play the role of standardized patients is not an effective model. Health professionals have a tendency to give clues and unintentionally assist the students who are being evaluated on a task. Laypersons are much more authentic in the role of a patient.

The skills lab is an essential environment to teach nursing skills. However, the space can also be used for teaching previously learned skills. After a long scholastic break, skills may be forgotten by students due to lack of practice (Roberts, Vignato, Moore, & Madden, 2009). Knowledge of psychomotor skills decreases after as little as 2 weeks and may have to be relearned after 2 months. Course faculty can schedule the lab space for skills reintroduction to the students. Having a daylong skills session before the semester commences is an effective strategy to refresh, practice, and critique skills in time for the beginning of actual patient care delivery. Skills must be sufficiently practiced to support retention of the skills and permit the student to gain the ability to transfer the skill knowledge to the clinical area competently (Oermann et al., 2011). These intensive skill sessions promote the performance of learned skills and also develop confidence in the nursing students.

Video recording may be used as an adjunct to learning or evaluation of skills. This method of assessment offers findings that are very objective when used for grading purposes. Students can learn by video-recording and critiquing their own performance or viewing the video and discussing their performance with a faculty member. They can also video-record and submit their videos for evaluation and feedback by a faculty member. In a study by Brimble (2008), skills assessment using video analysis in a simulated environment was found to be an effective evaluation tool. The nursing students completed a questionnaire before, during, and after videotaping a simulation in the skills lab. The most common positive theme that students expressed was the ability to learn from their mistakes by watching the reenactment of their performance on video. Subjects indicated that the visual feedback they received from viewing their actual performance complemented the verbal critique offered by the faculty member. Negative themes included feelings of anxiety, being judged by others, and being embarrassed. However, Miller, Nichols, and Beeken (2000) found that students prefer faculty member presence during skill demonstrations and immediate feedback rather than video recording and delayed feedback.

■ Potential Problems

Major problems inherent in the development of the modern skills laboratory are the cost to provide the needed technology and supplies, and the physical space to house them. In order for students to practice with the equipment used in the profession, it must be purchased from medical vendors. Supplies are very expensive, especially when they are the most recent equipment used by the clinical agencies. Needles with integral safety devices are often more costly than traditional needle systems. Students must see and practice with the tools that they will use in their clinical experiences, which requires frequent equipment revision in the laboratory. According to Gantt (2010), a well-administered skills lab should be guided by a strategic plan that is visionary and intentional. A strategic planning process is important to clarify goals, to direct expenditures to the highest priorities, and to increase the efficiency of operation. It also serves to inform administrators of the critical importance of sustained funding of the unit and the integral role that the skills lab plays in the education of students. As enrollment in schools of nursing increases due to shortage mandates, the skills lab provides cost-effective learning space that is available from early morning to late in the evening for student use.

Skills labs have typically been large rooms with multiple beds and static mannequins. Large numbers of students often practice the same skill at the same time. Although this type of space and instruction present a good beginning, additional smaller simulation rooms are needed for the more costly high-fidelity human patient simulators with all of the equipment, technology, and added supplies needed for implementing simulations. In addition, some labs have a small control room with a one-way mirror attached to each simulation room.

Other problems include lack of faculty willingness to embrace new technology and other services offered by the skills lab. Implementation of high-fidelity simulation, evidence-based case scenarios, and the additional time it takes to have three to five students at a time complete the skills within the case scenarios requires dedicated faculty participation. Learning new simulation teaching strategies and management of the simulators requires additional faculty time and energy. Writing evidence-based scenarios that contain the necessary skills is another time-intensive faculty activity, unless these are purchased. According to Childs (2002), faculty and students must be interested and motivated to use the skills lab for the multiple teaching opportunities that are possible. Often, a core group of faculty members uses the services of the skills lab on a routine basis, but all instructors should be informed about the applicability of skills lab services to augment the delivery of the curriculum content. In return, the skills lab must be responsive to the faculty and their needs, to maximize the use of available technology.

A discussion has emerged recently regarding the taking of photos and videos in the skills laboratory by the students. Students often wish to remember situations or procedures learned in the lab by taking a photo of equipment or videotaping a procedure performed by an instructor or other peer. Faculty members must remember that these images may be posted on the Internet or social media sites. The faculty must consider the university's guidelines concerning the use of images taken while at the campus. Also, no images of students should be generated without a signed photo consent on file with the university.

Communication with faculty and students about the skills lab services is a critical element of an effectively functioning lab. This challenge is often addressed through the use of web-based software. Currently, most colleges and universities support a web-based framework such as Blackboard or WebCT. The skills lab should offer a website directed to students and faculty where policies and procedures, calendar events, and contact information for lab personnel are posted. A schedule of open lab times and remedial sessions should be easily accessible for students who need those services. Communication is an essential key to allow users to take full advantage of all the services offered by a well-equipped skills lab.

Every skills laboratory must be a safe environment for faculty, students, and staff. Skills labs are required to follow strict safety procedures to protect personnel and students in the lab from injury or spills. Needles, sutures, and performance of certain procedures pose daily threats. Adherence to federal and local government regulations may prove costly, but is a necessary component of a safe and effective skills lab.

■ Conclusion

The skills laboratory provides an enriched teaching and learning atmosphere that encourages active and involved exploration and mastery of new knowledge and skills to develop competent graduate nurses. Theory is applied to practice and validated in the skills lab through teaching and technology. The faculty member can use unlimited strategies to educate students who have a spectrum of learning needs in order to foster clinical reasoning. In the protected environment of the skills lab, students learn, make mistakes, question conceptual ideas, practice psychomotor skills, and expand knowledge and understanding to new levels. Students learn by doing through experimentation that would be impossible and dangerous in direct patient care situations. Faculty members must engage in direct observation and supervision of all student activities, which is often difficult in a busy clinical agency. Transition to the role of graduate nurse is enhanced by effective and innovative use of the new skills laboratory.

Teaching Examples:

Comprehensive Nursing Skills Experiences

In a fundamental skills course offered by various disciplines, skills are a primary focus requiring didactic instruction and demonstrations first given in lecture and then reinforced in the skills lab. Skills that are appropriate for beginning nursing students include the complex task of medication administration, which includes obtaining or understanding healthcare provider orders; learning the appropriate dosages and where to research information about the drug; calculating dosages from the correct amount of drug available; safely and competently handling the syringe during drawing up of medication, administration; disposal of the syringe; recognizing appropriate sites for administration (subcutaneous or intramuscular); performing the five rights prior to administration; and recording the medication in the permanent patient record. All these basic skills must be understood and practiced repeatedly by the student. To meet the wide range of learning styles, instruction should include verbal and written material as well as audiovisual demonstrations and one-on-one interactions and demonstrations with the students. Kinesthetic learning is provided by the use of different types of syringes, vials, and pills; and solitary practice is combined with discussion, reflective observation, and active experimentation.

Administration of insulin and digoxin can be used as examples for student practice. Sliding-scale insulin orders could be written in a mock chart, and students could be given various blood glucose results so that different amounts of insulin would have to be drawn up. In the lab, students practice drawing up insulin, selecting an appropriate site, administering the medication on a mannequin, discarding the syringe, and documenting on the mock chart. They should also practice giving oral medications such as digoxin correctly, which would include auscultation of the apical pulse. Not only must they be able to perform the skill of giving the medication correctly, but they would also need to recognize that an apical pulse rate must be taken before administration, know under which circumstances the medication should be withheld based on current literature, and recognize when the healthcare provider must be notified for future actions.

Once the skills have been practiced, three or four students are introduced to the high-fidelity simulator. They are presented with the history and physical findings of a patient who is hospitalized with selected clinical problems. A mock chart is available with healthcare provider orders, which include treatment and medication orders. Medications are noted on the medication administration record, including insulin sliding scale, oral medication, and prn medication orders. The students are made aware of the time of day and results of lab studies such as blood glucose readings. Students at this point are assigned selected skills to perform, such as wound dressing change, urinary catheterization, administration of pain medication via the intramuscular route, application of bandages, or performance of a basic head-to-toe assessment. The skills are embedded in the scenario and must be performed according to patient need and healthcare provider orders. The students must prioritize their actions based on the dynamic events unfolding in the patient scenario. This complex situation cultivates clinical reasoning and problem solving to meet patient demands. The faculty member acts as facilitator to encourage competent participation by individual students and provides immediate feedback to correct problems in cognition and performance of skills. As the students progress in level of learning ability across the curriculum, the faculty member offers less prompting to increase the independence exhibited by the students. By applying adult learning principles, the students are allowed to demonstrate more creativity in a learning environment that supports personal knowledge and meets immediate learning goals.

Evaluation of required skills is an important function of the skills lab. The lab provides unlimited opportunities for faculty to observe and test acquisition of psychomotor skills as well as cognitive processing. For example, the evaluation process in the form of a formalized checkoff can be implemented at the end of a semester to determine mastery of required skills. Before the checkoff is completed, students receive detailed procedural (step-by-step) information or criteria regarding the skills that they must master. By knowing the exact expectation before the evaluation, the anxiety level experienced by the students is decreased, and the faculty member can more easily determine the skill level of an individual student unclouded by psychological barriers. Practice opportunities are provided to reinforce skills the week before checkoff. The lab is arranged to represent the hospital setting with a patient in bed, a medication room, and a supply area. The student receives an assigned skill, reviews the patient's mock chart, assembles the necessary equipment to perform the skill, and prepares the patient for the procedure. The interaction with the mannequin should appear as authentic as possible. This situation can be achieved by encouraging the student to communicate with the patient in a normal manner. The faculty member observes the performance of the skill based on the criteria previously provided to the student. A checkoff form is used to document and evaluate the student's actions in relation to the criteria. The faculty member does not interact with or prompt the student in any manner. If the student fails to follow the criteria, points are deducted, affecting the final score. The criteria contain selected critical behaviors that must be accomplished successfully to pass the evaluation. Examples of critical behaviors are contamination of a sterile field or recapping of a used needle. If the student fails to acquire sufficient points or neglects to perform critical behaviors, the student fails the checkoff and is provided the opportunity for remediation and a repeated attempt. Failure of the course is possible if the student is unable to successfully master performance of the skill. The skills lab is an excellent venue to assess competency and determine learning needs. By utilizing theory combined with innovative teaching approaches and technological advances in the skills laboratory, faculty members optimize learning opportunities.

Discussion Questions

1. Research supports the theory that all students learn in different ways. Choose one psychomotor skill that is taught in a skills laboratory (such as nasogastric tube placement or intravenous catheter insertion) and develop a teaching plan for an auditory, visual, and kinesthetic learner that can be implemented in the skills environment.

2. As clinical placement sites decrease in availability for undergraduate students, what role will the skills laboratory play to fill the gaps in learning from lack of clinical experiences and facilitate students' transition to a level of competency in clinical skills upon graduation? Discuss the strengths and weaknesses of utilizing the skills laboratory for an increasing percentage of clinical learning.

3. Discuss ways in which the skills laboratory can be utilized and marketed to the community to optimize university lab personnel and year-round use of potentially vacant facilities as an external source of revenue.

References

Benner, P. (2001). *From novice to expert: Excellence and power in clinical nursing practice.* Upper Saddle River, NJ: Prentice-Hall.

Billings, D. M., & Halstead, J. A. (2011). *Teaching in nursing: A guide for faculty.* St. Louis, MO: Elsevier Saunders.

Brimble, M. (2008). Skills assessment using video analysis in a simulated environment: An evaluation. *Pediatric Nursing, 20*(7), 26–31.

Childs, J. C. (2002). Clinical resource centers in nursing programs. *Nurse Educator, 27*(5), 232–235.

Clarke, D., Davies, J., & McNee, P. (2002). The case for a children's nursing skills laboratory. *Pediatric Nursing, 14*(7), 36–39.

Curl, E., Smith, S., Chisholm, L., Hamilton, J., & McGee, L. (2007). Multidimensional approaches to extending nurse faculty resources without testing faculty's patience. *Journal of Nursing Education, 46*(4), 193–195.

Dobbin, K. R. (2001). Applying learning theories to develop teaching strategies for the critical care nurse: Don't limit yourself to the formal classroom lecture. *Critical Care Nursing Clinics of North America, 13*(1), 1–11.

Gantt, L. (2010). Strategic planning for skills and simulation labs in colleges of nursing. *Nursing Economics, 28*(5), 308–313.

Godson, N. R., Wilson, A., & Goodman, M. (2007). Evaluating student nurse learning in the clinical skills laboratory. *British Journal of Nursing, 16*, 942–945.

Gonzol, K., & Newby, C. (2013). Facilitating clinical reasoning in the skills laboratory: Reasoning model versus nursing process-based skills checklist. *Nursing Education Perspectives, 34*(4), 265–267.

Infante, M. S. (1985). *The clinical laboratory.* New York, NY: John Wiley & Sons.

Knowles, M. (1989). *The making of an adult education: An autobiographical journey.* San Francisco, CA: Jossey-Bass.

Lapkin, S., Levett-Jones, T., Bellchambers, H., & Fernandez, R. (2010). Effectiveness of patient simulation manikins in teaching clinical reasoning skills to undergraduate nursing students: A systematic review. *Clinical Simulation in Nursing, 6*(6), 207–222.

McNett, S. (2012). Teaching psychomotor skills in a fundamentals laboratory: A literature review. *Nursing Education Perspectives, 33*(5), 328–333.

McWilliam, P. L., & Botwinski, C. A. (2010). Developing a successful nursing objective structured clinical examination. *Journal of Nursing Education, 49*(1), 36–41.

McWilliam, P. L., & Botwinski, C. A. (2012). Identifying strengths and weaknesses in the utilization of objective structured clinical examination (OSCE) in a nursing program. *Nursing Education Perspectives, 33*(1), 35–39.

Miller, H., Nichols, E., & Beeken, J. (2000). Comparing video-taped and faculty-present return demonstrations of clinical skills. *Journal of Nursing Education, 39*, 237–239.

Oermann, M., Kardong-Edgren, S., Odom-Maryon, T., Hallmark, B., Hurd, D., Rogers, N. . . . Smart, D. (2011). Deliberate practice of motor skills in nursing education: CPR as exemplar. *Nursing Education Perspectives, 32*(5), 311–315.

Oranye, N. O., Ahmad, C., Ahmad, N., & Bakar, R. A. (2012). Assessing nursing clinical skills competence through objective structured clinical examination (OSCE) for open distance learning students in Open University Malaysia. *Contemporary Nurse, 41*(2), 233–241.

Pravikoff, D. S., Tanner., A. B., & Pierce, S. T. (2005). Readiness for US nurses for evidence-based practice. *American Journal of Nursing, 105*(9), 40–52.

Roberts, S. T., Vignato, J. A., Moore, J. L., & Madden, C. A. (2009). Promoting skill building and confidence in freshman nursing students with a "skills-a-thon." *Journal of Nursing Education, 48*(8), 460–464.

Schroeder, C. C. (2004). *New students–New learning styles.* Retrieved from http://www.virtualschool.edu /mon/Academia/KierseyLearningStyles.html

Tarnow, K., & Butcher, H. K. (2005). Teaching the art of professional nursing in the learning laboratory. In M. E. Oermann & K. T. Heinrich (Eds.), *Annual review of nursing education* (Vol. 3, pp. 375–392). New York, NY: Springer.

Tracey, D., DiStefano, M., Morris-Hackett, N., & Steefel, L. (2013). Using quick response codes to facilitate self-directed learning in a nursing skills laboratory. *Journal of Nursing Education, 52*(11), 664.

Vyas, D., Ottis, E. J., & Caligiuri, F. J. (2011). Teaching clinical reasoning and problem-solving skills using human patient simulation. *American Journal of Pharmaceutical Education, 75*(9), 1–5.

CHAPTER 17

Human Patient Simulation

Catherine Bailey

Human patient simulations (HPSs), sometimes called *high-fidelity patient simulations*, have been used by health professional educators for more than 50 years (Rosen, 2008). In addition to high-fidelity patient simulations, various other types of simulated experiences have supported the educational needs of healthcare professionals. The term *fidelity* has been classified according to the degree to which a simulated experience approaches reality (Meakim et al., 2013). In other words, the level of fidelity increases as the realism or authenticity of the circumstances of the simulation increase. Low-fidelity simulations help to immerse the participants in a clinical situation or practice of a skill by using case studies or role-playing experiences with the use of partial task trainers or static mannequins (Meakim et al., 2013). Task trainers, designed to represent specific anatomic areas of the body, have been useful for the acquisition and validation of complex psychomotor, assessment, and diagnostic skills (Decker, Sportsman, Puetz, & Billings, 2008). Task trainer arms have been recognized as the traditional method for teaching peripheral vascular catheter insertions (Alexandrou et al., 2012).

Moderate or mid-level fidelity is associated with experiences that are more technologically sophisticated than those practiced with a static mannequin (Meakim et al., 2013). "Computer-based self-directed learning systems simulations in which the participant relies on a two-dimensional focused experience to problem solve, perform a skill and make decisions" are an example of a mid-level fidelity experience (Meakim et al., 2013, p. S7). A learning system that permits nurses to practice their cardiopulmonary resuscitation skills with automated feedback would be identified as a mid-level fidelity experience.

High-fidelity experiences are those that use "full scale computerized simulators, virtual reality or standardized patients that are extremely realistic and provide a high level of interactivity and realism for the learner" (Meakim et al., 2013, p. S6). Virtual simulation (VS) is a pedagogy that provides clinical experiences for participants by using avatars in a three-dimensional setting that are located on web-based platforms (Foronda, Lippincott, & Gattamorta, 2014). The VS technology simulates real-life scenarios and provides students with opportunities to develop their knowledge, to engage in decision making, and to improve learning and communication skills. A *standardized patient* is a person who is trained to consistently portray a patient in a scripted scenario for the purpose of instruction, practice, or evaluation (Meakim et al., 2013). This chapter focuses on HPS experiences with the use of full-scale computerized simulators, otherwise known as high-fidelity patient simulators.

■ Definition and Purposes

High-fidelity patient simulators (HFPSs) are computerized, life-sized mannequins with complex, interrelated, multisystem physiologic and pharmacologic models that generate observable responses from the mannequin and allow students to interact with the simulator as they would with an actual patient in the clinical environment (Decker et al., 2008). The first human patient simulators were developed in the 1960s, and their use became widespread when anesthesia educators and researchers used simulators to improve education and study clinical performances (Gaba & DeAnda, 1988; Good & Gravenstein, 1989). By the late 1990s, the use of HFPSs evolved from the management of anesthesia to include other types of patient-related care within emergency medicine (Fritz, Gray, & Flanagan, 2008), Armed Forces medicine, pediatrics, surgery, trauma, cardiology, intensive care medicine, dentistry, and military medicine triage (Rosen, 2008). In 2005, computerized infant mannequins were introduced to assist with neonatal resuscitation. Applications of high-fidelity patient simulator use among healthcare providers have included training for procedures and communications, evaluations for individual responses to critical incidents and deteriorating patients, equipment evaluations, task analyses, and team training (Aebersold & Tschannen, 2013; Lupien, 2007; Merchant, 2012). Common educational applications of simulation have included theme-based workshops on ventilation, pharmacology, airway management, conscious sedation, disaster response, ongoing skills development, and the practice of clinical decision making.

The first nurse-specific uses of HFPSs were introduced to nurse anesthetists (Fletcher, 1995). After 2000, the use of HFPSs expanded to include the educational activities of prelicensure nursing students, licensed nurses returning to practice, and the validation of clinical judgment and competencies of nurses in the practice setting (Hoffman & Burns, 2011). Areas of focus have included the development of procedural skills, critical thinking, and patient safety; the development of safer patient and nurse environments; competency testing of skills; and comprehensive models for the development of the graduate nurse from novice to expert and enhanced teamwork and crisis management skills of healthcare providers (Merchant, 2012; Nehring, 2010).

In the United States, HPSs are supported by the use of automated human patient simulators such as METIman, iStan, Human Patient Simulator (HPS), PediaSim, BabySim, and Caesar; Lucina, a childbirth simulator from CAE Healthcare (2015); SimMan 3G, SimMan G Trauma, SimMom, SimBaby, SimJunior, SimMom, and SimNewB from Laerdal (2015); and various models of Hal (a standard simulator and a trauma simulator), Noelle (a maternal and neonatal birthing simulator, including preemie and newborn), and Suzi (a nursing simulator) from Gaumard Scientific (2015). The simulators typically include the following four components: a lifelike mannequin, a freestanding enclosure that contains many of the simulator's components, a computer to integrate the function of the simulator components, and an interface that allows the user to control the simulation and modify physiologic parameters.

Depending on the sophistication of the specific HFPS, features may include a functioning cardiovascular system with synchronized palpable pulses, heart sounds, measurable blood pressures (by palpation or auscultation), electrocardiographic waveforms, and invasive parameters such as arterial, central venous, and pulmonary artery pressures that may be displayed on a physiologic computer monitor (CAE Healthcare, 2015; Gaumard, 2015; Laerdal, 2015). Respiratory system components include self-regulating spontaneous ventilation, measurable exhaled respiratory gases, and breath sounds. Other simulator features include bowel sounds; speech; pharmacologic systems capable of responding to administered drugs; a urologic system; blinking and reactive pupils; tongue swelling; bronchial occlusion; jugular vein distention; and the ability to accept defibrillation, use of a transthoracic pacemaker, needle cricothyroidotomy, jet ventilation, needle thoracentesis, chest tube insertion, IV fluid administration, intraosseous infusion capability, and pericardiocentesis.

Examples of some modifiable physiologic parameters include changes in heart rates or sounds, respiratory rates or breath sounds, and the quality of bowel sounds. Most of the simulators have both a portable interface allowing instructors to control simulations from either the mannequin's bedside or a remote location where changes can be made without the participant's knowledge. To initiate a simulation, the user selects a patient profile, such as a healthy adult male or female. If desired, a clinical scenario, such as a case that progresses to anaphylaxis, can be superimposed on the physiology of the healthy adult profile. Once the scenario has been initiated, the instructor may allow the simulation to run as programmed or make on-the-fly modifications to individualize learning opportunities and emphasize specific teaching points.

■ Conditions for Learning

A well-planned HPS can replicate high-risk clinical situations, while providing a safe and reproducible platform for the student to demonstrate clinical competencies under realistic conditions in real time with actual clinical supplies (Hooper, Shaw, & Zamzam, 2015). Other observable practical advantages of simulation include the ability to allow learner-driven management errors to develop, to allow multiple treatment options to be explored without injury or discomfort to a real patient, and to manipulate time as a factor in managing nursing care (Larew, Lessans, Spunt, Foster, & Covington, 2006).

Educational advantages of simulation include opportunities for learners to improve competence and clinical judgment; to practice communication skills; to gain self-confidence, knowledge, and perceptions of being prepared to practice (Fisher & King, 2013; Kim, Lee, Avila, Ouyang, & Walker, 2015); and to also reinforce learning with constructive feedback during debriefing or reflective sessions following the simulation (Fanning & Gaba, 2007). The application of mental health-based simulation techniques has provided opportunities to identify biases, anxieties, and fear as well as knowledge deficiencies among nursing students (Brown, 2015).

Because of the ability to create customized learning scenarios, HPSs can be used in a wide variety of situations for all types of students. Simulation may be useful to precede, complement, or replace actual clinical experiences. For example, prior to clinical experiences, simulation has been used to orient students to care on an unfamiliar unit. Meyer, Connors, Hou, and Gajewski (2011) prepared student nurses with a 6-hour curriculum over 4 days of caring for pediatric patients in an HPS setting prior to entering their clinical rotation. During the simulations, they practiced taking vital signs; administering medications; communicating with healthcare providers, the child, and the child's parents; and documentation. When compared to their peers who did not participate in these simulations, students who did participate demonstrated more significant and positive effects on therapeutic skills, scores in documentation, and interpersonal communication during their clinical rotations (Meyer et al., 2011).

Used concomitantly with clinical practice, simulation provides students and faculty with the opportunity to replicate real clinical experiences and then use the simulator for reflection to explore more useful alternative management strategies. Students could also create customized patients based on their knowledge of physiology and pathophysiology and then compare the responses of their simulated patients to patients observed in clinical practices (Register, Graham-Garcia, & Haas, 2003).

Although the fidelity of HPSs is not sufficiently developed to replace the practice of caring for human patients, simulation can be used to create learning opportunities that are not ordinarily available in most clinical environments. For example, students can practice high-risk technical procedures such as defibrillation, using actual equipment in real time, or provide patient care during cardiopulmonary resuscitation or anaphylactic reactions on the simulator. In the field of anesthesiology, programs such as Anesthesia Crisis Resource Management (ACRM; Gaba, Howard, Fish, & Smith, 2001) and Team Oriented Medical Simulation have focused on the actions of all members of a healthcare team, with the goal of improving team performance (Baker, Gustafson, Beaubien, Salas, & Barach, 2005).

Following an analysis of the documented effects of HPS in hospital-based education programs, Merchant (2012) concluded that simulation offered nurse educators enhanced learning opportunities with an ability to measure clinical performance during certain aspects of nursing care. Specifically, efforts that focused on teamwork-related competencies and crisis management demonstrated positive clinical outcomes that included error reduction, decreased mortality rates, cost reductions, and increased patient safety in high-risk circumstances.

In addition to its uses as an instructional tool, simulation has been recognized for its potential to evaluate student cognitive or behavioral skills from a formative or summative perspective. Techniques for formative evaluation of student performances include using simulation as a mechanism for providing feedback on current skills and decision-making processes or for observing progression of a student's competencies. Instruments that are useful for formative evaluation capture students' perceptions about their learning and self-confidence, and provide faculty with insights associated with the pedagogy of simulations (Elfrink Cordi, Leighton, Ryan-Wenger, Doyle, & Ravert, 2012).

Summative evaluations offer opportunities to determine the competency of a participant engaged in an activity at the end of a time period, and use of the HPS may be associated with an assigned grade (Meakim et al., 2013).

One of the difficulties associated with integrating HPSs into a program is the costs associated with the initial setup. They include the purchase of the simulators and their associated support systems; the maintenance of the simulation lab and all of the necessary supplies; the supporting lab personnel, which could include instructional, administrative, and clerical roles; and insurance costs (Fletcher & Wind, 2013). Following the startup phase of an HPS program, the costs of maintaining the program can be challenging. There is an ongoing need to support these efforts, from those in administrative positions with budgetary authority to the personnel who must participate in the program activities.

■ Theoretical Foundations

The landmark Flexner Report to the Carnegie Foundation in 1910 established the dominant paradigm for healthcare education in the 20th century (Beck, 2004). Two key components of the model were to practice scientific medicine while the learner was also engaged in laboratory experimentation and hands-on care at the bedside. The scientific curriculum had historically featured lecture-based instruction during the first 2 years of training, where students were passive recipients of factual scientific knowledge (Papa & Harasym, 1999). Information was imparted by domain experts according to a predetermined timetable. Although the lecture format assured that the important educational material had been disseminated, the learner was at risk of lacking the conceptual links necessary for retention of the information. By contrast, the clinical practicum more effectively engaged students with a contextual experience for the facts that they had learned.

Achieving a successful balance between academic and clinical education has challenged educators, who must prepare graduates for healthcare institutions with both broad-based knowledge and technologically current specialty clinical skills (Manuel & Sorenson, 1995). These expectations have in the past created a sense of placing classroom learning, viewed as the foundation of academic priorities, in competition with the need for clinical experiences, a workplace priority. From the perspective of situated cognition, both classroom and clinical experiences are equally necessary, as knowledge is believed to be situated as a product of the activity, context, and culture in which it is used and not just something that happens inside of a person's head (Brown, Collins, & Duguid, 1989).

Situated Cognition

Situated cognition, sometimes called *situated learning*, is recognized as a learning theory propsing that learning is influenced by the situation within which it occurs (Onda, 2012). In a high-fidelity simulation environment, situated cognition emphasizes the necessity of higher-order thinking skills over the retrieval of memorized facts. When students face a complex or ill-defined task within the context of a high-fidelity simulation scenario, they are afforded an opportunity to recall information that is relevant to the situation as they problem-solve and practice skills that are appropriate for situations similar to those in a clinical setting.

The principles of the situated cognitive framework include:

1. Thinking and learning as measures of knowledge make sense only within particular situations.
2. People act and construct meaning within communities of practice.
3. Knowledge depends on the use of a variety of artifacts and tools.
4. Situations make sense within a historical context. (Paige & Daley, 2009, p. e99).

With the synthesis of the situated cognition principles and the characteristic needs of nursing education, three interacting components have been used to support learners in their quest for knowledge (Paige & Daley, 2009). The interacting components of a situated cognitive framework may be viewed as people (including the community, or more specifically patients, families, nurses, physicians, and ancillary personnel), ingredients or tools (including prior knowledge or concepts), and activity (including participation in real-life events). **Figure 17-1** shows a graphic representation of the situated cognition framework.

Learning that is structured within the situated cognition framework and the application of HPS offers nursing educators a strategy to bridge a student's advancement from theory-based knowledge to practice and social integration into professional nursing (Paige & Daley, 2009). For explanation purposes, Paige and Daley described a case of the care of a patient experiencing unstable angina. An HPS provided students with opportunities to transfer knowledge, which was enhanced by an environment

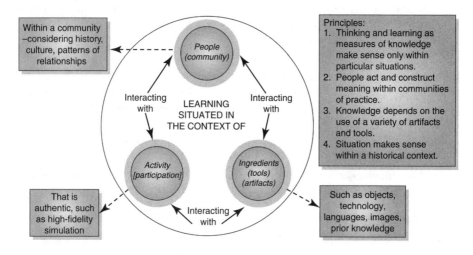

■ **Figure 17-1**   Situated cognition framework.

Reproduced from Paige, J. B., & Daley, B. J. (2009). Situation cognition: A learning framework to support and guide high-fidelity simulation. *Clinical Simulation in Nursing, 5*, e97–e103. doi:http://dx.doi.org/10.1016/j.ecns.2009.03.120. Copyright (2009), with permission from Elsevier.

in which they needed to page the physician, provide a status report, take verbal orders, and prepare a drug for administration. The construction of meaning within the community of practice was exemplified by the necessity to meet the needs of the simulated patient, which included answering the patient's questions about chest pain and interventions to reduce pain and anxiety. The ingredients or tools included the student's prior knowledge of the concept of pain, which demanded an understanding of pain that was tailored to the unique needs of a patient with cardiac tissue ischemia. Finally, the principle of the historic context that encompassed cultural practices, values, and strategies of thinking and perceiving was viewed as enculturation into the healthcare environment with a review of the roles and responsibilities of professional nurses.

■ Nursing Resources for the Use of HPS

The desire to promote the most appropriate and efficacious use of HPS associated with the education and evaluation of nurse-related health care has prompted a need to provide empirically supported guidance for these efforts. Two major nursing resources that provide this type of support are the International Nursing Association for Clinical Simulation and Learning (INACSL) and the National League for Nursing (NLN).

The INACSL is a professional organization whose mission is to promote research and disseminate evidence-based practice standards for clinical simulation methodologies and learning environments (INACSL, 2015a). INACSL's stated vision is to be nursing's portal to the world of clinical simulation pedagogy and learning environments (INACSL, 2015b). *Clinical Simulation in Nursing*, an international, peer-reviewed journal published online monthly, is the official journal of the INACSL. The INACSL has published INACSL *Standards of Best Practice: Simulation*[SM] for the purpose of advancing the science of simulation, sharing best practices, and providing evidence-based guidelines for implementation and training (INACSL, 2015a). These *Standards of Best Practice: Simulation* address the terminology used, professional integrity of participants, participant objectives, facilitation methods, the simulation facilitator, debriefing processes, participant assessment and evaluation, simulation-enhanced interprofessional education, and simulation designs (Sittner et al., 2015). Each standard is supported by rationales, outcomes, criteria, and guidelines for its application during simulation. Readers are invited to visit the INACSL website at https://inacsl.org for a more detailed understanding of the value of the INACSL contribution to simulation.

The National Council of State Boards of Nursing Simulation Study (NCSBNSS) used the *Standards of Best Practice: Simulation* in its national multisite study to quantify empirical support for replacing clinical hours with simulation experiences in prelicensure nursing education (Hayden, Smiley, Alexander, Kardong-Edgren, & Jeffries, 2014). In 2015, an expert panel determined that the findings from the NCSBNSS provided confidence that a substitution of 50% of simulation time promoted outcomes similar to traditional clinical experiences (Alexander et al., 2015). The panel additionally developed a set of simulation guidelines for prelicensure programs that promote the use of the INASCL *Standards of Best Practice: Simulation* as well as the resources that are supported by the National League for Nursing.

The National League for Nursing (NLN) promotes excellence in nursing education to build a strong and diverse nursing workforce to advance the health of our nation and the global community (NLN, 2015). The NLN has been an advocate for simulation and technology. Through a collaborative relationship with leaders in simulation, the NLN has created simulation scenarios for use across curricula, pioneered nursing education webinars, and established an annual technology conference that supports the integration of technology into its initiatives (Tagliereni, 2015). The NLN supports the Simulation Innovation Resource Center (SIRC), an online e-learning site where nursing faculty can learn how to design, implement, and evaluate the use of simulation in nursing education (NLN, 2015). *Nursing Education Perspectives* is the peer-reviewed, bimonthly research journal of the NLN. It provides an evidence base for best practices and a forum for the exchange of information regarding teaching and learning with simulation technology, among other issues important to nursing education. Online access to NLN-promoted courses and research on simulation strategies can be found at http://sirc.nln.org/.

NLN Jeffries Simulation Theory

Following a systematic process involving rigorous research, a thorough synthesis of the literature, and discussions among nurses immersed in simulation activities, the simulation framework originally developed by Jeffries (2005, 2007) has been revised and is now endorsed as the NLN Jeffries Simulation Theory (NLN-JST) (Jeffries, 2016). Jeffries describes *clinical simulation* as "a phenomenon defined as a perceived situation, a process, a group of events, and/or a group of situations" (2016, p. xi). To understand the phenomenon of clinical simulation, this mid-range theory is intended to provide guidance for the implementation of simulation and future research in studying simulation phenomena, and also to contribute to the science of nursing education (Jeffries, 2016).

The concepts of the NLN-JST include the context (which encompasses all of the contextual factors that impact every aspect of the simulation), the background, the design elements, the simulation experience (SE), the facilitator and educational strategies, the participant attributes, and the outcomes of the simulation (Jeffries, Rodgers, & Adamson, 2016). The outcomes of the simulation may relate to the participant, the patient, and the system. (Jeffries et al., 2016). **Figure 17-2** provides a graphic representation of the NLN Jeffries Simulation Theory.

Context

The contextual factors of the simulation have been identified as the circumstances and the setting of the SE (Jeffries et al., 2016; Jeffries, Rodgers, & Adamson, 2015). The context may include the overarching purpose of the SE, which could be for instructional or evaluative purposes, and also the place, which could be an academic or practice setting.

Although a design for best practices in simulation facilities has not been established, planners have been advised to focus on the intended function of the environment by integrating the concepts of clinical, educational, and theatrical environments

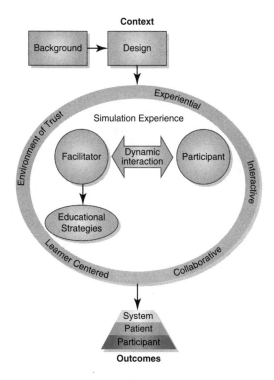

Figure 17-2   NLN Jeffries Simulation Theory.

Reproduced from Jeffries, P. R., Rodgers, B., & Adamson, K. (2016). NLN Jeffries Simulation Theory: Brief narrative description. In P. R. Jeffries (Ed.), *The NLN Jeffries Simulation Theory* (p. 40). New York, NY: National League for Nursing. Copyright © 2016 by the National League for Nursing, New York, NY. Reprinted with permission.

(Seropian & Lavey, 2010). For example, the types of rooms to consider would include an open learning area; a simulation theater; a control room; a room for debriefing, observations, or conferencing; a supply room; preparation areas; medication rooms; server rooms; rest rooms; offices; and reception areas.

The most basic critical aspect of a successful simulation program is the designation of dedicated physical space for the simulator and its support equipment. To accommodate the simulator, instructor, and four to six students requires approximately 250 square feet of floor space. A sample floor plan for a simple simulation room is presented in **Figure 17-3**.

High-fidelity patient simulators require electricity and, in the case of student anesthetists, gas sources, which could include oxygen, carbon dioxide, nitrogen, and nitrous oxide. Electricity requirements include two to four outlets for the simulator plus additional sources of power for patient care equipment. Depending on the type of simulation selected, patient care equipment may include physiologic monitors, infusion pumps, ventilators, anesthesia machines, and a defibrillator. Support equipment

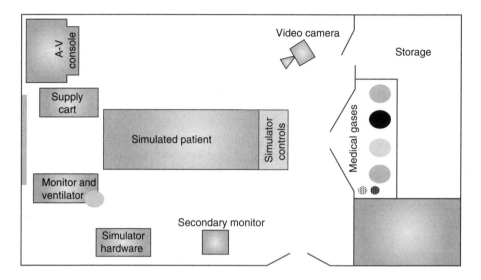

■ **Figure 17-3**   Sample floor plan for a simple simulation room.

includes airway devices, needles and syringes, dressings, chest tubes, intravenous and urinary catheters, scrub wear, gloves, and surgical masks, caps, and gowns.

The efficacy of simulation can be enhanced through video recordings of sessions with subsequent debriefing. Recording systems range from a single video camera to complex recording systems that allow multiple camera views, superimposed physiologic waveforms, and audio recordings from participants and faculty. Dedicated simulation centers may include a debriefing room where the videotapes can be reviewed or an observation room for the purpose of simultaneous instruction of other students.

Simulation centers also include a control room adjacent to the training room. One-way glass windows between the rooms allow individuals in a control room to observe simulation sessions as the operator and faculty communicate via headsets with microphones. In this type of room arrangement, a technician or faculty member in the control room is responsible for monitoring the simulation, making adjustments to the scenario as necessary, and selecting video and audio sources for recording.

Background

The background includes the goals and expectations that influence the design of the SE (Jeffries et al., 2015, 2016). The theoretical perspective for the specific SE and how it fits within the curriculum are important elements that inform the design and implementation of the activity. According to Jeffries et al., the background also includes the resources of time and equipment and how they will be allocated.

Design

The design includes the elements that must be considered before the HPS is implemented. The design includes the measurable learning objectives that guide the selection of activities and clinical scenarios in terms of content and problem complexity (Jeffries et al., 2015, 2016; Lioce et al., 2015). The elements of the physical, conceptual, and psychological aspects of fidelity include the decisions related to the necessary equipment, the moulage, and the predetermined roles and responses of the facilitator as they relate to the participants' interventions. Other considerations for the design include the participant roles, the progression of the activities, the briefing and debriefing strategies, and decisions associated with video recordings of the SE. *Briefing*, used synonymously with *prebriefing*, describes the activities that include an orientation to the equipment, environment, mannequin, roles, time allotment, objectives, and patient simulation (Meakim et al., 2013). *Debriefing* describes the activities that follow the simulation experience to permit the participants to explore emotions, question and reflect, and provide feedback to one another (Meakim et al., 2013).

Successful simulation sessions depend on carefully planned scenarios and clearly defined roles of the participants. Depending on one's expertise level, the facilitator may be responsible for selecting the scenario, guiding students through the simulation, providing important information and clinical cues that are not immediately available from the simulator (such as skin temperature), providing transition cues, modeling behaviors, monitoring student performance, and troubleshooting in the event of an unexpected simulator issue. In complex situations, the facilitator may be assisted by another faculty member or technician who may serve as the simulator operator. In this case, the operator's responsibilities would include activating the simulation system, starting the patient software, overlaying the clinical scenarios, monitoring the progress of a scenario, and adjusting the scenario as it was intended to play out by the primary facilitator. Additional faculty, students, or assistants may also role play as members of the healthcare team and family.

Simulation Experience

The HPS is characterized by an environment that supports an experiential, interactive, collaborative, and learner-centered situation (Jeffries et al., 2016). According to Jeffries et al., there should also be a shared responsibility of trust between the facilitator and participants of the experience. Within the HPS, there is a dynamic interaction between the facilitator and the participants. The attributes of the facilitator include skills, preparation, and educational techniques. The educational strategies, which may be adjusted as the experience advances, include the timing of activities and use of feedback, identified as cues during the experience or debriefing toward the end of the SE. Participant attributes that affect the SE have been identified as age, gender, levels of anxiety, and self-confidence, as well as the state of preparedness for roles of the activity (Jeffries et al., 2015, 2016).

Outcomes Evaluation

The outcomes of the simulation may relate to the participant, the patient, and the system (Jeffries et al., 2015, 2016). Participant outcomes could include satisfaction, self-confidence, learning, and translation of learning into the clinical environment;

patient outcomes could relate to the health outcomes of recipients whose caregivers were trained using simulation; system or organizational outcomes could be associated with cost-effectiveness and improved changes in practice. A first consideration regarding the outcomes associated with simulation relates to a clear conceptual definition of the selected phenomena (Adamson & Prion, 2015). The next concern is with an operational definition that provides a valid and reliable measurement of the selected outcome. A few examples of outcomes that have been operationalized for evaluating participants after HPS are the Lasater Clinical Judgment Rubric (LCJR), the Simulation Effectiveness Tool-Modified (SET-M), and the Creighton Competency Evaluation Instrument (CCEI).

The Lasater Clinical Judgment Rubric (LCJR)

The LCJR was developed by Lasater in an attempt to provide a measure of clinical judgment skills (Lasater, 2007). The LCJR is based on the conceptual framework of the Clinical Judgment Model (CJM), which describes the variety of reasoning processes that nurses employ as they provide care in complex patient care situations (Tanner, 2006). As clinical learning is one of the outcomes of clinical judgment, the model implies that nurses are continually learning as they develop their expertise through experiences and reflection. Components of the model include noticing, interpreting, responding, and reflecting. These components suggest that the nurse must be aware of the patient's needs, make sense of the situation, and respond with the best course of action, which will be submitted to reflection after outcomes are realized and evaluated. **Figure 17-4** displays the Clinical Judgment Model developed by Tanner (2006).

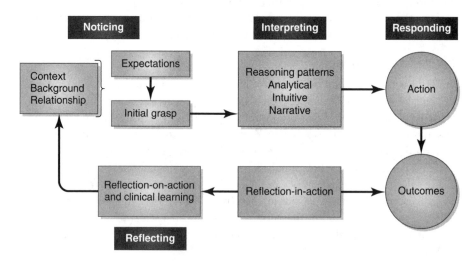

■ **Figure 17-4**   Clinical judgment model.

Reproduced from Tanner, C. A. (2006). Thinking like a nurse: A research-based model of clinical judgment in nursing. *Journal of Nursing Education, 45*(6), 204–211. Retrieved from http://www.healio.com/nursing/journals/jne. Reprinted with permission from Slack Incorporated, copyright 2009.

The LCJR provides the four phases of the CJM—noticing, interpreting, responding, and reflecting—with 11 dimensions (Lasater, 2007). Effective noticing involves focused observations, recognizing deviations from expected patterns, and information seeking. Effective interpreting involves prioritizing data and making sense of data. Effective responding involves a calm, confident manner; clear communication; well-planned intervention/flexibility; and skillfulness. Effective reflecting involves evaluation/self-analysis and commitment to improvement. The rubric offers participants an opportunity to reflect on their performance for each dimension and rate themselves as exemplary, accomplished, developing, or beginning following a simulation experience. It should be noted that the LCJR is only appropriate for actively involved participants; it is not useful for examining the thinking of observers (Shelestak, Meyers, Jarzembak, & Bradley, 2015).

The LCJR has reportedly met the criteria for instrument validity and intrarater and interrater reliability during HPS through the efforts of three research teams (Adamson, Gubrud, Sideras, & Lasater, 2012). Adamson and Kardong-Edgren (2012) used a database of standardized, validated, video-archived simulations that depicted nursing students performing at three different scripted levels of proficiency, while nurse educator observers rated the student behaviors as below expectations, at level of expectations, and above expectations. Gubrud-Howe (2008) reported acceptable interrater reliability of observations with the LCJR during rater training and also following a pretest and posttest design when pairs of students working as registered nurses were observed during 50-minute-long simulations. Sideras (2007) demonstrated that four observers, who were not informed of the educational levels of the nursing students, could apply the LCJR and accurately differentiate between the clinical judgment performance of graduating seniors and end-of-junior-year-level student abilities from three recorded simulation cases as a type of validity for known groups. Despite the reported achievement of instrument reliability, Adamson et al. (2012) suggested that researchers still need to (1) identify the locations of variability in reliability of the LCJR under different conditions of use, (2) identify the true ranges of students' clinical judgment abilities, (3) avoid cases of complex simulation scenarios where floor and ceiling effects influence rating responses, and (4) establish standards of rater training for the instrument.

The Simulation Effectiveness Tool–Modified (SET-M)

The SET-M is a modified version of the Simulation Effectiveness Tool that was originally designed to assess how well the simulation experience met the student learner's needs (Leighton, Ravert, Mudra, & Macintosh, 2015). According to Leighton et al., the SET-M provides a better reflection of the *Standards of Best Practice in Simulation* as well the Quality and Safety Education for Nursing (QSEN) competencies. The instrument contains 20 items (with 3-point ordinal scales) that are divided into four subscales that address prebriefing, learning, confidence, and debriefing. Exploratory factor analysis testing supported the existence of the four subscales. Internal consistency reliability testing for the subscales of prebriefing, learning, confidence, debriefing and the overall instrument demonstrated acceptable to good Cronbach's alphas of .833, .852, .913, .908, and .936, respectively (Leighton et al., 2015).

Creighton Competency Evaluation Instrument (CCEI)

The CCEI is a modified version of the Creighton Simulation Evaluation Instrument (C-SEI) that was developed to evaluate clinical competencies among students within both associate and baccalaureate nursing programs for the National Council of State Boards of Nursing Simulation Study (NCSBNSS) (Hayden, Keegan, Kardong-Edgren, & Smiley, 2014). As there was a belief that competencies observed in the simulation setting would also be demonstrated in the clinical environment, the items within the CCEI were reframed to reflect the core competencies found in the documents associated with the QSEN and the American Association of College of Nurses Essentials (Hayden et al., 2014).

The major concepts within the revised CCEI were categorized as assessment, communication, clinical judgment, and patient safety, with a total of 23 items (Hayden et al., 2014). Content validity of the CCEI was determined by 35 faculty members who used a Likert-type scale with scores ranging from 1 (strongly disagree) to 4 (strongly agree) to rate the items according to necessity, fitness to reflect the corresponding category, and ability to understand the behaviors within the category. The mean scores for content validity were 3.89, 3.86, and 3.78, respectively. Interrater reliability was supported by 31 faculty and staff who viewed and rated videos of the same simulation scenario at three levels of proficiency. The responses of each of the 31 faculty were then compared with those of an expert rater. The overall agreement with the expert rater was 79.4%; Cronbach's alphas were above .90 and considered highly acceptable. When the CCEI was used by clinical instructors, the instrument was rated to be easy to use, easy to understand, and useful to rate performance and learning among students in both the simulation and clinical environments.

The use of summative evaluations during an HPS has met with controversy. As the aim of HPS is to prepare the student to safely and effectively care for patients in the actual clinical setting, investigators have not been able to measure an empirical relationship between the performance of the student in a simulated environment and the actual clinical setting. This is related to the limited numbers of valid and reliable psychometric measurements that can be used for this purpose. Adamson, Kardong-Edgren, and Willhaus (2013) have reported that the literature is full of low-level participant evaluations that address how learners reacted to a learning process. Adamson and colleagues stressed that there is a serious need to measure what really matters from a perspective of translational research and to identify how simulation affects not only learners and their behaviors, but also patient outcomes. These types of goals suggest that more researchers should focus on developing measurement instruments that are appropriate for the specific populations and activities that they are intended to measure, in addition to having sufficient reliability and validity scores.

An Example of Scenario Development

To develop and implement a new simulation scenario, the following process is recommended:

1. *Determine educational objectives or goals.* For example, the simulation may be intended to promote the advancement of technical, cognitive, or behavioral

abilities or a combination of these competencies. Decide how the attainment of the objectives will be evaluated and measured. Determine in advance whether the progression of the simulation will be constrained to unfold with a predetermined sequence or to develop spontaneously.

2. *Construct a clinical scenario to facilitate attainment of educational objectives.* Although the scenario should be clinically realistic, it should be customized to the student's level of expertise and designed to promote the student's successful progression toward a higher level of decision making and demonstration of competencies.

3. *Define underlying physiologic concepts to be manifested throughout the scenario as they relate to the patient's responses to various events as they occur.* Determine which essential elements of the clinical scenario are to be represented in the simulation experience, which elements may be absent or overlooked, and which missing elements should be integrated into the experience. For example, as a patient develops a progressive hypoxemia, tachypnea and decreasing hemoglobin saturation, as measured by pulse oximetry, are expected to occur. Although a real patient would also eventually become cyanotic, the designer of the HPS experience must decide whether the observation of skin color changes should be a necessary part of the educational objectives. When considering the fidelity of the clinical situations, it is also essential to decide whether changes must be technically accurate or just sufficiently realistic and prominent to elicit the intended response from the learners.

4. *In the case of high-fidelity human simulators that have preprogrammed patients and scenarios, modify the scenario as necessary.* Program modification generally includes specifying the baseline physiology and clinical condition of the underlying patient, preparing the scenario to include optional modifiable states, and defining transitions between various patient states as the scenario evolves.

5. *Identify required equipment.* Decide which devices will be displayed prominently or stored (as they might be in the clinical environment); whether learners will have the opportunity to inspect, assemble, and test equipment prior to the experience; and if the student will have options among multiple devices for use in the simulation. Decide whether additional personnel will be required to implement the clinical scenario, the qualifications (both actual and the role played) of the additional participants, and how the participants will be able to access/involve the supplemental personnel resources.

6. *Develop questions to guide an environment of reflective debriefing after the simulation.*

7. *Run the program and collect feedback.* Prior to use with students, the scenario should be run to establish that the simulation scenario unfolds as designed, with the intended levels of instructor and faculty participation.

8. *Reiterate steps until satisfied.* The simulation scenario is continuously refined until it unfolds as intended, without unintentional ambiguous details that distract from attainment of the educational objectives, and the faculty is able to concentrate on observing and evaluating the student's performance while maintaining a positive, effective learning environment.

Once the simulated scenario begins, the instructor may participate in a variety of ways. The instructor may function as a role model who demonstrates critical thinking, decision making, and therapeutic interventions; as a coach who is available to help students when necessary; or as a passive bystander observing the scenario with minimal involvement. Regardless of the level of participation during the simulation, one of the instructor's key responsibilities is to facilitate the debriefing session afterward to reinforce the objectives of the scenario and to ensure that the intended learning occurred. During an ideal debriefing session, through reflective thinking, the students should have opportunities to describe and interpret the scenario, clarify their thoughts and actions as they occurred during the simulation, critique their performance in a nonthreatening way, and generate alternative decisions and plans of actions that would improve future performances.

■ Limitations of HPS

Although HPS offers educators in the health professions numerous opportunities to prepare students for the clinical setting, there are some limitations that should be recognized and addressed. One limitation to HPS is its incomplete or inaccurate presentation of reality. Participants in a simulation are expected to suspend disbelief and respond to the patient according to what they observe. Although simulators provide lifelike representations of human beings, they are not capable of exhibiting a complete range of signs and behaviors. Thus, instructors need to identify cues that contradict the intended signs within the simulator or be prepared to provide the critical cues that are necessary for appropriate advancement of the scenario.

Another limitation relates to the fact that most simulation-based learning experiences tend to focus on the needs of deteriorating patients who need emergent care. Onello and Regan (2013) have warned that this emphasis may place students at risk of being biased to anticipatory and reactionary responses that may be inappropriate for the longitudinal care needs of patients in the clinical setting. An example of this type of bias observed in the simulation lab occurred when the participants in an HPS became hypervigilant and wanted to administer epinephrine before the patient presented any signs of anaphylaxis.

■ Conclusion

Simulation has become a popular topic among academic communities that are promoting it as a strategy to facilitate learning in healthcare education. Following the National Council of State Boards of Nursing (NCSBN) Simulation Study, the NCSBN reported that high-quality simulation experiences could be used to substitute for up to 50% of traditional clinical experiences (Alexander et al., 2015). In order to meet the criteria of high-quality SEs, the NCSBN has published *Simulation Guidelines for Prelicensure Nursing Programs*, which are intended to provide guidance for evaluating the readiness of the program to substitute simulation for traditional clinical experiences and also for establishing evidence-based simulation programs (Alexander et al., 2015). Then, the publication of the NLN-JST as a mid-range theory has shown support for the theoretical thinking and testing that has been done to promote simulation as a learning methodology among nursing education researchers (Jeffries, 2015). Now the challenge for nursing is to test and use the theory to guide research in studying the phenomenon of HPS and use it to contribute to the science of nursing education (Forneris & Fey, 2016).

While recognizing the challenge of studying simulation-based learning, research should be systematically developed using rigorous research standards that reflect the state of the science (Franklin, Leighton, Cantrell, & Rutherford-Hemming, 2015). For example, the research questions should be aligned with the evidence-based guidelines outlined in the INACSL *Standard of Best Practice: Simulation* (2013) and also guided by the relationships of the concepts within the NLN-JST framework. As there is an ongoing challenge to develop valid and reliable methods to evaluate the effectiveness of HPS interventions, there is a need to develop measurement instruments that are useful for specific patient situations. In order to bridge the gaps between classroom-based instruction and the dynamic, unpredictable clinical environment, there is also a need to investigate the translation of knowledge from the simulation environment to the clinical setting among students as well as newly graduated nurses (Weaver, 2011).

Teaching Example:
Using High-Fidelity Simulation in an Undergraduate Critical Care Nursing Course

This example[1] illustrates how simulation was used to reinforce concepts of respiratory assessment and nursing care as part of a critical care nursing elective for senior-level undergraduate nursing students.

The course included 40 didactic hours and was designed to complement a 200-hour clinical practicum. The course focused on pulmonary, cardiovascular, and neurologic critical care; advanced hemodynamic monitoring; and critical care pharmacology. The respiratory care section of the course included lectures on respiratory gas exchange, advanced assessment techniques, arterial blood gas analysis, airway management, and ventilatory support. To complement the lectures, a simulation session was developed.

1. Determine educational objective.
   The simulation session was designed so that the student would be able to achieve the following objectives:
   - Complete and continuously revise the assessment of a patient who is acutely and dynamically ill.
   - Select appropriate oxygen therapy devices for a specified clinical situation.
   - Collect and prepare the appropriate equipment and medications for emergent tracheal intubation.
   - Administer appropriate medications to facilitate emergent tracheal intubation and assess the drug effects.

[1]Scenario developed by Beverly George-Gay, MSN, CCRN, assistant professor and coordinator of distance and continuing education, Department of Nurse Anesthesia, Virginia Commonwealth University, Richmond, VA.

(continues)

- Perform airway management procedures, as indicated, to include bag-valve-mask ventilation, tracheal intubation, and insertion of an endotracheal tube.
- Confirm appropriate placement of an endotracheal tube.
- Prepare an unstable patient for transport from an inpatient unit to a critical care unit.
- Initiate positive-pressure ventilatory support for an acutely ill patient and adjust ventilatory parameters (to include mode, FiO_2, tidal volume, respiratory rate, and positive end-expiratory pressure) as indicated by patient condition, arterial blood gases, capnography, and spirometry.
- Although the scenario involved only nursing students, it can easily be expanded to include respiratory and emergency care providers. The instructor was actively involved in the session as a coach who provided interactive feedback to students and helped them clarify clinical observations.

2. Construct a clinical scenario.

   Students were told that they were going to evaluate a patient with pneumonia hospitalized on an inpatient medical unit. A brief patient history was provided.

   Students were given the opportunity to assess the patient, including observation of respiratory effort, lung auscultation, estimation of arterial oxygenation by pulse oximetry, and measurement and analysis of arterial blood gases. At the time of initial contact, the patient demonstrated signs of moderate hypoxia to include rapid, shallow breathing, mild oxyhemoglobin desaturation, and rales on chest auscultation. Upon a signal from the instructor to the simulator operator, the patient experienced significant oxyhemoglobin desaturation.

   The scenario was designed so that the patient initially would require oxygen therapy and then require more aggressive treatment, including tracheal intubation and positive-pressure ventilation using a bag-valve device with both face mask and tracheal tube. Once the patient was transferred to the critical care unit, ventilatory support using various modes such as assist control, intermittent mandatory ventilation, positive end-expiratory pressure, and pressure support ventilation could be explored.

3. Define underlying physiologic concepts to be manifested through the scenario—patient and events.

   The physiologic concepts underlying pneumonia include decreased lung compliance and increased shunt. Manifestations of these alterations include an adaptive respiratory pattern with increased rate and smaller tidal volume, increased peak inspiratory pressure, hypoxemia, mild hypercarbia, rales, tachycardia, and cardiac dysrhythmias. Patient deterioration within the scenario resulted from progressive reductions in lung compliance and increases in shunt. For this exercise, it was determined that sufficient physiologic changes to induce learner critical thinking, decision making, and action were more important than technical accuracy.

4. Modify programmed patient and scenarios, as necessary.

   A geriatric model developed by faculty and master's-level nursing anesthesia students was used.[2] To exhibit signs of pneumonia, rales were introduced, lung compliance was decreased, shunt fraction was increased, and the CO_2 set point was increased slightly (to produce mild hypercarbia). Temperature was increased slightly to reflect an underlying infective process. As a result of these changes, tidal volume decreased automatically and respiratory rate increased to compensate for the reduced tidal volume. Physiologic alterations were also manifested automatically through changes in heart rate and arterial blood gases.

---

[2]Development of the geriatric model was supported, in part, by a grant from the Division of Nursing, U.S. Department of Health and Human Services, Bureau of Health Professions.

So that the patient would initially appear to be stable and then deteriorate upon the instructor's command, baseline and decompensation states were created. Although an automatic transition could have initiated the decompensation at a predetermined time, a manual transition was selected to assure that the destabilization occurred when intended by the instructor.

5. Assemble required equipment.

Because the patient was not physically transported from the medical unit to the critical care unit, the simulation lab was originally configured with equipment available to acute care personnel. Items included a resuscitation cart with cardiac monitor and defibrillator, an oxygen source, oxygen therapy devices, and various airway management devices such as a bag-value-mask device, pharyngeal airways, endotracheal tubes, laryngoscopes, and suction equipment. Once the scenario shifted to the critical care unit, a positive-pressure ventilator was also available for student use.

6. Run program and collect feedback.

Prior to use with students, the scenario was run several times to observe the rate of change for physiologic variables and the effects of various therapeutic options.

7. Reiterate steps 2–6 until satisfied.

Physiologic parameters were modified incrementally so that the patient would appear stable, but with sufficient respiratory compromise to entice the learner to initiate oxygen therapy. Once the deterioration sequence was initiated, the decompensation had to be sufficient to warrant more aggressive therapy yet progress at a rate such that novice nurses with limited skills and therapeutic options could stabilize the patient.

To implement the simulation, the instructor selects the customized geriatric patient from the Patient Options menu of the user interface and respiratory exercise from the Scenario Options menu. The simulator immediately begins emulating the pneumonia patient in the stable baseline state. Progression to the decompensation state requires only one additional keystroke or mouse click.

Careful testing of the simulated patient and clinical scenario reduces the likelihood of unanticipated events during the educational session; however, the instructor should be prepared to help students with assembling and using unfamiliar equipment as well as performing advanced technical skills, such as effective bag-valve-mask ventilation and tracheal intubation. Careful coordination with the simulator operator will allow the patient to deteriorate at a rate appropriate for the experience of the learners, with pauses in the deterioration (if desired) during specific teaching moments or as technical maneuvers are performed.

For this exercise, evaluation of the learner achievement was formative and informal. After the simulated patient's condition was stabilized, the faculty and students reflected on clinical signs observed and how the patient's condition, clinical setting, and events affected decision making and actions; medications, devices, and procedures used to stabilize the patient; and potential alternative solutions that would have led to more rapid or improved outcomes.

Discussion Questions

1. You are responsible for developing a human patient simulation for student nurses who have completed a pharmacology and a physical assessment course. You plan to allow the students an opportunity to demonstrate the nursing skills associated with taking vital signs before they administer a patient's heart

medications in the simulation lab. Discuss how you would design this experience. For example, identify your learning objectives, list which modifiable physiologic features on the simulator would be useful as the students assess the patient, what type of equipment you will need to create a realistic environment, what kind of scenario you will develop, and how you will evaluate the students' performances.

2. You are in the beginning stages of developing a plan for human patient simulations in your medical-surgical nursing course. The first scenario will include an opportunity for students to recognize and respond to signs of deterioration in a patient with asthma. Access the INASCL *Standards of Best Practice: Simulation* at the INASCL website (https://inacsl.org). While referring to the standards for professional integrity of the participant and the facilitator, create a working document that will guide the attitudinal and behavioral expectations for both students and faculty members. Explain how these expectations relate to the NLN Jeffries Simulation Theory.

3. You are designing a human patient simulation for students who will be providing care for a patient with unstable angina that may progress into a myocardial infarction. Develop a guide for the activities of facilitation for the simulation. Refer to the INASCL *Standards of Best Practice: Simulation*. Link your plans with the relationships of the concepts within the NLN Jeffries Simulation Theory.

References

Adamson, K. A., Gubrud, P., Sideras, S., & Lasater, K. (2012). Assessing the reliability, validity, and use of the Lasater Clinical Judgment Rubric: Three approaches. *Journal of Nursing Education, 51*(2), 66–73. doi:10.3928/01484834-20111130-03

Adamson, K. A., & Kardong-Edgren, S. (2012). A method and resources for assessing the reliability of simulation evaluation instruments. *Nursing Education Perspectives, 33*(5), 334–339. Retrieved from http://www.nln.org/nlnjournal/index.htm

Adamson, K. A., Kardong-Edgren, S., & Willhaus, J. (2013). An updated review of published simulation evaluation instruments. *Clinical Simulation in Nursing, 9,* e393–e400. http://dx.doi.org/10.1016 /j.ecns.2012.09.004

Adamson, K. A., & Prion, S. (2015). Making sense of methods and measurement: Defining the latent variable. *Clinical Simulation in Nursing, 11,* 392–393. http://dx.doi.org/10.1016/j.ecns.2015.03.009

Aebersold, M., & Tschannen, D. (2013). Simulation in nursing practice: The impact on patient care. *Online Journal of Issues in Nursing, 18*(2), Manuscript 6. doi:10.3912/OJIN:.Vol18No02Man06

Alexander, M., Durham, C. F., Hooper, J. I., Jeffries, P. R., Goldman, N., Kardong-Edgren, S. . . . Tillman, C. (2015). NCSBN simulation guidelines for prelicensure nursing programs. *Journal of Nursing Regulation, 6*(3), 39–42. Retrieved from http://www.journalofnursingregulation.com

Alexandrou, E., Ramjan, L., Murphy, J., Hunt, L., Betihavas, V., & Frost, S. A. (2012). Training of undergraduate clinicians in vascular access: An integrative review. *Journal of Vascular Access, 17*(3), 146–158. http://dx.doi.org/10.1016/j.java2012.07.001

Baker, D. P., Gustafson, S., Beaubien, J. M., Salas, E., & Barach, P. (2005). Medical team training programs in health care. In Agency for Healthcare Research and Quality, *Advances in patient safety: From research to implementation* (AHRQ Publication No. 050021-4, pp. 253–267). Rockville, MD: AHRQ. Retrieved from http://www.ahrq.gov/downloads/pub/advances/vol4/Baker.pdf

Beck, A. H. (2004). The Flexner Report and the standardization of American medical education. *Journal of the American Medical Association, 291*(17), 2139–2140. Retrieved from http://jama.jamanetwork .com/journal.aspx

Brown, A. M. (2015). Simulation in undergraduate mental health nursing education: A literature review. *Clinical Simulation in Nursing, 11*, 445–449. http://dx.doi.org/10.1016/j.ecns.2015.08.003

Brown, J. S., Collins, A., & Duguid, P. (1989). Situated cognition and the culture of learning. *Educational Researcher, 18*, 32–42. Retrieved from http://edr.sagepub.com

CAE Healthcare. (2015). *Simulators.* Retrieved from http://www.caehealthcare.com/eng/patient-simulators

Decker, S., Sportsman, S., Puetz, L., & Billings, L. (2008). The evolution of simulation and its contribution to competency. *Journal of Continuing Education in Nursing, 39*(2), 74–80. Retrieved from http://www.slackinc.com/subscribe/jcen.asp

Elfrink Cordi, V. L., Leighton, K., Ryan-Wenger, N., Doyle, T., & Ravert, P. (2012). History and development of the Simulation Effectiveness Tool (SET). *Clinical Simulation in Nursing, 8*, e199–e210. doi:10.1016 /jecns.2011.12.001

Fanning, R. M., & Gaba, D. M. (2007). The role of debriefing in simulation-based learning. *Society for Simulation in Healthcare, 2*(2), 115–125. doi:10.1097/SIH.0b013e3180315539

Fisher, D., & King, L. (2013). An integrative literature review on preparing nursing students through simulation to recognize and respond to the deteriorating patient. *Journal of Advanced Nursing, 69*(11), 2375–2388. doi:10.1111/jan.12174

Fletcher, J. D., & Wind, A. P. (2013). Cost considerations in using simulations for medical training. *Military Medicine, 178*, S37–S46. doi:10.7205/MILMED-D-13-00258

Fletcher, J. L. (1995). AANA journal course: Update for nurse anesthetists—Anesthesia simulation: A tool for learning and research. *Journal of the American Association of Nurse Anesthetists, 63*, 61–67. Retrieved from http://www.aana.com/newsandjournal/Pages/aanajournalonline.aspx

Forneris, S. G., & Fey, M. (2016). NLN Vision: Teaching with simulation. In P. R. Jeffries (Ed.), *The NLN Jeffries Simulation Theory* (pp. 43–49). New York, NY: National League for Nursing.

Foronda, C., Lippincott, C., & Gattamorta, K. (2014). Evaluation of virtual simulation in a master's-level nurse education certificate program. *CIN: Computers, Informatics, Nursing, 32*(11), 516–522. doi:10.1097/CIN.0000000000000102

Franklin, A. E., Leighton, K., Cantrell, M. A., & Rutherford-Hemming, T. (2015). Simulation research for academics: Novice level. *Clinical Simulation in Nursing, 11*, 214–221. http://dx.doi.org/10.1016 /j.ecns.2015.01.007

Fritz, P. Z., Gray, T., & Flanagan, B. (2008). Review of mannequin-based high fidelity simulation in emergency medicine. *Emergency Medicine Australasia, 20*, 1–9. doi:10.1111/j.1742-6723.2007.01022.x

Gaba, D., & DeAnda, A. (1988). A comprehensive anesthesia simulation environment: Recreating the operating room for research and training. *Anesthesiology, 69*, 387–394. Retrieved from http://anesthesiology.pubs.asahq.org/journal.aspx

Gaba, D. M., Howard, S. K., Fish, K. J., & Smith, B. E. (2001). Simulation-based training in anesthesia crisis resource management (ACRM): A decade of experience. *Simulation & Gaming, 32*(2), 175–193. Retrieved from http://sag.sagepub.com

Gaumard. (2015). *Gaumard Simulators: Innovating Health Care for the Future.* Retrieved from http://www.gaumard.com/aboutsims

Good, M. I., & Gravenstein, J. S. (1989). Anaesthesia simulators and training devices. *International Anesthesiology Clinics, 27*, 161–166. Retrieved from http://journals.lww.com/anesthesiaclinics/pages /default.aspx

Gubrud-Howe, P. M. (2008). *Development of clinical judgment in nursing students: A learning framework to use in designing and implementing simulated learning experiences* (Unpublished dissertation). Portland State University, Portland, OR.

Hayden, J., Keegan, M., Kardong-Edgren, S., & Smiley, R. A. (2014). Reliability and validity testing of the Creighton Competency Evaluation Instrument for use in the NCSBN National Simulation Study. *Nursing Education Perspectives, 35*(4), 244–252. doi:10.5480/13-1130.1

Hayden, J. K., Smiley, R. A., Alexander, M., Kardong-Edgren, S., & Jeffries, P. R. (2014). The NCSBN National Simulation Study: A longitudinal, randomized, controlled study replacing clinical hours with simulation in prelicensure nursing education. *Journal of Nursing Regulation, 5*(2), S4–S41. Retrieved from http://www.journalofnursingregulation.com

Hoffman, R. L., & Burns, H. K. (2011). Using high-fidelity simulation as a teaching strategy with baby boomers returning to the RN workforce. *Journal of Nurses in Staff Development, 27*(6), 262–265. doi:1097/NND.0b013e31823097e9

Hooper, B., Shaw, L., & Zamzam, R. (2015). Implementing high-fidelity simulations with large groups of nursing students. *Nurse Educator, 40*(2), 87–90. doi:10.1097/NNE.0000000000000101

International Nursing Association for Clinical Simulation and Learning (INACSL). (2013). Standards of best practice: Simulation. *Clinical Simulation in Nursing, 11*(4), 214–221. Retrieved from https://inacsl.org

International Nursing Association for Clinical Simulation and Learning (INACSL). (2015a). *INACSL standards of best practice: Simulation*[SM]. Retrieved from http://www.inacsl.org/i4a/pages/index.cfm?pageid=3407

International Nursing Association for Clinical Simulation and Learning (INACSL). (2015b). *Mission and vision of INASCL.* Retrieved from https://inacsl.org/about/mission

Jeffries, P. R. (2005). A framework for designing, implementing, and evaluating simulations used as teaching strategies in nursing. *Nursing Education Perspectives, 26*(2), 96–103. Retrieved from http://www.nln.org/newsroom/newsletters-and-journal/nursing-education-perspectives-journal

Jeffries, P. R. (2007). *Simulation in nursing education: From conceptualization to evaluations.* New York, NY: National League for Nursing.

Jeffries, P. R. (2015). Guest editorial: Signs of maturity . . . Simulations are growing and getting more attention. *Nursing Education Perspectives, 36*(8), 358–359. Retrieved from http://nlnjournals.org/doi/pdf/10.5480/1536-5026-36.6.358

Jeffries, P. R. (2016). Preface. In P. R. Jeffries (Ed.), *The NLN Jeffries Simulation Theory* (pp. x–xi). New York, NY: National League of Nursing.

Jeffries, P. R., Rodgers, B., & Adamson, K. (2015). NLN Jeffries Simulation Theory: Brief narrative description. *Nursing Education Perspectives, 36*(5), 292–293. doi:10.5480/1536-5026-36.5.292

Jeffries, P. R., Rodgers, B., & Adamson, K. (2016). NLN Jeffries Simulation Theory: Brief narrative description. In P. R. Jeffries (Ed.), *The NLN Jeffries Simulation Theory* (pp. 39–42). New York, NY: National League of Nursing.

Kim, K. H., Lee, A., Avila, S., Ouyang, A., & Walker, A. (2015). Applications of high fidelity simulation for acquisitions of nursing skills: Nursing students' perspective. *International Journal for Innovation Education and Research, 3*(1), 78–95. Retrieved from http://www.ijier.net

Laerdal. (2015). *Patient simulators.* Retrieved from http://www.laerdal.com/us/nav/207/Patient-Simulators

Larew, C., Lessans, S., Spunt, D., Foster, D., & Covington, B. (2006). Innovations in clinical simulation: Application of Benner's theory in an interactive patient care simulation. *Nursing Education Perspectives, 29*(1), 16–21.

Lasater, K. (2007). Clinical judgment development: Using simulation to create an assessment rubric. *Journal of Nursing Education, 46*(11), 496–503. Retrieved from http://www.healio.com/nursing/journals/jne

Leighton, K., Ravert, P., Mudra, V., & Macintosh, C. (2015). Updating the simulation effectiveness tool: Item modifications and reevaluation of psychometric properties. *Nursing Education Perspectives, 36*(5), 317–323. doi:10.5480/15-1671

Lioce, L., Meakim, C. H., Fey, M. K., Chmil, J. V., Mariani, B., & Alinier, G. (2015). Standards of best practice: Simulation Standard IX: Simulation design. *International Nursing Association for Clinical Simulation and Learning, 11*(6), 309–315. http://dx.doi.org/10.1016/j.ecns.2015.03005

Lupien, A. (2007). High fidelity patient simulation. In M. J. Bradshaw & A. J. Lowenstein (Eds.), *Innovative teaching strategies in nursing and related health professions* (4th ed., pp. 197–214). Sudbury, MA: Jones & Bartlett.

Manuel, P., & Sorenson, L. (1995). Changing trends in healthcare: Implications for baccalaureate education, practice, and employment. *Journal of Nursing Education, 34*(6), 248–253. doi:10.3928/0148-4834-19950901-04

Meakim, C., Boese, T., Decker, S., Franklin, A. E., Gloe, D., Lioce, L., . . . Borum, J. C. (2013). Standards of best practice: Simulation standard I: Terminology. *Clinical Simulation in Nursing, 9*, S3–S11. http://dx.doi.org/10.1016j.ecns.2013.04.001

Merchant, D. C. (2012). Does high-fidelity simulation improve clinical outcomes? *Journal for Nurses in Staff Development, 28*(1), E1–E8. doi:10.1097/NND.0b013e318240a728

Meyer, M. N., Connors, H., Hou, Q., & Gajewski, B. (2011). The effect of simulation on clinical performance: A junior nursing student clinical comparison study. *Simulation in Healthcare, 6*, 269–277. doi:10.1097/SIH.0b013e318223a048

National League for Nursing (NLN). (2015). Retrieved from www.nln.org/home

Nehring, W. M. (2010). History of simulation in nursing. In W. M. Nehring & F. R. Lashley (Eds.), *High-fidelity patient simulation in nursing education* (pp. 3–26). Sudbury, MA: Jones & Bartlett.

Onda, E. L. (2012). Situated cognition: Its relationship to simulation in nursing education. *Clinical Simulation in Nursing, 8*(7), e273–280. doi:10.1016/j.ecns.2010.11.004

Onello, R., & Regan, M. (2013). Challenges in high fidelity simulation: Risk sensitization and outcome measurement. *Online Journal of Issues in Nursing, 18*(3). doi:10.3912/OJIN.Vol18No03PPT01

Paige, J. B., & Daley, B. J. (2009). Situation cognition: A learning framework to support and guide high-fidelity simulation. *Clinical Simulation in Nursing, 5*, e97–e103. doi:http://dx.doi.org/10.1016/j.ecns.2009.03.120

Papa, F. J., & Harasym, P. H. (1999). Medical curriculum reform in North America, 1765 to the present: A cognitive science perspective. *Academic Medicine, 74*(2), 154–164. Retrieved from http://journals.lww.com/academicmedicine/Abstract/1999/02000/Medical_curriculum_reform_in_North_America,_1765.15.aspx

Register, M., Graham-Garcia, J., & Haas, R. (2003). The use of simulation to demonstrate hemodynamic response to varying degrees of intrapulmonary shunt. *American Association of Nurse Anesthetists Journal, 71*, 277–284. Retrieved from http://www.aana.com/newsandjournal/Pages/aanajournalonline.aspx

Rosen, K. R. (2008). The history of medical simulation. *Journal of Critical Care, 23*, 157–166. doi:10.1016/j.jrc.2007.12.12.004

Shelestak, D. S., Meyers, T. W., Jarzembak, J. M., & Bradley, E. (2015). A process to assess clinical decision-making during human patient simulation: A pilot study. *Nursing Education Perspectives*, 185–187. doi:10.5480/13-1107.1

Seropian, M., & Lavey, R. (2010, December). Design considerations for healthcare simulation facilities. *Simulation in Healthcare, 5*, 338–345. doi:10.1097/SIH.0b013e318ec8f60

Sideras, S. (2007). *An examination of the construct validity of a clinical judgment evaluation tool in the setting of high-fidelity simulation* (Unpublished dissertation). Oregon Health & Science University, Portland, OR.

Sittner, B. J., Aebersold, M. L., Paige, J. B., Graham, L. L. M., Parsons Schram, A., Decker, S. I., & Lioce, L. (2015). INACSL standards of best practice for simulation: Past, present, and future. *Nursing Education Perspectives, 36*(5), 294–298. doi:10.5480/15-1670

Taglereni, E. (2015). *NLN Center for Innovation in Simulation and Technology.* Retrieved from http://www.nln.org/centers-for-nursing-education/nln-center-for-innovation-in-simulation-and-technology

Tanner, C. A. (2006). Thinking like a nurse: A research-based model of clinical judgment in nursing. *Journal of Nursing Education, 45*(6), 204–211. Retrieved from http://www.healio.com/nursing/journals/jne

Weaver, A. (2011). High-fidelity patient simulation in nursing education: An integrative review. *Nursing Education Perspectives, 32*(1), 37–40. Retrieved from http://www.nln.org/nlnjournal/index.htm

CHAPTER 18

Innovations in Facilitating Learning Using Patient Simulation

Kim Leighton

Nearly two decades have passed since faculty in the healthcare industry began facilitating learning with high-fidelity human patient simulation, a technique that continues to grow in sophistication. Educators often struggle with the realization that they are unable to prepare students adequately to assume the role of the healthcare provider. The vast amount of content, technical and interpersonal skills, and professional role expectations, coupled with the increased number of incoming students and decreased availability of clinical placements (Nehring, 2010), have created a frustrating and sometimes dangerous situation that has not abated. Clinical sites, which once were the primary place of learning, now restrict student activities, leading to suboptimal experiences for content integration and mastery. Many healthcare facilities have restricted the number of students per unit, causing the clinical instructor to divide time between units and floors, thereby decreasing observation and interaction time with learners. Students also have been restricted, at some facilities, from giving intravenous medication, accessing and administering narcotics and other critical medications, as well as documenting in the electronic health record (EHR). Additionally, today's hospitalized patients have medically complex needs that are often situated within challenging psychosocial circumstances that are beyond the capabilities of novice nursing students to manage. Observational experiences and mentor-apprenticeship are not always beneficial because preceptors are frequently preoccupied with pressing patient problems and are not as invested in student learning. Using human patient simulation as a teaching strategy provides opportunities for educators to fill gaps in students' knowledge and experience that are a result of limitations posed by traditional clinical environments.

The use of simulation, situated in a learning environment that has been manipulated to closely resemble any clinical setting, can present learners with almost any situation they might find in a patient care setting. Although the technology still intimidates many, the techniques of facilitating learning are at the essence of this pedagogy. For those who embrace this pedagogy, teaching with simulation, using realistic scenarios, is exciting and rewarding.

This methodology provides an environment for educating learners without risk to human life and increases confidence and ability to transfer knowledge and skills into actual clinical practice (Weaver, 2011). This chapter is intended to present innovative ways of utilizing patient simulation.

■ Definitions

Simulation-based learning experiences and patient simulators are commonly referred to as low, medium, and high fidelity. *Fidelity*, or "the degree to which a simulated experience approaches reality" (Meakim et al., 2013, p. S6), follows a continuum beginning with low-fidelity simulation experiences, such as use of role play, or may incorporate a static mannequin that does not respond to intervention. Medium-fidelity simulations build on the degree of realism presented and may involve task trainers or medium-fidelity simulators that provide a degree of feedback to the participant. At the upper range of the continuum lie high-fidelity simulations that provide for more immersive simulation-based learning experiences (SBLEs), using realistic and sophisticated computer technology to enhance the abilities of the patient simulator to provide feedback to learners. Many believe standardized patients (SPs) to be the highest level of fidelity, as humans are trained to portray a patient with specific medical issues. Standardized patients, also known as simulated patients (SiPs), have commonly been used by medical schools but have recently gained traction in nursing education, particularly in graduate programs. There is ongoing discussion about the definitions of these roles, but agreement that this person "takes on the characteristics and persona of another person and portrays that person in a simulation or staged event" (Churchouse & McCafferty, 2012, p. e364). The SP may also be trained to provide feedback to learners from the perspective of the patient. In some cases, hybrid simulations are created in which various levels and types of simulation are combined. While early focus was on the fidelity of the simulator, educators now categorize the fidelity of the physical dimension (including environment and equipment), the psychological dimension (including task and function), and the conceptual dimension (Paige & Morin, 2013).

An example of using different levels of fidelity to achieve various outcomes surrounding the same skill follows. Task trainers or low-fidelity trainers and mannequins allow repeated skill practice, such as catheter insertion. The catheter is inserted and removed according to a defined order of skill demonstration. Higher-fidelity simulations challenge students to reach higher-level objectives by prioritizing care and promoting clinical reasoning and judgment. Students must critically think about why the catheter is important to the patient's care, its correlation to the illness or disease process, and expected outcomes, in addition to planning for additional care and safety needs of the patient as the scenario proceeds. The addition of communication enhances fidelity, as the patient simulator or the patient's family may question the student, asking for an explanation of the procedure. Although the skill of catheterization is the same, it has not occurred in isolation, but in context as a part of the total care of the patient. An overview on background and use of the high-fidelity patient simulator is presented in Chapter 17.

■ Purpose

The purpose of integrating simulation into any curriculum is to provide students with beneficial learning experiences that will assist in meeting course and program objectives while promoting safe patient care. The focus of the SBLE is on the needs of the learner, rather than on the needs of the patient, in contrast to what it must be in the hospital or other clinical environment. However, the overall goal of SBLE is to improve patient outcomes. Carefully chosen SBLEs provide the opportunity for multiple objectives to be met by multiple learners at the same time.

Following the seminal report *To Err Is Human* (Kohn, Corrigan, & Donaldson, 2000), the Institute of Medicine (IOM) identified five core competencies for integrating safety and quality into nursing education, all of which can be addressed in the simulation laboratory. The competencies are (1) provide patient-centered care, (2) work in interdisciplinary teams, (3) employ evidence-based practice, (4) apply quality improvement, and (5) utilize information (Greiner & Kneble, 2003). In 2006, the Quality and Safety Education for Nurses (QSEN) initiative was created based on these five initiatives plus an additional focus on safety, with the goal to decrease preventable patient deaths by improving education (Sherwood & Barnsteiner, 2012). Simulation is one of the methodologies promoted to enhance clinical learning when used in addition to traditional learning experiences (Finkelman & Kenner, 2012). Examples of how the QSEN competencies can be included in SBLE are shown throughout this chapter.

■ Educator Development in Simulation Pedagogy

In the fall of 2014, the National Council of State Boards of Nursing (NCSBN) published the results of a landmark national simulation study (Hayden, Smiley, Alexander, Kardong-Edgren, & Jeffries, 2014). The findings of this study led to the conclusion that up to 50% of traditional clinical hours can be replaced by SBLE in all prelicensure nursing courses if the following conditions are met:

1. "Faculty members are formally trained in simulation pedagogy,
2. An adequate number of faculty members support the student learners,
3. Subject matter experts conduct theory-based debriefing, and
4. Equipment and supplies [are available] to create a realistic environment" (p. S38).

The release of these findings led to a concern that nursing schools may decide to replace their traditional clinical hours without having adequately trained faculty. The NCSBN recommended incorporation of best practices into simulation programs through use of the *Standards of Best Practice: Simulation*^SM (International Nursing Association for Clinical Simulation and Learning [INACSL], 2013).

The INACSL developed its first seven Standards in 2011, made revisions and added Guidelines in 2013, and added two more Standards in 2015. The Standards include:

I. Terminology: defines terms used within the Standards
II. Professional Integrity of Participant: outlines the responsibilities of the learners (e.g., confidentiality, professionalism, respect)

III. Participant Objectives: describes how to develop SBLE around cognitive, psychomotor, and affective objectives

IV. Facilitation Methods: identifies the variety of methods that can be chosen based on learner needs and experience level

V. Simulation Facilitator: describes appropriate ways to guide learners toward meeting learning objectives

VI. The Debriefing Process: identifies the need for a theory-based process to facilitate learning

VII. Participant Assessment and Evaluation: identifies the criteria for using simulation for formative and summative evaluation (INACSL, 2013)

VIII. Simulation-Enhanced Interprofessional Education (Sim-IPE): offers guidelines for collaborative opportunities (Decker et al., 2015)

IX. Scenario Design: outlines what to include in a well-designed scenario (Lioce et al., 2015)

The NCSBN provided further guidance through the release of simulation guidelines for prelicensure nursing programs to use as they prepare and plan for successful use of simulation in their programs (Alexander et al., 2015). These guidelines include the need for administrative commitment, appropriate facilities, educational and technological resources, and qualified faculty and personnel (p. 40). Preparation checklists are provided for faculty and programs to use to determine their level of preparedness.

There are currently no published methods to objectively evaluate simulation facilitator competency. However, a rubric has been created, based on Benner's Novice to Expert theory (Benner, 1984), and has been evaluated by an expert panel of nursing simulationists. Data collection is under way to test the psychometric properties of this tool, which will be made widely available when it is deemed valid and reliable.

The remainder of this chapter outlines the steps involved in creating effective SBLEs, while providing ideas for innovative ways to manage this pedagogy within the guidelines and standards described.

■ Using the Method

Designing the Simulation-Based Learning Experience

Deciding on appropriate SBLEs to integrate into any curriculum takes careful thought and planning. Above all, decisions should be made based on the objectives of the program and the course in which the SBLE is to take place. Major curricular threads also should be considered when selecting SBLEs to include. All clinical courses and many didactic classes, such as pathophysiology, pharmacology, and cultural issues, can incorporate simulation. A review of the program's specific strengths and limitations will assist in choosing SBLEs that will best meet student needs. Concepts that seem hard for students to grasp or that are difficult to teach are excellent choices for SBLEs. Test scores and item analysis, such as from the National Council Licensure Examination–Registered Nurse or Practical Nurse (NCLEX-RN; NCLEX-PN),

Assessment Technologies Institute (ATI), Health Education Systems, Inc. (HESI), or faculty-developed tests for specific courses, give indications of content and concepts that students often do not comprehend well. SBLEs that address these areas should be chosen to facilitate learning in weak areas.

When choosing SBLEs, there are two lines of thought: (1) choose conditions or illnesses that are not readily available in the clinical agencies, so that all students will have the opportunity to care for that type of patient; and (2) choose conditions or illnesses that are most commonly seen in clinical practice, so as to provide the opportunity for repetition that may lead to earlier recognition of deteriorating conditions. SBLEs that prepare students for specific clinical experiences, for high-risk situations, or for complex patients also are excellent choices. The timing of the simulation is yet another important consideration. Didactic material corresponding to the SBLE should have been covered prior to the learning experience so that students have the necessary foundation upon which to base their decision making. Some schools incorporate simulation at the beginning of each course to assist with preparation for entering a new clinical rotation and again at the end of the rotation as a capstone experience. Test scores after simulation may reflect a deeper understanding of the content than before simulation. Each course within a program will have its own needs and objectives that can be addressed through carefully planned SBLEs.

Using standardized templates when designing simulations will help to ensure that all relevant information is included, such as objectives, the patient story, health history, healthcare provider orders, lab results, needed supplies and setup information, method of evaluation, preparation questions and materials for students, and a debriefing plan. Numerous template examples are available online. Another option is to use scenarios outlined in various simulation books and journals or to adopt/adapt scenario packages from simulation vendors.

Scheduling Students in the Simulation Laboratory

Scheduling of the SBLE is often a major hurdle for faculty to overcome. For most educational institutions, class scheduling is part of a complex process that includes many departments, faculty, resources, and buildings. Making even one change can be very disruptive to the system. Therefore, it is important to consider a variety of options when integrating simulation into the curriculum, beginning with a critical look at current teaching methods and clinical experiences. Often health education programs have been challenged to increase enrollment but have limited clinical resources. As a result, experiences that do not provide the best opportunity to meet learning objectives for the student may have been added to the clinical rotation schedule. The site's experiences may be too complex, or too easy, for a given level of learner. Available hours, such as those in the evening or on weekends, may not fit easily into the course schedule. Occasionally, professional behaviors at the clinical site do not mesh with those taught in the nursing program. Faculty are encouraged to critically review all clinical placement sites to determine if needs are being well met in those environments. If not, consideration should be made for moving the experience to the simulation lab.

A question is often raised about the number of clinical hours that can be provided in the simulation lab. While the NCSBN has suggested that up to 50% of clinical time can be replaced with simulation (Hayden, Smiley et al., 2014), the actual number of hours allowed remains dependent upon the regulations of the program's licensing organization in each state. States vary widely on this issue; all allow simulation as a supplement to traditional clinical hours, but fewer allow substitution of simulation for clinical experiences. At least one state does not allow any substitution of simulation for traditional clinical experiences, whereas others allow as much as 50%. Other states leave discretion to the faculty as long as program outcomes continue to be met. A more difficult question is, "How many hours of simulation are needed to replace the same number of clinical hours?" "Does 1 hour of simulation equal 1 hour of clinical?" Some simulation experts believe that, due to the concentrated nature of learning in the simulation lab and the continuous presence of and observation by a faculty facilitator, a ratio such as 1 hour of simulation for 3 hours of clinical could be considered. This question is challenging to answer, and the answer has to be supported by research.

Scheduling simulation throughout the curriculum is best achieved by using a variety of scheduling methods. This allows for increased simulation use with less disruption to the course schedule. Several methods can be utilized: stations in a lab, set blocks of time, postclinical conference, entire day, and class time. It is important to remember that the students will always take longer to make decisions and perform skills than faculty expect, as this is part of their learning process. To decrease frustration and the need for catching up during the day, allow more time than thought necessary to schedule SBLEs.

Stations

Using stations works well for integrating SBLEs into assessment and fundamental skills courses. These courses are often designed so that students work in pairs and small groups to practice psychomotor skills, communication techniques, and critical thinking. Students often rotate through different learning activities during lab time. A short SBLE that allows the students to apply what they have learned within the context of a patient situation can be added. Using this method may result in adding time to the existing lab, but more often, another (perhaps less effective) learning station can be deleted.

Blocks of Time

This method creates a set period of time for self-determined groups or faculty-assigned groups to participate in an SBLE. All blocks of time might be scheduled together during a specific week of the course, or the blocks of time could be distributed throughout the semester until everyone has completed their time. Blocks of time must be long enough and filled with enough activity to make it worth the students' time to come to campus for the experience. For programs with set amounts of student contact hours, some faculty have decreased their time at the traditional clinical site by 10 minutes/week over a 15-week semester, resulting in the ability to reassign that time (150 minutes) to simulation.

Clinical Post Conference

A scheduling method involving a conference at the end of each clinical practice experience can be planned in advance or done impromptu based on activities of the clinical day. Typically, clinical post conferences last approximately 1 hour and occur at the end of the clinical day. They are designed to serve as a time to reflect on the day's activities, but they are often used for various other activities as well, such as topical review of difficult theoretical concepts, as review prior to exams, or even as time to remain on the clinical unit to observe an unusual activity. This time frame is included in the schedule of the clinical day, and some faculty facilitators have found that simulated clinical experiences, designed to include concepts unique to their clinical unit, are a valuable use of this time. For example, a postoperative unit may have several patients with chest tubes, but not every student has the opportunity to care for those patients. Managing a chest-tube patient in the simulation laboratory provides an opportunity for every student to care for that type of patient.

Entire Day

In this scheduling method, a clinical group participates in various SBLEs over an entire day. Rather than going to a hospital unit or clinical agency for a clinical experience, the students report to the simulation laboratory. The simulation laboratory is placed on the clinical schedule rotation instead of an agency site. A typical day's schedule should begin and end at the usual clinical times. Students can provide care for a variety of patient types, depending on the length of the scenarios, or they can provide care to one patient over a simulated period of time, perhaps over days or even months. It is helpful to assign rotating roles to keep students engaged. Expectations for preparation, care, resource use, and documentation should be the same as on the clinical unit.

During Class

Simulations can be conducted during class time by either moving a portable simulator to the classroom, using two-way interactive video (e.g., Skype™) to transmit from the simulation laboratory to the classroom, or incorporating an SP or role-playing experience. Portable simulators are designed for ease of movement and can be placed in the front of the classroom to demonstrate various concepts. Students can be chosen to participate in caring for the simulated patient either randomly, based on skill level, or based on identified learning needs. Students remaining in the audience can participate in directing the care, prioritizing care, or observing for various aspects of care, such as communication techniques. Using video, especially two-way interactive video, provides the same in-class learning advantage without moving the simulator. Another learning opportunity is provided when both an adult and a pediatric simulator are moved into the classroom, setting the stage for comparing and contrasting the care of an adult patient and pediatric patient with the same illness or disease process.

An additional in-class learning opportunity exists through use of the simulation software. The computer running the simulation software can be connected to the classroom LCD projector, allowing all students to see the patient parameters. After orienting students to the various parameters, the faculty member can demonstrate the hemodynamic changes that occur with hypervolemia, hypovolemia, pneumothorax, pericardial tamponade, different cardiac rhythms, and numerous medications. The simulator does not have to be connected to this computer in order to demonstrate these features. Further discussion of classroom use of simulation is provided in the "Implementing the Simulation-Based Learning Experience" section of this chapter.

Fidelity of the Simulated Clinical Experience

Realism of the simulated clinical experience is commonly referred to as *fidelity*. There is no consensus as to how much fidelity is necessary for learning to occur, but historically, many simulationists believed that the closer to reality a scenario was, the more engaged students became and the more opportunities there were for learning to occur. As the concept of fidelity has matured, it has become clearer that the highest level of fidelity is unnecessary for many SBLEs (Paige & Morin, 2013). Cook et al. (2013) found that they were unable to adequately evaluate fidelity as a design feature due to the diversity of meanings and variety of ways in which the term was used in the literature. Another analysis found that in nearly all studies reviewed, there was no significant advantage related to fidelity when evaluating performance outcomes (Norman, Dore, & Grierson, 2012). The literature is now replete with studies of fidelity levels within a variety of courses, with different levels of students, and its impact on characteristics such as anxiety and confidence. Gaba's advice from more than a decade ago (2004) is unchanged: It is important to match the level of fidelity to the desired learning outcomes, as some simulated clinical experiences require higher levels of fidelity than others.

The learning can be positive or negative, and while it is hoped that only positive learning is transferred to real patient care, the potential for negative transfer of learning also exists. Therefore, it is important that processes and procedures in the simulation laboratory mimic reality as closely as possible. For example, it is not appropriate to have students pretend to wash their hands prior to providing care to the simulated patient. Having them pretend repeatedly over time increases the risk of carrying this implanted behavior to the patient care area. As outlined earlier in the chapter, there are a variety of ways to classify fidelity. This section focuses on three common areas where educators can have an impact when designing the SBLE: the patient, holistic aspects of the patient, and the environment.

Physical Patient

Fidelity of the simulated patient's physical condition should involve as many of the student's senses as possible, including sight, smell, touch, and hearing. This involves significant creativity on the part of the faculty member, but can often be accomplished at little cost. Creating this type of fidelity is often referred to as *moulage*. Examples of low-cost solutions to create physical conditions are provided in **Table 18-1**. Always test new moulages in an inconspicuous area if there is a risk that staining could occur.

Table 18-1   Physical Fidelity of the Simulated Patient

Sense	Physical Condition or Disease	Moulage
Sight	Vomit	Egg white whisked with fork; streak with yellow food coloring with toothpick tip
Smell	Blood clots	Thick, lumpy tapioca with red food coloring; partially gelled sugar-free red gelatin
Touch	Incontinence	Water with yellow food coloring and ammonia
	Vomit	Add grated parmesan cheese to vomit
Hearing	Clammy skin	Spray with water bottle
	Hospital sounds	Loop MP3 recording and play back
	Hospital pages	Announce random overhead pages via microphone

Holistic Aspects of the Patient

Nursing care of the patient involves not only physical care, but developmental, cultural, psychosocial, and spiritual care as well. These important aspects are often left out of the SBLE, leading students to report that learning needs related to holistic care were better met in the traditional clinical environment (Leighton, 2014). Simulation does provide an environment where students can learn to identify and address patient concerns outside of the physical realm (Cordeau, 2012).

Positively impacting these learning needs is easy to do in the simulation lab and costs little or no money to do so. In most cases, adding more information to the patient's story or health history can add this dimension. **Table 18-2** outlines several ways in which holistic patient care can be added to the SBLE.

A variety of props can be added to the simulated patient's room to help prompt students to address holistic aspects of care. A picture frame with a family picture including several children might be placed at the bedside to see if students address the patient's role in the family. A Bible, Koran, or other religious book or icon can be placed at the bedside to shift the focus to spiritual aspects of care. It is helpful to have resources available to students so they can look up information about different cultural and religious beliefs while caring for the simulated patient.

Environment

Simulation centers or laboratories come in all shapes and sizes, from the corner of a skills lab to a large, free-standing space with individual patient rooms. Whatever the space, it is important to make that space appear as realistic as possible to the intended clinical environment. While this is typically a patient's hospital room, many SBLEs can occur in other settings, such as a patient's home, an outpatient setting, or in the recovery room. Having the equipment and props characteristic of the desired environment will help learners to be engaged and learn the use of appropriate equipment and supplies.

Obtaining supplies and equipment can be a costly endeavor. Consider discussing simulation needs with clinical nurse managers who may be able to divert opened

Table 18-2   Holistic Care of the Simulated Patient

Aspect	Patient	Concern
Developmental	45-year-old male with heart attack	He and wife have five children, and he is unable to return to construction job.
	14-year-old with abdominal pain	Patient is sexually active and has contracted a sexually transmitted disease.
Cultural	26-year-old female speaks only Vietnamese	The only available person who knows Vietnamese is the hospital's maintenance man.
	88-year-old Native American patient urgently needs medication	The patient prefers to wait for a tribal medicine elder.
Psychosocial	8-year-old boy requires appendectomy	Parents recently moved to the area and the family's health insurance has not yet taken effect.
	72-year-old patient with COPD requires several medications	The patient is unable to afford medications with current finances.
Spiritual	52-year-old female requires abdominal surgery	The patient refuses to remove jewelry with religious icons.
	66-year-old patient who was just diagnosed with cancer	The patient refuses treatment because he believes the illness is a result of past sins.

sterile kits to the simulation laboratory if they cannot be used with human patients. Many hospitals have warehouses where unused or overstocked equipment is stored. Simulation laboratories are often able to purchase at a discount or borrow equipment. Many pharmacies now return expired medications for account credit; however, simulation personnel may be able to obtain these medication vials or ampoules. Great care must be taken to dispose of real medications according to policy and to note that the fluid in the vials must not be used for real patients. Different regions of the country have differing rules and regulations as to disposal of expired items. Some simulation laboratories have reported obtaining syringes and expired intravenous fluids from veterinarians and from patients who no longer require home-care services. Be creative in seeking out solutions to supply and equipment needs. Depending on the location of the simulation lab, it may be necessary to provide clear signage stating that all equipment and supplies are not to be used for real patients, and access to those outside the employ of the lab should be limited and monitored.

Student Preparation/Professional Expectations

It is recommended that students prepare for SBLE in the same manner and to the same degree as they do for traditional clinical experiences. Providing the students with focused preparation activities is more efficient than the time spent seeking out information from the chart, the patient, the family, and other caregivers, as is often the case when preparing to care for human patients. Preparation activities contribute to learning and allow the simulation facilitator to answer questions, clarify misconceptions, enhance the knowledge base, and facilitate learning rather than teach. Time in the simulation lab is therefore likely to be focused and intense.

Professional behavior and dress are important to the learning experience in the simulation laboratory. In fact, observations have been made that students behave more professionally when in uniform than when in street clothes (Ravert, 2010). While learning to manage a variety of patient types and conditions, students are also learning professional behaviors and communication techniques. Providing an environment in which professional behaviors are modeled and practiced may enhance professionalism. As simulation activities continue to replace traditional clinical teaching methods, efforts should be made to ensure that the experiences in the simulation laboratory are as realistic as possible.

Prebriefing

Facilitators are encouraged to conduct a prebriefing to begin the SBLE. During this time, assigned preparatory work may be reviewed and questions answered. Misconceptions are clarified, and facilitators determine whether students are prepared to provide care to the simulated patient. If not prepared, a student might be dismissed from the lab experience to return at another scheduled time when he or she has prepared better. After preparation is evaluated, the students will be given report on their patient, and they may be asked to determine which types of care are needed and how that care will be prioritized. This ensures that students know where to begin upon entering the patient's room. Roles may be predetermined, and facilitators should ensure that the students are oriented to the simulator, environment, and expectations.

■ Implementing the Simulation-Based Learning Experience

Faculty Roles

Faculty roles during simulation are primarily facilitative. Although the role varies somewhat depending on the level of the students, the faculty may choose to provide the learners with prompts and cues. These are most often in the form of carefully crafted questions that stimulate critical thinking and problem solving and assist the students in taking necessary actions with appropriate interventions. As students progress through the program, fewer prompts and cues are required or are given. One way to manage cues is to stay in character and voice cues and questions via the patient's voice. For example, the simulated patient could ask, "Are there any side effects I should watch for?" when receiving a medication; or "I've heard I can get AIDS from a blood transfusion," requiring students to provide explanations. The facilitator can then evaluate the students' knowledge based on their responses.

In the absence of EHRs, critical thinking, problem solving, and planning care are aided in simulation when a large flip chart or whiteboard is utilized. One person is assigned to be the documenter/recorder for the simulation. Beginning with report, the documenter writes down pertinent information and continues to record as assessments, new data, and interventions occur. The information can then be easily viewed by all participants and is constantly referred to. This documentation can be utilized as the student calls the healthcare provider, as the patient (facilitator) asks questions about the meaning of newly acquired lab data, or as students plan care based on new orders. If a flip chart is used, the paper can easily be removed and taken to debriefing for further evaluation and discussion of care. This method is also useful for concept mapping or nursing process development. The use of the EHR is further discussed later in the "Charting" section of this chapter.

The Dreyfus and Dreyfus model of skill acquisition (1980), adapted for use in nursing by Benner (1984), supports learning on a continuum beginning with novice and progressing through the advanced beginner, competent, proficient, and expert stages. This model has implications for faculty who facilitate sessions in the simulation laboratory. Learning the skill of facilitation is a new challenge for most faculty, and they begin at a novice level. It is important for faculty to recognize this and to not attempt an SBLE that is overly complex and detailed for their first effort. They should begin with simple scenarios, as these simulations can often have as much impact as those that are complex. As the level of comfort with facilitation grows, so will creativity and willingness to attempt more complex scenarios. Trying to do too much at the beginning will only frustrate the facilitator and the students, making the next attempt at simulation more of a challenge.

The novice-to-expert approach has also been used to help determine the role of facilitators when interacting with students in the simulation laboratory. The current trend is for the facilitator to observe the scenario from a separate control room, as it is believed that students can then perform autonomously and without interference. However, other options have also proven successful, and offer options for labs that do not have a separate control space. In addition, the level of the learner should be considered. Novice students may experience increased stress or anxiety when placed in an unfamiliar environment and given new expectations to care for a simulated patient. They have little to no experience to draw from, and it may be of value for the faculty to be present at the bedside, to assist in proper assessment techniques and respond to questions immediately.

As the students progress to advanced beginner, the facilitator can play the role of a family member. Continued presence in the room provides a level of comfort and reportedly decreases anxiety among students. The facilitator asks questions of students while in the family member role and is able to determine if students understand the care that they are providing and can provide appropriate education and responses to the patient and family.

When learners reach the proficient stage, the facilitator becomes further removed, although (depending on the laboratory setup) he or she might remain in the room with the students. However, at this point, the facilitator only observes unless it is essential to intervene and redirect the students. While some educators advocate for students to experience the results of their indecision or incorrect decisions, this must be weighed in light of whether the learning objectives will be met satisfactorily. At the expert stage, the facilitator is completely removed from the simulated patient room, when possible, and observes through a one-way window or via audiovisual technology.

Student Roles

One of the biggest challenges facing faculty in the simulation laboratory is that of group size. Defining roles for each individual student brings focus to the experience and decreases confusion. A variety of roles can be utilized, depending on the SBLE objectives. Roles can be chosen at random or purposefully assigned based on identified student weaknesses. Suggestions of roles and responsibilities utilized by many simulation laboratories are provided in **Table 18-3**.

Facilitators are encouraged to utilize roles that are nurse-specific, as outlined in Table 18-3. Assigning roles of other healthcare providers, such as laboratory technician, respiratory therapist, or physician, is often troublesome, as the students do not have the background to know the roles of those providers. It is also challenging to have students play the role of the family member, again because most lack that type of experience, but also because they have to perform in front of their peers. Those who are shy or introverted tend to struggle in these types of roles, whereas extroverts often go off script or may break out in laughter at inappropriate times.

Facilitators often express concern that the students in the observation role will not learn as much as those actively caring for the simulated patient. In Phase III of the NLN/Laerdal project *Designing and Implementing Models for the Innovative Use of Simulation to Teach Nursing Care of Ill Adults and Children: A National, Multi-Site, Multi-Method Study*, researchers reported that there were no significant differences in knowledge gain, satisfaction, or self-confidence based on the role of the student (Jeffries & Rizzolo, 2006). However, students prefer to have an active role in a primary position, rather than observe or have a supporting role (Harder, Ross, & Paul, 2013).

Table 18-3   Roles for Students in the Simulation Laboratory

Role	Responsibilities
Primary nurse	• Assessment: final decision
	• Consider two primary nurses so one student is not responsible alone if a poor outcome is experienced
Secondary nurse	• Backs up primary nurse if two-primary-nurse system not used
	• Assists the primary nurse in assessment and decision making
Medication nurse	• Administers medications safely according to orders
Documentation nurse	• Documents on paper or electronically to maintain a patient record
	• Documents on flip chart or whiteboard to keep all informed of assessment findings and care provided
Healthcare communicator	• Provides information to healthcare provider in person or via phone calls; contacts ancillary departments for test results
Observer	• Provide a focused role for the observer, such as observing for communication between nurse and patient, identification of cultural care, patient education provided by nurse, recognition of psychosocial care, overall management of care

Use of Resources in the Simulation Lab

Mobile devices, such as phones with Internet service, and electronic tablets and notebooks are being incorporated into simulation experiences. During the SBLE, students can immediately access textbook information and can look up diseases, care plans, drug and laboratory guides, medical dictionaries, procedural guidelines, and literature databases. It is important in today's constantly changing healthcare environment that students learn where to access needed information rather than expecting to always rely on memory. Point-of-care access is vital so that nurses can rely on the latest evidence-based information to make decisions. These tools are invaluable as students move from performing skills to making decisions about care based on the latest knowledge available. Clinical calculators are also utilized in simulation laboratories to more safely determine drug dosing and intravenous drip rates, and for other physiological calculations.

The Joint Commission (TJC) identified communication breakdown as one of the top three leading root causes of sentinel events in the United States between 2013 and the second quarter of 2015. Between 2004 and the second quarter of 2015, communication was among the top five causes in every category of sentinel event types that resulted in death or permanent injury (TJC, 2015). These sentinel events resulted in unintended harm to patients and prompted recommendations for standardized handoff communications. The mnemonic SBAR (Situation-Background-Assessment-Recommendation) is used by hospitals across the country to improve communication. During the SBLE, students can get valuable practice in communication skills by giving handoff reports, by calling healthcare providers, and by interacting with the interdisciplinary team utilizing the SBAR format. Use of the format assists students in becoming more organized and confident in their thinking and reporting.

Charting

Types of documentation can range from paper charting, using blank forms obtained from a local facility or creating one's own, to electronic charting comparable to a full hospital-grade EHR. The level of complexity in the design of these documentation systems is up to the faculty. Some faculty create realistic systems using Microsoft Office™ products such as Word and Excel. There is no known research indicating whether one method is better than another. The underlying principles and concepts of documentation are the important focus.

Charts and forms for all aspects of patient care should be constructed for each SBLE. Additional forms that might be appropriate for the SBLE, such as emergency department records, blood transfusion and blood bank forms, and incident reports, for example, should also be available. Documentation forms should be as similar as possible to those the students utilize in their clinical areas. Unfortunately, a large variety of documentation systems exist, and many students have to learn a different system at each clinical site.

Various methods are utilized in simulation laboratories to create documentation opportunities for students. While it is helpful to utilize a system as close to what students see on the traditional clinical unit as possible, many simulation laboratories do not have the resources to do this. Several existing commercial products are available, but many simulation facilitators create their own system.

Multidisciplinary/Interdisciplinary Team Simulations

As a result of the prominence of the QSEN competencies mentioned earlier in the chapter, nursing faculty are collaborating with other healthcare specialties to incorporate SBLEs that foster an interdisciplinary team approach with other healthcare students. The Institute of Medicine has said that "all health professionals should be educated to deliver patient-centered care as a member of an interdisciplinary team, emphasizing evidence-based practice, quality improvement approaches, and informatics" (IOM, 2003, p. 3). As the population ages and lives with multiple comorbidities and chronic health needs, the care for that population requires the collaboration of multiple healthcare professionals. Therefore, simulation provides the perfect opportunity for students to work together on complex patient care problems. Pharmacy, respiratory therapy, social work, seminary, and medical practitioners or students have all collaborated with nursing students during SBLEs. Students learn the knowledge, roles, responsibilities, and frame of reference that each person brings to the patient situation. They learn to work together as a team, to share the information they have about the patient, and to communicate and resolve differences related to care.

Many hospitals and schools of nursing are utilizing the TeamSTEPPS program developed by the Department of Defense's Patient Safety Program in collaboration with the Agency for Healthcare Research and Quality (AHRQ). This program provides materials and a training curriculum for an evidence-based teamwork system to improve communication and teamwork skills. Information about this program can be obtained at http://teamstepps.ahrq.gov/. The goal of TeamSTEPPS and all interdisciplinary training is to assist in providing higher-quality, safer patient care through more effective communication among health professionals.

Classroom Use of Simulation

Most faculty think of a laboratory space when envisioning the use of human patient simulation in their courses; however, simulation can be added to the classroom experience as well. Three common methods of integrating simulation into classroom teaching follow.

Simulator in Classroom

Many patient simulators are portable and can be moved easily into a classroom. Although this may seem overwhelming the first one or two times, it is not difficult to learn with repetition and can be accomplished in only a few minutes. Once the simulator is in the classroom, the instructor can place it at the front of the class and, at the desired time, invite two or three students to care for the patient, who should be designed to facilitate learning of concepts currently being taught. Students often hesitate to volunteer for this role and may have to be assigned.

The simulated patient's condition or illness may be cared for to resolution during one time frame of the class, or the care can be divided into sections corresponding to the didactic material as it is presented. Another option is to simulate two different but similar conditions, such as heart failure and COPD. Selected students care for each patient, and the subsequent patient management is subjected to contrast and comparison analysis.

Simulation via Two-Way Interactive Video

Some simulators and their environs are not designed for easy transport and are difficult to remove from the laboratory. In such instances, simulation via two-way interactive video can be used. The simulated patient remains in the laboratory and the designated number of students leave the classroom to care for the patient there. This interaction is broadcast to the classroom using existing interactive video capabilities. Many schools do not have the resources for this type of equipment, but many free or low-cost options are now available via the Internet. One effective method is to place a laptop on a bedside table, or similar surface, at the foot of the bed. If there is not a built-in camera, an inexpensive webcam can be attached. From the laptop, a Skype call can be placed for free to the larger classroom and the simulation can be broadcast via an existing liquid crystal display (LCD) projector. Placing the phone on speaker mode and augmenting with a portable microphone allows the class members to communicate with each other.

Simulation Software

The laptop that runs the simulation software can be connected to an overhead LCD projector in the classroom in the same manner that a computer is connected to project PowerPoint presentations. Once the laptop is connected, the students are oriented to the instructor view and instructed on which visible parameters to monitor. Simple to complex material can be visually presented using the following examples:

- Administer the same medication and dose to a young, healthy simulated patient and to a simulated patient with cardiovascular disease. Observe changes in blood pressure and heart rate (novice students) or mean arterial pressure and central venous pressure (advanced students).
- Provoke a pneumothorax through the software and have learners monitor the respiratory rate and oxygen saturation levels for changes.
- Create a pericardial tamponade through the software and have learners monitor hemodynamic changes with various amounts of fluid.
- Remove 2–3 liters of blood through the software and have students monitor hemodynamic changes. Conversely, administer 2–3 liters of crystalloids and monitor the same hemodynamics.

After the Simulated-Based Learning Experience

Debriefing

Debriefing is essential to the simulation experience. It is during this time, when students have the opportunity to reflect on the experience, that much of the learning occurs. Faculty function as facilitators in the debriefing by stimulating students to consider what they were thinking during the simulation, how they were feeling, what they did, what occurred as a result, and how they can apply what they have learned to their care of real patients. It is important for students to be able to follow the fast-paced simulation with a quiet time away from the simulator where they can cognitively process and reflect on what occurred (Groom, Henderson, & Sittner, 2013).

Several different methods are popular with those facilitating simulation. Plus/delta places actions into a positive column and a column designated for actions or activities that could be done differently. Another method is advocacy/inquiry, which uses comments such as, "I saw you do _____ assessment and wondered what other assessments might provide more information," to provoke further discussion. Debriefing models with varying levels of complexity and overlap have been developed in recent years, including Debriefing for Meaningful Learning©, Promoting Excellence and Reflective Learning in Simulation (PEARLS), Debriefing with Good Judgment, the 3D (Defusing, Discovering, and Deepening) Debriefing Model, the Gather-Analyze-Summarize (GAS) Method, and the Outcome Present State-Test (OPT) Model. Though each model has its own specific components, the overall goals of debriefing are the same: to understand, analyze, and synthesize thoughts, feelings, and actions; ensure that the experience is interpreted correctly by all participants regardless of their role; ensure that learning objectives are met; link classroom content to clinical practice; and positively change behaviors or practice.

The facilitator has many responsibilities for guiding the debriefing, beginning with a review of the expectations—including respectful communication without distractions such as cell phones. A trusting environment should be established to promote confidentiality and freedom to become engaged. The facilitator should keep a learner-centered focus based on the learners' level of engagement by maintaining eye contact and practicing active listening. Using open-ended questions with a Socratic style in conjunction with advocacy/inquiry technique is a common way to help learners reflect on the experience and what has been learned. Audiovisual records of the experience may be judiciously used for deeper analysis. It is the facilitator's responsibility to provide constructive feedback, ensure that the learning objectives are met, and help the learners identify how to take what has been learned and apply it to their clinical practice (Dreifuerst & Decker, 2012).

Debriefing should be conducted immediately following the SBLE to capture the initial reactions of the learners; however, debriefing may also occur during the scenario if needed. If a critical error has occurred, an important teaching moment arises, or the students have gone down a path that will never meet the learning objectives, then it would be appropriate to pause the SBLE to debrief what is happening, and then resume the scenario. In general, following the scenario, debriefing should take place away from the bedside in order to separate the actions of patient care from the reflective activity of debriefing. There has also been considerable discussion about how long debriefing should last, but there are no research-based decisions. The length of debriefing is dependent upon the objectives, the level of the learners, and the actions or decisions that occurred during the SBLE (Dreifuerst & Decker, 2012). As with the scenario itself, educators should err on the side of planning for more time than believed necessary.

After a Simulated Patient Death

A special circumstance exists when the SBLE involves the death of the simulated patient. There continues to be controversy surrounding simulation of death, especially when it is not tied to the learning objectives of the SBLE. Many simulation facilitators are fearful that simulated death experiences will cause the students to believe they killed the simulated patient or are responsible for its death, leading to feelings of guilt. There is also concern that buried feelings may rise to the surface, leading to psychological trauma. The facilitator is charged with recognizing and managing psychological stress of participants (Leighton, 2009a).

Recommendations for managing simulated death have been developed: they include the need to assess the comfort level of the facilitator when dealing with death, provide adequate prebriefing, save simulator death for more advanced learners, prohibit punitive use of simulator death, balance emotions, provide careful debriefing, and assure psychological safety (Corvetto & Taekman, 2013). The debriefing process is vital to managing the psychological stress, as students are given the opportunity to talk about their feelings and explore the events that occurred during the SBLE in a safe, nonjudgmental environment. The facilitator may consider involving a chaplain or mental health practitioner in the scenario or during the debriefing. In some cases, the facilitator may need to refer the student for further psychological assistance (Leighton, 2009a). Anecdotally, many students have reported that experiencing death in the simulation lab helped them to better understand previous real-life experiences.

■ Evaluation/Assessment

Over the past several years, the number of valid and reliable tools available for use in SBLE has grown dramatically. Adamson, Kardong-Edgren, and Wilhaus (2012) provided an updated list of these tools, but numerous additional psychometrically sound options have been published since then. For this section, the terms *assessment* and *evaluation* are used interchangeably. Four areas of SBLE should be assessed: the experience, the participants, the curriculum, and the facilitator. (The lack of a valid, reliable tool to evaluate facilitators was discussed earlier in the chapter.)

Evaluating the Experience

Despite an educator's best efforts, it is possible to create SBLEs that do not meet the learning needs of the students; therefore, it is vital to evaluate the effectiveness of the experience. An early tool developed by the National League for Nursing, the Simulation Design Scale, assesses the students' perception of the objectives, fidelity, problem solving, student support, and debriefing constructs (Franklin, Burns, & Lee, 2014). There are two tools that specifically address the debriefing construct of the SBLE. The Debriefing Experience Scale (Reed, 2012) consists of 20 items within four subscales: analyzing thoughts and feelings, learning and making connections, facilitator skill in conducting the debriefing, and appropriate facilitator guidance. The Debriefing Assessment for Simulation in Healthcare (DASH) tool (Brett-Fleegler et al., 2012) considers six elements related to the behaviors of the facilitator. These tools can be completed by students to provide valuable feedback to faculty about their debriefing skills. A tool that evaluates the SBLE from prebriefing through the scenario and debriefing is the Simulation Effectiveness Tool-Modified (SET-M). This tool is an update of the SET that was developed in 2005 (Elfrink Cordi, Leighton, Ryan-Wenger, Doyle, & Ravert, 2012) and evaluates items on four subscales: Prebriefing, Confidence, Learning, and Debriefing (Leighton, Ravert, Mudra, & Macintosh, 2015). Students should complete evaluations of the SBLE at the end of the experience. These evaluations can provide valuable information about what was most helpful to the students and what might be changed to make the SBLE an even better learning experience.

Evaluating the Participants

It is important to measure outcomes following SBLE. Knowledge gains are often evaluated through the use of pretests and posttests, while checklists are used by observers to evaluate completion of skills; however, these are rarely evaluated for reliability and validity prior to use. Several psychometrically sound tools are available now for use in evaluating different outcomes of SBLE. The Creighton Competency Evaluation Instrument (CCEI) was developed as an evaluation instrument for use in both traditional and simulated clinical environments. It includes four categories—assessment, communication, clinical judgment, and patient safety—along with items designed to rate student performance (Hayden, Keegan, Kardong-Edgren, & Smiley, 2014). The Simulation Thinking Rubric (Doolen, 2015) and Lasater Clinical Judgment Rubric (Adamson, Gubrud-Howe, Sideras, & Lasater, 2011) can be used to evaluate higher-order thinking following establishment of evaluator interrater reliability. The Spielberger's State-Trait Anxiety Inventory (STAI) (Spielberger, 1985) is also commonly used to evaluate anxiety levels of learners under different conditions. Surveys used for the purpose of establishing student satisfaction with simulation as a teaching strategy provide results that can be used internally to garner support for simulation; however, studies related to satisfaction have saturated the literature.

Simulation as a Part of the Curriculum

The Clinical Learning Environment Comparison Survey (CLECS) (Leighton, 2015) was created to compare how well undergraduate nursing students believed their learning needs were met in the traditional and simulation learning environments. This tool was developed to help clarify the similarities and differences between the two environments and was used in the NCSBN simulation study. This valid and reliable tool has six subscales: nursing process, teaching-learning dyad, communication, self-efficacy, holism, and critical thinking. This tool can be used at the end of the semester for course evaluation, or at program end to provide valuable information about how well learning needs were met in the traditional and simulation learning environments throughout the students' course of study. The tool can also be used as part of a comprehensive evaluation of simulation lab faculty and staff, as well as to evaluate individual SBLEs.

High-Stakes Testing

The use of high-stakes testing with simulation for nursing has been under a microscope for several years. A roundtable discussion held at the 2009 International Nursing Association for Clinical Simulation and Learning conference led to general agreement that while a worthy goal, nursing education was not yet ready for high-stakes testing, due to a variety of reasons, including the fact that not all nursing programs are teaching with simulation (due to budgetary reasons). Another concern of significant proportions was the lack of consistent methods of facilitation and use of standardized scenarios (Kardong-Edgren, Hanberg, Keenan, Ackerman, & Chambers, 2011). *High-stakes evaluation* was defined as a process "that has major academic, education, or employment consequence" (Meakim et al., 2013, p. S7).

The National League for Nursing (NLN) undertook a 3-year multi-site project to investigate the use of simulation for high-stakes evaluation (Schultz, 2010). Experts worked to develop scenarios that were appropriate for this type of evaluation, while noting that facilitator differences can still alter outcomes (Willhaus, Burleson, Palaganas, & Jeffries, 2014).

In 2014, a second town hall meeting was held at that year's INACSL conference to revisit this topic. In a poll of the audience prior to discussion, approximately 50% of attendees responded in favor of high-stakes testing. This was followed by a robust discussion among the membership about concerns, as well as favorable opinions, related to this type of evaluation. Following this dialogue, a follow-up poll indicated that favor toward high-stakes testing had dropped 20%, indicating a distinct need for work to continue in this area before sweeping changes are made (Rutherford-Hemming, Kardong-Edgren, Gore, Ravert, & Rizzolo, 2014).

On a campus level, it is imperative that nursing programs identify their philosophy related to evaluation or assessment in the simulation laboratory. To begin, definitions must be determined. During meeting discussions, participants use a variety of different terminology to describe evaluation, assessment, and testing. It is clear that many of these conversations are attempting to compare apples to oranges.

Questions that should be considered during discussions about evaluation, testing, and assessment could include:

- "Is the simulation lab better suited for facilitating learning or for evaluating students? Is it possible to do both?
- Is it fair to test students if they have not had significant exposure to SBLE?
- Are faculty all competent in their roles? How is this variable controlled for evaluation purposes?
- How do we account for the variety of student responses and interventions that are inherent in simulations?
- Are we sending mixed messages when we tell students that simulation is a safe environment to learn in and then use that same environment for evaluation?
- Do we test students in the traditional clinical environment? Is it then fair to test in the simulation lab?
- If the focus is on testing, will the experience become an experience about performing rather than about learning?

- What can you learn about your students in the simulation environment without formal evaluation or testing?
- If we say that most of the learning occurs in debriefing, can we fairly evaluate students before that debriefing occurs?" (Leighton, 2009b, p. e57).[1]

■ Research and Advancement Opportunities

It should be clear to the reader of this chapter that a wide variety of research opportunities exist for the users of simulation. Outcomes-based simulation research has grown exponentially as facilitators have become more sophisticated in their understanding of this pedagogy.

Conducting research in the simulation laboratory has several advantages over research in the traditional clinical environment—first and foremost, there is no risk to patients. Facilitators are also able to control the scenario, patient responses, communication with healthcare providers, and equipment made available. However, those same faculty are also difficult to control as a variable. Faculty have different levels of education for their role of facilitator, respond in different ways to students' efforts to communicate, and often need to step outside of the planned script to respond to unpredictable student actions (Alinier, 2008). The lack of standardization for educating faculty to the facilitator role continues, as a variety of mechanisms for education are used: train-the-trainer sessions, attending webinars, reading books and journals, using resources on websites, and attending conferences, to name but a few (Nehring, Wexler, Hughes, & Greenwell, 2013). Coupled with the current lack of tools to evaluate facilitator competency, this variability creates many challenges for researchers.

It is a responsibility of each of us as simulation facilitators and proponents to help move the field forward through well-designed research studies and documentation of best practices and standards of excellence. It is no longer enough to document that students like simulation or that they prefer this method to another. The time has come to document that learning occurs and study the transferability of that learning to traditional patient care. As the competition for clinical sites continues to increase, simulation will take a vital role in the future of nursing education. The INACSL has outlined the following priorities for research in 2016:

- Translational research
- Evaluation methods
- Validity and reliability of instruments
- Ratio of clinical time to simulation time
- Prebriefing and briefing
- Use of theory in simulation
- Measurement of higher-order thinking (e.g., clinical reasoning)
- Faculty development
- Facilitator competence
- Communication

---

[1] Reproduced from Leighton, K. (2009). What can we learn from a LISTSERV? *Clinical Simulation in Nursing*, 5(2), e57–e58. Copyright (2009b), with permission from Elsevier

Two international simulation organizations have taken the lead on furthering the competency of faculty and the overall management of simulation programs: INACSL and the Society for Simulation in Healthcare (SSH). Both organizations include members of all types of healthcare educators, although the INACSL has a narrower focus to nursing in general. The two organizations affiliate with each other, and members can avail themselves of numerous benefits, including ongoing education, annual conferences, and academic journals.

The Society for Simulation in Healthcare has created a certification program for simulation educators that now includes an advanced level. In addition, SSH has developed an accreditation program for simulation centers and laboratories. Following a self-study and site visit, centers around the world have been accredited.

The Association of Standardized Patient Educators (ASPE) provides support and education for those who work with this type of simulation. Numerous other simulation organizations exist around the world and for specific audiences, such as the International Pediatric Simulation Society. In addition to the resources offered by these organizations, the National League for Nursing hosts the Simulation Innovation Resource Center (SIRC), an online repository of course offerings, forums, and databases with information to support simulationists.

■ Conclusion

This chapter has provided information intended to help those who take on the challenge of facilitating learning in the simulation laboratory. While many nursing programs have managed to obtain funding for simulation equipment, there continues to be little forethought given to how faculty will manage to learn this type of teaching strategy and where the time will come from for that purpose. This chapter was intended to aid the process of faculty development by providing realistic ideas that can be easily implemented by facilitators of learning in simulation laboratories. The simulator and its features have little value if faculty do not know how to effectively teach with the technology.

Teaching Example

Strategy

The strategy involves the incorporation of fidelity, role of faculty, and holistic aspects of patient care for a beginning assessment course using an SBLE. Participants in the simulation laboratory include the course faculty member and up to eight students.

Expectations

The students are expected to obtain subjective and objective assessment data and inform the healthcare provider of their findings. Prerequisite knowledge should include anatomy and physiology of the cardiovascular system and corresponding assessment techniques. The example involves a young, morbidly obese female patient whose symptoms are precipitated by a systolic heart murmur. Guidelines for the instructor follow.

Setting

Place the simulator on a bed or stretcher and inform students the "patient" has not been seen by a healthcare provider. Place two individual breast models (often used to teach palpation for lumps) on the chest of the simulator. The patient's obesity can be simulated by placing a pillow over the abdomen and securing it with an elastic wrap or gauze roll. Put female clothes appropriate for the weather on the simulator (to make it easier to dress the simulator, cut the shirt up the back, leaving the collar intact; cut the pants along the back to the inseam) and add a woman's wig to the head. Makeup can be applied to the simulator after it is tested in a nonvisible place for staining. Personal effects such as a magazine, cell phone, and purse can be placed on the bedside table next to a bottle of sugary carbonated beverage.

Simulator Settings

Set systolic murmur (or other preferred abnormal heart sound). All other settings are normal.

Faculty Role

If this is the first SBLE for students, they are at a novice level and will need faculty assistance. Orient students to the simulator and its applicable features prior to starting the scenario. Only tell students what they need to know to care for this patient, as providing information on IV sites, defibrillation, or monitoring is above their knowledge level and will be extraneous information.

Begin outside of the simulator's room and brief students on the patient who has just arrived at the healthcare provider's office. Report is as follows: "This is a 38-year-old female with complaints of fatigue, orthopnea, and palpitations. She is 5 feet, 2 inches tall and weighs 100 kilograms."

Student Expectations

- Knock on the door and announce entry
- Introduce self and role to patient
- Wash hands
- Ask subjective questions to obtain more information from the patient, such as the following (with answers in parentheses):
  - How long ago did your symptoms start? (6 months ago; gradually worsening)
  - Any associated symptoms? (no shortness of breath or chest pain)
  - What makes the symptoms worse? (walking and exercise)
  - What makes the symptoms go away? (rest)
  - How many pillows do you use at night? (three)
  - Do you have any history of medical problems? (no)
  - Do you have any family history of medical problems? (no cardiac disease)
  - Do you smoke, drink alcohol, or use drugs not prescribed for you? (no)
  - How much do you exercise in a week? (none)
  - Has there been any change in your weight recently? (gained 40 pounds past 4 months)
  - What is your typical diet? (fast food, soda)
  - Do you take any medications? (ibuprofen as needed for back pain)
  - When was the last time you saw a healthcare provider? (2 years prior for PAP smear)

Questioning may continue until the facilitator believes that enough data have been collected. The facilitator then prompts the beginning of the physical assessment.

Student Expectations

- Wash hands upon entering the room
- Explain what will be done to patient
- Conduct general survey
- Provide for privacy

(continues)

- Complete head-to-toe physical assessment with emphasis on cardiovascular system
- Wash hands after assessment of the patient is complete
- Make sure personal items are in reach
- Ensure safe environment

During the physical assessment, the students will discover an abnormality in the heart sounds. Although it may be beyond their scope to recognize and define a heart murmur, they should be able to identify that an abnormality exists. All other findings, including vital signs, are normal.

Holistic Aspects (one or more may be included)

- *Psychosocial.* Patient does not have health insurance and voices concern about how to pay for office visit, follow-up tests, or prescriptions.
- *Spiritual.* Patient may be anxious and ask student to pray with her.
- *Cultural.* Patient may be from a culture other than that of most of the students.
- *Developmental.* Patient may blame weight gain on a recent life experience, such as a divorce.

Anticipated and Unanticipated Events and Consequences

Nervousness

As this is often the first SBLE for the students, they are prone to nervousness and have trouble getting started. The facilitator may need to ask each student to pose a subjective question to the patient. The person responding as the patient should allow time for questions to be formulated, not rushing the students.

Scattered Thought Processes

Novice students tend to randomly ask subjective questions without organization. Following subjective questioning, the facilitator can help them to prioritize their completed assessment questions and findings.

Incorrect Assessment Techniques

The facilitator is at the bedside with this novice group and can correct technique as problems occur. Unless the SBLE is recorded, learners at this level may not recall what they did right or wrong by the time debriefing occurs.

Failure to Recognize Abnormality

The novice student may fail to recognize an abnormality due to lack of experience to draw upon. If this is the case, the facilitator should point it out and have all students listen to the heart sounds. The respiratory rate may be lowered on the simulator and the heart sound volume increased to facilitate hearing of abnormal heart sounds.

Evaluation of Learner Attainment

The intent of this SBLE is to provide an introductory-level experience for the student who has not yet interacted with a real patient and is just beginning to learn physical assessment techniques and concepts. The facilitator will often be surprised by the learner's inability to formulate subjective questions and conduct a basic physical assessment. Remembering that novice learners have no experiences to draw upon will keep expectations in perspective. Learners should be able to demonstrate physical assessment techniques learned in class; however, they often need help in refining their technique and need reassurance that they are doing the assessment correctly.

Discussion Questions

1. You are responsible for ensuring that faculty who will be facilitating learning in the simulation lab are qualified. What faculty development opportunities will you consider providing so as to meet the conditions set by the National Council of State Boards of Nursing guidelines?
2. When designing a simulation-based learning experience, what resources are available to help you determine what the focus of the experience should be?
3. You have been asked to address the faculty at the monthly faculty senate meeting. The purpose is to try to gain support for integration of simulation throughout the curriculum. What information will you convey in the 5 minutes you have been given?

References

Adamson, K., Gubrud-Howe, P., Sideras, S., & Lasater, K. (2011). Assessing the reliability, validity, and use of the Lasater Clinical Judgment Rubric: Three approaches. *Journal of Nursing Education, 51*(2), 66–73. doi:10.3928/01484834-20111130-03

Adamson, K., Kardong-Edgren, S., & Willhaus, J. (2012). An updated review of published simulation evaluation instruments. *Clinical Simulation in Nursing, 9*(9), e393–e400. doi:10.1016/j.ecns.2012.09.004

Alexander, M. A., Durham, C. F., Hooper, J. I., Jeffries, P. R., Goldman, N., Kardong-Edgren, S., Tillman, C. (2015). NCSBN simulation guidelines for prelicensure nursing programs. *Journal of Nursing Regulation, 6*(5), 39–42.

Alinier, G. (2008). Pitfalls to avoid in designing and executing research with clinical simulation. In R. R. Kyle, Jr., & W. B. Murray (Eds.), *Clinical simulation: Operations, engineering and management* (pp. 515–516). New York, NY: Elsevier.

Benner, P. (1984). *From novice to expert: Excellence and power in clinical nursing practice.* Menlo Park, CA: Addison-Wesley.

Brett-Fleegler, M., Rudolph, J., Eppich, W., Manuteaux, M., Fleegler, E., Cheng, A., & Simon, R. (2012). Debriefing assessment for simulation in healthcare. *Simulation in Healthcare, 7,* 288–294.

Churchouse, C., & McCafferty, C. (2012). Standardized patients versus simulated patients: Is there a difference? *Clinical Simulation in Nursing, 8*(8), e363–e365.

Cook, D. A., Hamstra, S. J., Brydges, R., Zendejas, B., Szostek, J. H., Wang, A. T. . . . Hatala, R. (2013). Comparative effectiveness of instructional design features in simulation-based education: Systematic review and meta-analysis. *Medical Teacher, 35,* e867–e898.

Cordeau, M. A. (2012). Teaching holistic nursing using clinical simulation: A pedagogical essay. *Journal of Nursing Education and Practice, 3*(4), 40–50. doi:10.5430/jnep.v3n4p40

Corvetto, M., & Taekman, J. (2013). To die or not to die? A review of simulated death. *Simulation in Healthcare, 8*(1), 8–12.

Decker, S. I., Anderson, M., Boese, T., Epps, C., McCarthy, J., Motola, I., . . . Scolaro, K. (2015). Simulation standard VIII: Simulation-enhanced interprofessional education (Sim-IPE). *Clinical Simulation in Nursing, 11*(6), 293–297.

Doolen, J. (2015). Psychometric properties of the Simulation Thinking Rubric to measure higher order thinking in undergraduate nursing students. *Clinical Simulation in Nursing, 11*(1), 35–43.

Dreifuerst, K. T., & Decker, S. I. (2012). Debriefing: An essential component for learning in simulation pedagogy. In P. R. Jeffries (Ed.), *Simulation in nursing education: From conceptualization to evaluation* (2nd ed., pp. 105–129). New York, NY: National League for Nursing.

Dreyfus, S. E., & Dreyfus, H. L. (1980). *A five-stage model of the mental activities involved in directed skill acquisition.* Washington, DC: Storming Media. Retrieved from http://www.dtic.mil/cgi-bin/GetTRDoc?AD=ADA084551&Location=U2&doc=GetTRDoc.pdf

Elfrink Cordi, V. L., Leighton, K., Ryan-Wenger, N., Doyle, T., & Ravert, P. (2012). History and development of the Simulation Effectiveness Tool (SET). *Clinical Simulation in Nursing, 8*(6), e199–e210.

Finkelman, A., & Kenner, C. (2012). *Teaching IOM: Implications of the Institute of Medicine reports for nursing education* (3rd ed.). Silver Spring, MD: American Nurses Association.

Franklin, A. E., Burns, P., & Lee, C. S. (2014). Psychometric testing on the NLN Student Satisfaction and Self-Confidence in Learning, Simulation Design Scale, and Educational Practices Questionnaire using a sample of pre-licensure novice nurses. *Nurse Education Today, 34,* 1298–1304.

Gaba, D. (2004). A brief history of mannequin-based simulation & application. In W. F. Dunn (Ed.), *Simulators in critical care education and beyond* (pp. 7–14). Des Plaines, IL: Society of Critical Care Medicine.

Greiner, A. C., & Kneble, E. (Eds.). (2003). *Health professions education: A bridge to quality.* Washington, DC: The National Academies Press.

Groom, J. A., Henderson, D., & Sittner, B. J. (2013). NLN/Jeffries Simulation Framework state of the science project: Simulation design characteristics. *Clinical Simulation in Nursing, 10*(7), 337–344.

Harder, N., Ross, C., & Paul, P. (2013). Student perspective of role assignment in high-fidelity simulation: An ethnographic study. *Clinical Simulation in Nursing, 9,* e329–e334. doi:10.1016/j.ecns.2012.09.003

Hayden, J., Keegan, M., Kardong-Edgren, S., & Smiley, R. A. (2014). Reliability and validity testing of the Creighton Competency Evaluation Instrument for use in the NCSBN national simulation study. *Nursing Education Perspectives, 35*(4), 244–252.

Hayden, J. K., Smiley, R. A., Alexander, M., Kardong-Edgren, S., & Jeffries, P. R. (2014). The NCSBN national simulation study: A longitudinal, randomized, controlled study replacing clinical hours with simulation in prelicensure nursing education. *Journal of Nursing Regulation, 5*(2), C1–S64.

Institute of Medicine (IOM). (2003). *Health professions education: A bridge to quality.* Washington, DC: National Academies Press.

International Nursing Association for Clinical Simulation and Learning (INACSL), Board of Directors. (2013). Standards of best practice: Simulation. *Clinical Simulation in Nursing, 9*(6 suppl.), S1–S32.

Jeffries, P. R., & Rizzolo, M. A. (2006). Final report of the NLN/Laerdal simulation study. In P. R. Jeffries (Ed.), *Simulation in nursing education* (pp. 145–158). New York, NY: National League for Nursing.

The Joint Commission. (2015). *Sentinel event data: Root causes by event type 2004–2Q 2015.* Retrieved from http://www.jointcommission.org/sentinel_event_statistics/

Kardong-Edgren, S., Hanberg, A. D., Keenan, C., Ackerman, A., & Chambers, K. C. (2011, January). A discussion of high-stakes testing: An extension of a 2009 INACSL conference roundtable. *Clinical Simulation in Nursing, 7*(1), e19–e24. doi:10.1016/j.ecns.2010.02.002

Kohn, L. T., Corrigan, J., & Donaldson, M. S. (2000). *To err is human: Building a safer health system.* Washington, DC: National Academy Press.

Leighton, K. (2009a). Death of a simulator. *Clinical Simulation in Nursing, 5*(2), e59–e62.

Leighton, K. (2009b). What can we learn from a LISTSERV? *Clinical Simulation in Nursing, 5*(2), e57–e58.

Leighton, K. (2014). *Learning needs in the traditional clinical environment and the simulated clinical environment: A survey of undergraduate nursing students.* Saarbrucken, Germany: Scholar's Press.

Leighton, K. (2015). Development of the Clinical Learning Environment Comparison Survey. *Clinical Simulation in Nursing, 11*(1), 44–51. doi:10.1016/j.ecns.2014.11.002

Leighton, K., Ravert, P., Mudra, V., & Macintosh, C. (2015). Updating the Simulation Effectiveness Tool: Item modifications and reevaluation of psychometric properties. *Nursing Education Perspectives, 36*(5), 317–323. doi:10.5480/15-1671

Lioce, L., Meakim, C. H., Fey, M. K., Chmil, J. V., Mariani, B., & Alinier, G. (2015). Simulation standard IX: Simulation design. *Clinical Simulation in Nursing, 11*(6), 309–315.

Meakim, C., Boese, T., Decker, S., Franklin, A. E., Gloe, D., Lioce, L., . . . Borum, J. C. (2013). Standards of best practice: Simulation standard I: Terminology. *Clinical Simulation in Nursing, 9,* S3–S11. Retrieved from http://dx.doi.org/10.1016/j.ecns.2013.04.001

Nehring, W. M. (2010). History of simulation in nursing. In W. M. Nehring & F. R. Lashley (Eds.), *High-fidelity patient simulation in nursing education* (pp. 3–26). Sudbury, MA: Jones & Bartlett.

Nehring, W. M., Wexler, T., Hughes, F., & Greenwell, A. (2013). Faculty development for the use of high-fidelity patient simulation: A systematic review. *International Journal of Health Sciences Education, 1*(1), 1–36.

Norman, G., Dore, K., & Grierson, L. (2012). The minimal relationship between simulation fidelity and transfer of learning. *Medical Education, 46*(7), 636–647.

Paige, J. B., & Morin, K. H. (2013). Simulation fidelity and cueing: A systematic review of the literature. *Clinical Simulation in Nursing, 9*(11), 3481–e489. doi:10.1016/j.ecns.2013.01.001

Ravert, P. (2010). Developing and implementing a simulation program: Baccalaureate nursing education. In W. M. Nehring & F. R. Lashley (Eds.), *High-fidelity patient simulation in nursing education* (pp. 59–74). Sudbury, MA: Jones & Bartlett.

Reed, S. J. (2012). Debriefing Experience Scale: Development of a tool to evaluate the student learning experience in debriefing. *Clinical Simulation in Nursing, 8*(6), e211–e217. doi:10.1016/j.ecns.2011.11.002

Rutherford-Hemming, T., Kardong-Edgren, S., Gore, T., Ravert, P., & Rizzolo, M. A. (2014). High-stakes evaluation: Five years later. *Clinical Simulation in Nursing, 10*(12), 605–610. doi:10.1016/j.ecns.2014.09.009

Schultz, C. M. (2010). High-stakes testing!? Help is on the way. *Nursing Education Perspectives, 31*(4), 205.

Sherwood, G., & Barnsteiner, J. H. (Eds.). (2012). *Quality and safety in nursing: A competency approach to improving outcomes.* Hoboken, NJ: Wiley.

Spielberger, C. D. (1985). Assessment of state and trait anxiety: Conceptual and methodological issues. *Southern Psychologist, 2*(4), 6–16.

Weaver, A. (2011). High-fidelity patient simulation in nursing education: An integrative review, *Nursing Education Perspectives, 32*(1), 37–40.

Willhaus, J., Burleson, G., Palaganas, J., & Jeffries, P. (2014). Authoring simulations for high-stakes student evaluation. *Clinical Simulation in Nursing, 10*(4), e177–e182. doi:10.1016/j.ecns.2013.11.006

CHAPTER 19

Interprofessional Education Strategies

Jenn Salfi

The delivery of safe and quality care in today's complex and ever-changing healthcare system relies on effective interprofessional communication and team functioning. Role clarity among team members also has been declared essential in collaborative relationships, as well as a mutual and ongoing focus on person-centered care. Interprofessional education (IPE) aims to develop these competencies of role clarity, communication, team functioning, and person-centered care, which serve as the foundation for a collaborative workforce that is better prepared to respond to the challenges and complexities of the current health care environment (World Health Organization, 2010).

■ Interprofessional Education

Interprofessional education occurs when students of "two or more professions learn with, from, and about each other to improve collaboration and the quality of care" (Centre for the Advancement of Interprofessional Education [CAIPE], 2002, para 1). CAIPE (2008) uses the term *interprofessional education* to include learning in both academic and clinical settings, before and after qualification, certification, or licensure. Some of the benefits of exposing prelicensure students to IPE are that it helps to cultivate mutual trust and respect, confronts misconceptions and stereotypes, and dispels prejudice and rivalry between professional groups (CAIPE, 2010).

Effective Interprofessional Education

A few key points should be upheld when designing and implementing activities and opportunities for IPE. Effective IPE (1) reinforces and provides the opportunity for students to develop and refine essential team-based skills; (2) provides students with the opportunity to learn about their own scope of practice, while learning the skills, languages, and perspectives of others' professional roles; and (3) is grounded in mutual respect, honoring the distinctive experiences and expertise that all participants bring to the healthcare team from their respective backgrounds (CAIPE, 2010). Embedded within these principles of effective IPE are several competencies (knowledge, skills, and behaviors) that are required for interprofessional collaborative practice. The

The author wishes to thank Patricia Solomon for her review and contributions to this chapter.

number and specificity of interprofessional competencies may vary across academic institutions, but overall they can be summarized into four core areas:

1. Knowledge of and the ability to clearly articulate one's professional role and responsibilities.
2. Knowledge of the roles and responsibilities of other health professionals, and knowledge of when to refer and/or collaborate with others, in order to provide optimal person-centered care.
3. Possession of the skills required for collaboration, and the ability to collaborate with others to establish common goals (i.e., demonstrates effective communication, including skills in effective listening, shared decision making, giving/receiving feedback, and conflict management).
4. Contribution to team function by consistently exhibiting the following behaviors: upholding values and ethics that are person-centered and reflect a shared commitment to delivering safer, more efficient, and more effective systems of care; respecting others' opinions; demonstrating flexibility and open-mindedness; and demonstrating the ability to trust others within the team (Canadian Interprofessional Health Collaborative [CIHC], 2010; Interprofessional Education Collaborative of the United States [IPEC Expert Panel], 2011).

These four competency domains are embedded in three levels of IPE: exposure level, immersion level, and mastery level (Charles, Bainbridge, & Gilbert, 2008).

Exposure Level

Exposure-level IPE strategies are primarily knowledge based, with a strong emphasis on the first two competencies of role clarity. These strategies are typically of short-term duration, and enhance awareness of the scopes of practice of all health and social care professions within a team. Some examples of exposure-level IPE strategies might include interviewing and shadowing other professionals, as well as observing multidisciplinary panel discussions.

Immersion Level

Immersion-level IPE strategies are typically of longer duration than exposure activities and require higher levels of interaction between the student groups. All four competencies may be addressed through these strategies. Students are required to communicate and collaborate with other health professional students, share in decision making, and solve problems together. A couple of examples of immersion-level IPE strategies are communication skills labs and gross anatomy dissection courses (both of which are described in greater detail later in this chapter).

Mastery Level

Mastery-level IPE strategies are the most complex and integrative group of activities. At the mastery level, students integrate their interprofessional knowledge and skills in a team environment. Typically, these IPE strategies are of long-term duration, and students have the opportunity to build relationships in a team environment and be actively engaged in team decision making about client care. Although mastery-level strategies are primarily clinical practice experiences, some extended courses or student projects may also be considered mastery-level activities.

■ Theoretical Foundation

IPE introduces a pedagogy with its own classification that aims to recontextualize traditional and distinct bodies of professional knowledge into the knowledge of collaborative practice. Most prelicensure education is uniprofessional, in which students learn together as a single group and do not learn with or alongside other professional groups. IPE attempts to sensitize students to the roles of other healthcare professionals and teach the delivery of interprofessional care (Schmitt, 1994).

Social psychology theories such as contact theory (Carpenter & Hewstone, 1996) have been used in the interprofessional literature. Originally developed by Allport (1954), contact theory proposes that the most effective way to reduce tension between groups is to bring them together. Allport (1954) believed that simply placing people together was not enough to effect positive change, so he proposed the following three conditions: (1) equality of status between groups; (2) groups that work on common goals; and (3) cooperation of the groups during their contact.

This form of teaching can overcome the traditional ways of knowing about how to be a professional practitioner, and it has the potential to result in more effective relations within the healthcare team. The most predominant philosophical argument for IPE is that when IPE is offered at the prelicensure level, improvements will be made in interprofessional communication and collaboration in practice and, ultimately, will result in improved delivery of care and health outcomes for patients (Salvatori & Solomon, 2005).

■ Types of Learners

Some prelicensure programs are at the undergraduate level (e.g., nursing). The introduction of IPE at the undergraduate level remains controversial. One of the arguments against the introduction of IPE at the undergraduate level is that most students at this level have not acquired a sense of their own professional characteristics or sufficient practical experience to be able to experience the full benefits of IPE (Fraser, Symonds, Cullen, & Symonds, 2000). Some believe that premature introduction of IPE could have negative repercussions for undergraduate students because it might interfere with the establishment of a distinct professional identity (Miller, Ross, & Freeman, 1999). Conversely, students at the postgraduate level are able to take full advantage of the learning opportunities available through IPE, because they possess background professional knowledge and practical experience on which to base their insight and discussions (Barr, Freeth, Hammick, Koppel, & Reeves, 2000).

Currently, there are no studies demonstrating that early exposure to IPE hinders the ability to acquire or develop one's professional identity. Some advantages associated with integrating IPE within undergraduate curricula include the opportunity to overturn negative stereotypes at an early stage in an individual's professional socialization (Barr et al., 2000); and to improve the student's overall attitudes, behaviors, and confidence necessary to be an effective member of a healthcare team upon graduation (Salfi, Solomon, Allen, Mohaupt, & Patterson, 2012).

■ Using the Method: Interprofessional Education Strategies

Communication Skills Lab

The ability to communicate in a respectful manner facilitates connectedness among members of a team, as it demonstrates an awareness of equal power and fosters shared decision making, responsibility, and authority (Sele, Salamon, Boarman, & Sauer, 2008). One example of an immersion-level IPE strategy is the communication skills lab, which was originally developed in 2004 and designed to address core IPE competencies (Salvatori, Mahoney, & Delottinville, 2006). It has been suggested that students need to be challenged with complex, realistic healthcare problems using cooperative learning as part of the learning process, such as using a paper-based healthcare scenario or, better yet, a simulated patient (D'Eon, 2004).

Developing the Scenario

The scenario provides the starting point for learning in a communication skills lab. Well-constructed scenarios provide a focus for learning, stimulate interest in the content, and provide a meaningful context within which prior learning is activated and new knowledge is gained (Drummond-Young & Mohide, 2001). The design and development of a patient scenario are composed of several steps. Using a design similar to that of Drummond-Young and Mohide (2001), the framework shown in **Figure 19-1** was constructed to illustrate the steps of development used to create a scenario for an interprofessional communication skills lab.

1. *Identify the who, what, why, and how of the scenario.*
   a. *Who will be the audience experiencing the scenario? Make sure the scenario has something to offer each profession.* In creating the scenario referred to in this chapter, the author first had to identify who the audience was going to be, so that the scenario could be designed to offer each student (profession) opportunities for learning in terms of knowledge, skills, and dispositions (Drummond-Young & Mohide, 2001). A scenario involving an older adult in the community setting was chosen, both for its complexity and for the number of health, and social care professionals who could potentially be involved in the delivery of care.
   b. *Why is this scenario being developed? What is the purpose?* The main purpose of this scenario was to provide an opportunity for communication and collaboration among students from across a variety of professional programs. Effective communication skills (sharing information, listening attentively, respecting others' opinions, demonstrating flexibility, using a common language, providing feedback to others, and responding to feedback from others) are critical in a healthcare team and are the main focus of these interprofessional labs.

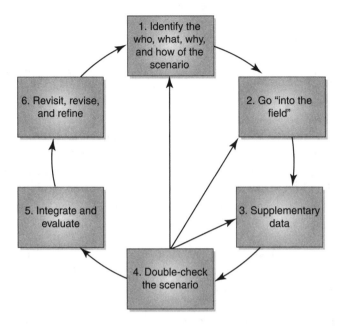

■ Figure 19-1   The cyclical nature of developing a scenario. Multiple steps are involved in creating a scenario for an interprofessional communication skills lab.

Example Scenario:

The Case Manager's Home Visit

Mrs. Cooke is a 74-year-old woman who lives with her small dog in a one-bedroom apartment. Because Mrs. Cooke was recently widowed, her community case manager came to reassess her ability to function on her own. Prior to this visit, Mrs. Cooke was receiving 1 hour of personal care per week to assist with her bath. Upon the case manager's arrival, the door to the apartment was wide open, Mrs. Cooke was wandering around without stockings, and her blouse was half-open. Bruises were visible on her legs. Her wallet sat open on the kitchen table, next to an empty medication dosette.

c. *What are the main concepts/issues of the scenario?* A scenario about an older adult in a community setting could present several topics for exploration (for example, safety in the home, elder abuse, depression/suicide, caregiver burden, and long-term care placement). Effective communication and efficient collaboration within a team of healthcare professionals are critical in order to deliver a holistic plan of care that is person-centered.

d. *How will it play out? What is your vision for execution?* The author wanted to develop a scenario that would mimic a common situation in the community setting: caregiver burden and long-term care placement. The vision for the scenario involved a recently widowed woman and a very tired and worried daughter, whose relationship had become very tense since the daughter suggested assessment for long-term care placement. To play out the scenario, it was envisioned that there would be two standardized patients—a mother and daughter dyad—so that the students could gain practice assessing and communicating with both individuals, as well as observe the dynamics of the relationship and communication patterns between an older adult and her daughter.

2. *Go into the field.* If possible, go into the field and retrieve/develop a scenario based on a real clinical case(s). To further enhance the authenticity of the scenario, have a professional who has had experience with a similar case provide detail and feedback. Authenticity and customization of an interprofessional event so that it reflects relevant healthcare delivery and settings are important for a positive experience for the participants (Hammick, Freeth, Koppel, Reeves, & Barr, 2007).

3. *Provide supplementary data.* The scenario itself should be brief, with enough detail to stimulate critical thinking and encourage hypothesis generation. Previous research indicates that students prefer and appreciate a complex scenario (Salvatori et al., 2006). Create supplementary resource material—for example, lab results or chart data—to offer additional details of the scenario.

A community case manager was selected as the lead professional in this case, as case managers are the individuals who primarily assess and coordinate home care services, and potentially initiate the process for long-term care assessment. They also tend to be one of a variety of healthcare professionals (e.g., nurse, physical therapist, occupational therapist, social worker, dietitian, or speech-language pathologist).

The example scenario was created with enough information to steer the interprofessional group of students toward the author's intended focus for the scenario: an older woman with a decreased ability to function safely at home, and possibly a potential candidate for long-term care placement. However, the scenario also included a few extra details to stimulate brainstorming and critical thinking. For example, the following topics could be explored from this scenario:

- What is the cause of her current state?
- Polypharmacy?
- Disease?
- Other sources of confusion: Diabetes? Urinary tract infection?
- What else could be going on?
- Depression? Grief and bereavement? Potential for suicide?
- Was there an intruder?
- Falls? Other safety concerns?
- Is she able to stay in her own home with increased home care service?

4. *Double-check the scenario.* After the scenario has been created, seek feedback, preferably from other healthcare professionals with similar experiences. Once

feedback has been received and adjustments made as necessary, recruit and train standardized patients for the scenario. *Standardized patients* are individuals who "are specially trained, by a specific yet not complex method similar to 'method acting' to simulate an actual patient in every detail" (Barrows & Tamblyn, 1980, p. 63). In the example scenario, two standardized patients were trained: an older woman as the mother and another woman as the daughter. In training this dyad, the author simply narrated her vision of the scenario, describing in detail the personalities of each individual, the relationship between the mother and daughter, and the communication (verbal and nonverbal) techniques to be acted out by each individual. Another detail that was included in the author's vision for the scenario was the appearance of the standardized patient; in this case, the elderly woman was to appear a bit disheveled, indicating probable difficulty in completing activities of self-care.

Once details and plausibility of the scenario have been checked out and the standardized patients have been trained, test the scenario to observe how it unfolds. Does it unfold as you had envisioned it? Does it meet the objectives of the skills lab and have something to offer each discipline in the group? Does the scenario promote communication, teamwork, and collaboration? Make adjustments and add information to the scenario as necessary.

5. *Integrate and evaluate.* Integrate the scenario into the program, and continue to evaluate the content and process of the scenario. Gather feedback on a regular basis from multiple sources, including faculty, students, and standardized patients. Students, faculty, and standardized patients all bring a unique perspective to the scenario, which can elicit valuable comments and suggestions for change.

6. *Revisit, revise, and refine on a regular basis.* Scenarios grow old and outdated, so to remain current in the field of health care and continue to offer exciting new challenges for the students, scenarios must be revisited on a regular basis. Review the scenario and determine whether it should be refined, revised, or re-created.

The composition of a small group in a communication skills lab may vary from week to week (depending on the availability of students), but generally consists of five to eight students, with representation from at least three professional groups (Salvatori et al., 2006). A week prior to class, students are asked to complete some key readings to provide some context for the IPE event. They are also asked to review their scope of professional practice, because this is information that they will be required to share during the lab.

The initial interview with a standardized patient is 20–30 minutes in duration. When the interview is over, the patient leaves the room, and the student team meets to discuss its findings and treatment and/or discharge plan. Once this task has been completed, the patient returns to the room, and a follow-up meeting is conducted to discuss the interprofessional plan of care. The entire session typically runs for approximately 3 hours in length, with a 15- to 20-minute break midway.

Gross Anatomy Dissection Course

Interprofessional education can take place at any place or at any time within a health or social professional curriculum—it should not be limited by location—so long as the previously stated principles of effective interprofessional education are upheld. Effective IPE should not be viewed in isolation, but rather as a continuum over a prelicensure curriculum, which is continuously reinforced as the student develops as a professional. This continuum should be planned with specific and shifting goals for each level of the learner, and should use a variety of pedagogical methodologies (Thibault, 2011). That being said, a dissection course in anatomy presents yet another venue for offering an effective immersion-level IPE strategy.

Anatomy is typically a content-intensive course. A qualitative study from Sweden exploring the experiences of medical students with their anatomy courses revealed that learners acquire knowledge of anatomy in three ways: through memorizing; by contextualizing, and through experiencing. It was suggested that both contextualization and experiential learning were most effective in helping students retain knowledge of anatomy and physiology (Wilhelmsson et al., 2010).

Contextualization and linkage to clinical problems are commonly achieved through case-based learning experiences (Thistlethwaite et al., 2013). Case-based learning may also serve as a venue for interaction, fostering teamwork, communication skills, professionalism, and respect for one another (Thomas, Denham, & Dinolfo, 2011). Recognizing the potential for learning gross anatomy while developing competencies in interprofessional collaboration, a novel interprofessional case-based gross anatomy dissection course was designed and implemented in a large university in southern Ontario. The 10-week-long course is offered annually to students from a variety of health professional programs, providing them with the opportunity to communicate and collaborate while working through gross anatomy clinical cases and dissection. The weekly 3-hour course is divided into segments: two presentations, a case-based discussion in interprofessional teams; and hands-on dissection in the same interprofessional teams. Prior to each class, students use their course guide to review cases and anatomy. To open each session, anatomy relevant to the week's dissection and case study is presented. Next, a student coordinator from one of the represented professions outlines the scope of practice of her or his discipline. Students then complete case studies in their assigned interprofessional teams (six to eight students). This provides the opportunity to discuss the roles of their profession in managing the case, and to learn about the roles of others. The session ends with hands-on dissection in their interprofessional teams (Fernandes, Palombella, Salfi, & Wainman, 2015). Over the course of 10 weeks, students acquire knowledge of nine body systems of human anatomy, as well as knowledge of other professional roles within a healthcare team. The nature of this immersion-level IPE strategy also affords students the opportunity to develop the skills and positive attitudes required for effective interprofessional team functioning.

Evaluation of IPE Strategies

Interprofessional Communication Skills Lab

Interprofessional activities are generally well received by participants, especially when the context for learning reflects the students' current or future practice (Hammick et al., 2007). In one mixed-method study, students from a variety of health professional programs ($n = 96$) rated their satisfaction with the communication skills labs as high. Students enjoyed the opportunity to interact with colleagues from other professions in an intensive, yet realistic, educational event. It was revealed that the students learned about each other's scopes of practice and became more confident in their communication skills. The skills of the facilitator and preparation for the experience were perceived to promote the success (Solomon & Salfi, 2011).

Gross Anatomy Dissection Course

In order to assess what students learned about interprofessional collaboration, teamwork, and anatomy in an interprofessional dissection course, a sequential explanatory mixed-methods study design was conducted, collecting data from class cohorts spanning from 2011 to 2014 ($n = 97$). Quantitative results revealed that both the "perception of actual cooperation" and "competency and autonomy" subscales within the Interdisciplinary Education Perception Scale (IEPS; McFadyen, Maclaren, & Webster, 2007) demonstrated statistically significant positive change ($P < 0.05$). Similar results were seen within the Readiness for Interprofessional Learning Scale (RIPLS; McFadyen et al., 2005), where the "teamwork and collaboration," "positive professional identity," and "roles and responsibilities" subscales showed statistically significant positive change ($P < 0.05$). Qualitative findings mimicked these results, highlighting key themes of (1) learning about self and others, (2) learning about anatomy, (3) experiencing the benefits of a long-duration IPE initiative (developing pride and faith), and (4) going forward (commitment to future interprofessional practice) (Fernandes et al., 2015).

Small-Group, Case-Based Learning Approach

Both the communication skills labs and the gross anatomy dissection courses rely on the formation of small interprofessional groups. Small-group learning allows students to develop a sense of responsibility for their learning progress. Small-group learning in an interprofessional environment further enhances learning as students develop a sense of responsibility for accurately representing the knowledge and skills base of their profession. Furthermore, students in a group environment learn about human interaction, develop interpersonal skills, and may become more aware of their own emotional reactions and moral standing. Learning how to listen and provide and receive evaluative feedback, all of which are essential in a healthcare environment, are also skills that small-group learning helps to cultivate (Neufeld & Barrows, 1974).

The interprofessional nature of the group provides an opportunity to learn about each other's roles and skills set, and the students learn to respect the distinctive experiences and expertise that each participant brings from his or her individual professional fields (CAIPE, 2008). Working in student teams establishes mutual respect and enhances collaboration, and the relatively equal status of students contributes to a sense of safety, allowing them to take risks that they normally would not be ready to take in clinical practice (O'Neill & Wyness, 2004). Finally, the experiential learning associated with the communication skills lab and the gross anatomy dissection course reinforces the importance of communication and teamwork in providing safe and quality care in the healthcare setting (Barnsteiner, Disch, Hall, Mayer, & Moore, 2007).

■ Potential Problems

There are many barriers to interprofessional education strategies, despite the many benefits associated with this style of learning. IPE is "complex and time consuming to arrange and sustain" (Kilminster et al., 2004, p. 719). It can be very challenging to identify available time for IPE initiatives within prelicensure programs (Hammick et al., 2007). Incompatible clinical shifts and timetables, as well as rigid curriculum, were identified as the most significant barriers in establishing IPE (Morison, Boohan, Jenkins, & Moutray, 2003).

Another barrier to the delivery of IPE in health science programs includes faculty interest and expertise in IPE. As identified by Hammick and colleagues (2007), a key mechanism for effective IPE involves faculty development. Unfortunately, funding to support the initiation of IPE opportunities for students has diminished, as has the number of faculty interested in IPE. Faculty need to be knowledgeable, competent, and confident if they are to be effective in implementing interprofessional core competencies into the health sciences curricula. Faculty also need to be proficient in applying principles of adult learning, as this has also been cited as essential for well-received IPE (Hammick et al., 2007).

Even though skills and content may be similar across professional programs in health sciences, there still tends to be minimal interaction between the students in each professional program. This lack of attention to IPE could lead to undervaluing or misinterpreting each profession's contributions, with the potential of impairing communication, collaboration, and teamwork in the clinical environment after graduation. Thus, in order to address the calling for competent healthcare teams that are adequately prepared to respond to the challenges and complexities of the current healthcare environment, IPE still has to be endorsed and mandated by programs, with full support from senior administration, and faculty champions who are committed to exploring a variety of approaches and venues for interprofessional education.

■ Conclusion

Students in healthcare and social care programs do not acquire interprofessional competencies from sitting side by side in lecture halls, and they do not develop skills in communication and collaboration by simply observing or shadowing a different health professional. Both the communication skills lab and the gross anatomy dissection course provide unique opportunities to communicate and collaborate with students from a variety of prelicensure programs, which has been shown to promote both role understanding and the importance of working together as a team, which are critical in preparing a collaborative, practice-ready workforce.

Discussion Questions

1. What interprofessional education strategies could you realistically implement in your clinical and/or academic setting that would allow your students to learn with, from, and about other health professionals? What interprofessional competencies would you be developing?
2. How would you evaluate an IPE strategy to determine whether or not the strategy has been effective?
3. Are there obstacles in your setting that might prevent or hinder your ability to initiate, implement, and/or sustain IPE strategies? What could you do to overcome some of these obstacles?

References

Allport, G. (1954). *The nature of prejudice*. Reading, MA: Addison-Wesley.

Barnsteiner, J., Disch, J., Hall, L., Mayer, D., & Moore, S. (2007). Promoting interprofessional education. *Nursing Outlook, 55*(3), 144–150.

Barr, H., Freeth, D., Hammick, M., Koppel, I., & Reeves, S. (2000). *Evaluations of interprofessional education: A United Kingdom review for health and social care*. Retrieved from http://www.caipe.org.uk/publications.html

Barrows, H., & Tamblyn, R. (1980). *Problem-based learning*. New York, NY: Springer.

Canadian Interprofessional Health Collaborative (CIHC). (2010). *A national interprofessional competency framework*. Vancouver, BC: Author.

Carpenter, J., & Hewstone, M. (1996). Shared learning for doctors and social workers: Evaluation of a programme. *British Journal of Social Work, 26*, 239–257.

Centre for the Advancement of Interprofessional Education (CAIPE). (2002). *Interprofessional education: A definition*. Retrieved from http://www.caipe.org.uk/about-us/defining-ipe

Centre for the Advancement of Interprofessional Education (CAIPE). (2008). *Interprofessional education: A definition*. Retrieved from http://www.caipe.org.uk/about-us/defining-ipe

Centre for the Advancement of Interprofessional Education (CAIPE). (2010). *Defining IPE*. Retrieved from http://www.caipe.org.uk/about-us/defining-ipe

Charles, G., Bainbridge, L., & Gilbert, J. (2008). *The college of health disciples and the UBC model of interprofessional education*. Vancouver, BC: University of British Columbia.

D'Eon, M. (2004). A blueprint for interprofessional learning. *Journal of Interprofessional Care, 19*, 49–59.

Drummond-Young, M., & Mohide, E. A. (2001). Developing problems for use in problem-based learning. In E. Rideout (Ed.), *Transforming nursing education through problem-based learning* (pp. 165–193). Sudbury, MA: Jones & Bartlett.

Fernandes, A., Palombella, A., Salfi, J., & Wainman, B. (2015). Dissecting through barriers: A mixed-methods study on the effect of interprofessional education in a dissection course with health care professional students. *Anatomic Science Education (ASE) Journal, 8*, 305–316.

Fraser, D., Symonds, M., Cullen, L., & Symonds, I. (2000). A university department merger of midwifery and obstetrics: A step on the journey to enhancing interprofessional learning. *Medical Teacher, 22*(2), 179–183.

Hammick, M., Freeth, D., Koppel, I., Reeves, S., & Barr, H. (2007). A best evidence systematic review of interprofessional education (BEME Guide No. 9). *Medical Teacher, 29*(8), 735–751.

IPEC Expert Panel. (2011). *Interprofessional Education Collaborative: Core competencies for interprofessional collaborative practice: Report of an expert panel* (1st ed.). Washington, DC: Interprofessional Education Collaborative. Retrieved from http://www.aacn.nche.edu/education-resources/ipecreport.pdf

Kilminster, S., Hale, C., Lascelles, M., Morris, P., Roberts, T., Stark, P., . . . Thistlethwaite, J. (2004). Learning for real life: Patient-focused interprofessional workshops offer added value. *Medical Education, 38*, 717–726.

McFadyen, A. K., Maclaren, W. M., & Webster, V. S. (2007). The Interdisciplinary Education Perception Scale (IEPS): An alternative remodelled sub-scale structure and its reliability. *Journal of Interprofessional Care, 21*, 433–443.

McFadyen, A. K., Webster, V., Strachan, K., Figgins, E., Brown, H., & McKechnie, J. (2005). The Readiness for Interprofessional Learning Scale: A possible more stable sub-scale model for the original version of RIPLS. *Journal of Interprofessional Care, 19*, 595–603.

Miller, C., Ross, N., & Freeman, M. (1999). *Shared learning and clinical teamwork: New direction in education for multiprofessional practice.* London, UK: English National Board of Nursing Midwifery and Health Visiting.

Morison, S., Boohan, M., Jenkins, J., & Moutray, M. (2003). Facilitating undergraduate interprofessional learning in healthcare: Comparing classroom and clinical learning for nursing and medical students. *Learning in Health and Social Care, 2*(2), 92–104.

Neufeld, V., & Barrows, H. (1974). The "McMaster philosophy": An approach to medical education. *Journal of Medical Education, 49*(11), 1040–1051.

O'Neill, B., & Wyness, M. (2004). Learning about interprofessional education: Student voices. *Journal of Interprofessional Care, 18*(2), 198–200.

Salfi, J., Solomon, P., Allen, D., Mohaupt, J., & Patterson, C. (2012). Overcoming all obstacles: A framework for embedding interprofessional education (IPE) into a large, multi-site BScN program. *Journal of Nursing Education, 51*(2), 106–110.

Salvatori, P., Mahoney, P., & Delottinville, C. (2006). An interprofessional communication skills lab: A pilot project. *Education for Health, 19*(3), 380–384.

Salvatori, P., & Solomon, P. (2005). Interprofessional education. In P. Solomon & S. Baptiste (Eds.), *Innovations in rehabilitation sciences education* (pp. 95–111). Berlin, Germany: Springer.

Schmitt, M. (1994). USA: Focus on interprofessional practice, education, and research. *Journal of Interprofessional Care, 8*, 9–18.

Sele, K., Salamon, K., Boarman, R., & Sauer, J. (2008). Providing interprofessional learning through interdisciplinary collaboration: The role of modelling. *Journal of Interprofessional Care, 22*(1), 85–92.

Solomon, P., & Salfi, J. (2011). Evaluation of an interprofessional education communication skills initiative. *Education for Health, 11*, 616. Retrieved from http://www.educationforhealth.net

Thibault, G. (2011). Interprofessional education: An essential strategy to accomplish the future of nursing goals. *Journal of Nursing Education, 50*, 313–317.

Thistlethwaite, J. E., Bartle, E., Chong, A. A., Dick, M. L., King, D., Mahoney, S., . . . Tucker, G. (2013). A review of longitudinal community and hospital placements in medical education: BEME Guide No. 26. *Medical Teacher, 35*, e1340–e1364.

Thomas, K. J., Denham, B. E., & Dinolfo, J. D. (2011). Perceptions among occupational and physical therapy students of a nontraditional methodology for teaching laboratory gross anatomy. *Anatomy Science Education, 4*, 71–77.

Wilhelmsson, N., Dahlgren, L. O., Hult, H., Scheja, M., Lonka, K., & Josephson, A. (2010). The anatomy of learning anatomy. *Advances in Health Science Education in Theory and Practice, 15*, 153–165.

World Health Organization (WHO). (2010). *Framework for action on IPE & collaborative practice.* Geneva, Switzerland: Author.

SECTION V

Teaching in Unstructured Settings

The teaching–learning strategies in this section are intended to encourage new ways of thinking, application of concepts, and use of imagination or visualization as applied in practice settings. By stretching their thinking, students realize that they can independently and successfully approach and solve problems. Games and communication exercises enable the students to visualize themselves in realistic settings and increase insight into individual responses to situations. Learning is most effective when students assume a participatory role, occasionally counter to roles held previously. The teacher assumes the part of a facilitator, encouraging interaction among students and holding an advisory, rather than leading, role.

Clinical experience has been the mainstay of a health professional's education. Students need foundational experiences specific to their practice roles, in some form of a skills lab, and then they need opportunities to combine or broaden use of both technical and communication skills. Chapters on simulation detail a prescribed amount of control of the learning environment, which is therefore safer than the clinical setting. Another advantage of a controlled setting is that it provides needed learning opportunities that are not always available or possible in practice settings. Simulation experiences bring together application of content, hands-on care, and professional, interdisciplinary communication, to represent the actual practice setting as closely as possible. Such learning opportunities strengthen students for future practice opportunities.

CHAPTER 20

Philosophical Approaches to Clinical Instruction

Martha J. Bradshaw

■ Introduction

The purpose of clinical instruction is to give the student opportunities to bridge didactic information with the realities of practice. Clinical learning within the realm of health professions education is best achieved when there is consistent and meaningful interaction between the student and a clinical instructor who is part of an educational institution. In guided situations, students blend theoretical knowledge with experiential learning, in order to effect a synthesis and understanding of those endeavors known collectively as *good clinical practice*. Clinical learning is directed by an educator who operationalizes his or her practical knowledge about teaching. Through use of this practical knowledge, the instructor translates the didactic content into application for use in health care.

Clinical instruction in all health professions has become more challenging because of changes in the healthcare environment and the need for health professionals to fulfill increasingly diverse roles. Instructors need to examine their personal philosophy (underlying beliefs) about teaching, especially considering the changes in traditional models of clinical learning. The need for clinical judgment or clinical reasoning, especially in complex patient settings, calls for dual competence: content-specific knowledge and an ability to use the information for clinical practice and decision making. However, constant changes in the practice settings make competence elusive and demanding (Little & Milliken, 2007).

■ Role of the Clinical Instructor

The goal of the clinical learning experience is for the instructor to guide novices in what constitutes safe practice and to help them develop clinical reasoning abilities. In the clinical setting, planning and selection of clinical learning activities tend to be instructor driven. Depending upon the instructor's amount of experience and sense of self-efficacy, the nature of clinical learning may become more student centered. In either case, the teacher guides the students in applying theory to patient care.

The faculty role in clinical instruction is as diverse and demanding as are the settings. The instructor is expected to be competent, experienced, knowledgeable, flexible, patient, and energetic. The instructor should be capable of balancing structure with spontaneity. Clinical learning is aimed at knowledge application, skill acquisition, and professional role development. The instructor must be aware of didactic information the students are studying, in order to provide parallel opportunities for application. In nursing, students are led in practicing and improving patient care skills, and need guidance in valuing the skills (Clark, Owen, & Tholcken, 2004). By recognizing the importance of a skill and performing it safely and efficiently, students will increase confidence in their abilities to provide direct patient care. Clinical instructors also help students understand and respect the uniqueness of each client and family in order to individualize holistic care (Northington, Wilkerson, Fisher, & Schenk, 2005). Nursing students have indicated that their most successful clinical experiences (over time, such as a semester or rotation) are ones in which the instructor uses strategies to improve self-confidence, foster responsibility, and encourage critical thinking (Etheridge, 2007). In summary, the role of the clinical instructor is to direct the student to think like a health professional (physical therapist, nurse, dentist, etc.).

Typically, two approaches to clinical instruction exist: technical or task focus and outcomes focus (Forbes, 2010). Task mastery instruction is based on the instructor's decisions about what behaviors and ways of thinking are important for care providers and, therefore, should be reproduced in students. In essence, clinical instructors are gatekeepers, allowing students to enter the profession once they have demonstrated their ability. With the outcomes approach, the instructor serves as a mentor, guiding students in patient-centered decision making, actions, and evaluation that serve as the framework for comprehensive care. The technical approach may be suitable with novice students or in technical programs, but the outcomes-focused approach has a more far-reaching effect on students as they progress in their educational program.

The successful student clinical experience—measured in terms of learning outcomes and an internalized sense of fulfillment—is largely influenced by the planning and selection of learning activities available to the students. Selection of activities, as well as actual teaching, is value-laden and reflects the faculty member's philosophical approach to clinical learning and the role or roles the instructor chooses to fulfill. The roles in which individual instructors see themselves may include interaction with students, serving as a role model, or functioning as an expert reference. Roles that students see as important for clinical instructors to fill have been identified as being knowledgeable and professionally competent; being able to be encouraging and supportive; being providers of helpful feedback, having organizational skills, and showing respect for others, especially students (Cook, 2005; Hanson & Stenvig, 2008). Once this self-image is determined, teachers consciously or subconsciously shape situations that enable them to enact their various roles. This action enhances teacher effectiveness because the instructor is most comfortable in fulfilling preselected roles.

There is some indication that background knowledge and preferences for orientation to practice strongly influence planning and decision making by teachers

(Yaakobi & Sharan, 1985). Therefore, an instructor with a concrete, structured practice background (such as surgical nursing) may select or plan patient assignments that are more structured than those selected by an instructor from a less structured background (such as psychiatric nursing). A potential conflict exists between teacher and student regarding learning and practice preferences. Consequently, an effective clinical instructor is one who has the knowledge and practice experience plus understands students' learning preferences and educational needs. Furthermore, new graduates report that their best learning opportunities in clinical occurred when they had a variety of patient care experiences (Etheridge, 2007).

■ Foundations for Selection of Clinical Activities

Another philosophical perspective that governs clinical learning is the instructor's view of the *purpose* of the clinical learning experience. The three most common purposes are for students to (1) apply theoretical concepts, (2) experience actual patient situations, and (3) see and implement professional roles. Based on the chosen perspective, the instructor selects the agency or unit and plans the type of clinical assignment that is best suited for the identified purpose. The realism of clinical activities brings added benefit to any of the three types of experiences.

The planning and supervising of clinical learning call for the instructor's own philosophical stance to be blended with the selected goal(s) of the clinical experience. Student assignments may have one of the following goals:

- Learn the **patient**: provide one-to-one total care
- Learn the **content area**: practice a variety of care activities in one setting
- Learn **role(s)**: function as a staff or team member, as a practitioner, as an administrator, or in other selected role(s)

The instructor who selects a student focus for clinical assignments may value empowerment as part of his or her philosophical approach to teaching. The aims of this approach are the cultivation of responsibility, authority, and accountability in novice practitioners (Manthey, 1992). Selected clinical activities directed toward empowerment could include:

- **Analytic nursing**: use of actual experiences (instructor or student based) to define and solve problems
- **Change activities**: develop planned change and identify resources to effect this change
- **Collegiality**: professional interactions (instructor–student, student–student, student–staff) to solve problems and promote optimal care
- **Sponsorship**: collaboration and interaction with preceptors, administration; analysis of bureaucratic system (Carlson-Catalano, 1992)

Within the framework of the assignment, the instructor then makes decisions about which activities will enhance learning outcomes. This process again reflects the teacher's values, beliefs about how learning should take place, and how teacher role fulfillment will influence this learning. For example, the instructor who values participatory learning and role modeling will be actively involved in many aspects of the student's activities, and his or her presence will be felt by the student—at the bedside or interacting with staff members. Role modeling, an encouraging attitude, and serving as a resource person are attributes that decrease student anxiety about the clinical experience and strengthen the instructor–student relationship (Cook, 2005; Hanson & Stenvig, 2008). The instructor who wishes to foster independence in students may take on the role of resource person and become centrally available to students as needed. The instructor who places emphasis on organization and task accomplishment will oversee numerous student activities and facilitate completion of the assignments within a designated period. Many instructors value all of these activities as a part of student learning. Accomplishing all of these activities calls for a great deal of diversity and planning by the teacher. There are clear advantages for students to be engaged in more than one type of learning experience from one clinical day or week to the next. This broadens the possibilities for learning and also strengthens understanding of multiple roles and diversity of settings. Students who experienced multiple clinical placements described themselves as more adaptable in new environments (Adams, 2002).

Some philosophical approaches to teaching and role assumption by educators are more subtle, yet promote more complex, higher-order learning. More specifically, the teacher who values empowerment and accountability in students will take on a less directive role and assume one that is more enabling for each student. Bradbury-Jones, Sambrook, and Irvine (2007) point out that the concept of empowerment is associated with decision making, ability to express one's own needs, and ability to negotiate. Personal empowerment is closely aligned with self-esteem, a much needed characteristic for self-confidence. A sense of self-confidence and empowerment develops through positive experiences and reflection of self during the experience. A student who has the freedom and opportunity to advocate for the patient, volunteer a plan of care, and give an opinion about decisions of care will feel more empowered. The instructor who wishes to promote independence in students must be willing to release a certain amount of control, in order to give students freedom to learn and grow.

Periodic, timely feedback is essential. Students can only recognize strengths and areas for improvement when they are given objective, constructive feedback. Feedback should be not only evaluative, but also encouraging in order to bolster confidence and independence. Augustine (1992) investigated feedback by clinical instructors and discovered that, in addition to group feedback, such as in conferences or orientation, students felt the need for personal feedback from the instructor until they were certain what the instructor wanted from them. This need indicates both the value of the instructor as a guide and also the emphasis students place on feedback for clinical success or failure. Furthermore, feedback is an opportunity for the student to refine his or her practices by gaining insight from an experienced clinician (the instructor). The topic of feedback and clinical evaluation is addressed in depth in Chapter 28.

■ Clinical Activities and Clinical Reasoning

The instructor who promotes clinical reasoning in students fashions learning activities to meet this goal. Discovery learning is one way in which student autonomy, problem solving, and clinical reasoning can be enhanced. Students can have opportunities to realize, or discover, patient responses to certain aspects of care, or experience how structuring an activity differently is more time-saving. These discoveries boost self-esteem when students see what they have learned on their own, or that they have the ability to resolve certain problematic situations. The instructor then is rewarded by seeing growth take place in the students.

According to a meta-analytic review conducted by Alfieri, Brooks, Aldrich, and Tenenbaum (2011), a discovery learning task can range from implicit pattern detection, to the elicitation of explanations and working through manuals, to conducting simulations. Discovery learning can occur whenever students are not provided with an exact answer, but instead get the resources so that they can find the answer themselves. Detection of implicit patterns can occur with beginning students by having them assume an observational role. By watching the practitioner conduct routine responsibilities, learners develop an "Ah-ha" understanding about the role. The next step, then, is seeking explanations for actions and a description of decision making. This can be accomplished particularly well in a student–preceptor relationship. These observations and thought processes can be applied in simulated, then actual, patient situations as students continue to grow in knowledge and expertise.

Another approach to promoting growth of problem-solving abilities is to emphasize the clinical, or patient, problem, rather than the clinical setting. Student assignments that take place in familiar, repetitive settings enable students to deal with patients *in that setting*. In addition to learning how to deal with clinical problems, students in new or unexpected settings also experience professional socialization through role discontinuity. In making the transition from instructor-directed, structured, familiar assignments to empowering, unstructured, undefined patient problems, students experience new ways of defining their own roles and responsibilities as practitioners. The chapter on clinical pathways (Chapter 27) describes how to structure and evaluate students in a one-time clinical setting.

■ Student-Centered Learning

The strategy of reciprocal learning not only meets clinical learning needs, but promotes collegiality as well. Reciprocal learning usually takes the form of peer teaching, or student-to-student instruction. This learning occurs informally within most clinical groups and can become more purposeful and goal-directed through instructor planning. By pairing students for specific learning activities, the student learner gains information, experience, and insight in new ways. Learners receive individualized, empathetic instruction and may feel more relaxed with a peer than with a faculty teacher. The student teacher also learns about instruction, helping, and working with others. Peer support is useful for building student self-confidence, providing a mechanism for feedback from someone other than the clinical instructor, and initiating students into the collaborative role (Brooks & Moriarty, 2009).

From the viewpoint of the instructor, student-centered learning increases student accountability and independence. This is especially beneficial for students who are closer to graduation and need to break ties to the instructor. As students increase independence, the instructor can receive satisfaction from this new level of student performance. Students appreciate the trust that the instructor conveys to them. In fact, the promotion of cooperative learning, active involvement, and the recognition of diverse ways of learning are attributes that students rank highly in effective teachers (Wolf, Bender, Beitz, Weiland, & Vito, 2004).

■ Faculty Development

The powerful influence of the instructor as a person should not be overlooked. Development of an effective clinical instructor and the evolution of a meaningful, positive clinical learning experience are based on insight, planning, and implementation by the faculty member. Therefore, individual teachers need to cultivate an appropriate self-image as a teacher. In addition, the clinical instructor should indulge in periodic self-reflection: Is my own clinical competence being maintained? Are my own views on the profession and the teaching–learning process congruent with student perspectives and needs? Should teaching strategies, types of assignments, or communication skills be revised? Just as encouraging self-reflection in students guides them in viewing their clinical experience as a success (Hanson & Stenvig, 2008), self-reflection by the instructor will also bring about synthesis of the experience and evaluation of successes and failures. The effective faculty member then may need to reshape his or her own teaching perspectives to better blend with the perspectives held by the clinical students.

■ Conclusion

The philosophical approach to teaching is the foundation on which the instructor operationalizes his or her own practical knowledge. The responsibilities for the instructor are great, calling for clinical expertise, role modeling, and understanding of teaching and learning principles for a variety of students, settings, and clinical experiences.

Carlson-Catalano (1992) pointed out that much of the instruction that takes place is related to how the instructor has internalized professional values and developed a self-image as a practitioner and role model. The instructor who wishes to promote empowerment in students must see himself or herself as empowered to do so. Only then can needed socialization and empowerment take place. The empowered instructor is able to visualize the potential learning opportunities in the clinical environment (Chally, 1992). The nature of clinical practice has been redefined, as must the nature of clinical learning experiences.

Effective clinical instruction emerges from conscious efforts by the instructor. These efforts should be based on background knowledge, strongly formed values, and a well-defined self-image as a nurse teacher. Applying these personal resources enables the teacher to bring about effective clinical instruction. Formal and personal learning outcomes then are achievable.

Discussion Questions

1. Give examples of how nursing theories can be applied to patient care situations.
2. When a clinical instructor pairs students for reciprocal learning, should the students be asked to evaluate each other's performance?
3. How can an instructor promote independence and empowerment in a student who lacks confidence?

References

Adams, V. (2002). Consistent clinical assignment for nursing students compared to multiple placements. *Journal of Nursing Education, 41*, 80–82.

Alfieri, L., Brooks, P. J., Aldrich, N. J., & Tenenbaum, H. R. (2011). Does discovery-based instruction enhance learning? *Journal of Educational Psychology, 103*(1), 1–18. doi:10.1037/a0021017

Augustine, C. J. (1992). Dimensions of feedback in clinical nursing education. *Dissertation Abstracts International,* 54-02A:0433.

Bradbury-Jones, C., Sambrook, S., & Irvine, F. (2007). The meaning of empowerment for nursing students: A critical incident study. *Journal of Advanced Nursing, 59*(4), 342–351.

Brooks, N., & Moriarty, B. (2009). Implementation of a peer-support system in the clinical setting. *Nursing Standard, 23*(27), 35–39. http://dx.doi.org/10.7748/ns2009.03.23.27.35.c6836

Carlson-Catalano, J. (1992). Empowering nurses for professional practice. *Nursing Outlook, 40,* 139–142.

Chally, P. S. (1992). Empowerment through teaching. *Journal of Nursing Education, 31,* 117–120.

Clark, M. C., Owen, S. V., & Tholcken, M. A. (2004). Measuring student perceptions of clinical competence. *Journal of Nursing Education, 43,* 548–554.

Cook, L. J. (2005). Inviting teaching behaviors of clinical faculty and nursing students' anxiety. *Journal of Nursing Education, 44,* 156–161.

Etheridge, S. A. (2007). Learning how to think like a nurse: Stories from new nursing graduates. *Journal of Continuing Education in Nursing, 38*(1), 24–30.

Forbes, H. (2010). Clinical teachers' approaches to nursing. *Journal of Clinical Nursing, 19,* 785–793.

Hanson, K. J., & Stenvig, T. E. (2008). The good clinical nursing educator and the baccalaureate nursing clinical experience: Attributes and praxis. *Journal of Nursing Education, 47,* 38–42.

Little, M. A., & Milliken, P. J. (2007). Practicing what we preach: Balancing teaching and clinical practice competencies. *International Journal of Nursing Education Scholarship, 4,* 1–14.

Manthey, M. (1992). Empowerment for teachers and students. *Nurse Educator, 17,* 6–7.

Northington, L., Wilkerson, R., Fisher, W., & Schenk, W. (2005). Enhancing nursing students' clinical experience using aesthetics. *Journal of Professional Nursing, 21,* 66–71.

Wolf, Z. R., Bender, P. J., Beitz, J. M., Wieland, D. M., & Vito, K. O. (2004). Strengths and weaknesses of faculty teaching performance reported by undergraduate and graduate nursing students: A descriptive study. *Journal of Professional Nursing, 20,* 118–128.

Yaakobi, D., & Sharan, S. (1985). Teacher beliefs and practices: The discipline carries the message. *Journal of Education for Teaching, 11,* 187–199.

CHAPTER 21

Crafting the Clinical Experience: A Toolbox for Healthcare Professionals

Stephanie S. Allen
Lyn S. Prater

Clinical teaching is where it happens, and the clinical teacher needs to be able to know what to do to make it happen. Healthcare education historically has been based upon the expert–novice or mentor–protégé model. Optimal learning outcomes are not achieved when the teacher is just an authority figure and content expert. Rather, optimal clinical learning is best achieved when the teacher is a true educator. In order for expert clinicians to become effective teachers in their professional programs, an additional knowledge base and skill set are required. The clinical experience is a time in which the student applies theory to practice. It is the role of the clinical instructor to facilitate this application and evaluate learner outcomes. Establishing and maintaining professional boundaries with students, while remaining current in practice, teaching, and implementing evidence-based practice, is both an art and a science. This chapter provides a framework for implementing the use of best teaching practices in the areas of clinical teaching and evaluation.

■ Role Preparation

Role preparation for health professions faculty typically came from graduates completing educational preparation in order to practice in their chosen professions, gaining clinical experience, and showing an interest in teaching. It is thus incumbent upon the educational institution to provide the necessary mentoring for new faculty so that not only the scholarship of discovery can be implemented, but also the scholarship of integration, application, and teaching can be developed. These roles identified by Boyer (1990) provide a pathway for faculty to develop and flourish in the structure of higher education.

The scholarship of *discovery*, as noted by Boyer (1990), is the need for scientific inquiry into the discipline of healthcare professions, and this faculty research role is imperative in higher education. In addition, the Institute of Medicine core competencies are being utilized as the foundation for nursing program evaluation (Morris & Hancock, 2013). The scholarship of *integration* is that part of the faculty role where the making of meaning, perspective, and connections across disciplines, and the placement of the specialties in a broader context, can be explored and applied. Bartels (2007) reminds us that "nursing faculty must be prepared to assume this role of interdisciplinary integration, finding ways to connect not only with evidence discovered within the profession, but also with evidence generated across professions" (p. 156). The scholarship of *teaching* is the heart of health professions education, but is often not a part of the basic education for entry into practice. The scholarship of *application* is relevant in the healthcare professions because it calls for the educator to maintain competency in the clinical field. Remaining current in practice heightens the educator's ability to blend academic and practice roles. Teaching will likely be the primary activity of most nursing faculty, so it is imperative that this role be articulated and developed in new faculty.

Clinical teaching is especially challenging, as the clinical sites can vary greatly from institution to institution and faculty must help students assimilate into their role of caregiver in an increasingly acute setting. Ongoing changes in technology, along with a generation of students who must learn to conform to an intense, highly regulated, and highly standardized system for healthcare delivery, make the clinical teaching event both challenging and rewarding. Clear objectives, professional boundaries, and collegial relationships with healthcare staff are all important components for clinical faculty to realize a successful clinical experience for students. This area of scholarship is especially pertinent for nursing faculty, as nursing is an applied practice. The scholarship of application is invaluable as faculty members prepare and guide their students for the practice arena of the future. An ongoing process for evaluating the effectiveness of the clinical instructor is an important aspect of performance assessment and feedback for professional development. Input from a variety of evaluators, including students, agency personnel, and the academic clinical coordinator, will provide comprehensive feedback (Buccieri, Brown, & Malta, 2011).

In addition to incorporating Boyer's model into a personal teaching style, the clinical educator must be aware of and able to implement effective clinical teaching behaviors. Esmaeili, Cheraghi, Salasali, and Ghiyasvandian (2014) found three main themes related to effective clinical education: (1) appropriate communication, (2) incorporation of theory into practice, and (3) instructors with specialty-specific knowledge. The open collegial relationship is maintained by providing clear and consistent expectations. Adapting the experience to the student requires student participation in determining learning goals and needs. "Mentors must strive to develop their knowledge and clinical behaviors according to students' needs in clinical settings" (Esmaeili et al., 2014, p. 460). An important category of facilitating clinical reasoning is utilizing thinking out loud with the student. The benefit of receiving environmental support lies in feeling valued. According to Esmaeili et al. (2014), respectful and caring interpersonal relationships between the instructor and the student result in supportive and approachable communication. Also, students view faculty as positive role models if they are current in their specialty.

An additional aspect of role preparation, according to Wetherbee, Peatman, Kenney, Cusson, and Applebaum (2010), is for the clinical and academic stakeholders to mutually agree on standards and outcomes, so that all work toward a common goal. Role preparation is critical to the success of the healthcare professional as an educator. Utilizing resources available and garnering support from seasoned faculty will make the implementation of the educator role easier.

■ Implementing the Role

Students recognize and respond to clinical instructors who exhibit passion and enthusiasm for their work. Passion is contagious and promotes the development of a positive learning environment. According to Spurr, Bally, and Ferguson (2010), there are five dimensions of passion that can provide a framework for clinical teaching:

1. Commitment
2. Achievement
3. Trust
4. Caring
5. Collaboration

A recent international study found that the instructor's caring behaviors positively influenced nursing students' caring behaviors. This study of 586 student nurses from four countries provided a cross-cultural perspective on the importance of faculty role modeling the competence of caring as an effective teaching strategy (Labrague, McEnroe-Petitte, Papathansiou, Edet, & Arulappan, 2015). As clinical faculty define and develop their teaching approaches, these passions may be used as a framework for building their philosophy of teaching and supporting their values.

Clinical Orientation: How to Get Off to a Good Start

It is the responsibility of the clinical instructor to complete all required agency orientation and be knowledgeable of agency policies and procedures. Good rapport will be maintained between the instructor and clinical site when students and faculty follow agency guidelines. This both shows respect for the agency and allows an opportunity for professional development in the students. Instructors cannot just drop off students on a unit or at a clinical agency and expect the staff to provide all of the teaching. Staff nurses appreciate an instructor who is present, acts as a team member, has experience, is relaxed, and is organized. A component of orientation will be the identification for the staff of what their responsibilities will be. Frequently, clinical staff as agency employees are called upon to participate in the educational experience. Clinical staff are familiar with their role as patient care providers and in teaching patients and family members, but they may not have been provided any formal instruction about teaching or serving as preceptor of students. Consequently, clinical instructors need to communicate to the healthcare system clinical liaison clear expectations for each clinical experience. Unless the educational institution provides a structured orientation for this process, the clinical instructor will be responsible for this process as well. If this formal process does not take place, each student's clinical experience will differ due to the varying quality of instruction provided by the instructor/preceptor within each clinical setting.

Establishing rapport with the clinical management and staff takes time and dedication. Refer to **Figure 21-1**, which is a typical schedule for new faculty orientation.

New Faculty Orientation

Room 407

Lyn Prater, PhD, RN, Undergraduate Clinical Coordinator

1. Welcome and introductions

2. Baylor mission, philosophy, and curriculum

3. Human needs framework

4. Intranet

5. Care plans

6. Learning contract

7. Midterm evaluations

8. Final evaluations

9. Clinical evaluation tool

10. Schedule

11. Workroom, secretary, and communications

12. Clinical expectations

13. Dress code

14. Questions and answers

■ **Figure 21-1**   Orientation for new clinical faculty.

An additional consideration for ensuring a positive experience for faculty and students related to clinical placement is to ensure that the faculty members have consistent placement on clinical units from semester to semester. This provides organizational familiarity, continuity, and a positive sense of belonging for students (Newton, Cross, White, Ockerby, & Billett, 2011).

Crafting the Clinical Experience

Once faculty have oriented themselves and the students to the clinical site, it is critical to craft the clinical experience so that the assignments match the course objectives and are congruent with the theoretical concepts. For example, the instructor would assign patients who have fluid and electrolyte deficits during the time frame the students are learning about this concept in their theory course. Additional practice with calculating maintenance fluids and analyzing lab values will help the students make the connections between theory and practice. More background on the selection of clinical activities can be found elsewhere in this text.

In clinical settings in which the patient care activity is very specific, the clinical instructor might want to use an assignment sheet or form. This communication tool provides an easy reference for the unit staff to know which students will be caring for which patients. Because this assignment sheet contains sensitive information, it must be posted away from public access. Outlining clearly, on the assignment sheet, which student is doing what and when helps the staff know which experiences to save for a student and which ones they themselves are responsible for. At the beginning of the clinical day, the instructor will review the student's preclinical preparation and determine whether there are any gaps or inconsistencies for care. The student will receive report from the primary caregiver assigned to his or her patient and assume care within the context of the agency guidelines and clinical assignment. "Oral shift reporting can stimulate learning if it includes consultation and discussion between nursing students and the nursing staff" (Skaalvik, Normann, & Henriksen, 2010, p. 2300). In order for the clinical instructor to organize a number of students within a clinical setting, he or she must negotiate and communicate the student's responsibility. As an example, even if a student has read the procedure for lab blood draws, he or she will benefit from watching it done at least once before attempting it on the patient.

It is imperative to follow agency policies regarding the procedures in which students may and may not participate. Please refer to **Figure 21-2**, which is an example of an agency schedule for student orientation. Credibility as a clinical instructor may initially be tested by staff members as well as by students. This is not unusual and should not threaten the instructor's sense of clinical competence. Once trust is established, the clinical instructor will find that this testing dissipates. Purposeful assignments should, in addition, be congruent with the evaluation tool. Clinical instructors can improve their students' satisfaction while in the clinical setting by providing specific instructions, delivering individualized attention, and maintaining organization. (Lovecchio, DiMattio, & Hudacek, 2015). Keeping detailed anecdotal notes and documenting the student's progress or lack thereof in meeting the course objectives make the final evaluation process less subjective. Providing students with specific, positive examples as well as examples of omissions or errors helps guide them in reflective practice. An important question that is worth discussing is: "What would you do differently next time?" In addition to focusing on the nursing role, interprofessional socialization opportunities should be taken advantage of in the clinical setting. According to DiVall et al. (2014), "interprofessional education is the cornerstone of providing future healthcare providers" (p. 576).

Clinical Rounds

Clinical rounds provide an opportunity to observe students interacting with their patients and patients' family members. Introductions by either the student or the instructor are important to facilitate ongoing rapport. Rounds also provide the opportunity for spontaneous learning by using the teachable moment. An astute clinical instructor will use these teachable moments as she or he encounters the student engaged in the delivery of real-time care. Guidance and/or gentle prompting regarding additional resources for the teaching/learning event can be given, and role modeling by the instructor can be provided at the bedside. The clinical instructor may observe a student assuming responsibility in the role or having difficulty and becoming an onlooker. The "onlooker" may describe himself or herself as being excluded from delivering care, unable to overcome obstacles, and feeling insecure in his or her role.

Guidelines and Expectations for Students: Presbyterian Hospital Dallas Nursing Clinical Experience/Rotation

PHD Nursing Staff/Support	Nursing Institution/Instructor	Students
• RNs/all patient care staff will ultimately maintain responsibility for patients.	• Faculty must always be on assigned units and be available for students' learning experience.	• Responsible for action with patients.
• Nursing staff will show a positive attitude and willingness to mentor students and be role models.	• Faculty must be proficient and qualified in the area of teaching experience/clinical assignment.	• Responsible for reporting to the nursing staff information concerning patients.
• Nursing staff will share objective observations regarding students' clinical performance with faculty.	• Disseminate and post clinical assignments (length, dates, hours of clinical experience) and phone/pager numbers as appropriate for each service area/unit and NPD (include student/faculty names and numbers).	• Be prepared for clinical assignments; show initiative in learning and work as a partner with the staff nurse.
• Provide cooperation to promote the success of the student clinical rotation.	• Arrange own conference space as needed.	• Exhibit professional and courteous behavior with patients and staff.
• Designate an individual on unit as a student contact.	• Supervise students' *first* time using clinical skills with patients on units.	
• RNs may observe students do procedures with patients *only* after instructors have checked off students.	• Notify unit personnel and NPD of student objectives for the learning experiences in writing.	• Notify the unit if unable to be onsite for the assigned day.
• NPD is the department responsible for coordinating all student affiliation educational rotations; *any changes* of rotation *must be approved* by NPD.	• Clinical assignment changes must be approved by NPD.	• Always report/check out with the RN assigned to patients before leaving the unit either for a break or for the conclusion of the clinical day.
	• Seek information from RNs about student performance.	
	• Provide NPD with proof of malpractice/liability insurance and CPR certification of both faculty and students prior to the beginning of the semester (day of orientation).	• Complete end-of-semester PHD evaluation regarding the learning experience at PHD.
• Maintain professional and courteous behavior with instructors and students.		
• Maintain standards of patient care.	• Provide NPD with Texas Nursing Registration number of each faculty member assigned to PHD.	
• NPD provides orientation for faculty and students to hospital and assigned units.	• Maintain professionalism and courtesy with both staff and students.	• Be vaccinated for HBV; the series of injections must begin prior to the beginning of the semester and proof must be provided to NPD.
• Nursing staff provides orientation on the assigned unit.	• Obtain approval from NPD for any faculty/substitute on the clinical schedule throughout the rotation.	
• Recommend a maximum faculty-to-student ratio of 1:10.	• Conduct end-of-semester PHD evaluation with students regarding the learning experience at PHD and return to NPD.	• Maintain confidentiality of patient information.
• NPD provides an evaluation tool for completion by students and gives results to staff.	• Be vaccinated for HBV; the series of injections must begin prior to the beginning of the semester and proof must be provided to NPD.	
• PHD requires faculty and nursing students to be vaccinated for HBV.	• Maintain confidentiality of patient information.	

■ **Figure 21-2**   Agency orientation schedule.

CPR, cardiopulmonary resuscitation; HBV, hepatitis B virus; NPD, nursing professional development; PHD, Presbyterian Hospital Dallas; RN, registered nurse.

Used with permission from Texas Health Resources, Presbyterian Hospital Dallas.

In this situation, the clinical instructor must recognize and intervene for the patient's safety and well-being and must provide timely feedback to promote independence and increase confidence (Hellstrom-Hyson, Martensson, & Kristofferzon, 2012). Timely feedback may prevent students from making incorrect assumptions about clinical competence and allows for improvement in future performance (Hauer & Kogan, 2012; Nottingham & Henning, 2010). Melo, Williams, and Ross (2010) stated:

> To best support students in a rigorous and demanding program of study[,] faculty development should include strategies and tools to assist clinical tutors with assessing students for signs of psychological distress. Early intervention through psychological counseling may provide much needed support for students who are highly anxious. (p. 773)

Ongoing care and teachable moments are excellent occasions for challenging students to grow by using directed questioning. An example of this type of questioning is when the instructor asks the student to discuss the rationale for use of a medication as a treatment modality that differs from the drug's primary action (e.g., nifedipine in the preterm labor patient). According to Hoffman (2008), clinical instructors should be utilizing higher-level questions to facilitate critical thinking skills in the clinical setting. "These questions require the student to correlate clinical findings with textbook descriptions and apply this content to the care of their patients" (p. 234). It is important to avoid spoon-feeding the answers. Make the student look up policies and procedures and medical terminology. This provides an opportunity to utilize resources and to become self-directed in their pursuit of knowledge in the profession.

One of the goals of the clinical teaching experience is to provide the students with an experience that keeps them engaged and places them in the role of a total patient care provider. By eliciting feedback from both the student and the staff members, the instructor will be able to determine whether the assignment is too challenging or is not keeping the student engaged, and thus will be able to adjust it accordingly. Developing self-awareness in students is a professional priority. It is important to share observations made by the staff and instructor that promote a positive professional demeanor as well as those that detract from a student's professional demeanor. When a student is overly focused on programming an IV pump and not making eye contact with a family member who is asking a serious question, the establishment of a therapeutic relationship is affected. Actions by students, such as washing hands in the patient's room and then running those hands through their hair before putting on sterile gloves for a central line dressing change, may diminish trust when observed by patients and family members. At these times, the instructor must redirect the student to ensure safety, using a professional approach.

Clinical Decision Making

Baxter and Boblin (2007) have provided insight into the types of clinical decisions students make depending upon the level of placement within their program. Students' progress from assessment decision making to interventional decision making, with the capability of appraisal, incurs risk to themselves as well as to the patients. It is important, then, for the clinical instructor to monitor and support the student throughout the clinical day and semester by being present and providing feedback for the decisions the student makes. One method of providing this feedback for students, related to their critical thinking, is through reflective writing. Naber, Hall, and Schadler (2014) determined that students' critical thinking was improved by having students participate in reflective writing assignments based on Paul's model of critical thinking.

In addition to clinical rounds, preclinical and postclinical conferences provide a rich opportunity for clarification and teaching. There are advantages and disadvantages to preplanned conference activities. An instructor should have a planned conference activity, but should also be able to be flexible and spontaneous when the need arises. Both instructor and student may be exhausted by this point in the learning process, so it is important for the clinical instructor to utilize innovative strategies to assist the students to find meaning in their recent clinical experience (Megel, Nelson, Black, Vogel, & Uphoff, 2013). Student–nurse dyads and group activities are proven strategies designed to create a supportive learning environment that enables students to meet the clinical learning objectives (MacGowan, 2010; Ruth-Sahd, 2011). Closure at the end of the clinical experience is an important last step for both students and clinical instructors. Some examples of activities to use in postclinical conferences are discussed next.

Postclinical Conferences

Example One: Taking Action Based on Analysis of Patient Information

Analyzing patient information guides the students in cultivating analytical abilities and assuming accountability for action.

Step 1.   Each student identifies abnormal assessment findings.
Step 2.   Each student analyzes which nursing implications those abnormalities have for patient care.
Step 3.   Each student shares with the group how patient care was altered and the team process for implementation of the changes.

Example 2: Applying Evidence-Based Research to Practice

Applying evidence-based research to practice prompts students to examine current evidence regarding practices in which they have participated during the clinical day. Exercises such as this will enable the practicing professional to remain current in practice.

Examples of these activities include using current clinical situations from the day's experiences and pulling the current theory content threads out to interact with away from the bedside. This provides a nonthreatening atmosphere that is not time dependent and allows exploration in greater detail. For example, the week that fluid and electrolyte content is covered in class, the instructor could use the following steps.

Step 1.   Assign each student to look up abnormal lab values for every patient cared for.

Step 2.   Print the lab data and remove all patient identifiers.

Step 3.   Lay the lab data out on the table and ask each student to identify which are their patient's data.

Step 4.   Provide 10 minutes to do research before asking the students to report back to the group the implications these abnormalities have for the care they provided.

It will be instantly clear who included lab preparation within their preclinical preparation.

Example 3: Incorporating Evidence-Based Practice

Another example for postclinical conference learning and discussion would be incorporating evidence-based practice (EBP) into students' care for the day.

Step 1.   Students are instructed to bring an evidence-based research article that is related to some aspect of their patient's care.

Step 2.   Students present the research findings along with an example of how they incorporated the findings into their patient care with the clinical group.

Example 4: Peer-to-Peer Feedback

A fourth example for postclinical conference is peer-to-peer feedback. Guiding students through the process of critiquing each other's documentation emphasizes the significance of attention to detail and provides a model for future communication with professional peers. The ability to give and receive peer-to-peer feedback as students is a rehearsal for future practice as we prepare students for entry into peer interaction within their practice. Lundberg (2008) states:

> Relating clinical experiences to others helps students develop realistic expectations of their clinical skills and allows for immediate feedback from others, thus reinforcing their perceived abilities to function as a nurse. Shared stories are another form of peer modeling where other students can witness how their peers work through difficult situations. (p. 88)

Step 1.   Have students sit next to one another in pairs.

Step 2.   Provide each pair with a tool to analyze the written documentation they have completed during that clinical experience.

Step 3.   The students hand over their documentation to their peer; the peer evaluates it using the standardized tool.

Step 4.   Once the evaluation is complete, the peers share their findings and make suggestions for additions and corrections to the documentation. An innovative way to facilitate EBP learning by students is a more formal academic–clinical agency partnering process described by Susan Moch and colleagues (Moch, Quinn-Lee, Gallegos, & Sortedahl, 2015). This approach helps busy staff engage with students on a common project that ultimately benefits both agencies.

FIDeLity

Constructive feedback regarding the students' performance is an important part of the clinical educator's role. Fink (2003) provides an acronym, *FIDeLity*, to guide educators in providing this much-needed feedback.

FIDeLity:
*F*requent
*I*mmediate
*D*iscriminating (based on criteria and standards)
*D*one *L*ovingly (or supportively) (Fink, 2003)

As the instructor of record provides feedback to clinical students, she or he may wish to integrate the FIDeLity acronym as a communication tool.

F—Frequent

Fink (2003) describes the widespread practice of giving feedback only in the form of a midterm and a final grade as being insufficient. No matter how often feedback is provided, the students may request more. It is worth the instructor's time to elicit whether the feedback provided is meeting the students' needs or whether they require additional information.

I—Immediate

Utilizing a broad, open-ended question upon exiting the patient's room, such as "How do you think that went?," will allow the student the opportunity to reflect on his or her clinical performance. For instance, if the instructor has observed a break in sterile technique and the student did not self-correct, the instructor has to intervene at the bedside. If the student required excessive prompting during a procedure, the instructor needs to clearly articulate that the student is not performing up to speed. At this point it is the instructor's responsibility to design remediation activities away from the clinical site to provide additional opportunities for instruction and practice.

The problem with delayed feedback is that students cease to care about why their answer or activity was good or not. When the feedback comes a week or more after the learning activity, they just want to know, "Wha'd I get?" (Fink, 2003, p. 96).

D—Discriminating

Discriminating and distinguishing features of good and poor performance in ways that are clear to students are imperative. One way to accomplish this is in postclinical conference with the instructor asking the question, "What was the best part of your day, and what was the worst part of your day?" This will give students the opportunity to hear about their peers' issues and will provide a milieu for open sharing and debriefing. It is not uncommon for some experiences among students to be similar, and this provides opportunity for peer-to-peer feedback and support. This situation may result in confidence building in the growing professional. As Anderson and Kiger (2008) point out about students, "their experiences of managing in different situations [serve] to enhance their belief in themselves and their abilities" (p. 445). In addition, when giving feedback regarding written assignments, the instructor must provide detail as described by Fink (2003): "Knowing that their organization was good but their use of evidence and reasoning was poor provides more discriminating and useful feedback than either 'OK' or a 'B'" (p. 96).

L—Lovingly

Feedback delivered lovingly, with empathy and personal understanding, is an essential component in providing the feedback. Providing feedback by acknowledging students' feelings in their attempts to be successful communicates the instructor's personal empathy and understanding. There are times when the consequences of students' unsafe actions will result in their removal from the clinical setting. This may be one of the most challenging aspects of the clinical instructor role. An example of this type of feedback provided by the instructor to the student is, "I know you are trying, but you performed three unsafe actions in 3 hours, and I am dismissing you from clinical practice for the day."

Conducting the Clinical Day

Every instructor should develop a purposeful, organized method for conducting the clinical day. Typically, the structure is based on a plan for both instructor and students. Patient care assignments for each clinical experience must be tied to course objectives. The instructor will map his or her day by using a master sheet for jotting notes. This tool, which includes all aspects of patient care, helps the clinical instructor track and plan times for specific interventions such as medications and treatments. To ensure that interventions and medications are administered in a timely manner, restrictions will have to be placed on the number of students participating in direct patient care activities at one time. For instance, during a 12-hour shift, all eight students will have a medication administration experience; however, four students will give medications at the beginning of the shift while the remaining students will administer medications during the last 6 hours of the shift.

During this process, it is the responsibility of the student to keep the instructor and staff informed of the outcome(s) of the interventions implemented. Documentation is an important aspect of the learning activity and may be regulated by the clinical institution. Regardless of whether the student or the staff actually document in the medical record, it is the responsibility of the student to provide accurate and timely patient status reports. An additional responsibility of the instructor is to keep accurate anecdotal notes during the clinical day for use in formative and summative evaluations.

Anecdotal notes are an important tool for the clinical educator, as they can be used to evaluate the student's progress and are a critical component in the documentation process of formative and summative evaluation. A word of caution regarding written notes was given by Indar-Maraj (2007): "Teachers must carefully examine their value systems, philosophies and beliefs and not allow these to influence their evaluation of students" (p. 8). Recordkeeping of clinical student behaviors over time is captured in the form of instructor-generated anecdotal notes. Instructors may wish to develop a tool to be used during each clinical experience and that is directly related to the institution's formal clinical evaluation tool. (Refer to the sample formats for anecdotal notes shown in **Figures 21-3** and **21-4**.)

Pediatric Clinical Anecdotal Notes Form

Absences _____ Makeup work _____ Name _____

	WEEK 1	WEEK 2	WEEK 3	WEEK 4	WEEK 5	Family Assessment	Denver Developmental Screening Test	Physiological	Psych	Social	Spiritual

■ **Figure 21-3** Anecdotal notes form.

N4435 Level III Nursing Practicum

Clinical Evaluation: Daily Data Form

Student _____

Date _____ Unit _____

Assessment: Interaction(s) _____ Use of time _____ Activities _____

Use of standardized clinical tools _____ Thoroughness and depth in assessment _____

Evidence of preclinical prep _____ Level of thrp. comm. tech. _____

Adapts comm. to pt's state _____ Presentation of data at post conference _____

Meds: Name _____ Action _____ Dosage _____ S/E _____ S/E Obs _____ Nsg. Implic _____ **Lab** _____

Analysis: Level of clinical decision making _____ ID of Nsg. Dx/interventions/priorities _____

Planning: Realistic and measureable goals _____ Can formulate an in-depth plan of care _____

Takes initiative in planning pt/family education based on specific needs _____

Implementation: Ability to thrp. comm. _____ Awareness of specialty standards of practice _____

Communicates accurately verbally and in writing _____ Collaborates _____

Nursing actions evident today _____

Evaluation: Evaluates care provided and client outcomes _____

Evaluates all interventions for client and family response _____

Develops alternative interventions and goals when needs not/partially met _____

Professional Behaviors: Arrived on time _____ Compliance with dress code _____ Self-initiative/self-direction _____

Shows interest in learning _____ Seeks out learning experiences _____

Asks pertinent questions _____ Supportive/respectful of peers _____

Respects client confidentiality _____ Assumes responsibility for actions _____

Comments:

■ **Figure 21-4** Anecdotal note format.

Courtesy of Judy Howden, RN, PhD.

331

■ Student Issues

A hallmark of a good clinical educator is knowledge of the student's background and learning needs (Hanson & Stenvig, 2008). Emerging workforce generation characteristics were discussed in Chapter 3. In addition, instructional strategies must be tailored to the cognitive style of the student. This requires the educator to be flexible and adapt his or her teaching style to the needs of each student in the clinical setting (Noble, Miller, & Heckman, 2008). Cognitive styles were discussed previously in this text.

Hopkins (2008) found that early identification of at-risk nursing students is related to success and retention in their academic program. This early identification begins with the admissions process, where academic and nonacademic predictors can be utilized for student selection. Stinson (2009) recommends early intervention with students who are not doing well in clinical practice to improve their performance. It is prudent to have a clinical faculty member serve on the admissions committee, as the admission criteria can make or break the clinical experience for students. "Admission policies can either promote success or facilitate failure in a baccalaureate nursing program" (Newton, Smith, & Moore, 2007, p. 440). Once the program identifies which predictors of success are valid, the next step is to develop a model of student support. Academic institutions may have this additional support in the form of a success center or additional student services.

At times the clinical instructor may be called upon to manage a challenging student situation. The purpose of the following material is to address some issues that may challenge the clinical instructor. Setting and enforcing boundaries is a key element in establishing the instructor–student relationship. Although codes of ethics may initially be introduced in a theory course, it is in the clinical setting where students are bound to practice by these codes of ethics. Having students describe their ethical responsibilities during a certain clinical situation or having them discuss how they protected their patients' confidentiality are examples of integrating this concept into the clinical experience (Numminen, Leino-Kilpi, van der Arend, & Katajisto, 2010). By defining and maintaining clear boundaries, the instructor is role modeling behavior that will be expected in future practice. Setting emotional boundaries with the student will facilitate the educator's role in managing the clinical experience. Maintaining this professional boundary prevents the clinical instructor from ceding his or her power and getting off track with the student. Realize that maintaining this balance will require focus, vigilance, and self-awareness.

Unprofessional Behavior

One challenging student situation involves unprofessional behavior on the part of the student. This may be something that the clinical instructor observes while it is occurring, or it may be reported by someone else. This could range from a minor infraction such as nontherapeutic communication to a major issue such as a Health Insurance Portability and Accountability Act (HIPAA) violation. "Students should be engaged early-on in the significance of professional accountability for security and confidentiality related to information technology" (Day & Smith, 2007, p. 141). It is within the instructor's role to enforce compliance with professional issues such as tardiness, absence, and dress codes. Consistency among faculty related to enforcing policies such as these provides the student with a standardized approach and allows for integration of these professional behaviors over time. Infractions involving unprofessional behavior must be dealt with immediately: the student must be confronted with the issue and given the opportunity to problem-solve future prevention strategies. This is an appropriate time to explore with the student the question, "What would you do differently next time?" Many evaluation tools include professional behavior as a grading criterion, and any infraction may cause lowering of the final clinical grade.

Incivility

Incivility is a form of unprofessional behavior. Entry into professional practice requires individuals to conduct themselves with a professional demeanor. The instructor must role model these professional behaviors at all times. Defining clear guidelines and setting boundaries should begin on the first day of the clinical experience, as this will set the tone for the entire instructor–student interaction. Regardless of the instructor's clear expectations for professional behavior, there may be a student who is unable to conform. Uncivil acts such as challenges to faculty knowledge or credibility, general taunts or disrespect to faculty or other students, inappropriate e-mails or telephone conversations, vulgarity, harassing comments, and threats of physical harm are issues that require addressing and reporting through appropriate institutional channels. If the clinical instructor's interventions with the student are unsatisfactory, seeking the guidance of a more seasoned faculty member is a prudent strategy. One should never feel as though one is faced with decisions in isolation. According to Clark and Springer (2007), "Evidence suggests that incivility on American college campuses, ranging from insulting remarks and verbal abuse to violence, is a serious and growing concern" (p. 7).

> Emerging evidence suggests that incivility in the workplace has significant implications for nurses, patients, and health-care organizations. Because today's students are tomorrow's colleagues, conversations regarding how to address incivility and bullying should include specific aspects of nursing academia and the preparation of new nurses. (Luparell, 2011, p. 92)

Uncivil encounters disrupt the teaching–learning environment; therefore, it is incumbent upon clinical faculty members to help students learn to cope with conflict in healthy and constructive ways. Additionally, Clark (2010) points out that incivility can be inflicted upon a student by his or her instructor, which may result in long-term consequences such as fractured self-esteem. In her paper "Why Civility Matters," Clark (2010) states: "Civility is an authentic respect for others that requires time, presence, willingness to engage in genuine discourse and intention to seek common ground. Civility matters because treating one another with respect is requisite to communicating effectively, building community and creating high-functioning teams" (p. 7). More recently, Clark has developed a workplace civility index (2013b), a faculty civility index (2013a), and a student civility index (2013c), all of which can be utilized in the clinical setting for data collection and evaluation.

Two predictors of student satisfaction in the clinical learning environment found by Lovecchio et al. (2015) were task orientation and individualization. Faculty have the responsibility to plan specific assignments to meet clinical objectives, which then provides students with a structured work allocation. Individualization of students' clinical experiences as they advance in the program enhances independence and transition to professional practice.

Academic Dishonesty and Unethical Behavior (Honor Code)

Most institutions have an honor code. It is the responsibility of the clinical instructor to be familiar with and comply with the policy, as well as to report violations in a timely manner. Subsequently, when students choose to behave in an academically dishonest way, it becomes the educator's duty to assess whether the student can learn to think with a moral compass. If the answer is no, the student cannot behave ethically, so permitting the student to graduate and enter into the nursing profession should not be an option (Laduke, 2013, p. 405).

Altering charts or failing to report a mistake may result in patients experiencing negative outcomes. At times these aberrant behaviors may be a symptom of a more serious problem, such as chemical dependence, which may contribute to unsafe patient care. Reporting guidelines and testing of students for chemical usage may be covered by both agency and educational institution policies. For healthcare professionals, it is crucial that this moral development be examined for entry-level practice.

Safety

Safety in the clinical setting is imperative and is receiving unprecedented attention on several fronts. Due to the ethical imperative of "first, do no harm," the integration of quality and safety content into the clinical curriculum is paramount. Safety issues related to patient care center on near-misses and adverse events and require healthcare professionals to comply with a code of ethics. Reporting, investigating causal systems failures, and revealing the primary error to the physician and possibly the patient is a primary role of the healthcare professional (Lachman, 2007). It is the instructor's responsibility to assess each student's preparation for delivering safe patient care prior to the beginning of the clinical experience. If the instructor determines that the student is inadequately prepared, he or she may choose to dismiss the student from the clinical setting to prevent a breach in patient safety.

A breach in patient safety is commonly a critical point for failure in the clinical course. An example of this type of breach of safety is a student coming inadequately prepared for medication administration. As Harding and Petrick (2008) remind us, "The practice of purposefully incorporating medication safety knowledge throughout connected theory and practice courses" is beneficial to student learning (p. 47). Medication administration is an opportunity for the student to incorporate theory into practice. It is incumbent upon the clinical instructor to document and provide feedback to the student who has had a breach of patient safety. The clinical instructor must also follow agency guidelines for reporting such incidents. "Educators should monitor student errors and incidents over time (i.e., quality assurance determinants) to identify how education structures and processes are contributing to potential and actual student error" (Gregory, Guse, Davidson, & Russell, 2007, p. 81).

■ Evaluation of Clinical Learning

The purpose of evaluation is to help the student grow in his or her profession. Traditionally, evaluation has been looked upon as a negative or punitive act, and thus may be viewed as adversarial between the student and faculty member. This, however, is not the case, because evaluation is an opportunity for growth. The evaluation of clinical performance should not be subjective, because it is based on a standardized evaluation tool, and the instructor must collect data sufficient to weigh the evaluation against the behavioral outcomes over time.

Even though the instructor should have given oral and written feedback during the clinical day, a formal midterm and final evaluation of the student's performance are necessary to provide formative feedback and act as a mechanism for grade assignment. The purpose of formative evaluation is to provide specific and detailed feedback to the student and observe his or her ability or inability to integrate this feedback into his or her clinical practice. One of the goals of this formative evaluation is to allow students the opportunity to internalize the processes of self-reflection and self-discovery in their personal practice. It is hoped that this ongoing communication between students and instructor will promote insight into the strengths and weaknesses of each student's professional practice. Susan Luparell (2007) makes a good point when she encourages clinical instructors to "Say what you mean and mean what you say" (p. 105). Luparell also states, "In addition, the use of the sandwich approach when providing feedback may interfere with the student hearing the true message."

Sample formats for midterm evaluations, as shown in **Figures 21-5** and **21-6**, can be utilized as a means to provide specific formative feedback on clinical performance. Figure 21-5 is a narrative response tool where the instructor details areas of strengths and weaknesses to this point in the clinical experience. Figure 21-6 is an example of a tool that describes specific behavioral outcomes that the student must display in order to be a safe and effective care provider. Often, once they see a letter grade, students ask, "What can I do to improve my grade?" By receiving a list of outcome behaviors, the student has the opportunity to incorporate them into his or her practice. "Be specific" was a common phrase used by a colleague during midterm evaluations. She often wrote "increase specificity" on assignments, and the students would

BAYLOR UNIVERSITY, LOUISE HERRINGTON SCHOOL OF NURSING

Nursing 3425 Level II Clinical

Faculty:

Student Midterm Progress Report

Student: [Student Name]

Preparation for clinical experiences:

Assessment skills

Analysis *(application of physiologic and pathophysiologic concepts to clinical practice)*

Planning for care

Implementation of nursing interventions

Medications/IVs knowledge and administration

Patient/family education

Communication skills

Evaluation of care

Professionalism

Student signature: **Date:**

■ **Figure 21-5**   Student midterm progress report.

question what that meant. By providing specific examples, the instructor helped students understand what to do differently before repeating the assignment.

Anecdotal notes are an important means by which the clinical instructor can provide specific details regarding the student's performance that will require remediation, as well as documenting areas of superior performance. Hall, Daly, and Madigan (2010) reported that the majority of clinical nursing faculty use anecdotal notes on a weekly basis as a means for collecting data for summative evaluation. Cooke, Mitchell,

Expected Clinical Performance Behaviors

The following behaviors are examples of the expectations of students in Practicum III, and are based on the Baylor University Louise Herrington School of Nursing (BULHSON) Clinical Performance Evaluation tool.

Assessment

1. **Collects data through appropriate physical assessment techniques**

   a. Assessment data is collected independently by student and reflects consistent application of principles taught in NUR 3314.

   b. Techniques and equipment are used correctly throughout collection of assessment data.

   c. Student demonstrates awareness of any deficiencies he or she may have in physical assessment skills and seeks opportunities/assistance to remedy these deficiencies.

   d. Physical assessment skills reflect an in-depth knowledge of anatomy and physiology.

   e. Physical assessment data collections are adapted correctly/appropriately for the client in the pediatric and psych settings.

2. **Collects data (subjective and objective) from available resources**

   a. All references/resources utilized for practicum experiences/written work are from appropriate, practice-specific professional nursing texts, journal articles, or resources recommended by faculty. References are recent (within past 5 years) and reflect current research.

   b. All references/resources used for practicum experiences/written work are specific to needs of assigned clients/families.

   c. Student uses agency policies and procedures as guidelines for data collection.

   d. Advanced interviewing skills are used to collect in-depth data from the client/family.

   e. Before utilizing data from staff, student will validate those findings in assessment of the client/family.

   f. Data collection from the chart reflects in-depth understanding of information recorded.

   g. All pertinent diagnostic/lab/screening values are noted and analyzed. Results not on chart are obtained from computer or lab via phone.

   h. The student is aware of all current medical and nursing orders for the patient.

   i. The student continuously assesses the patient/family environment.

   j. The student demonstrates an awareness of the nursing unit environment in terms of where supplies, equipment, and resources are located.

3. **Documents assessment data in a clear and organized manner**

   a. All documentation of data is obtained from student's own assessment.

   b. Documentation of assessment data is thorough and is entered in the chart in a timely/correct manner using charting standards for agency.

   c. The student takes the initiative to chart data on all unit-specific and client-specific flow sheets.

4. **Shows evidence of pre-clinical preparation**

   a. Student consistently has required database/worksheet completed prior to the beginning of each clinical day.

   b. Student can verbalize to instructor an appropriate plan of nursing care specific to the patient/family at the beginning of the clinical day.

   c. Student demonstrates in-depth knowledge of physiologic and pathophysiologic concepts applicable to assigned client.

   d. Student demonstrates knowledge of all medications (routine, one-time, as needed) ordered for the client or that the client has recently received at the beginning of the clinical day. Student only has to look up newly ordered medications during the practicum day.

■ **Figure 21-6**   Expected clinical performance behaviors.

(continues)

e. Student demonstrates preparedness for nursing procedures that he/she may perform for the patient.

f. Student has reviewed appropriate resources; that is, information from Baylor School of Nursing skills lab (NUR 3414), Medical City procedure manuals, skills discussed in required or reserved materials specific to this course, or other resources as designated by the instructor.

g. Student takes the initiative to obtain information from staff nurse (during report) needed to care for client/family.

h. Student comes prepared for clinical day with needed equipment.

Analysis

1. **Clinical decision making reflects an understanding of the relationships of assessment data to the client's problem/diagnosis**

   a. Student can verbalize or describe in written work an in-depth understanding of client/family condition/ status based on accurate synthesis of data collected in relation to nursing theory base.

   b. Student takes initiative during the clinical day to discuss with instructor the meaning of assessment findings and implications for clinical decisions. Student can analyze situation with minimal cues from instructor.

2. **Identifies priorities requiring nursing actions based on assessment and determines when reassessment is indicated**

   a. Student consistently verbalizes in clinical setting, or documents in written work, the most important client/family needs that require nursing action. This is based on sound nursing theory and nursing assessment/reassessment data, and incorporates collaboration with client/family.

3. **Formulates nursing diagnosis based on assessment data**

   a. All nursing diagnoses are based on active client/family problems that are pertinent while student is present in the clinical setting.

   b. Student utilizes appropriate format for writing nursing diagnoses, as taught in NUR 3310.

   c. Etiology portions of the nursing diagnoses are always based on problems that can be alleviated with nursing interventions.

   d. Student's written work or verbalization demonstrates accurate assessment data to support the diagnoses.

   e. Student comes prepared for the clinical day with appropriate nursing diagnoses as required.

Planning

1. **Formulates appropriate and measurable goals for self and client**

   a. Student verbalizes at the beginning of or during the clinical day (or includes in written work) measurable client/family goals based on data analysis. As data analysis fluctuates or changes, student can revise patient/family goals. Goals formulated by the student are realistic and achievable during the time period the student cares for the family.

   b. Student can consistently verbalize or document in written work personal goals that will enhance nursing care and contribute to own professional growth. Student takes initiative to actively achieve these goals.

2. **Plans care in a systematic, logical, organized manner**

   a. The student is able to articulate an in-depth plan of holistic nursing care to the instructor at any time during the clinical day. This is also consistently reflected in written work.

   b. The plan of care is flexible enough to meet patient/family needs in a timely manner and coincides with plans/activities of other healthcare personnel.

   c. The student is able to consistently verbalize rationale for each nursing activity within the plan of care.

   d. All plans of care are consistent with procedural guidelines for specific nursing units at the agency.

■ **Figure 21-6** Expected clinical performance behaviors. (*continued*)

3. **Plans health teaching based on identified learning needs and readiness of client**

   a. The student can independently interview client/family to determine/assess actual learning needs and plan to meet those needs.

   b. Patients/families under the student's care are consistently evaluated for readiness and understanding before nursing care activities are performed.

   c. The student demonstrates the ability to develop in-depth teaching plans for specific client/family learning needs, based on concepts taught in NUR 3222.

   d. Patient/family health teaching is an ongoing process during the care provided by the student.

   e. The student demonstrates preparation for anticipated client/family learning needs.

   f. All health teaching is based on current nursing theory and is planned at an appropriate developmental stage/knowledge base of the client/family.

   g. The student keeps the instructor informed of planned or incidental health teaching the instructor can observe.

   h. Student uses agency resources (computer programs, videotapes, teaching manuals) with clients and families.

4. **Communicates clearly regarding nursing care plan (NCP) with all appropriate individuals**

   a. The family is informed by the student of his/her plan of care at the beginning of the shift and on an ongoing basis. The client and/or family is informed of the student's scope of responsibility.

   b. The student informs the staff nurse of all assessment and care he/she will provide at the beginning of and throughout the clinical day.

   c. The student takes initiative on the unit to enhance learning experiences without compromising assigned patient care.

   d. The student consistently takes initiative to keep the staff and instructor informed of the plan of nursing care and changes in that plan.

Implementation

1. **Utilizes effective and appropriate verbal/nonverbal communication skills**

   a. Student communication with clients/families is consistently goal-oriented.

   b. Student demonstrates advanced skill in establishing rapport and effective communication with client/families who have complex/complicated interactive behaviors.

   c. Student is aware of and able to modify personal barriers/behaviors that can interfere with therapeutic communication.

   d. Student is able to maintain a level of objectivity while establishing rapport and trust with client/family.

   e. Student demonstrates behavior that promotes confidence of the patient/family in the student's skills.

   f. Student is able to continue therapeutic communication as appropriate with client/family in the presence of nurse, instructor, physician, or other health team members.

2. **Provides direct patient care in a safe, accurate, organized manner**

   a. Student's care consistently provides for client safety. The student demonstrates anticipation of patient behaviors that could compromise health/safety and plans care accordingly.

   b. All care provided reflects the nursing diagnosis and patient/family needs and is based on appropriate nursing theory.

   c. The student demonstrates an ability to anticipate supplies/equipment, etc., needed for care and has items needed readily available.

   d. The student demonstrates critical thinking skills in carrying out nursing care in a logical, patient-centered manner.

(continues)

  e. The student consistently calculates medication and intravenous (IV) fluid dosages correctly without assistance and in a timely manner. The student can determine safe dosage ranges without assistance.

  f. The student notifies the instructor of all procedures for which the instructor needs to be present.

  g. The student assumes responsibility for keeping the patient's environment orderly, safe, equipped with needed supplies, and esthetically appropriate.

3. **Administers medications safely according to established procedure**

  a. Student consistently observes "5 rights" in administering all medications, IV solutions, etc.

  b. Student notifies instructor of all medications to be administered.

  c. Student verbalizes to instructor, without prompting, the following information regarding medications the patient has recently received, medications the student is administering, or those the patient has ordered:

   i. Classification of drug

   ii. Purpose of medication for patient

   iii. Safe and correct dose

   iv. How drug acts/pharmacology of drug

   v. Potential drug interactions

   vi. Pertinent side effects the patient may experience and how the student will manage potential side effects

   vii. How the drug will be administered; that is, drip rate, type of syringe to be used, how client currently takes medication, etc.

   viii. Client/family teaching that will be needed regarding medication

   ix. Nursing implications for administration of drug

   x. Student's plan for monitoring drug effectiveness and side effects

   xi. Developmental considerations of medication

  d. Student demonstrates proficiency in all aspects of medication administration and documentation.

4. **Communicates accurately verbally and in writing (charting and reporting)**

  a. Student's charting provides thorough documentation of nursing care provided. The charting consistently reflects action taken when assessment is abnormal.

  b. All health teaching is consistently documented on appropriate forms.

  c. All charting reflects appropriate medical/nursing abbreviations, correct grammar, and correct spelling.

  d. Student consistently takes initiative to keep staff nurse informed of nursing interventions, patient/family status, etc. Student reviews his/her charting with staff nurse when reporting off.

  e. Student consistently reports off to appropriate staff nurse without being reminded.

  f. Student immediately reports to new nurse if there is a change in the patient's primary nurse assignment during the clinical day.

  g. The student's documentation follows agencies charting procedures.

5. **Collaborates with client/family/health team and other appropriate individuals**

  a. Student consistently informs nurse and instructor at outset and throughout shift of his/her plan for care, medication administration, charting, and referral needs.

  b. The student takes the initiative to discuss clarification of medical orders with the appropriate nurse and physician.

  c. The student takes the initiative as appropriate to consult with other health team members (e.g., physician, social worker, child life specialist, dietitian, etc.) to validate his/her plan of care.

■ **Figure 21-6**   Expected clinical performance behaviors.   (*continued*)

d. The student provides nursing care in which the client and family are active participants.

e. Care provided by the student consistently reflects an integration of individual family member needs to promote family growth.

Evaluation

1. **Uses evaluation appropriately in the nursing process (utilizes data to validate if identified goals are met)**

   a. Student consistently evaluates the results of the care provided in relation to the outcome criteria established for the patient/family goals. Student documents all data regarding outcomes.

   b. Student demonstrates objectivity in evaluation process.

2. **Evaluates effectiveness of specific interventions**

   a. Student consistently observes for side effects of and patient response to all medications and therapies the patient is receiving.

   b. Individual nursing actions are evaluated and documented on a consistent basis.

   c. Client/family response to care provided is observed and documented.

   d. Evaluation and documentation of client/family education is in measurable terms.

3. **Develops alternate interventions and goals when appropriate**

   a. The student demonstrates awareness of and planning for differing outcomes. The student can verbalize in advance alternate nursing interventions for these outcomes.

   b. Student demonstrates the proper course of action that should be taken if the client experiences ineffective response or adverse reaction to (1) specific therapies (e.g., medications, IV therapy, blood products, etc.), or (2) normal process of adaptation.

   c. The student can implement alternate interventions while demonstrating flexibility, objectivity, timely organization, and professionalism.

Professional Behaviors

1. The student demonstrates promptness in attendance at all clinical experiences, post-conferences, and seminars.

2. The student consistently demonstrates honesty and integrity in the provision of care and his/her clinical performance.

3. The student will adhere to professional behaviors as listed in the NUR 4435 syllabus.

4. The student's behavior in the clinical setting consistently reflects maturity; responsibility for own actions; and respect for patients, staff, instructors, and peers.

5. The student assumes responsibility for adherence to verbal and written guidelines set forth by individual faculty members in the pediatric, psych, and community settings.

6. The student consistently demonstrates professional behavior and a pleasant demeanor despite personal problems/concerns/issues.

Moyle, Henderson, and Murfield (2010) suggest the use of a clinical progression portfolio format to capture students' progress in clinical practice.

The final clinical evaluation allows the instructor to analyze and deliver to students the progress of their clinical performance over time. This summative event prepares students to move forward in their program with guided input regarding their current state of practice. Assigning a grade plays an important role in determining whether competencies have been met during directly supervised clinical experiences (Amicucci, 2012). Although the tools are standardized, it is important for the clinical instructor to individualize his or her evaluation comments.

Edgecombe and Bowden (2009) remind us that "[l]earning outcomes [are] expressed as both intrinsic and extrinsic" (p. 97). The summative evaluation will examine students' ability to meet the course objectives that were imposed by the program curriculum. The intrinsic objectives of each student's personal need to learn upon exposure to nursing practice in the clinical environment should also be documented and discussed. To prepare for final clinical evaluations, an appointment time should be scheduled, which is agreed upon with both the faculty member and each student. The meeting place should be private because the evaluation content and conversation should remain confidential. When a student arrives for the evaluation, a copy of the completed tool is provided for the student to read and sign, following any discussion of reflective practice, clarification of evaluative comments, and an opportunity for self-appraisal on the part of the student. When meeting with students to give midterm and final evaluations, it is a good practice to have two clinically based faculty members present. This could be two faculty members who have simultaneously taught the student during the evaluation period, or two faculty members from the same content domain. This practice validates for the student the significance of the evaluation comments and provides for physical and emotional safety of the primary instructor in case the evaluation becomes emotionally charged.

Learning contracts or clinical practice warning forms are documents used by clinical instructors to delineate unsafe clinical practice or a breach in professional practice. These contracts become a part of the evaluation process and typically include a remediation plan. The purpose of these learning contracts is to provide additional structure and clear communication as to what the student must do to be successful in the clinical course. Orientation for clinical faculty assists in their providing effective clinical instruction. For example, use of a clinical warning form to document inadequate, unsafe student performance may help with optimal formative and summative evaluation of a struggling student, in that it creates a paper trail for legal purposes and an educational wake-up call for the student (Beitz & Wieland, 2005, p. 44). As Barrington and Street (2009) found in their research regarding learner contracts, these tools improved learner–faculty communication and reflection on learning. For a sample document regarding safety in the clinical setting, refer to **Figure 21-7**. For an example of how to record a breach in professional behavior, refer to **Figure 21-8**.

Writing and delivering the learning contract to the student who is not performing at an acceptable level should not be a contentious process, but it should be presented in a clear and compassionate manner. The clinical instructor cannot ensure success solely through the use of the contract, but is responsible for designing the plan for success. The learning contract outlines the roles both instructor and student play in any additional remediation sessions that may take place outside the clinical setting. Part of the process for implementing the learning contract is to provide the student with feedback during each clinical experience. This may be referred to as meeting or not meeting the terms of the contract. If safety issues are not remediated,

BAYLOR UNIVERSITY LOUISE HERRINGTON SCHOOL OF NURSING STANDARDS OF SAFE CLINICAL PRACTICE

In all clinical situations students are expected to demonstrate responsibility and accountability as professional nurses with the ultimate goal being safe patient care. The Baylor University Louise Herrington School of Nursing (LHSON) believes that this goal will be attained if each student's daily clinical practice is guided by the Standards of Safe Clinical Practice that always includes, but is not limited to, the following behaviors.

The student will:

1. Know and conform to the Texas Nursing Practice Act and Texas Board of Nursing rules and regulations as well as all federal, state, or local laws, rules, or regulations.
2. Adhere to the American Nurses Association (ANA) Code of Ethics.
3. Adhere to Health Information Portability and Accountability Act (HIPAA) and institutional privacy practices.
4. Prepare for clinical learning assignments according to course requirements and as determined for the specific clinical setting.
5. Practice within the boundaries of the nursing student role as established by the LHSON and the assigned agencies.
6. Provide nursing care required to promote health and prevent illness or further complications.
7. Demonstrate the application of previously learned skills and principles in a safe manner while providing nursing care.
8. Administer medications and/or treatments in a safe manner according to guidelines provided by LHSON and the assigned clinical agency.
9. Promptly report significant client information in a clear, accurate, and complete oral or written manner to the appropriate person(s).
10. Comply with institutional policies and procedures when implementing nursing care.
11. Meet the clinical expectations as outlined in the course syllabus and the LHSON Clinical Performance Evaluation Tool.

I have read the Baylor University Louise Herrington School of Nursing Standards of Safe Clinical Practice, Texas Nursing Practice Act Rules 217.11 and 217.12, ANA Code of Ethics, HIPAA, and clinical course syllabus. I understand that these standards are expectations that guide my clinical practice and will be incorporated into the evaluation of my clinical performance in all clinical courses. Failure to meet these standards may result in my removal from the clinical area, which may result in clinical and course failure.

Student signature and date: _____

Student printed name: _____

■ **Figure 21-7**   Clinical safety contract.

the student may not be allowed to continue in the clinical setting, which may result in a course failure.

Nurse educators need to be fully present with students who are at risk of failing clinical courses in ways that foster personal and professional growth, rather than distancing themselves. This is not easy work. As educators, we are inclined to disconnect from students to protect our own vulnerability, particularly when performance issues arise (McGregor, 2007, p. 509). Ultimately the student must display the outcome behaviors necessary for success in the course, which are directly related to the

Baylor University Louise Herrington School of Nursing Professional Behaviors Student Counseling Record

Student: **Instructor:**
Date: **Course:**

Data Record and Statement of the Problem
Noncompliance with course expectations and performance standards for NXXXX, level XX related to professional behaviors

Date and time of occurrence: [Faculty comments added here.]

Description of occurrence: [Faculty comments added here.]

Course Expectations and Performance Standards
As professionals, students are expected to demonstrate professional behaviors as listed in the course syllabus.

- Project a positive image through the use of language, accountability, behavior, and appearance.
- Demonstrate professional behaviors at all times during the clinical experience (arrives on time, respects client confidentiality, assumes responsibility for own actions, is in appropriate uniform with pertinent equipment, etc.).
- Demonstrate an active role in own learning process (shows interest in learning experience, seeks out learning opportunities, and asks pertinent questions).

Student Goals
The student will adhere to professional behaviors. [Faculty comments added here.]

Student Responsibilities
1. The student will review professional behaviors in the NUR XXXX syllabus, Level XXX Clinical Evaluation Tool, LHSON Student Information Guide, and Baylor University Student Policies and Procedures found at http://www.baylor.edu/student_policies.
2. The student will implement chain of command as necessary.

Faculty/Instructor Responsibilities
The instructor will continue to be available during clinical and business hours to answer any questions concerning the clinical experience, which includes, but is not limited to, professional behaviors.

Evaluation
Failure to demonstrate any of the clinical professional behaviors outlined in the NUR XXXX syllabus, Level XXX Clinical Performance Evaluation Tool, LHSON Student Information Guide, Baylor University Student Policies and Procedures, and/or this Student Counseling Record may result in the lowering of the numerical grade and/or a failure of the course.

Instructor Comments

Student Signature: _____   Date: _____
Instructor Signature: _____   Date: _____

THE ORIGINAL COPY OF THIS FORM MUST BE GIVEN TO THE UNDERGRADUATE PROGRAM DIRECTOR WITHIN 24 HOURS OF COMPLETION.

■ **Figure 21-8**   Student counseling record.

standardized final clinical evaluation tool. The learning contract is signed by both clinical instructor and student, and a copy is placed in the student's academic file.

Clinical Practice Failure

Clinical practice failure is the lack of clinical competence and the inability of the student to meet the course objectives. Issues such as unsafe clinical practice, unprofessional behaviors, poor attendance, inability to implement appropriate interventions, falsification of patient records, omissions in documentation, nontherapeutic communication, and errors in medication administration are all examples of critical elements of practice that may result in clinical practice failure. "Not all nursing students can be successful, yet when failure is the outcome, students' dignity, self-worth and future possibilities must be preserved" (McGregor, 2007, p. 504). Some clinical practice failures indicate that the student needs more exposure or time in the clinical setting to be successful.

There are implications for clinical instructors as well as their students when clinical practice failures occur. From the student's perspective, the failure may result in a wake-up call that leads to revising his or her strategies for success throughout the remainder of the clinical experiences. A second outcome for the student may be the revelation that the particular health profession is not for him or her, at which time he or she may choose to revise his or her degree plan. At other times, the student may become angry and blame his or her failure on the clinical instructor. This student reaction will have implications for the clinical instructor, as he or she may become a part of an appeals process. Rutkowski (2007) reminds us that assessing nursing students' competence during practice placements may result in a clinical practice failure. Safeguarding the public is the goal of safe clinical practice. Each healthcare professional's code of conduct must be the standard against which competency is measured. McGregor (2007) summarizes the picture of clinical practice failure by stating: "In the face of a clinical failure, what really matters is how the student and the teacher interact. When tensions about clinical performance arise, teachers need to become partners who stand with, rather than against, vulnerable students who are struggling to become competent nurses" (p. 510). For more detailed information on an evaluation session, please see Chapter 28.

Clinical Practice Success

The ultimate goal of clinical teaching is clinical practice success for the student. This means the student has met the objectives of the course and is ready to progress in the program or into the workforce. Creating supportive clinical learning environments, utilizing interprofessional mentoring, infusing evidence-based practice at the bedside, honing interpersonal skills with patients and families, and incorporating reflective practice on a daily basis are all pillars that provide the foundation for the clinical professional to focus on and overcome challenges that are constantly present in the ever-changing healthcare environment. Students who have inherited a passion for lifelong learning from their clinical instructors will be well equipped and resilient to meet the demands as they grow in their professional roles.

■ Conclusion: Light at the End of the Tunnel

The outcomes of our teaching experience directly advance our chosen healthcare profession. It is continually rewarding to write letters of recommendation for students as they enter the clinical practice arena and prepare for graduate school. The ebb and flow of the academic calendar can provide a predictable schedule for those who like a beginning and ending point to their work. The clinical practice day may be unpredictable and the generation of learners may change, but clinical teaching still provides a stimulating and rewarding practice field.

Discussion Questions

1. What are the key components of a healthcare professional's clinical teaching role?
2. What tools can a clinical instructor utilize to evaluate a student's clinical decision making?
3. How can the keeping of anecdotal notes by the clinical instructor affect the summative evaluation process?

References

Amicucci, B. (2012). What nurse faculty have to say about clinical grading. *Teaching and Learning in Nursing, 7*, 51–55. doi:doi.org/10.1016/j.teln.2011.09.002

Anderson, E., & Kiger, A. M. (2008). "I felt like a real nurse": Student nurses out on their own. *Nurse Education Today, 28*(4), 443–449.

Barrington, K., & Street, K. (2009). Learner contracts in nurse education: Interaction within the practice context. *Nurse Education and Practice, 9*, 109–118.

Bartels, J. (2007). Preparing nursing faculty for baccalaureate-level and graduate-level nursing programs: Role preparation for the academy. *Journal of Nursing Education, 46*(4), 154–158.

Baxter, P. E., & Boblin, S. L. (2007). The moral development of baccalaureate nursing students: Understanding unethical behavior in classroom and clinical settings. *Journal of Nursing Education, 46*(1), 20–27.

Beitz, J., & Wieland, D. (2005). Analyzing the teaching effectiveness of clinical nursing faculty of full and part time generic BSN, LPN-BSN, and RN-BSN nursing students. *Journal of Professional Nursing, 21*(1), 32–45.

Boyer, E. L. (1990). *Scholarship reconsidered: Priorities of the profession.* New Youk: NY: Carnegie Foundation for the Advancement of Teaching.

Buccieri, K. M., Brown, R., & Malta, S. (2011). Evaluating the performance of the academic coordinator/director of clinical education: Developing tools to solicit input from program directors, academic faculty, and students. *Journal of Physical Therapy Education, 25*(2), 26–35.

Clark, C. (2010). Why civility matters. *Reflections on Nursing Leadership, 36*(1), 4.

Clark, C. (2013a). Clark Civility Index for faculty© Presentation at the 2013 Assessment Technologies Institute, LLC (ATI), Nurse Educator Summit, Las Vegas, NV.

Clark, C. (2013b). *Creating and sustaining civility in nursing education.* Indianapolis, IN: Sigma Theta Tau International Publishing.

Clark, C. (2013c). Two-part series: Fostering civility in nursing education and practice. Part II—Cindy's "Five RITES" for fostering student-driven civility. *Reflections on Nursing Leadership, 39*(1). Retrieved from http://www.reflectionsonnursingleadership.org/Pages/Vol39_1_Clark_5RITES.aspx

Clark, C., & Springer, P. J. (2007). Incivility in nursing education: A descriptive study of definitions and prevalence. *Journal of Nursing Education, 46*(1), 7–44.

Cooke, M., Mitchell, M., Moyle, W., Henderson, A., & Murfield, J. (2010). Application and student evaluation of a clinical progression portfolio: A pilot. *Nurse Education in Practice, 10*, 227–232.

Day, L., & Smith, L. (2007). Integrating quality and safety content into clinical teaching in the acute care setting. *Nursing Outlook, 55*(3), 138–143.

DiVall, M., Kolbig, L., Carney, M., Kirwin, K., Letzeiser, C., & Mohammed, S. (2014). Interprofessional socializations: A way to introduce collaborative competencies to first-year health science students. *Journal of Interprofessional Care, 28*(6), 576–578.

Edgecombe, K., & Bowden, M. (2009). The ongoing search for best practice in clinical teaching and learning: A model of nursing students' evolution to proficient novice registered nurses. *Nurse Education and Practice, 9*, 91–101.

Esmaeili, M., Cheraghi, M., Salasali, M., & Ghiyasvandian, S. (2014). Nursing students' expectations regarding effective clinical education: A qualitative study. *International Journal of Nursing Practice, 20*(5), 460–467.

Fink, L. (2003). *Creating significant learning experiences.* San Francisco, CA: Jossey-Bass.

Gregory, D. M., Guse, L. W., Davidson, D., & Russell, C. K. (2007). Patient safety: Where is nursing education? *Journal of Nursing Education, 46*(2), 79–82.

Hall, M. A., Daly, B. J., & Madigan, E. A. (2010). Use of anecdotal notes by clinical nursing faculty: A descriptive study. *Journal of Nursing Education, 49*(3), 156–159. doi:10.3928/01484834-20090915-03

Hanson, K. J., & Stenvig, T. E. (2008). The good clinical nursing educator and the baccalaureate nursing clinical experience: Attributes and praxis. *Journal of Nursing Education, 47*(1), 38–42.

Harding, L., & Petrick, T. (2008). Nursing student medication errors: A retrospective review. *Journal of Nursing Education, 47*(1), 43–47.

Hauer, M., & Kogan, J. R. (2012). Realizing the potential value of feedback. *Medical Education, 46*(2), 140–142. doi:10.1111/j.1365-2923.2011.04180.x

Hellstrom-Hyson, E., Martensson, G., & Kristofferzon, M. (2012). To take responsibility or to be an onlooker: Nursing students' experiences of two models of supervision. *Nurse Education Today, 32*(1), 105–110.

Hoffman, J. (2008). Teaching strategies to facilitate nursing students' critical thinking. In M. Oermann (Ed.), *Annual review of nursing education* (6th ed., pp. 225–236). New York, NY: Springer.

Hopkins, T. H. (2008). Early identification of at-risk nursing students: A student support model. *Journal of Nursing Education, 47*(6), 254–259.

Indar-Maraj, M. (2007). Clinical evaluation of nursing students: Challenges and solutions. *MedSurg Matters, 16*(4), 6–8.

Labrague, L., McEnroe-Petite, D., Papathansiou, I., Edet, O., & Arulappan, J. (2015). Impact of instructor's caring on students' perceptions of their own caring behaviors. *Journal of Nursing Scholarship, 47*(4), 338–346.

Lachman, V. (2007). Patient safety: The ethical imperative. *MedSurg Nursing, 16*(6), 401–403.

Laduke, R. (2013). Academic dishonesty today, unethical practices tomorrow. *Journal of Professional Nursing, 29*(6), 402–406.

Lovecchio, C., DiMattio, M., & Hudacek, S. (2015). Predictors of undergraduate nursing student satisfaction. *Nursing Education Perspectives, 36*(4), 252–254.

Lundberg, K. (2008). Promoting self-confidence in clinical nursing students. *Nurse Educator, 33*(2), 86–89.

Luparell, S. (2007). Managing difficult student situations: Lessons learned. In M. Oermann & K. Heinrich (Eds.), *Annual review of nursing education* (pp. 101–110). New York, NY: Springer.

Luparell, S. (2011). Incivility in nursing: The connection between academia and clinical settings. *Critical Care Nurse, 31*(2), 92–95.

MacGowan, M. (2010). Finding and integrating the best available evidence into the group work field practicum: Examples and experiences from MSW students. *Social Work with Groups, 33*(2–3), 210–228.

McGregor, A. (2007). Academic success, clinical failure: Struggling practices of a failing student. *Journal of Nursing Education, 46*(11), 504–511.

Megel, M., Nelson, A., Black, J., Vogel, J., & Uphoff, M. (2013). A comparison of student and faculty perceptions of clinical post-conference learning environment. *Nurse Education Today, 33*, 525–529.

Melo, K., Williams, B., & Ross, C. (2010). The impact of nursing curricula on clinical practice today. *Nurse Education Today, 30*(8), 773–778.

Moch, S., Quinn-Lee, L., Gallegos, C., & Sortedahl, C. (2015). Navigating evidence-based practice projects: The faculty role. *Nursing Education Perspectives, 36*(2), 128–130.

Morris, T., & Hancock, D. (2013). Institute of Medicine core competencies as a foundation for nursing program evaluation. *Nursing Education Research, 34*(1), 29–33.

Naber, J., Hall, J., & Schadler, C. (2014). Narrative thematic analysis of baccalaureate nursing students' reflections: Critical thinking in the clinical education context. *Journal of Nursing Education, 53*(9), S90–S96.

Newton, J. M., Cross, W., White, K., Ockerby, C., & Billett, S. (2011). Outcomes of a clinical partnership model for undergraduate nursing students. *Contemporary Nurse: A Journal for the Australian Nursing Profession, 39*(1), 119–127.

Newton, S., Smith, L., & Moore, G. (2007). Baccalaureate nursing program admission policies: Promoting success or facilitating failure? *Journal of Nursing Education, 46*(10), 439–511.

Noble, K. A., Miller, S. M., & Heckman, J. (2008). The cognitive style of nursing students: Educational implications for teaching and learning. *Journal of Nursing Education, 47*(6), 245–253.

Nottingham, S., & Henning, J. (2010). Provision of feedback to students, Part 1: Overview of strategies. *Athletic Therapy Today, 15*(5), 19–21.

Numminen, O. H., Leino-Kilpi, H., van der Arend, A., & Katajisto, J. (2010). Nurse educators' teaching of codes of ethics. *Nurse Education Today, 30*(2), 124–131. doi:doi.org/10.1016/j.nedt.2009.06.011

Ruth-Sahd, L. A. (2011). Student nurse dyads create a community of learning: Proposing a holistic clinical education theory. *Journal of Advanced Nursing, 67*(11), 2445–2454.

Rutkowski, K. (2007). Failure to fail: Assessing nursing students' competence during practice placements. *Nursing Standard, 22*(13), 35–40.

Skaalvik, M. W., Normann, H. K., & Henriksen, N. (2010). To what extent does the oral shift report stimulate learning among nursing students? A qualitative study. *Journal of Clinical Nursing, 19*(15–16), 2300–2308.

Spurr, S., Bally, J., & Ferguson, L. (2010). A framework for clinical teaching: A passion-centered philosophy. *Nurse Education in Practice, 10*, 349–354. doi:10.1016/j.nepr.2010.05.002

Stinson, S. (2009, Spring). Maximizing minority students' success in clinical. *Minority Nurse*, 1–5. Retrieved from CINAHL with full-text database.

Wetherbee, E., Peatman, N., Kenney, D., Cusson, M., & Applebaum, D. (2010, October). Standards for clinical education: A qualitative study. *Journal of Physical Therapy Education*. Retrieved from http://www.highbeam.com/doc/1P3-2279669081.html

CHAPTER 22

The Preceptored Clinical Experience

Brian M. French
Miriam Greenspan

The preceptored clinical experience provides an opportunity for students, new graduate clinicians, experienced clinicians new to a work setting or practice area, or others to work with an experienced staff member to begin socialization and role transition, as well as gain exposure to the healthcare arena. This experiential teaching and learning methodology provides clear benefits to the learner, preceptor, school, and healthcare setting.

■ Definition and Purposes

In 15th-century England, the word *preceptor* was first used to identify a tutor or instructor. The term first appeared in the nursing literature in the mid-1970s (Peirce, 1991). The more recent use of the term *preceptorship* denotes an experience lasting a designated period of time, during which an experienced clinician or preceptor enters into a one-on-one relationship with a novice clinician learner (the *student, preceptee,* or *orientee*) to assist the novice in the transition from learner to practitioner (Baggot, Hensinger, Parry, Valdes, & Zaim, 2005; Benner, Tanner, & Chesla, 1996; Marcum & West, 2004; O'Malley, Cunliffe, Hunter, & Breeze, 2000). The preceptorship is a process during which the preceptor, through role modeling, information sharing, coaching, and direction, teaches the preceptee the art of professional practice. The precepted clinical experience is a planned and organized instructional program with specific objectives and goals. It can be useful in supporting the learning process of students at all levels during a clinical, management, education, or research practicum. Other uses include orienting new graduate clinicians or experienced clinicians transferring between clinical areas. Visitors to the clinical area, such as clinicians from another country seeking exposure to the U.S. healthcare system and roles, can also benefit from being precepted.

Students' precepted experiences typically take place within a capstone clinical course during the latter part of the curriculum. Such a course might be designed to promote synthesis of theoretical knowledge, allow for more in-depth study of a specific patient population, and apply evidence-based research to the clinical practice area. In addition, preceptors can assist students to demonstrate leadership and collaborative skills and provide experiences to enhance understanding of organizational behavior as well as ethical, legal, economic, and political issues.

Preceptorship is often used as a way of facilitating the role transition of novice clinicians. Preceptorship can also be used as a methodology for orienting experienced clinicians who are new to a particular patient population or institutional setting. This offers the clinician learner the opportunity to apply previously acquired knowledge in an experiential manner while safely accumulating new knowledge and experiences for future reference (Benner et al., 1996). During the preceptorship, a partnership in which both the preceptor and the preceptee contribute to the outcome is formed (Godinez, Schweiger, Gruver, & Ryan, 1999; O'Malley et al., 2000). The partnership becomes an ongoing mutual exchange between the preceptor and the learner, in a mutually trusting, supportive environment. The preceptor offers information, direction, and feedback, and the preceptee offers insight about personal goals, learning needs, and learning styles. During the preceptorship, both the student and the graduate clinician learn the rules, language, and behaviors of the work environment (Godinez et al., 1999; Horsburgh, 1989; O'Malley et al., 2000; Tradewell, 1996).

The preceptored experience differs from spend-the-day shadowing experiences or informal pairing relationships that are typically geared toward providing a broad exposure to the healthcare environment or toward promoting individual career awareness or understanding of the clinician role. It also differs from the mentor–mentee experience, which is generally a long-term relationship designed to promote career growth and development and may be mutually supportive and collaborative in nature (Alspach, 2000).

The preceptorship is the opportune time for the novice to be socialized into the new work setting. In the case of students, it may be the first exposure to the roles, responsibilities, and accountabilities of the clinician role. For the graduate clinician, the preceptorship serves as a period of transition from the role of student to that of professional. The experienced clinician moving into a new work setting also requires assistance with socialization and must adjust previous experiences to fit into the new work setting with new rules, new languages, and new patient populations.

■ Theoretical Foundations

Socialization has been defined as the passing of a role from one person to the next, the process by which a person acquires and internalizes new knowledge and skills (Horsburgh, 1989; Santucci, 2004; Tradewell, 1996). Socialization enables the transition from previous roles to new roles and from familiar to unfamiliar work environments. Tradewell also states that socialization occurs through observing the preceptor role model behaviors and language, as well as by exposure to incumbent staff as they reflect on their practice through stories of their own work experiences. Santucci states that the socialization period involves the learning of work systems, staff roles, and employer expectations for students and new employees alike. The preceptor informs, guides, and supports the clinician in navigating the social mores of the workplace and applying knowledge gained from past clinical and classroom experiences to the technologic and physiologic aspects of patient care in the new setting.

During this period, preceptees may experience a loss of confidence in their abilities to perform skills and think critically. For experienced clinicians entering a new practice arena, the loss of their self-confidence is particularly difficult. In their previous work setting, they have been capable, experienced practitioners, relying on past experiences and intuition to function effectively. They were comfortable in their practice and felt knowledgeable about the expectations of the work environment, resources, and sources of support. In the new work environment, their self-image changes, as they find themselves unsure of how to behave or practice and lacking in knowledge regarding resources and support systems. This unfamiliarity engenders a self-image or vision that is difficult to accept, even if the period is transient.

During the transition, the preceptee begins to leave behind previously learned beliefs and behaviors and integrate new standards and expectations into his or her practice. Kramer (1974) described this difficult process as *reality shock*, a period in which the learner begins to recognize differences and inconsistencies in the new environment in comparison to the old environment. Students transitioning to the professional role are exposed to the realities and contradictions of the real world, as compared to the known and ordered world of academia. The preceptee may question the value of what was learned as well as the ethics of what is observed in the workplace. Finding a balance and learning to mesh the academic and work environments in a way that is acceptable for the learner may be difficult and emotionally stressful, as familiar support and social systems are left behind. The work of learning, performing in a new role, balancing new and old roles, and making meaning of new work is an exhausting process that requires high energy consumption by the learner and significant support from the preceptor.

Communication and feedback are the backbone of the preceptor–preceptee relationship. Open, honest, compassionate, and timely feedback is valued by the preceptee. Such communication requires mutual trust and respect. While it takes time to develop this trust, the reality of the preceptorship experience is that it is of the moment, existing only within a limited time frame. It is critical that an initial meeting between the learner and the preceptor include a discussion of their past experiences, expectations, and goals for the relationship, and personal, work, learning, teaching, and communication styles. This conversation sets the stage for a successful, sharing relationship.

The preceptor is called on to be teacher, counselor, and clinician to guide the preceptee through this complex transition (O'Malley et al., 2000). A safe, supportive, and informative environment is vital during this period (Goh & Watt, 2003). While the key relationships are between preceptor and preceptee, supportive faculty and unit staff are also critical. Faculty, managers, and clinical specialists must meet with preceptors to describe the course or orientation program objectives and enlist the assistance of other staff as necessary to assist in designing the preceptorship. In this way, there is an investment in and support for the program from the beginning. Consideration should be given to the kind of support that will be provided to the preceptors throughout the experience. Support can be in the form of public acknowledgment of their work; scheduled meetings with the preceptor to ascertain whether assistance is needed, or with the preceptor and preceptee to discuss progress; support for the types of assignments the preceptor selects; and possible schedule adjustments for the preceptor to enhance the learning experience.

Types of Learners

Whether the individual involved in the precepted experience is a student, new graduate, experienced clinician, or temporary visitor, he or she is an adult learner who actively participates on some level in the identification of individual learning needs and in designing or choosing learning experiences intended to meet those needs. The precepted experience takes place in a complex and dynamic clinical environment with the preceptor facilitating the learning. The experience is enhanced for learners who exhibit well-developed adult learning characteristics. This includes an independent self-concept, willingness to freely share their life experiences with others, active engagement in the process to meet learning goals, an openness to learning opportunities regardless of when they occur in the experience, and a problem-centered approach to learning.

Conditions for Learning

The two most commonly named goals for the preceptored learning experience reported in the literature are the facilitation of socialization into the work setting and role transition from student to graduate clinician or from newly hired orientee to staff member (Gaberson & Oermann, 1999; Guhde, 2005; Smith & Chalker, 2005). Gaberson and Oermann also reported benefits for students in terms of the ability to integrate classroom theoretical knowledge with actual clinical practice within a healthcare organization. In addition, the preceptor has the ability to provide individualized attention and guidance to the learner and improve the learner's clinical competence and confidence. The schools also benefit from preceptored experiences because students depend less on faculty, as preceptors serve in the educator role. In this way, a faculty member can more effectively manage a group of students through collaborative relationships with preceptors.

From the organizational perspective, student-preceptored clinical rotations may assist in meeting mission statement goals, such as a commitment to educating future clinicians. In addition, preceptorships may facilitate recruitment of employees because the learner has a relationship within the organization and is exposed to the workplace and staff. The supportive relationship between an orientee and a preceptor may also affect new employee recruitment, job satisfaction, and retention rates (Casey, Fink, Krugman, & Propst, 2004; Gaberson & Oermann, 1999).

Resources

Although the preceptored experience may take place in any organization that delivers health care, it is important to ensure that the clinical environment matches the goals of the experience from either the course and student or the program and orientee perspective. The length of the experience is dependent on the goals to be achieved. In short, the experience can be of any length, but must be long enough to provide the varied clinical exposure and experiences to ensure achievement of course or orientation objectives.

Whether it is a student or orientee experience, the preceptor and learner will benefit from contact and guidance from a faculty member or organization-based educator, clinical specialist, or manager. Preceptors should have access to a student's goals and objectives or an orientee's competency checklist to facilitate planning, track achievements, and evaluate performance.

Organizations that provide clinical placements to student clinicians require qualified staff to precept. In addition, they require qualified staff to precept new or transferring employees. Depending on the staff mix in a given clinical area, there may not be an adequate supply of interested, committed, and educationally prepared staff to serve in the preceptor role; this could be a limiting factor for the number of students or new hires a unit or department is able to absorb. This is particularly true if the unit or department also welcomes groups of students and a clinical instructor at the same time, thus creating competition for patient assignments. Staff may view the role of preceptor and the teaching and evaluation responsibilities as added work, and this may also limit the number of students or orientees for a given clinical area. All of these scenarios require commitment on the part of the unit or department manager, clinical specialists, educators, and faculty to create a learning environment that supports staff throughout the process so they are prepared to serve and feel valued in their role as preceptor.

Recognition for clinicians who are preceptors can take many forms. Schools may appoint preceptors to adjunct faculty status, provide access to continuing education programs, provide certificates of appreciation or recognition receptions, and, in some cases, offer vouchers for free or reduced tuition for selected courses. Although these recognition and reward efforts may have a budgetary impact on the academic institution, benefits may also be realized through recruitment of preceptors to enroll in academic programs. Healthcare organizations may or may not provide similar incentives for staff who are preceptors, including certificates of appreciation, preceptor awards, luncheons, less off-shift or weekend scheduling, lighter-than-usual patient assignments, or pay differentials. Again, these methods of recognizing staff for their role as preceptor may have a budget impact, but may also encourage staff to participate in this key role and contribute to job satisfaction and retention through recognition of their hard work. Speers, Strzyzewski, and Ziolkowski (2004) report that nonmaterial benefits had greater relative importance for staff in their decision to serve in the preceptor role.

■ Using the Method

Under the guidance of an experienced clinician preceptor, the student or novice clinician begins to apply the knowledge and theory learned in the classroom to the reality of patient care and begins to transition from learner to professional. It is equally important for the environment to be one in which the novice feels safe enough to ask questions and take risks. Having clear expectations for the precepting experience, for both the preceptor and the novice, further contributes to a successful experience.

Faculty should review the goals prior to the experience if the novice is a student. If the novice is a new graduate clinician or an experienced clinician new to a particular work setting, he or she should come with expectations for the precepting experience and be prepared to discuss them with the preceptor. The preceptor, working with unit-based leadership, should also develop a set of goals and expectations for the precepting experience. During the initial meeting between the preceptor and the preceptee, goals and expectations for the experience should be shared and reworked into a mutually agreed-upon plan with time frames for achievement.

The preceptor is the key to the success of this experience. When designing the precepting experience, time and attention should be paid to the selection, preparation, and ongoing support of the preceptor. Attention should also be given to the roles and responsibilities of the learner, the clinical faculty, and the unit leadership in this learning experience.

The Preceptor

Precepting requires an individual who is committed to nurturing and teaching the next generation of professionals—someone who is both caring and clinically competent. On occasion, preceptors are selected based on their availability, convenience, and clinical abilities, but an outstanding clinician does not always translate into a skillful preceptor. There are four criteria for selecting a qualified preceptor. The first criterion in selecting a preceptor should be the clinician's interest in and willingness to assume the role in addition to his or her patient care responsibilities.

The second criterion is ensuring a positive relationship between the preceptor and the preceptee. The relationship must include trust and understanding if learning is to take place. Factors that can facilitate this trusting relationship include ensuring that the preceptor reviews written goals and objectives for the experience, to facilitate upfront planning; reviewing preceptor and preceptee expectations for communication, behavior, and timelines for goal achievement; and providing time for meetings for discussion, reflection, and feedback throughout the experience. Other factors that influence the relationship include involving the potential preceptor in the interview process for a new staff member and having a manager or clinical specialist choose a preceptor who matches the perceptions of the preceptee based on his or her knowledge of both individuals, including such factors as communication, learning, and teaching styles.

Clinical knowledge, skill, and ability are the components of the third criterion for choosing an ideal preceptor. A practitioner with a depth of understanding of the patient population and a high level of technical skill is necessary when selecting a preceptor. Benner and colleagues (1996) state that the competent practitioner often provides the best guidance for the new clinician. The competent practitioner is adept at assessing and diagnosing patient needs in a step-by-step fashion. This attention to detail and use of a logical and orderly process are useful when teaching the student or novice practitioner. Proficient, expert clinicians have a breadth of knowledge and intuition not possessed by the competent practitioner, but their skill often proves to be too abstract for the novice, and therefore they may not be the best choice to serve as preceptor. As a task-focused learner, the novice is comfortable with the concrete precepts of the competent practitioner.

The ability to listen and communicate with respect describes the fourth criterion for the preceptor. During the transition from student or orientee to practitioner, the amount of new information, new experiences, and new responsibilities may be overwhelming. Students and orientees may experience a range of emotions, from excitement and eagerness to anger and frustration, during the transition period. The preceptor will need to be attuned to these reactions and adapt the learning experience accordingly. To manage this, the preceptor will need to be able to listen closely and assess the needs of the preceptee, much as the preceptor assesses the needs of the patient.

The preceptor's role will be multifaceted. As teacher and guide, the preceptor will be introducing the novice to clinical practice (Godinez et al., 1999). In the first meeting between preceptor and preceptee, the preceptor will discuss the goals for the precepting experience. The preceptor will also determine the preceptee's learning needs and learning style. This can be done by simply asking how the preceptee learns best (e.g., visual, auditory, audiovisual, verbal, or kinesthetic), or through a more formal assessment process using any of a number of standardized tools, such as Kolb's learning style inventory (Kolb, 2005; Kolb & Kolb, 2005).

Role modeling patient care skills, from interpersonal interactions to assessment and diagnosis, and finally to intervention and evaluation, will be the initial primary method of teaching. Ongoing explanations for each action will inform the learner of the reasons for the choices the preceptor makes. In addition to modeling practice at the bedside, the preceptor will model skills in communication with the interdisciplinary team involved in patient care, as well as with the patient and family.

In the early phase of the precepted experience, the novice will observe and listen to the preceptor role model. As the experience progresses, the role of the preceptor will move to that of teacher, as the preceptor instructs the learner in providing direct patient care, using technology, interacting with the multidisciplinary team, and accessing the resources available within the work environment.

The preceptor will spend time coaching the preceptee by role playing interactions before they occur. For instance, the preceptor may have the preceptee practice reviewing the plan for participating in patient care rounds before they occur or giving a clinician-to-clinician report before the shift ends. The skill of the preceptor will be called into action, including knowing when to hover close by the preceptee as he or she provides direct care and knowing when to allow the learner to practice independently. As the patient dynamic changes, so will the choices the preceptor makes relative to the autonomy of the novice. When the patient's condition is acute or changes unexpectedly, the preceptor will work closely with the learner as he or she provides care, makes assessments, and plans with other members of the healthcare team. When the patient is well known to the preceptor and learner, with a stable or improved condition, the preceptor may choose to review the care plan with the learner and then observe and evaluate the learner's ability to implement the plan.

Along with the responsibility for teaching at the bedside, the preceptor must introduce and socialize the preceptee to the work environment to assist in the transition from student or orientee to professional clinician. It is incumbent upon the preceptor to introduce the preceptee to the culture of the unit, the values of the staff, the formal and informal roles occupied by members of the staff, and the formal and informal rules by which the unit functions. Preceptors will need to explain basics such as how the schedule works and how to manage the hospital's communication system, as well as how to cope with the realities of the healthcare environment. The preceptor becomes a guide to the learner who has left behind familiar environments and support systems and must form a new and stable base on which to grow as a clinician.

When working with new clinicians, the preceptor, with support from unit leadership, should attempt to carve out some time for reflection. While this is challenging in today's fast-paced clinical environment, it does serve several important purposes. Time away from the clamor of the unit allows the preceptor and learner to review the patient experience and to discuss in greater depth how and why specific patient care decisions were made. Perhaps most importantly, this time provides a safe space for the learner to reflect on his or her own thoughts and feelings about what has occurred with the patient and how he or she has performed. Through these discussions, the relationship between preceptor and preceptee is built, trust is developed, and communication is enhanced. This is vital for later discussions, as the pair evaluate the success of the practicum or process of orientation and each person's behavior in the process. Most likely, students will be familiar with this time for reflection, as this is common practice in an instructor-led clinical practicum.

The Preceptee

The preceptee is an active participant in the precepting experience and must assume a leadership role in ensuring the success of the experience. In addition to the initial sharing of goals for the experience, the learner is responsible for informing the preceptor when the goals are not being met, when new lessons are not clear, or when he or she is uncomfortable performing a new skill. Feedback from the learner helps the preceptor adapt and adjust the experience in a meaningful way that leads to a successful outcome. Without feedback, the preceptor will only be making assumptions, which may not always be correct. The learner is also accountable for following through on the suggestions and recommendations made by the preceptor. This may include practicing a skill, researching an unfamiliar aspect of clinical care, or reading a suggested article or chapter about a particular patient condition.

The Faculty and Unit Leadership

A strong collaborative partnership between academic faculty and service providers, including both unit leadership and staff, is a critical factor in ensuring a successful experience for students (Corlett, Palfreyman, Staines, & Marr, 2003). The role played by faculty and unit leadership will vary depending on the level of experience of both the preceptor and the preceptee. If the preceptor is new to the role, then the faculty or unit leadership will play a mentoring role in the process and may have to provide more guidance to ensure success. As the preceptor gains experience in the role, faculty and unit leadership may need to meet with the preceptor and preceptee only occasionally to monitor the process or consult on more complex issues that the preceptor is unable to solve independently. Regardless of the experience level of the preceptor, faculty or unit leadership must maintain open communication and monitor the experience on some level to ensure that objectives are met, and intervene if issues arise in the preceptor–preceptee relationship. Such support can be offered in direct discussions that occur periodically throughout the preceptorship, or by phone or e-mail when specific questions or concerns arise.

Evaluating the Preceptored Clinical Experience

Ideally, evaluation should be a formative and ongoing process, part of the daily communication between preceptor and preceptee. Discussion and feedback about skill performance, assessment and diagnosis, and bedside interactions should be part of the regular communication of each day. By incorporating this process into the routine of the day, it becomes a respectful, helpful activity and one that moves the precepting experience continuously forward. Competency-based tools, timelines, or lists of objectives can serve as valuable guidelines for such discussions. If goals have been set at the beginning of the precepting experience, discussion can be based on how closely the experience has come to meeting those goals. Asking simple questions, such as "How do you think you performed today?" "Is there anything you would do differently?" and "How close are we to reaching each goal?," provides a basis for self-reflection and allows the preceptor to evaluate the learner's understanding of his or her performance. The preceptor can then compare his or her assessment of the preceptee's performance with the learner's self-assessment and provide constructive feedback to support or improve the preceptee's performance. If only summative evaluation is used to evaluate the precepting experience, the learner will not benefit from the preceptor's suggestions and recommendations, as they will not have been provided in a time-sensitive or event-sensitive manner. As the orientation is nearing the end of its prescribed timeline, the burden of evaluating the orientee becomes more acute. Many schools and clinical units have created evaluation tools that consider the preceptor's actions, the preceptee's actions, or both. In addition, both the American Association for Critical-Care Nurses (AACN) and the Center for Nurse Executives have used survey data and focus groups to determine lists of core competencies (Berkow, Virkstis, Stewart, & Conway, 2009; Hickey, 2009). Important generic competencies identified in these documents include basic knowledge application, assessment, technical skill attainment, time management, critical thinking, and communication. For the new clinician, such tools most often follow a competency-based format that covers the various aspects of caring for a particular patient population, including skill acquisition, problem solving, and decision making. For the student, tools generally focus on goal attainment and the overall clinical experience, including the effectiveness of the preceptor. Preceptors may use a self-evaluation model focusing on the various aspects of the preceptor role, or they may receive feedback from the preceptee, faculty, or unit leadership using a more inclusive method.

Faculty or unit leaders should participate in the evaluation process periodically during the precepting experience. They can offer objective insight into the progress being made and recommendations gleaned from their expertise in patient care and teaching. They can also serve as role models and support the preceptor in handling more complex feedback issues that might occur during the precepting experience. Preceptors take their role very seriously and may feel they are solely responsible for the outcome of the experience. Indicators of lack of readiness for independent practice have been identified through focus groups and individual interviews. Preceptors have listed a lack of basic knowledge, followed by the inability to perform frequently taught and demonstrated skills, as the most concerning general indicators of a preceptee's lack of readiness for practice; specific behaviors that raise red flags include an inability to develop organizational skills, an apparent lack of interest in engaging with patients, and an unwillingness to participate in self-reflection or critical self-assessment (Luhanga, Yonge, & Myrick, 2008; Modic & Harris, 2007). Active and timely faculty or unit leadership involvement will help the preceptor manage some of the perceived burden of the preceptor's sense of responsibility for the outcome of the experience.

Potential Problems

For a successful partnership to develop, consistent, interested, capable preceptors are necessary (Boychuck-Duchsher, 2001; Boyle, Popkess-Vawter, & Taunton, 1996; Casey et al., 2004; Oermann & Moffitt-Wolfe, 1997). On the other side of the equation, there must be an engaged, participative preceptee (O'Malley et al., 2000).

The challenges described by students and new graduates during this transition include being able to set priorities and organize patient care needs, acquiring time management skills, fearing communication with physicians, lacking confidence in their performance, and struggling with dependence and independence in the preceptor–preceptee relationship (Casey et al., 2004; Oermann & Moffitt-Wolfe, 1997). The issue of independent practice is a dilemma for preceptors as well as preceptees. Knowing when to allow the preceptee to practice more independently or when to step in and actively guide and participate in the patient care is subjective and varies from moment to moment. An event that can be handled by a preceptee in one instance may require the direct involvement of the preceptor in another case because of the impact of individual patient characteristics. This seeming inconsistency in preceptor behavior may contribute to the preceptee's issues of confidence and highlights the need for open, honest communication between preceptor and preceptee.

Potential problems can arise in the preceptorial experience because of factors related to the preceptor, the learner, or the process. The importance of formal training in preparing a staff member to function effectively as a preceptor is well documented in the literature (Alspach, 2000; Neumann et al., 2004; Speers et al., 2004).

Although clinicians chosen to be preceptors are typically well prepared to care for their patients, to be effective as staff preceptors they must also be knowledgeable regarding the principles of adult education and adult learning, learning styles, planning and implementing learning experiences, reality shock, and the principles of evaluation and provision of constructive feedback. Faculty, managers, clinical specialists, and staff educators must provide opportunities for advanced education in these areas to adequately prepare clinicians to serve in their assigned role and to maximize the potential success of the preceptor–preceptee relationship and achieve a positive outcome. In addition, staff preceptors should have periodic contact with faculty and their managers, clinical specialists, and educators throughout the preceptorship to enhance communication, problem solve, and continue their development as preceptors through evaluative feedback of their performance. For preceptors, the sense of responsibility they feel for the experience extends beyond the clinical teaching that occurs. They often feel responsible for diagnosing and resolving all problems, even those that are beyond their scope to manage. Frequent involvement of faculty or unit leadership helps to establish a relationship in which the preceptor feels comfortable sharing concerns and seeking an expert's advice.

Learners must receive clear, upfront communication regarding their responsibility for the learning process, achievement of outcomes, preceptor expectations, and what they can expect of their preceptor, as well as practical issues such as adhering to assigned schedules and completion of assignments. This helps avoid misunderstandings about their role as learner and the goals of the experience. It also removes the primary responsibility for the success of the experience from the preceptor and ensures that the preceptee is aware of his or her accountability for successful outcomes.

Beyond preparation of both preceptor and learner, other issues internal to the individual must be considered as affecting the relationship. There are many potential causes for perceived or real personality conflicts between a preceptor and a preceptee, but many can arise when there is a clash of values and beliefs that can occur between different age groups. The need to manage generational issues in the workplace is well documented in the literature (Gerke, 2001; Weston, 2001). Differing worldviews, personal motivating factors, preferred work environments, perceptions of work–life balance, and individual strengths and differences can create conflicts between a preceptor of one generation and a preceptee of another. Awareness and understanding of these different generational values, behaviors, and expectations is the first step in working toward a successful preceptor–preceptee relationship. Integration of this information into preceptor preparation programs is key to assisting with the teaching and learning challenges created by a multigenerational workforce.

Preparation of preceptors and preceptees requires a structure to support expected outcomes. Educational preparation of preceptors to serve in their role, orientation of learners as to what to expect in the clinical setting, written course or orientation program objectives, competency or skill checklists, articulated time frames for outcome achievement, appropriate matching of preceptor and learner, and appropriate scheduling and identification of resources to assist in the process are all aspects of a well-planned and organized preceptorship. Effective planning and creation of tools to support the process allow the preceptor and learner to focus on the learning process within the context of the busy clinical environment.

The acuity and pace of the current clinical environment provide unique challenges for the preceptor and the student or orientee. The preceptor is no longer serving in one role—that of caregiver and coordinator of care—but also fills the role of teacher of caregiving and care coordination (Alspach, 2000). The challenge of teaching while providing high-quality care requires the preceptor to balance these roles. Most often, the student or new orientee has less clinical knowledge and skill than the more experienced preceptor. The preceptor must consider the rights of the patients and adhere to the ethical standard of beneficence, the duty to help, to produce beneficial outcomes, or at least to do no harm within the context of the teaching and learning process (Gaberson & Oermann, 1999). Patients must be aware that a learner is involved in their care as part of informed consent, and preceptors should ensure that the learner has demonstrated the knowledge and skill to provide care safely prior to doing so independently. The challenge for the preceptor is to achieve not only the desired patient clinical outcomes, but also the desired educational outcomes for the student or orientee. The preceptor's judgment must be used exquisitely to determine when a learner can provide care safely and learn safely to achieve both goals.

■ Conclusion

The preceptored clinical experience is a valuable teaching and learning methodology with clear benefits for academic institutions and healthcare organizations alike. Students and orientees who are in the preceptee role benefit from the real-world experience of seasoned clinical staff preceptors. Preceptors benefit by adding this credential to their experience and learning new and valuable teaching, communication, and evaluation skills. Planning and communication are the keys to ensuring a successful period of socialization and role transition for the preceptee.

Teaching Example:
New Graduate Critical Care Program

The new graduate critical care program (Mylott & Ciesielski, 2003; Mylott & Greenspan, 2005) is a 6-month orientation and continuing education program designed to develop and support baccalaureate-prepared new graduate registered nurses (RNs) in the acquisition of experiential nursing knowledge and the application of theory and research in the care of critically ill patients. The program takes place at Massachusetts General Hospital. Using Benner's (1984) and Benner and colleagues' (1996) concepts explicating the development of novice nursing practice, the program combines participative and reflective didactic sessions with a preceptored clinical practicum in the intensive care unit of hire. Preceptor development is facilitated through group workshops and individual consultation as requested. Eight intensive care units participate in the program: medical, surgical/trauma, cardiac surgery, neurological, pediatric, burn, postanesthesia, and coronary care. A team of central and unit-based critical care nurse directors, clinical nurse specialists, educators, and human resources staff meets regularly to provide program oversight and development.

The majority of participants complete the program within the allotted time. Formal didactic instruction is completed within 5 months, and the last month is free of classes to allow for immersion in practice. This approach serves as a transition period to full professional responsibility. This time frame is consistent with the literature on similar programs, and the nursing leadership believes that a 6-month orientation is needed for the new graduate to acquire the experiential knowledge and clinical skills to practice safely and independently. Preceptors and leadership believe that much of the variation in readiness to practice occurs in the last 2 months, when the work is largely about becoming an independent clinician.

Participant Characteristics

Through experience, the leadership group has identified several attributes that are associated with success. These attributes include experience working as a nursing assistant in critical care, passing the NCLEX RN licensing exam on the first attempt, and a committed desire to practice in critical care.

The average age of the program's new graduate nurse participants is 24.5 years, as compared with an average age of over 46.8 years for the general nursing population in the United States (U.S. Department of Health and Human Services [HHS], 2004). Implications for a growing proportion of younger nurses in the practice environment are described within the literature (Nursing Executive Center, 2002). In response, the program planners implemented a workshop on generational differences as an intervention to facilitate communication and the development of positive relationships between preceptors and new graduates; this workshop is delivered as needed (Tyrrell, 2005). Program evaluations of this workshop have been positive to date.

To evaluate the professional development of the new graduate participants, e-mail surveys with questions targeted toward their achievements were sent to participants in the first four classes ($n = 24$) who were employed at the institution. An 88% response rate ($n = 21$) was achieved, and collated responses indicated that respondents had accomplished much professionally and were highly involved in professional development activities. In addition to the items cited in Table 22-1, five respondents had served as preceptors to subsequent new graduate program participants.

Curriculum

The curriculum addresses the learning needs of both the new graduate preceptees and the experienced nurse preceptors. For the preceptees, a variety of learning options and supports are offered

Table 22-1   Professional Development Survey Responses

Professional Development Indicators	Affirmative Response (%)	Number
Enrolled in graduate school	37	8
CWH competent	94	20
Serves as unit resource nurse	59	12
Has passed CCRN exam or completed review course with intent to take exam	37	8
Clinical advancement program participation	10	2
Project Hope humanitarian effort	6	1

CCRN, critical care registered nurse; CWH, continuous veno-venous hemofiltration.

(continues)

throughout the 6-month experience. The style of teaching is case based, including simulation, narrative, and discussion sessions. Topic areas cover pathophysiology encountered in critically ill children and adults and interventions for each illness discussed. Content focuses on managing the patient requiring mechanical ventilation, as well as patients requiring close cardiac monitoring, invasive hemodynamic monitoring, and neurologic monitoring. Simulation sessions include respiratory distress and failure, shock, dysrhythmias with hemodynamic consequences, and cardiopulmonary arrests. These sessions require participants to work as a team to assess the patient, identify actual and potential problems, communicate and collaborate with various members of the healthcare team to identify and initiate interventions, and evaluate outcomes.

The preceptors are offered a workshop prior to participating in the program. The content includes new graduate behavior as described by Benner and colleagues (1996), teaching strategies, learning styles, communication and feedback skills, and interventions for precepting challenges. Techniques include simulation, case-based discussions, reflection, and role modeling. There is a panel discussion with experienced preceptors. Throughout the course of the 6-month program, preceptors are offered the opportunity to meet and discuss challenges with their peers.

The program's effectiveness is evaluated using a variety of measures. A focus group of preceptors and orientees is held in the fifth month to review the effectiveness from the participants' perspective. An evaluation tool is given to both preceptors and orientees to determine program effectiveness and areas in need of change. The tool's elements require both preceptors and orientees to evaluate the orientees' readiness to practice independently. In addition, both preceptors and orientees complete self-evaluations of how they fulfilled their program roles, and also evaluate their partner's effectiveness in fulfilling program roles. Finally, a postprogram review of each orientee's capabilities is done using standards agreed to by the intensive care unit leadership. The standards include participants' ability to:

- Manage patients requiring invasive, closely monitored treatments such as continuous venous-to-venous hemodialysis.
- Serve as a resource nurse responsible for managing the flow of patients and staff during a work shift.
- Function as a program preceptor within 2 years of program completion.

New Graduate in Critical Care Preceptor Narrative

The following is an adaptation of a narrative written by an experienced staff nurse preceptor (Albert, 2004). It describes the events of a typical day spent orienting a new graduate nurse participating in Massachusetts General Hospital's new graduate critical care program. The narrative was submitted as part of a portfolio in support of the preceptor's nomination as the first Norman Knight Preceptor of Distinction award. Nominees are asked to submit a narrative that illustrates their abilities as a preceptor. The author of the narrative, Jennifer Albert, RN, BSN, a staff nurse in the surgical/trauma intensive care unit, received the award. Awardees receive funds to attend a graduate course of their choice or protected paid time to complete a course of study with a clinical nurse specialist in their area of interest. An annual ceremony is held to announce the award and is followed by a reception for the hospital community and invited guests. A plaque that describes the award's purpose and lists the names of awardees is prominently displayed on the first floor of the hospital. The names of the patient and preceptee used in the narrative have been changed to ensure anonymity.

I am a staff nurse in the surgical intensive care unit, where I have practiced for the past 7 years. My nursing career began in 1989, 6 months before graduating from nursing school. As part of my senior practicum, I spent 20 hours per week working one-on-one with an experienced nurse on the surgical/trauma floor. I was blessed with a preceptor who was warm and welcoming, patient and professional, and who, above all, had the desire to share her knowledge and expertise with me, the neophyte nurse. I credit this positive experience with my willingness to take the challenge of reciprocating 2 years later when I was approached about precepting a student nurse from my alma mater. I was a bit apprehensive, as I had no previous teaching experience. What I did have, however, was the desire to share my newly acquired knowledge and to make this a fulfilling experience for this student, just as had been done for me 2 years previously.

Since my first experience in 1991, I have had the opportunity and privilege to serve as a preceptor for over a dozen nurses, all with varied levels of experience. My intent here is not to sound boastful, but rather grateful. For it is I who have truly been enriched both professionally and personally by each of these individuals whom I've had the opportunity to precept over the years.

Presently, I am nearing the halfway mark in a 6-month orientation process with my preceptee, Sue, a new graduate nurse enrolled in the critical care program. The narrative that follows is a glimpse into one of our days together.

Andy is a 39-year-old with a history of psoriasis who had presented to an outside hospital with diffuse erythema extending from his thigh to his ankle, fever, and worsening renal failure and mental status, despite having received a dose of IV antibiotics in that hospital the previous night. His symptoms were most likely the result of either renal failure or profound sepsis. He was transferred to our hospital for further evaluation, and his admitting diagnosis was necrotizing fasciitis. Andy would most likely be the most challenging and complex patient Sue had cared for thus far. Yet, as a preceptor, I knew the circumstances couldn't be more ideal because Sue had already had some exposure to this patient, as she had had the opportunity to observe his surgery, as well as participate in admitting him to our unit.

We assembled outside of Andy's room at 7:00 AM with the flow sheet to get report from the night nurse. I made the calculated, but hopefully inconspicuous decision to move my seat, so that I was sitting next to Sue so that she was sandwiched between the night nurse and me. A few years ago, it never would have occurred to me that where I sat during report had any relevance. Yet, one of my former orientees commented to me one day, "Have you ever noticed that during report they (the nurses giving report) tend to always address you?" Frankly, I had never made this observation, but as I watched over the next few months, it became apparent that this was indeed true. My colleagues had the tendency to talk directly to me, almost turning their backs toward my orientee at times. To prevent this, I began to position myself directly next to my orientee, so that there was no confusion and we were both being addressed during report.

We were told that Andy was started on drotrecogin alfa. Other critical pieces of data we received during report were that his platelet level had fallen to 40,000, his hematocrit was trending down, and his leg dressing, which had not been bloody during the night, was saturated with blood, only 1 hour after the surgeons had changed it.

We entered the room together and Sue began the morning routine of zeroing and leveling transducers, setting alarms, and checking drug doses and infusion rates. I noted, but chose to not yet verbalize my own observation, that there was heparin in all of the

(continues)

transducer bags. I quietly wondered if Sue had made the same observation, and if she had, would she make the connection that even this small amount of heparin could be contributing to Andy's thrombocytopenia and therefore needed to be removed from the transducers? Sue began a thorough physical assessment. Andy's neurological status was difficult to assess since he was heavily sedated.

Recalling that with previous patients we had shut off the propofol drip to get a more thorough exam, Sue questioned whether we should do this with Andy. Sue's ability to incorporate previous experiences was becoming evident and I supported her plan but cautiously reminded her about what had been relayed to us in report—that Andy became dyssynchronous with the ventilator and tended to drop his oxygen saturation when awake or undersedated. My role as preceptor was to help Sue anticipate this potential instability and I did so by questioning her about how she planned to react and which interventions she planned to employ if Andy became unstable. With an action plan in place, Sue moved ahead.

Having completed her physical exam, Sue discussed her findings and observations. She was particularly concerned and focused on the continued bleeding from Andy's leg. His dressing was saturated with blood. At that point in her orientation, Sue had no previous experience to draw on that would allow her to differentiate normal from excessive bleeding. I attempted to coax from her what she might expect to see in a patient who had lost significant blood volume by asking, "How might the patient's hemodynamic profile change?" "Which lab values would be of particular concern?" and "Which medications might be contributing to this ongoing bleeding?" Together we explored the answers, examining the most recent vital signs, interpreting the reading from the Swan Ganz catheter, and discussing the signs of hypovolemia. Lastly, I prompted Sue about the medication that might have been contributing to the patient's condition. She reviewed Andy's medication list but was unable to identify the two drugs that I found concerning. I suggested that she take a close look at the transducer bags. I immediately saw the smile go across her face as she identified her earlier oversight, even before actually looking at the bags. Sue removed the heparin from the transducers and I recommended that she take a 10-minute break to read about drotrecogin alfa, knowing that once she did, she would be able to identify my second concern—that this medication increases the risk of bleeding and is contraindicated with acute bleeding.

Sue was far enough along in her orientation that she had begun to take an active and participatory role in rounds. That day I took a backseat role and allowed her the primary role of interacting with the physicians during rounds. In preparation for this, I assisted her in generating a list of questions in regard to the bleeding that she might want to have answered or addressed. Rounds began and I stepped back into the patient's room, far enough away so that I could hear the discussion, yet not be directly involved in it. This allowed Sue the opportunity to independently interact with the physicians, while providing her with the security of knowing I was close by should she need my assistance. Following rounds, I had Sue reiterate the plan for the day, which she might have thought was redundant, but I needed to know she had extrapolated the correct information from rounds and that she was clear on how we were to proceed. (Courtesy of *Caring Headlines*)

Unbundling the Narrative

Ms. Albert's narrative provides an insightful view into the thinking and practice of an expert preceptor. She chose to become a preceptor based on her own positive experience working with a caring and skilled preceptor, her wish to continue that experience for others, and finally her realization of the rewards of precepting through her own personal and professional sense of enrichment. Ms. Albert's passion for the role came through clearly in the course of the narrative.

The expertise of precepting is apparent from the way Ms. Albert introduced the patient she selected for the shift. She was thoughtful and goal directed in the choice of patient assignment and gave specific reasons for her selection. She also displayed her awareness of the level of acuity this patient presented and the challenge this would be for Sue, her preceptee. Ms. Albert's clinical expertise is woven throughout the narrative, as she was able to guide her preceptee while anticipating potential patient problems and possible interventions.

Ms. Albert described the importance of having a sharing, respectful relationship with a preceptee. When a preceptee she had worked with previously presented her with a critical observation regarding staff behavior toward preceptees during report, Ms. Albert felt compelled to follow up to confirm. This resulted in a decisive change in her personal placement during report, underscoring her openness as a preceptor. She mirrored this behavior later in the narrative when she described her placement in the background during rounds with the physician staff. Ms. Albert never left Sue completely alone, but choreographed her presence such that it would not prevent other healthcare team members from treating the preceptee as the patient's nurse.

Ms. Albert's awareness of the new graduate's need for routine was clear as she described the daily regimen Sue must follow when starting the shift. She was constantly aware of the patient and his needs and was thinking many steps ahead of the preceptee, but allowed the preceptee time to think through issues and problem solve for herself. Rather than specifically telling Sue directly what to look for, she coached, provided clues, and asked thoughtful questions to guide her. In so doing, Ms. Albert taught and informed the preceptee while preparing her to begin her own critical thinking process. Ms. Albert used this process several times during the shift to help Sue identify actual and potential clinical issues and also to help her devise a plan for intervention. The tactic was also utilized to prepare Sue to participate in rounds with the healthcare team. Prepping the preceptee is another example of how an expert preceptor teaches and helps build the new graduate's self-confidence and self-esteem.

Finally, Ms. Albert was tuned into her preceptee's own needs. When she provided time for Sue to review drotrecogin alfa, she was aware of her preceptee's informational needs and also her need to step back and consider all that had occurred to that point in the day. The same held true when Ms. Albert reviewed the discussion from rounds that created an opportunity for Sue not only to review the care plan, but also to ask questions or clarify the points discussed. Finally, Ms. Albert was aware of how Sue might have felt about this process and was prepared to explain her reasons for engaging in such a manner.

Ms. Albert's narrative exemplifies the characteristics of an expert preceptor, starting with her commitment to precepting, extending through her own clinical expertise, and concluding with her ability to teach, coach, and guide her preceptee in a compassionate, respectful, yet structured manner.

Discussion Questions

1. You are faculty for a precepted clinical course for several last-semester nursing students. One of your students is having a conflict with her preceptor and is worried that her classroom knowledge is in conflict with current nursing practice. Describe how you will address your student's concerns.

2. You are faculty for a precepted clinical course and one of your student's preceptors is concerned that the student is unsafe with medication administration and skills. Describe how you will address these concerns and what strategies you can employ to improve your student's performance.

3. Research the concept of imposter syndrome; describe how a preceptee (student nurse, new graduate nurse, or new employee) is prone to this phenomenon and how the preceptor can alleviate this situation.

References

Albert, J. (2004). Preceptor narrative. *Caring Headlines, 1,* 4–5.

Alspach, J. G. (2000). *From staff nurse to preceptor: A preceptor development program. Instructor's manual* (2nd ed., pp. 11–13). Aliso Viejo, CA: American Association of Critical Care Nurses.

Baggot, D., Hensinger, B., Parry, J., Valdes, M. S., & Zaim, S. (2005). The new hire/preceptor experience: Cost-benefit analysis of one retention strategy. *Journal of Nursing Administration, 35*(3), 138–145.

Benner, P. (1984). *From novice to expert: Excellence and power in clinical nursing practice.* Upper Saddle River, NJ: Prentice Hall.

Benner, P., Tanner, C., & Chesla, C. (1996). Entering the field: Advanced beginner practice. In P. Benner, C. Tanner, & C. Chesla (Eds.), *Expertise in nursing practice: Caring, clinical judgment, and ethics* (pp. 48–77). New York, NY: Springer.

Berkow, S., Virkstis, K., Stewart, J., & Conway, L. (2009). Assessing new graduate nurse performance. *Nurse Educator, 34*(1), 17–22.

Boychuck-Duchsher, J. (2001). Out in the real world: Newly graduated nurses in acute-care speak out. *Journal of Nursing Administration, 31*(9), 426–439.

Boyle, D. K., Popkess-Vawter, S., & Taunton, R. L. (1996). Socialization of new graduate nurses in critical care. *Heart and Lung, 25*(2), 141–154.

Casey, K., Fink, R., Krugman, M., & Propst, J. (2004). The graduate nurse experience. *Journal of Nursing Administration, 34*(6), 303–311.

Corlett, J., Palfreyman, J. W., Staines, H. J., & Marr, H. (2003). Factors influencing theoretical knowledge and practice skill acquisition in student nurses: An empirical experiment. *Nurse Education Today, 23*(3), 183–190.

Gaberson, K., & Oermann, M. H. (1999). *Clinical teaching strategies in nursing.* New York, NY: Springer.

Gerke, M. L. (2001). Understanding and leading the quad matrix: Four generations in the workplace: The traditional generation, boomers, Gen X, nexters. *Seminars for Nurse Managers, 9*(3), 173–181.

Godinez, G., Schweiger, J., Gruver, J., & Ryan, P. (1999). Role transition from graduate to staff nurse: A qualitative analysis. *Journal for Nurses in Staff Development, 15*(3), 97–110.

Goh, K., & Watt, E. (2003). From "dependent on" to "depended on": The experience of transition from student to registered nurse in a private hospital graduate program. *Australian Journal of Advanced Nursing, 21*(1), 14–20.

Guhde, J. (2005). When orientation ends . . . Supporting the new nurse who is struggling to succeed. *Journal for Nurses in Staff Development, 21*(4), 145–149.

Hickey, M. (2009). Preceptor perceptions of new graduate nurse readiness for practice. *Journal for Nurses in Staff Development, 25*(1), 35–41.

Horsburgh, M. (1989). Graduate nurses' adjustment to initial employment: Natural field work. *Journal of Advanced Nursing, 14*(8), 610–617.

Kolb, A. Y., & Kolb, D. A. (2005). *The Kolb Learning Style Inventory–version 3.1: 2005 technical specifications.* Boston, MA: Hay Resources Direct.

Kolb, D. A. (2005). *The Kolb Learning Style Inventory–version 3.1: Self scoring and interpretation booklet.* Boston, MA: Hay Resources Direct.

Kramer, M. (1974). *Reality shock: Why nurses leave nursing.* St. Louis, MO: C. V. Mosby.

Luhanga, F., Yonge, O., & Myrick, F. (2008). Hallmarks of unsafe practice. *Journal for Nurses in Staff Development, 24*(6), 257–264.

Marcum, E. H., & West, R. D. (2004). Structured orientation for new graduates: A retention strategy. *Journal for Nurses in Staff Development, 20*(3), 118–124.

Modic, M. B., & Harris, R. (2007). Masterful precepting: Using the BECOME method to enhance clinical teaching. *Journal for Nurses in Staff Development, 23*(1), 1–8.

Mylott, L., & Ciesielski, S. (2003). It takes a village: New graduate nurses enter critical care at Massachusetts General Hospital. *Advance for Nurses, 29*–30, 32.

Mylott, L., & Greenspan, M. (2005). *MGH-IHP new graduate in critical care program annual report.* Executive summary presented to the vice president for patient care and chief nurse, Massachusetts General Hospital, and the director, graduate program in nursing, MGH Institute for Health Professions, Boston, MA.

Neumann, J. A., Brady-Schluttner, K. A., McKay, A. K., Roslien, J. J., Twedell, D. M., & James, K. M. G. (2004). Centralizing a registered nurse preceptor program at the institutional level. *Journal for Nurses in Staff Development, 20*(1), 17–24.

Nursing Executive Center. (2002). *Nursing's next generation: Best practices for attracting, training, and retraining new graduates.* Washington, DC: Advisory Board Co.

Oermann, M. H., & Moffitt-Wolfe, A. (1997). New graduates' perceptions of clinical practice. *Journal of Continuing Education in Nursing, 28*(1), 20–25.

O'Malley, C., Cunliffe, E., Hunter, S., & Breeze, J. (2000). Preceptorship in practice. *Nursing Standard, 14*(28), 45–49.

Peirce, A. G. (1991). Preceptorial students' view of their clinical experience. *Journal of Nursing Education, 30*(6), 244–249.

Santucci, J. (2004). Facilitating the transition into nursing practice: Concepts and strategies for mentoring new graduates. *Journal for Nurses in Staff Development, 20*(6), 274–284.

Smith, A., & Chalker, N. (2005). Preceptor continuity in a nurse internship program: The nurse intern's perception. *Journal for Nurses in Staff Development, 21*(2), 47–52.

Speers, A. T., Strzyzewski, N., & Ziolkowski, L. D. (2004). Preceptor preparation: An investment in the future. *Journal for Nurses in Staff Development, 20*(3), 127–133.

Tradewell, G. (1996). Rites of passage: Adaptation of nursing graduates to a hospital setting. *Journal of Nursing Staff Development, 12*(4), 183–189.

Tyrrell, R. (2005). *Understanding and leading a multigenerational workforce.* Boston, MA: Massachusetts General Hospital.

U.S. Department of Health and Human Services. (2004). *The registered nurse population: Findings from the March 2004 national sample survey of registered nurses.* Retrieved from http://bhpr.hrsa.gov /healthworkforce/rnsurveys/rnsurvey2004.pdf

Weston, M. (2001). Coaching generations in the workplace. *Nursing Administration Quarterly, 25*(2), 11–21.

Recommended Reading

Baltimore, J. (2004). The hospital clinical preceptor: Essential preparation for success. *Journal of Continuing Education in Nursing, 35*(3), 133–140.

Flynn, J. P., & Stack, M. C. (Eds.). (2006). *The role of the preceptor: A guide for nurse educators, clinicians, and managers* (2nd ed.). New York, NY: Springer.

Johnson, S. A., & Romanello, M. L. (2005). Generational diversity: Teaching and learning approaches. *Nurse Educator, 30*(5), 212–216.

Yonge, O., & Myrick, F. (2004). Preceptorship and the preparatory process for undergraduate nursing students and their preceptors. *Journal for Nurses in Staff Development, 20*(6), 294–297.

CHAPTER 23

Learning in a Faculty-Mentored Student Practice Center

Jennifer E. Mackey
Marjorie Nicholas
Lesley Maxwell

■ Introduction

If we are to pursue excellence in any field, then we must go beyond knowledge and skills in our education of graduate students. We need to identify the qualities of mind that underlie excellence and leadership potential in our disciplines, and we need to build those qualities into the foundations of our educational programs.

What does it mean to have a "critical spirit"? Experts in the field of critical thinking use this metaphorical label to mean "a probing inquisitiveness, a keenness of mind, a zealous dedication to reason, and a hunger or eagerness for reliable information" (Facione, 2015). The faculty members of the Department of Communication Sciences and Disorders at the MGH Institute of Health Professions asked themselves this question: What are the foundational qualities of mind that excellence and leadership in the field are built upon, and how can they be identified and nurtured in our graduate students? The result has been the development of an enhanced clinical curriculum that emphasizes excellence and systematically develops critical thinking, innovation, collaboration, social perception, risk taking, and self-knowledge and reflection in our students (see **Table 23-1**).

Professional licensure and program accreditation standards form the basis of the academic and clinical curriculum of clinical education programs. The American Speech-Language-Hearing Association (ASHA) requires that the education of graduate students seeking to become speech-language pathologists include the acquisition of both *knowledge* and *skills* in a variety of content and disorder areas (ASHA, 2014). The breadth and depth of knowledge and skills that are required for recent healthcare graduates to practice effectively in current times is immense. Programs of all types are struggling to develop sophisticated knowledge and skills in their graduates to meet an enlarging scope of practice. So, why expand the demands on students and faculty by developing an extra set of requirements related to the esoteric ideas of "excellence" or "leadership"?

Table 23-1   Core Competencies for Six Key Clinical Excellence Areas

Core Excellence Skills	Core Competencies
1. Critical Thinking	1a. Demonstrates ability to think critically (interpret, analyze, infer, evaluate, explain, self-regulate)
	1b. Demonstrates curiosity by asking questions and is alert to opportunities to think critically
	1c. Demonstrates open-mindedness to alternative worldviews and opinions and is flexible in considering alternatives
2. Innovation	2. Demonstrates creativity and innovation
3. Collaboration	3. Communicates and collaborates effectively, recognizing the needs, values, and preferred mode of communication and cultural/linguistic backgrounds of patients/clients, caretakers, families, interprofessional team members, and relevant others
4. Social Perception	4. Communicates effectively and flexibly based on the communicative context using verbal and nonverbal pragmatic skills
5. Risk Taking	5. Demonstrates a growth mindset by taking reasonable risks, learning from errors, and seeking feedback
6. Self-Knowledge and Reflection	6a. Demonstrates strong self-reflection and accurate self-evaluation and is able to identify personal strengths and challenges
	6b. Initiates and uses self-evaluation to refine clinical skills and set personal goals for clinical growth

The reason is simple. In a world where knowledge is exploding and skill sets must keep pace, the most valuable education is one that teaches you to think critically, to be innovative, to collaborate effectively, to take the perspectives of others and modify your behavior accordingly, to understand the value of taking thoughtful risks, and to practice in a manner that is self-reflective. Education should teach students how to unlock their personal potential to spend a lifetime pursuing excellence and becoming leaders in their chosen field.

As in most healthcare programs, ensuring students gain the requisite knowledge base required by the accrediting body is accomplished primarily via academic coursework. And, like education models in many healthcare professions, most programs in speech-language pathology in the United States utilize a series of clinical externships in which students work in different healthcare and educational settings to acquire the clinical skills they will need to become professional practicing clinicians. Many also have on-site clinics in which students learn the preliminary clinical skills they need before venturing out to their externships. In this chapter we describe the MGH Institute of Health Professions' faculty-mentored student practice clinic, known as the Speech, Language and Literacy Center. The center operates as both an entry-level and an advanced practice clinic. Although the examples we provide will necessarily be related to speech-language pathology, we believe the lessons learned from this clinical educational model are pertinent to a broad range of healthcare fields.

The model of clinical education we describe in this chapter is based on the *teacher-practitioner model* (Meyer, McCarthy, Klodd, & Gaseor, 1995; Montgomery,

Enzbrenner, & Lerner, 1991; Peach & Meyer, 1996). We propose an enhancement of this model to also include scholarship, which we refer to as the teacher-practitioner-scholar (TPS) model. One of the important features of our implementation of this model, highlighted in this chapter, is the integration of academic (knowledge-based) with clinical (practical and excellence skills-based) education. We describe both our entry-level and advanced practice clinics and then discuss the positive outcomes of using this model.

■ Definition and Purpose of the Teacher-Practitioner-Scholar Model

The essential principle of the TPS model is that students learn best from individuals who have roles as teachers, scholars, and practicing clinicians. In this model, supervising faculty members teach in the classroom, engage in scholarly activities, and provide clinical education in the center. In one of the best-known models of supervision in speech-language pathology (Anderson, 1981; McCrea & Brasseur, 2003), a continuum of skill development is emphasized for both the student and the supervisor. Interaction between the two parties is also a key feature of the continuum model. This interaction and the continuum of skill development are also fundamental features of the TPS model. This model, which is used by many academic institutions, seeks to create a strong linkage between scholarly and professional roles of the supervisor. Students have opportunities to see first-hand how theory relates to their clinical work with individuals with communication disorders. This model is the foundation for our faculty-mentored student practice center, which operates as a site for the education of students and provides communication therapy services to the community.

In its main role as a setting focused on student learning, the center provides an atmosphere for the integration of academic knowledge and research-based practice in a clinical environment. As a place where faculty mentor beginning clinicians, an on-site clinical center is an ideal environment for linking clinical practice with theory and academic coursework. We use the term *supervisor* to represent a person in the professional role of clinical instructor or preceptor. This setting encourages the development of excellence skills, as well as the development of students' self-evaluation and self-reflection skills and the establishment of personal goals for clinical and professional growth. Superficially, it might appear that the "best" learning atmosphere is a real-world setting, such as a hospital, rehabilitation center, or specialty clinic. While these settings offer diverse, rich, and important experiences, the pressures of productivity, insurance issues, and medically complex patients make these environments exceptionally challenging for beginning clinicians. Like many healthcare professionals, speech-language pathologists face personnel shortages and increased requirements for documentation. External supervisors often struggle with the demands of high caseloads and productivity and not enough time to teach and support students who with limited knowledge and experience. Therefore, these settings are often best suited to advanced students who have already developed a solid basis in the understanding of intervention planning, diagnosis, and professional interaction.

The design of the TPS model at the MGH Institute is uncommon across graduate programs in speech-language pathology nationally. Due to institutional requirements related to tenure and financial pressures at many colleges, academic faculty rarely participate in clinical work; clinicians involved in supervising students within graduate school clinics are often not faculty and are not frequently involved with academic teaching and scholarship. Thus, the split between researcher/academic and clinician begins immediately in the educational process itself. Beginning students need clear paths drawn from the classroom to clinical application if they are to learn to think critically while developing a scholarly approach to practice based on evidence from research. Our model provides this bridge from the classroom to the clinic. It is a bridge that is crossed in both directions, because research in applied fields should be guided by questions that arise in the real world of practice.

A secondary purpose of the faculty-mentored student practice center is to provide diagnostic and therapeutic services to community members with communication disorders. Because the faculty-student practice center is an integral part of the educational program, our institution financially supports the center as a place for student learning. Therefore, the center is not dependent on outside sources such as state or governmental funding or payments from insurance or private-pay individuals. Clients are requested to pay a nominal "user fee" to support purchase of materials used in the clinic, such as books, diagnostic tests, treatment materials, and software. This fee can be waived or reduced depending on individual circumstances. No client is ever denied services due to the inability to pay this fee. Having a "free" clinic is possible because of the nature of the integration of academic and clinical resources, including teachers and supervisors. Furthermore, because the clinic is not dependent on outside funding, it is able to provide services to underserved and underprivileged populations.

■ Use of the Teacher-Practitioner-Scholar Model

The Entry-Level Clinical Center

The Speech, Language and Literacy Center was designed as a space for beginning graduate students to work with children and adults who have various speech and language disorders, as well as for experienced graduate students to work in an outpatient setting with adults who have acquired communication disabilities. The physical layout of the center includes 14 individual treatment rooms and one large group/conference room. A digital observation system allows parents, caregivers, students, and supervisors to observe and record sessions. All treatment rooms have video cameras that project to a third observation room equipped with television monitors. Supervisors can observe sessions in this room and also have the ability to operate the camera remotely from the computer on their office desk. This gives student clinicians independence in the therapy room even while they are being carefully observed by a supervisor.

Students are supervised by licensed speech-language pathology faculty members with advanced expertise in their field. These supervisors are faculty members in the Communication Sciences and Disorders Department and are promoted on the basis of excellence in teaching and scholarship. This integration of academic and clinical expertise allows for a unique learning atmosphere for the students, and a rich collegial environment for faculty.

Students in their first year of the graduate program will have two semesters of clinical experience in the Speech, Language and Literacy Center. During one of these semesters, students work with children who have spoken language disorders, such as toddlers, preschoolers, or early school-age children who demonstrate difficulties in the areas of expressive or receptive language, articulation or phonology, or social communication. These children might also present with a specific diagnosis such as autism, cerebral palsy, or Down syndrome, but most often do not have a specific diagnosis. Students also spend one semester with school-age children and adults who have reading and writing disorders. Some of these clients may have a diagnosis of dyslexia.

These two semesters of clinical experience occur during the first and second semesters of the students' graduate program. Each student is paired with another student as a dyad partner. Dyad partners share two clients who are each seen twice a week for individual sessions. Each partner is responsible for the creation of weekly lesson plans as well as participation in diagnostic and therapeutic activities. This experience of working with a partner was designed to explicitly facilitate the development of professional collaboration skills. Beginning clinical work is often highly stressful for novice clinicians. Some students may have experienced some type of clinical environment during their undergraduate education or prior employment, but many see the clinical world as foreign and daunting. Pairing each student with another beginning graduate student fosters a feeling of companionship and collegiality. Because speech-language pathologists rarely work independently in the healthcare and educational fields, learning how to function on a collaborative team is a crucial skill. In addition, working in a partnership provides students with direct experiences with more than one client. This diversity of clients leads students to a greater understanding of a variety of disorders and fosters clinical growth in a manner that working independently with only one client would not allow.

In addition to the dyad partnership, students also participate in a weekly clinical team (CT) meeting. Students are provided written documentation of CT group expectations and responsibilities. These include examples of behaviors demonstrating the core clinical excellence skills as well as process requirements for case presentation. For example, students are expected to actively participate in group discussions by asking questions that demonstrate critical thinking, giving examples of innovative approaches they have developed, taking the risk to discuss and analyze errors, reflecting upon and assessing their performance, thinking from the perspective of the client, and communicating in a professional manner.

Each week, students spend 2 hours with a small group of students in a discussion format, facilitated by a faculty member. Therapy sessions are recorded so that students can then select a digital segment to present to the group. For example, students might select a clip of a therapy activity that yielded unexpected results, a positive outcome, or perhaps led them toward a question about the client and the therapeutic process. Each student is given time to discuss issues pertaining to his or her client, and is also required to participate in discussions regarding other clients. This forum engages each student in a learning process that expands his or her knowledge base beyond a single client. Because multiple clients are represented, students learn about therapy techniques and treatment planning for a variety of disorders. This type of "peer group supervision" allows students to expand their perspectives to include different viewpoints and to learn from their peers as well as their supervisor (Williams, 1995).

A clinical discussion group syllabus guides the faculty member in facilitating the group. The syllabus includes the core excellence skills to be targeted each week and the knowledge and skill objectives and activities for the week. Faculty use a questioning hierarchy based on Bloom's revised taxonomy (Anderson & Krathwohl, 2001) to facilitate growth in critical thinking. Students are provided with both the hierarchy and Bloom's taxonomy, which are also used to guide written feedback in planning documentation. Students are given explicit information about how to advance through the hierarchy of critical thinking toward advanced skills and self-supervision (Anderson, 1988), and how that progress is facilitated by supervisory scaffolding and the use of facilitative questions. Encouraging active engagement in the learning process as a group facilitates critical thinking and self-evaluation in all members. Expectations for clinical team meetings should be clear and openly discussed with students (see **Table 23-2**).

The development of self-knowledge and reflection is foundational to excellence in clinical practice. Active engagement in one's own learning encourages students to maintain an inquisitive nature and nurtures the development of critical thinking (Facione, 2015).

The concept of a continuum of competency utilizes a mastery approach to clinical learning and gives the students a feeling of acceptance of current skills, while

Table 23-2   Expectations for Clinical Team Meetings

Purpose of CT Meetings	Role of Students	Role of Supervisors
• Facilitate the development of core clinical excellence skills: 1. Critical thinking 2. Collaboration 3. Innovation/creativity 4. Risk taking 5. Advanced social perspective-taking 6. Active learning 7. Self-knowledge and reflection • Create a community of collaborative learners • Expose students to a broad range of clients • Provide information • Provide teaching context for learning and practicing new skills	• Pursue knowledge actively. Ask questions! Look things up! Read! • Think critically. Analyze and synthesize information. Integrate and apply information from courses. • Learn collaboratively with your peers. Offer ideas and resources, ask questions, seek to support the progress of all clients seen by your group. • Risk making mistakes! • Reflect thoughtfully and honestly about your performance and development. • Come to group having prepared to use the learning time actively, efficiently, and effectively.	• Provide information • Model core skills • Scaffold student development • Facilitate the development of critical thinking • Facilitate collaboration • Encourage, model, and reward risk taking and innovation • Require active learning • Facilitate the development of self-knowledge • Provide opportunities for self-evaluation • Evaluate student progress and participation

creating a mentorship relationship between faculty and student. Students are asked to self-evaluate and identify strengths and areas of growth in the beginning of the first term in the form of a narrative reflection on excellence. Students complete a reflective, competency-based self-assessment of skills during mid-term and final clinical evaluations. Supervisors use this assessment to assist students in developing clinical growth goals. It is common for students to either overestimate or underestimate their skill level at particular stages during the clinical learning process. Discussions between supervisors and students about perceived skills allow for the self-evaluation process to become foundational to growth in clinical excellence. Supervisors can then guide students in determining appropriate goals and objectives for growth. Students are required to take this self-assessment into advanced practice experiences in order to continue the reflection and growth process.

■ The Advanced Practice Clinical Center

The clinical excellence curriculum and the TPS model provide the base for clinical education across terms. In keeping with the philosophy of the entry-level clinical center, clinical education is provided in the advanced practice center by faculty members who also teach and conduct research in the area of acquired communication disorders. Students in the advanced practice clinical center are expected to further develop their clinical excellence and critical thinking skills to a more advanced level.

The advanced practice clinical center specializes in providing diagnostic and treatment services to adults with acquired neurogenic speech and language disorders such as aphasia, dysarthria, alexia, agraphia, and other cognitive-linguistic disorders resulting from brain damage. The center was started to provide a site for a subset of the second-year graduate students to gain clinical experience working with adults. It is operated as an outpatient rehabilitation center that provides speech-language pathology services to people who have acquired communication disorders. The advanced practice center operates simultaneously with the entry-level clinical center, so that both first- and second-year students are seeing clients in the center at the same time. Many other speech-pathology graduate programs throughout the country operate on a similar model.

In addition to providing a clinical practicum experience, the advanced practice center also allows students to learn several important realities of the larger health-care arena. With the high costs of health care in the United States and the limited availability of funds to pay for services, many adults with communication disorders no longer qualify for services. The reasons for this are varied, but generally arise from severe limitations in coverage for chronic conditions such as aphasia. Although a variety of therapies are generally covered by insurance plans in the first few months after a stroke or injury, many insurance plans no longer cover treatments for communication disorders in the chronic phase. As they enter the post-acute period, many people with brain injuries from stroke or head trauma are denied further treatment. This is particularly true for individuals with limited means or those without family members to advocate for extended coverage beyond the acute period.

Settings such as the advanced practice clinical centers in universities and other healthcare education institutions can serve as bridges across this gap in service. Patients can receive the treatments they require while students gain valuable insights into both the nature of chronic impairments and how variably people respond to their chronic conditions.

The clinical supervisors in the advanced practice clinic manage all new referrals and discharges of clients. Clients may continue to receive services in the clinic for as long as they are benefiting from the intervention provided. Following the World Health Organization *International Classification of Functioning* (ICF) model (WHO, 2001), both impairment-based and life-participation-based treatments are incorporated into the clinical practice model. *Impairment-based therapies* are those that would be considered standard treatments to improve a specific speech or language deficit that is interfering with communication to some extent. For example, direct treatment targeting impairments in syntax (the rules for combining words in language) would be a type of impairment-based therapy that could be provided. Life-participation-based treatment approaches are attempts to take a step further to address the effects the communication impairment has on an individual's quality of life and ability to participate in desired life activities. This approach also considers the environment as a potent factor in determining outcomes for post-stroke patients. By creating a supportive communication and social environment in the center, some of the environmental barriers that are routinely experienced by people with aphasia are lessened. Students also learn about a patient-centered orientation to care provision whereby each individual they are working with is more fully understood as a person living in an environmental context and not seen simply as a collection of impairments.

In their academic coursework covering acquired adult language disorders, students learn about the Life Participation Approach to Aphasia (LPAA; Chapey et al., 2008). A group of practitioners adhering to the LPAA has published a set of core values, which stress that services should be provided to people with aphasia as long as they are needed, the explicit goal of intervention should be the enhancement of life participation, and both personal and environmental factors should be the targets of intervention. Students learn about this approach and other recent advances in their academic coursework, but experiencing them first-hand in the advanced practice clinic makes them come alive for students. In this way, students learn to take on an advocacy role that they will be able to extend into and expand upon in other clinical contexts.

Along with faculty, students may participate in research in either the entry-level or advanced practice clinic. They have an option to complete a master's thesis during their 2-year program, and many have completed projects either fully or partially within the on-site clinic. Individual case studies, small-group assessment studies, and short-term treatment studies are possible types of projects that can be conducted within the center. In planning and conducting their research, students become familiar with the process necessary to complete a research project, from the initial step of getting approval from an Institutional Review Board (IRB) to the final stages of data analysis and interpretation. Although students are not required to do their research projects in the clinic, the on-site availability of subjects of all ages with a variety of communication disorders makes the process easier to accomplish for many students.

As the advanced practice center has grown to provide services to more than 60 people each semester, there have been increasing opportunities for graduate students to participate in interprofessional service delivery, an orientation strongly supported by all of the Institute's graduate programs. Students are not only educated in their own professions, but are also exposed in coursework and clinical experiences to the scope of practice for the occupational therapy, physical therapy, nursing, and physician assistant students.

One example of this was an intensive comprehensive aphasia program (ICAP) that was offered to eight participants with aphasia in collaboration with a nearby rehabilitation hospital. Participants attended the program all day for four full days a week. Each morning they received 2 hours of individual or dyad speech and language therapy, followed by an activity-oriented occupational therapy group. They were then transported to the rehabilitation hospital a half-mile away, where they were provided lunch and socialization time. The afternoon programming was a mix of adaptive sports activities (biking, boating), music therapy, group communication treatment, harmonica group, mindfulness meditation sessions, and a weekly swim group. Students provided all of the morning treatment, and they were required to monitor the participants' performance in terms of communication and participation in activities for all afternoon activities. Students worked directly with the professional staff members who were providing most of the afternoon programming, learning first-hand about what music therapists or adaptive sports trainers, for example, do in their clinical practice. In addition, they were helping to educate these other professionals about how to adapt their communication styles to people with different types and severities of aphasia. Both participants and students found the program challenging and inspirational.

Finally, the mix of clients in our waiting areas, who are attending either the entry-level or the advanced practice clinic, has presented some interesting learning experiences pertaining to living with disabilities among our students, faculty, clients, and their families. For example, we observed children attending the clinic reading books with an adult with aphasia in the waiting room. Young children have direct observation of individuals with disabilities and adult clients have opportunities to interact with young people in a social communication situation that might not otherwise be available to them. Similarly, students, faculty, and staff members benefit from the environment. For example, students in the entry-level clinic have the opportunity to interact with adults who have aphasia in the social environment of the waiting room before they have the course on aphasia. This gives students of all programs initial exposure to a population that they will learn about later in their education.

■ Types of Learners

A faculty-mentored student practice clinic can support a wide range of student learning styles and needs, including students who have little experience with clinical application as well as those who are moving toward independence. Using the TPS model, supervisors can often be matched to students with specific needs. For example, an instructor who is an expert writer might supervise a student who needs assistance with the development of clinical writing skills. This model also facilitates the learning styles of students who lack confidence, as well as those who appear overconfident.

It is common for students facing their first clinical encounter to feel unprepared, anxious, and frightened. Although many of these students find that they are able to move beyond this fear and quickly become acclimated to the clinical environment, some students continue to lack confidence in their clinical and interpersonal skills. The model allows the instructor to approach this type of student in a positive, supportive manner. Supervisors might spend time in the therapy room with the student clinician in order to model techniques and strategies before moving outside of the room to observe via camera. Students are also encouraged to use self-evaluation and peer discussion as means of improving self-confidence and awareness of areas of strength.

Likewise, students who have exaggerated perceptions of their knowledge and clinical skills (Brasseur, McCrea, & Mendel, 2005; Dowling, 2001) can also be supported in a faculty-mentored student practice clinic. It is for these students that the development of self-evaluation skills is most critical prior to going into an external placement. Analysis of a video after the session can be useful in order for the student to have a more objective view of what occurred in the session. For example, a supervisor might assist a student in analyzing a video clip of a session where a client's desired behavioral objective was not met. The supervisor can then help the student identify clinical and personal skills that should be further developed.

Recently, institutions of higher education have increasingly been moving in the direction of competency-based education models. In an environment where the costs of higher education to the student are coming under increasing scrutiny with respect to the eventual benefit of that education, using a competency-based model makes sense. The excellence curriculum that we devised for use in our onsite clinical centers can serve as a model for developing competencies that students across all programs are expected to develop over the course of their education.

■ Conclusion

Many positive outcomes have emerged as a result of this clinical education model. First, the TPS model has allowed our students to be highly prepared when entering external practicum experiences. Skills learned in the entry-level center are referred to as "portable skills" in that they are the key components of clinical excellence in all professional settings where a speech-language pathologist may practice, including clinics, hospitals, schools, and home environments. As a result, our students receive multiple job offers upon graduation and have become highly successful professionals in the field. The emphasis on excellence throughout the program allows students to become lifelong learners who see their professional growth as a continuum of development. Many alumni currently volunteer to precept our students in their clinical setting, and several former students have returned to our program to teach courses and supervise students in our on-site clinic.

Use of the teacher-practitioner-scholar model in a faculty-mentored student practice clinic allows the integration of academic knowledge, the development of clinical skills, and the beginning preparation for a lifetime of excellence. Leadership and the pursuit of excellence are not something that universities "train into" students. Students sit before us with the potential for a lifetime of excellence in service; it is our job to facilitate the unfolding of that potential.

Discussion Questions

1. How might the TPS model enhance a student's clinical education skills in various environments? What would be the benefits and challenges of this model for faculty and staff in a university setting?
2. The idea of clinical excellence is found in many fields in the healthcare professions. What do you see as the primary role(s) of a clinical educator in the development of these skills in your area of expertise?
3. Given that clinical centers in university settings can be costly, in your opinion, do the possible benefits of the faculty-mentored student practice center model outweigh the financial and workload challenges? Why or why not?

References

American Speech-Language-Hearing Association (ASHA). (2014). *2014 standards and implementation procedures for the certificate of clinical competence in speech-language pathology.* Retrieved from http://www.asha.org/Certification/2014-Speech-Language-Pathology-Certification-Standards

Anderson, J. (1981). Training of supervisors in speech-language pathology and audiology. *American Speech-Language-Hearing Association, 23,* 77–82.

Anderson, J. L. (1988). *The supervisory process in speech-language pathology and audiology.* Boston, MA: College-Hill Press.

Anderson, L., & Krathwohl, D. (2001). *A taxonomy for learning, teaching and assessing: A revision of Bloom's Taxonomy of Educational Objectives.* New York, NY: Longman.

Brasseur, J., McCrea, E., & Mendel, L. L. (2005). Remediating poorly performing students in clinical programs. *Perspectives on Issues in Higher Education, 9*(2), 20–26.

Chapey, R., Duchan, J. F., Elman, R. J., Garcia, L. J., Kagan, A., Lyon, J. G., & Simmons-Mackie, N. (2008). Life participation approach to aphasia: A statement of values for the future. In R. Chapey (Ed.), *Language intervention strategies in aphasia and related neurogenic communication disorders* (5th Ed.) (pp. 279–289), Philadelphia, PA: Lippincott Williams & Wilkins

Dowling, S. (2001). *Supervision: Strategies for successful outcomes and productivity.* Boston, MA: Allyn & Bacon.

Facione, P. A. (2015). *Critical thinking: What it is and why it counts.* California Academic Press, Insight Assessment. Retrieved from http://www.insightassessment.com/Resources/Select-Tools-For-Teaching-For-and-About-Thinking/Critical-Thinking-What-It-Is-and-Why-It-Counts/Critical-Thinking-What-It-Is-and-Why-It-Counts-PDF

McCrea, E. S., & Brasseur, J. A. (2003). *The supervisory process in speech-language pathology and audiology.* Boston, MA: Allyn & Bacon.

Meyer, D. H., McCarthy, P. A., Klodd, D. A., & Gaseor, C. L. (1995). The teacher-practitioner model at Rush-Presbyterian-St. Luke's Medical Center. *American Journal of Audiology, 4,* 32–35.

Montgomery, L., Enzbrenner, L., & Lerner, W. (1991). The practitioner-teacher model revisited. *Journal of Health Administration Education, 9,* 9–24.

Peach, R. K., & Meyer, D. H. (1996, April). The teacher-practitioner model at Rush University. *Administration and Supervision Newsletter,* 9–13.

Williams, A. L. (1995). Modified teaching clinic: Peer group supervision in clinical training and professional development. *American Journal of Speech-Language Pathology, 4,* 29–38.

World Health Organization (WHO). (2001). *International classification of functioning, disability and health.* Geneva, Switzerland: Author.

CHAPTER 24

Service Learning

Hendrika Maltby

Students in clinical placements are expected to acquire skills, solve problems, and prepare for future employment in professional fields. Many courses also require students to reflect on their practice—what went well, what did not, and how practice could be improved for the future. Experiential learning and reflection are two of the components of service learning. The involvement of the agency as a true partner in the meeting of agency needs and student learning adds the third component. The focus must be on both the students and the recipients of care in partnership (Bailey, Carpenter, & Harrington, 2002). That is, meeting community needs, students' learning objectives, and formal reflection on the experience are the components of service learning. This chapter describes the use of service learning in the health professions.

■ Definition and Purpose

The Community-Campus Partnerships for Health (CCPH, 2013) organization has defined service learning as:

> A structured learning experience that combines community service with preparation and reflection. Students engaged in service-learning provide community service in response to community-identified concerns and learn about the context in which service is provided, the connection between their service and their academic coursework, and their roles as citizens.

Using this definition, healthcare professionals have discovered that there are many opportunities to work with communities in enhancing health, as well as to work with each other. "Service-learning not only connects theory with application and practice but also creates an environment where both the provider of service and the recipient learn from each other" (Norbeck, Connolly, & Koerner, 1998, p. 2). This ties in with the philosophy of a liberal education, common in North American universities:

> Liberal education has always been concerned with cultivating intellectual and ethical judgment, helping students comprehend and negotiate their relationships with the larger world, and preparing them for lives of civic responsibility and leadership. It helps students, both in their general-education courses and in their major fields of study, analyze important contemporary issues like the social, cultural, and ethical dimensions of the AIDS crisis or meeting the needs of an aging population. (Schneider & Humphreys, 2005, p. B20)

Service learning operationalizes liberal education. Its purpose is to involve students in the community to provide a service that is determined by the community and connected to learning objectives in a course. Students begin to "understand that the people of a community are the true experts in knowledge of their community, because both the problems and the assets belong to them" (Mayne & Glascoff, 2002, p. 194).

■ Theoretical Foundations

Service as a concept in the community has been implemented since ancient times when people provided support and care to families (Cohen, Johnson, Nelson, & Peterson, 1998). Dewey was one of the first champions of service learning in the early 1900s, when service and educational goals were connected (Bailey et al., 2002). Over the years, various American presidents have established a variety of organizations that provided service to communities, such as the Peace Corps, VISTA volunteers, the Foster Grandparents program, and the Office of National Service.

Increasingly, community partnerships and interdisciplinary education are coming to the forefront of health professional education. In the Pew Health Commission's 1998 final report, a number of recommendations were made, and a set of 21 competencies for the 21st-century health professional were outlined that transcend disciplinary differences (Bellack & O'Neil, 2000). A main recommendation of this report was the requirement that all health professionals have interdisciplinary competence. This incorporates the competencies of partnering with communities to make health-care decisions and working in interdisciplinary teams. More recently, the Institute of Medicine (IOM) has made recommendations for education of public health professionals for the 21st century, noting that "effective interventions to improve the health of communities will increasingly require community understanding, involvement, and collaboration" (2003, p. 15). Service learning is part of this education.

CCPH is a nonprofit organization founded in 1996 that assists in fostering health-promoting partnerships between communities and health professional schools (Seifer & Vaughn, 2002). It is a "network of over 1000 communities and campuses throughout the United States and increasingly the world that are collaborating to promote health through service-learning partnerships for improving health professional education, civic engagement and the overall health of communities" (CCPH, 2009). Seifer (1998) also clarifies the differences between service learning, traditional clinical education, and volunteerism. In service learning, there is a balance between service and learning objectives and an emphasis on reciprocal learning, the development of citizenship skills and achievement of social change, reflective practice, addressing of community-identified needs, and the integral involvement of community partners. Seifer emphasizes that service learning is not required volunteerism, which lacks reciprocity and reflection and may not be connected to course objectives.

Using service learning in nursing and other health professions enables the development of perceptions and insight as described in cognitive learning theories in the opening chapter of this book. Devising a variety of teaching strategies to complement student learning styles is necessary to enhance this development. Students in health professions are usually practice oriented and want to do something, which relates to the adult learning principles of Knowles (1975) about recognizing the meaning or usefulness of the information learned. Cultural understanding can be a key element of this learning, as students work with a variety of populations. Service learning allows the student to implement classroom learning objectives while providing a wanted service to a community.

■ Types of Learners

Service learning is suitable for any level of student in any health education program. One resource, Campus Compact, a national coalition, is "committed to fulfilling the civic purposes of higher education" (Campus Compact, 2013b, first para.) by assisting faculty to integrate service learning into the classroom with institutional commitment to community engagement. To date, almost 600 colleges and universities have become signatories to the Presidents' Declaration on the Civic Responsibility of Higher Education (Campus Compact, 2013a), which challenges higher education to become engaged with the community so that the knowledge gained by the students can benefit society. Service learning (SL) has been added to courses and programs outside of health care as well, such as geography, political science, education, environment, and mathematics. At the University of Vermont, for example, 75 courses now have the SL designation so that students can easily find a course in which they can engage with the community (University of Vermont, 2013). These are at all levels and include undergraduate and graduate courses.

Examples in health care include a variety of professions in multiple settings. Cashman, Hale, Candib, Nimiroski, and Brookings (2004) had medical and nurse practitioner students provide depression screening at a community clinic through the application of service learning, providing a mutually beneficial opportunity. Chabot and Holben (2003) integrated service learning into dietetics and nutrition education. Health law students travel from the University of Maryland to Mississippi to partner with the Mississippi Center for Justice to examine hospital charity policies and debt collection practices (Rowthorn, 2012). Graduate rehabilitation students worked with inner-city seniors to provide primary prevention through service learning and also learned about interdisciplinary roles and advocacy for those in need (Hamel, 2001). Occupational and physical therapy students provided service at a child care facility (Hoppes, Bender, & DeGrace, 2005).

The nursing profession uses service learning in partnership with many community agencies. Much of the recent literature involved community/public health nursing clinical rotations focusing on the Veterans Administration Medical Center (Hudson, Gaillard, & Duffy, 2011), homeless individuals and families (Loewenson & Hunt, 2011), a sheriff's department (Fuller, Alexander, & Hardeman, 2006), a tuberculosis screening clinic (Schoener & Hopkins, 2004), an adult day-care center (Ross, 2012), a Community Health Improvement Center (Carter & Dunn, 2002), and a variety of community health agencies (Mallette, Loury, Engelke, & Andrews, 2005; Redman & Clark, 2002; Riedford, 2011). Additionally, service learning has been used as a tool for developing research skills (Janke, Pesut, & Erbacker, 2012), facilitating leadership and management skills (DeDonder, Adams-Wendling, & Pimple, 2011; Groh,

Stallwood, & Daniels, 2011), learning about health policy (O'Brien-Larivée, 2011), and increasing cultural awareness with prenursing students in a first-year experience course (Worrell-Carlisle, 2005).

All of the examples cited here used service learning: students provided a necessary service that was tied into the coursework they were undertaking. Reflection on the service and the process was a key element. Students were able to examine issues such as homelessness in the elderly (Hamel, 2001), disabled children (Hoppes et al., 2005), social justice (Groh et al., 2011; Redman & Clark, 2002), mental health in the community (Riedford, 2011), the financially disadvantaged (Scott, Harrison, Baker, & Wills, 2005), and culture (Worrell-Carlisle, 2005). Moreover, students had their worldview challenged and often changed their view in the process.

■ Conditions for Learning

Service learning courses can be placed anywhere in the curriculum, and students can be partnered in groups or as individuals working with homeless people, with those who have diabetes, in residential living centers, in health departments—in fact, almost anywhere and with anyone. The learning environment becomes very broad, especially when not bound by classroom walls. The first step is to build partnerships with community agencies that match course goals and objectives. Dunlap, Marver, Morrow, Green, and Elam (2010) discuss some of the variables that can affect campus/community partnerships and so must be considered, such as leadership, the academic calendar, and changing student cohorts. The CCPH website has a tool that can be used to inventory current partnerships to make decisions about future partnership work.

Prerequisites include teaching students what service learning is and how it differs from volunteerism. Outlining reflection requirements and how to incorporate this component is essential because reflection helps students to connect the service to course objectives and to understand why service is important. Reflection can be done in a variety of ways, such as in-class writing assignments, final papers, presentations, and journals.

■ Resources

Resources can be as much or as little as needed, depending on partnerships. Many placements are able to provide necessary supplies for projects, whereas others may rely on students providing the materials they need. For example, the agency may be able to fund clinics (e.g., screening for tuberculosis, influenza immunizations, cholesterol); other funding may be found through other sources such as area health education centers (AHECs) or the college/university. AHECs were begun by the U.S. government in the late 1970s "to address health staffing distribution and the quality of primary care through community-based initiatives designed to encourage universities and educators to look beyond institutions to partnerships that promote solutions which meet community health needs" (University of Vermont, College of Medicine, 2013). Research grants can also be applied for to incorporate service learning into the curriculum and to evaluate partnerships.

One of the major requirements is time, particularly when developing partnerships. Partners can be found anywhere. This may be through a partnership-type office at the educational institution (such as the Community-University Partnerships and Service-Learning office at the University of Vermont) that keeps a list of partners and their needs (e.g., a town planning office looking for geography students). Faculty members may have contacts via other courses, clinical experiences, service, or research in which they are involved.

Students also need time to provide the service. For example, a 3-credit-hour course takes about 9 hours of preparation time for students outside of class; therefore, the service can be a part of the 9 hours. Time can range from 10 to 15 hours over a semester to a concentrated 90 to 135 hours. The revision of assignments for the course can also incorporate the service learning projects. Suggested websites that can serve as a resource for faculty are listed at the end of this chapter.

■ Using the Method

Health seldom takes place in a vacuum. It requires the efforts of the individual, family, group, university, and community working in partnership. Service learning works to address the needs identified by a partner. Therefore, one of the first essential steps is to identify a partner. This can be done over a summer, during the semester prior to the service learning, or at the beginning of the course. Maurana, Beck, and Newton (1998) have outlined some principles of good partnerships, including common goals, mutual trust and respect, building on strengths, clear communication, and continuous feedback. They list three key themes in building successful partnerships: "1. Always remember that community members are experts in their community; 2. Promise less and deliver more; and 3. Be committed for the long haul" (p. 51). Once the partner has been identified, the contract can be as informal as a verbal agreement ("students will help . . .") or can be a formal written agreement outlining the roles and responsibilities of faculty, students, and partners. Websites identified in the "Notes on Resources" section at the end of this chapter provide examples of different types of contracts. Partnerships can become one of the strengths of the course and can be utilized each time the course is offered.

The course syllabus should incorporate service as part of the course and not as a "mere sidebar" (Heffernan, 2001, p. 1). Heffernan goes on to describe six models of service learning (**Box 24-1**). The model of service learning chosen for the course will depend on the goals and objectives that students need to meet.

Decisions on the partners and model of service learning lead to the other required components that should be included in the syllabus. How are the students going to engage with the partner? Will students work individually or in groups? Will the partner be a guest speaker in the class? Will students meet partners on their own, or will the faculty arrange formal meetings? Will projects be outlined in the syllabus, or will the partner and student(s) decide on this together? Will the projects be presented?

The reflection on service in conjunction with course objectives has to be clear. How are these reflections going to be done (e.g., in-class writing assignments that are announced or unannounced, final paper)? How will they be graded? Are there

---

Box 24-1   Models of Service Learning

1. Pure service learning where the service is the course content.
2. Discipline-based service learning that makes the link between content and experience explicit.
3. Problem-based service learning in which students may act as consultants.
4. Capstone courses usually offered to students in their final year.
5. Service internships—intense experiences with regular and ongoing reflection.
6. Community-based action research (or community-based participatory research) using research to act as an advocate for the community.

Data from Heffernan, K. (2001). *Fundamentals of service-learning course construction.* Providence, RI: Campus Compact.

---

specific criteria to be used? Will students have a grading rubric? Ash and Clayton (2004) provide an articulated learning structure for reflection through four questions: What did I learn? How did I learn it? Why does this learning matter? In what ways will I use this learning? Similarly, Kuiper (2005) suggests prompts for reflection such as "The problems I encountered . . . ; I think I solved them by . . . ; When I had difficulty I . . ." (p. 353). Using prompts guides students to critically reflect on the experience and how it affects both the partner and themselves. **Box 24-2** provides two examples of grading rubrics. More tools are available at http://www.ccph.info.

Finally, how will reciprocity be accomplished? Usually evaluations by and of all partners (the community, the students, the faculty) are necessary. These can be formal or informal. Shinnamon, Gelmon, and Holland (1999) developed evaluation of service learning tools for students, faculty, and community partners and asked questions about attitude, experiences, and influence on future work using a Likert scale. Evaluations help to create better relationships and a stronger experience. Other evaluation tools for student, partner, and faculty assessments are available on the CCPH website. Showcasing service learning projects during class presentations or a campus-wide poster presentation contributes to reciprocity by recognizing the work of the students and the partners.

International Service Learning

Another option for service learning is study abroad—immersion experiences of living and learning in another culture. This has several advantages, including increased student awareness of their own beliefs, values, practices, and behaviors and how that affects care; ability to learn from clients and provide culturally appropriate care; and ability to cope with factors affecting health and living conditions (Lipson & Desantis, 2007). A number of authors have described study-abroad experiences, including preparation of students and faculty (Doyle, 2004; Robinson, Sportsman, Eschiti, Bradshaw, & Bol, 2006), descriptions of the study-abroad opportunities (Anders, 2001; Bentley & Ellison, 2007; Harrison & Malone, 2004; Johanson, 2006; Tabi & Mukherjee, 2003), and learning cultural competence through these types of experiences (Caffrey, Neander, Markle, & Stewart, 2005;

Box 24-2 Sample Grading Rubrics for Reflection

Public Health Nursing (undergraduate-level) study-abroad course:

Community teaching projects to include elementary school and "teach the teachers" project (details to come). You will also participate in a variety of activities such as hospital visits, village clinic participation, and a community health fair. Other activities will be determined in-country as the opportunity arises. (P/F)

Journal: You will be keeping a written journal throughout your trip, in addition to reflection sessions while in country. During the trip, explore your thoughts, feelings, judgments, and an evaluation of your experience (not just a record of what you did each day). There is no right or wrong way to tell your "story." Make daily entries.

Criteria for a "pass" grade

Daily entries are made

Thoughts, feelings, judgments, and an evaluation of experiences are explored

Public Health Nursing (graduate-level), on-campus course:

Considerations on Practice: Questions based on readings, lectures, and clinical experiences with your project partners will be posted as an assignment under "Course Materials" (on Blackboard) on a class day. Reponses are to be submitted via Blackboard and will be due by midnight in 48 hours [can put specific day].

Criteria for a "pass" grade

500-750 words maximum

Question is answered

Linked to readings/lectures (with references)

Linked to clinical experiences

Perspective of the partner is included

Koskinen & Tossavainen, 2004; Maltby & Abrams, 2009; Walsh & DeJoseph, 2003; Warner, 2002). Readers are encouraged to explore the literature concerning these experiences.

Service learning during study-abroad experiences requires a long-term commitment (at least 5 years) for both learning and service with a partner outside of the country. Chisholm (2003) outlines the following three principles for international partnerships: trust, mutuality of benefit, and open communication. Trust entails being clear about goals, budgets, and limitations and includes being sure promises made can be kept. There must be a benefit for both partners (inherent in service learning). Open and complete communication is essential, ranging from the formal evaluation plans to the more informal check-ins. Adaptability is indispensable in the process. All principles of service learning still hold for international experiences, including linking community needs, students' learning objectives, and formal reflection on the experience. McKinnon and Fealy (2011) outline the core principles for developing global service learning programs in nursing, which "are based on the Seven Cs of Best Practice: Compassion, Curiosity, Courage, Collaboration, Creativity, Capacity building, and Competence" (p. 95).

Faculty interested in this type of experience for their students are encouraged to contact their office of international education (or equivalent), as it will provide logistical support. Many times it is the faculty themselves who have contacts in another country that are further developed for study-abroad opportunities. As Bosworth and colleagues (2006) state, "it began with one professor of nursing . . ." (p. 34).

■ Potential Problems

Teaching in, and the facilitation of, a service learning course take time, so a major potential problem is lack of time. Time is required to form partnerships, prepare students, and involve partners in the design and implementation of the course. Another potential problem is the lack of preparation of the students (partnerships, reflection). The information has to be in the course syllabus, and class time must be devoted to describing service learning, reflection, and the process of partnership. It is recommended that faculty teach only one service learning course at a time.

Lack of involvement of community partners in the design and implementation of the service learning projects can be a potential problem. As one of the components of service learning is reciprocity, involvement of community partners is mandatory. This can be remedied by clear and open communication. Regular contact with faculty is necessary so that issues can be dealt with early.

Another potential issue that has arisen is presenting service learning and the associated community-based participatory research work for promotion and tenure. There are now a number of resources available to faculty to support this work with communities and students. Nyden (2003) outlines some strategies that faculty can use, such as developing faculty networks, modifying tenure and promotion guidelines, and mentoring faculty and students. CCPH has developed a resource kit (available on its website) to provide health professional faculty with a set of tools to carefully plan and document their community-engaged scholarship and produce strong portfolios for promotion and tenure.

■ Conclusion

Service learning provides students the opportunity to develop transferable skills such as "the ability to synthesize information, creative problem solving, constructive teamwork, effective communication, well-reasoned decision making, and negotiation and compromise . . . and an increased sense of social responsibility" (Jacoby, 1996, p. 21). Service learning fits well with health professional education. Students need to get out of the classroom and become more involved in the community and with each other to make knowledge come alive. This strategy can provide students with insight into community conditions; community collaboration is lived, not just talked about in class.

■ Notes on Resources

One excellent resource on service learning is the CCPH website (http://www.ccph .info). It contains a plethora of information, including discipline-specific sample syllabi and other resources that include service learning, to provide assistance to faculty who want to use this methodology. Additionally, the site contains sample partnership agreements, strategies for assessment (student, faculty, partner perspectives), and suggestions for how to institutionalize service learning on your campus and access to electronic discussion groups. The other important piece of this type of teaching scholarship, which is also available on the website, is how to incorporate this work into the reappointment/promotion/tenure process.

There is a National Service-Learning Clearinghouse (NSLC, 2013) website (http://www.servicelearning.org), which has a range of information for elementary, high school, and tertiary education settings. It includes information on national and international conferences, e-mail discussion lists, service learning ideas and curricular examples, sample forms and templates, and technical assistance staff. This site has a link to the Corporation for National and Community Service (CNCS, 2013), which lists opportunities in a variety of organizations (http://www.nationalservice.gov /about). Access to the CNCS strategic plan is available through this website, which has further information on service learning from kindergarten to graduate school.

Service learning is being used for international projects such as faculty-led study-abroad courses. The International Service Learning (ISL) organization (http://www .islonline.org/about) provides medical and educational teams of primarily student volunteers to provide services for the underserved populations of Central and South America, Mexico, and Africa. The goal of ISL is to partner student and professional teams from developed countries with service opportunities in developing countries. The International Partnership for Service-Learning and Leadership (IPSL, 2009) is another organization that links academic programs and volunteer service, giving students a fully integrated study-abroad experience. IPSL (http://www.ipsl.org) promotes the theory and practice of service learning and development and promotion of service learning in institutions of higher education around the world. Faculty who want to incorporate service learning into study-abroad options will need to consult with their own institutions' international offices.

Teaching Example:
Public Health Nursing (Fourth Year, Spring Semester)

An example of a service learning project is one in which we partnered with *Living Well*, an organization on campus whose mission is to "create opportunities for accessing information, identifying resources, developing skills, and making healthy choices . . . through innovative programming, collaborating with and supporting campus partners, and advocating for individual and community health" (http://www.uvm.edu/~chwb/livingwell). The center director approached the course faculty member to see if nursing students could be involved in a university-wide health fair. That fair, titled *Spring into Health*, was held about a month before final examinations and took place in the student center, which is centrally located.

Following enthusiastic support, nursing students were involved in all aspects: planning, marketing, budgeting, organizing and purchasing, implementation, and evaluation. Outreach to the community was made for donations from area businesses for give-aways (e.g., passes for fitness

(continues)

classes, cheese, water bottles, sunscreen). The nursing students also reached out to other professional groups on campus: the Communication Sciences and Disorders students provided a table on dyslexia, nutrition students helped to develop and staff a Healthy Eating table, and the Women's Center set up an information table. They also enlisted the second-year nursing students to offer blood pressure screenings. Outside agencies, such as the American Red Cross, Therapy Dogs, and RU12 Community Center (dedicated to advancing community and the health and safety of the lesbian, gay, bisexual, transgender, and queer [LGBTQ] Vermonters), were invited to set up displays with information and activities. Other tables, staffed by the nursing students, included smoking cessation, get moving, stress relief, and handwashing (disease prevention). Not only were information about the topic and give-aways provided, participants were also engaged in activities. For example, at the handwashing table, participants rubbed their hands with Glo-Germ (a product that makes surface bacteria visible under special lighting), then washed their hands and put them under a "black light" to see how well they did. At the stress relief table, participants were able to have a neck massage; at the "get moving" table, participants did 1 minute of an exercise in order to obtain their prizes. There was a trivia question wheel to check nutrition facts. As participants visited each table, they received stamps on a "health passport" to obtain tickets for grand prizes (e.g., Cabot Creamery cheese basket, Ben and Jerry's gift basket).

Throughout the day of the fair, the nursing students also kept track of numbers of participants and provided pens so that participants could make comments on the table coverings. They also compiled a resource guide to planning a health fair for future nursing students. A debriefing meeting was held with the *Living Well* staff. The nursing students met the course objectives of implementing a population-based intervention, engaging in partnerships, and using professional communication skills. The *Living Well* center was able to hold a health fair, and the population of university students was educated on a variety of topics in a creative and engaging manner. The nursing students also completed reflections based on their work, making this an ideal service learning project.

Gerontological Nursing (third year, fall semester); Jason Gabarino DNP, RN-BC, CNL

At the University of Vermont (UVM), service learning is incorporated into an undergraduate course in gerontological nursing. This activity provides students with the opportunity to work with older adults who reside at a local assisted living facility. Each week, a group of seven to eight students formulates and delivers a unique Reminiscence Therapy session suitable for older adults with various cognitive and physical abilities.

The service learning activity provides a mutual benefit for both the student participants and residents at the assisted living facility. For the students, it serves as direct insight into the lived experience of elders in the community setting. Students are provided the opportunity to practice communication skills, exercise their creativity, and gain an understanding of the multitude of diverse needs within this population. Students report a wealth of knowledge gained from the older adults, including life advice and suggestions for successful aging. Older adults who volunteer to participate in the activity have reported enjoying the opportunity to speak to and actively engage with students of a younger generation. Reminiscence therapy encourages older adults to talk about previous experiences and events, and has shown the ability to improve mood, cognitive levels, and social engagement (Haslam et al., 2013).

Following the Reminiscence Therapy, each student is paired with an older adult; the two then return to adult's room for an individual, hour-long conversation. This allows the resident and student to become better acquainted and share more intimate life stories and experiences. To conclude the experience, students participate in a faculty-led debriefing session and are responsible for completing a reflection paper that evaluates and summarizes the activity. The majority of students have found this to be a very positive experience, and many share a new or increased interest in pursuing a career in caring for older adults.

Discussion Questions

1. How would you add service learning to one of the courses that you teach? Think about who would be a partner, how the partner would be engaged in the process, what students would be involved, and how many hours students would have to complete this activity.

2. Find out if there is a service learning office on your campus. What can that office provide to help you incorporate this learning strategy into your course/ curriculum?

3. Choose one of the models of service learning outlined in the chapter. Describe the pros and cons of using this model.

References

Anders, R. L. (2001). A nursing study abroad opportunity. *Nursing and Health Care Perspectives, 22*(3), 118–121.

Ash, S. L., & Clayton, P. H. (2004). The articulated learning: An approach to guided reflection and assessment. *Innovative Higher Education, 29*(2), 137–154.

Bailey, P. A., Carpenter, D. R., & Harrington, P. (2002). Theoretical foundations of service-learning in nursing education. *Journal of Nursing Education, 41*(10), 433–452.

Bellack, J. P., & O'Neil, E. H. (2000). Recreating nursing practice for a new century: Recommendations of the Pew Health Professions Commission's final report. *Nursing and Health Care Perspectives, 21*(1), 14–21.

Bentley, R., & Ellison, K. J. (2007). Increasing cultural competence in nursing through international service-learning experiences. *Nurse Educator, 32*(5), 207–211.

Bosworth, T., Haloburdo, E., Hetrick, C., Patchett, K., Thompson, M. A., & Welch, M. (2006). International partnerships to promote quality care: Faculty groundwork, student projects, and outcomes. *Journal of Continuing Education in Nursing, 37*(1), 32–38.

Caffrey, R. A., Neander, W., Markle, D., & Stewart, B. (2005). Improving the cultural competence of nursing students: Results of integrating cultural content in the curriculum and an international immersion experience. *Journal of Nursing Education, 44*(5), 234–240.

Campus Compact. (2013a). *Signatories*. Retrieved from http://www.compact.org/resources-for-presidents /presidents-declaration-on-the-civic-responsibility-%20of-higher-education/signatories

Campus Compact. (2013b). *Who we are*. Retrieved from http://www.compact.org/about/history-mission -vision

Carter, J., & Dunn, B. (2002). A service-learning partnership for enhanced diabetes management. *Journal of Nursing Education, 41*(10), 450–452.

Cashman, S. B., Hale, J. F., Candib, L. M., Nimiroski, T. A., & Brookings, D. R. (2004). Applying service-learning through a community–academic partnership: Depression screening at a federally funded community health center. *Education for Health, 17*(3), 313–322.

Chabot, J. M., & Holben, D. H. (2003). Integrating service-learning into dietetics and nutrition education. *Topics in Clinical Nutrition, 18*(3), 177–184.

Chisholm, L. A. (2003). Partnerships for international learning. In B. Jacoby & Associates (Eds.), *Building partnerships for service-learning* (pp. 259–288). San Francisco, CA: Jossey-Bass.

Cohen, E., Johnson, S., Nelson, L., & Peterson, C. (1998). Service-learning as a pedagogy in nursing. In J. S. Norbeck, C. Connolly, & J. Koerner (Eds.), *Caring and community: Concepts and models for service-learning in nursing* (pp. 53–63). San Francisco, CA: American Association for Higher Education.

Community-Campus Partnerships for Health (CCPH). (2009). *Promoting health equity and social justice* (home page). Retrieved from http://ccph.info/CCPH

Community-Campus Partnerships for Health (CCPH). (2013). *Service-learning: Definition*. Retrieved from http://ccph.info/CCPH

Corporation for National and Community Service. (2013). *About CNCS*. Retrieved from http://www .nationalservice.gov/about

DeDonder, J., Adams-Wendling, L., & Pimple, C. (2011). A service-learning project facilitating leadership and management skills. *Journal of Nursing Education, 50*(7), 423–424.

Doyle, R. M. (2004). Applying new science leadership theory in planning an international nursing student practice experience in Nepal. *Journal of Nursing Education, 43*(9), 426–429.

Dunlap, R. K., Marver, D., Morrow, B. J., Green, B. R., & Elam, J. (2010). A community health service-learning roundtable: Nursing education partnership for community health improvement. *Journal of Nursing Education, 50*(1), 44–47.

Fuller, S. G., Alexander, J. W., & Hardeman, S. M. (2006). Sheriff's deputies and nursing students: Service-learning partnership. *Nurse Educator, 31*(1), 31–35.

Groh, C. J., Stallwood, L. G., & Daniels, J. J. (2011). Service-learning in nursing education: Its impact on leadership and social justice. *Nursing Education Perspectives, 32*(6), 400–405.

Hamel, P. C. (2001). Interdisciplinary perspectives, service learning, and advocacy: A nontraditional approach to geriatric rehabilitation. *Topics in Geriatric Rehabilitation, 17*(1), 53–70.

Harrison, L., & Malone, K. (2004). A study abroad experience in Guatemala: Learning first-hand about health, education, and social welfare in a low-resource country. *International Journal of Nursing Education Scholarship, 1*(1), Article 16.

Haslam, C., Haslam, S., Ysseldyk, R., McCloskey, L., Pfisterer, K., & Brown, S. (2013). Social identification moderates cognitive health and well-being following story- and song-based reminiscence. *Aging & Mental Health, 18*(4), 425–434.

Heffernan, K. (2001). *Fundamentals of service-learning course construction.* Providence, RI: Campus Compact.

Hoppes, S., Bender, D., & DeGrace, B. W. (2005). Service learning is a perfect fit for occupational and physical therapy education. *Journal of Allied Health, 34*, 47–50.

Hudson, C. E., Gaillard, S., & Duffy, N. (2011). Developing a community health clinical practicum service-learning model: An academic and VA medical center partnership. *Nurse Educator, 36*(1), 7–8.

Institute of Medicine (IOM). (2003). *Who will keep the public healthy? Educating public health professionals for the 21st century.* Washington, DC: Author.

International Partnership for Service-Learning and Leadership. (2009). *International service-learning programs.* Retrieved from http://www.ipsl.org

Jacoby, B. (1996). *Service-learning in higher education: Concepts and practices.* San Francisco, CA: Jossey-Bass.

Janke, R., Pesut, B., & Erbacker, L. (2011). Promoting information literacy through collaborative service learning in an undergraduate research course. *Nurse Education Today, 32*, 920–923.

Johanson, L. (2006). The implementation of a study abroad course for nursing. *Nurse Educator, 31*(3), 129–131.

Knowles, M. (1975). *Self-directed learning: A guide for learners and teachers.* New York, NY: Cambridge.

Koskinen, L., & Tossavainen, K. (2004). Study abroad as a process of learning intercultural competence in nursing. *International Journal of Nursing Practice, 10*(3), 11–120.

Kuiper, R. A. (2005). Self-regulated learning during a clinical preceptorship: The reflections of senior baccalaureate nursing students. *Nursing Education Perspectives, 26*(6), 351–356.

Lipson, J. G., & Desantis, L. A. (2007). Current approaches to integrating elements of cultural competence in nursing education. *Journal of Transcultural Nursing, 18*(1 suppl.), 10S–20S.

Loewenson, K. M., & Hunt, R. J. (2011). Transforming attitudes of nursing students: Evaluating a service-learning experience. *Journal of Nursing Education, 50*(6), 345–349.

Mallette, S., Loury, S., Engelke, M. K., & Andrews, A. (2005). The integrative clinical preceptor model: A new method for teaching undergraduate community health nursing. *Nurse Educator, 30*(1), 21–26.

Maltby, H. J., & Abrams, S. (2009). Seeing with new eyes: The meaning of an immersion experience in Bangladesh for undergraduate senior nursing students. *International Journal of Nursing Education Scholarship, 6*, Article 33.

Maurana, C. A., Beck, B., & Newton, G. L. (1998). How principles of partnership are applied to the development of a community-campus partnership. *Partnership Perspectives, 1*(1), 47–53.

Mayne, L., & Glascoff, M. (2002). Service learning: Preparing a healthcare workforce for the next century. *Nurse Educator, 27*(4), 191–194.

McKinnon, T. H., & Fealy, G. (2011). Core principles for developing global service-learning programs in nursing. *Nursing Education Perspectives, 32*(2), 95–100.

National Service-Learning Clearinghouse (NSLC). (2013). *America's most comprehensive service-learning resource*. Retrieved from http://www.servicelearning.org

Norbeck, J. S., Connolly, C., & Koerner, J. (1998). *Caring and community: Concepts and models for service-learning in nursing*. San Francisco, CA: American Association for Higher Education.

Nyden, P. (2003). Academic incentives for faculty participation in community-based participatory research. *Journal of General and Internal Medicine, 18,* 576–585.

O'Brien-Larivée, C. (2011). A service-learning experience to teach baccalaureate nursing students about health policy. *Journal of Nursing Education, 50*(6), 332–336.

Redman, R. W., & Clark, L. (2002). Service-learning as a model for integrating social justice in the nursing curriculum. *Journal of Nursing Education, 41*(10), 446–449.

Riedford, K. B. (2011). Bridging the gap between clinical experience and client access: Community engagement. *Journal of Nursing Education, 50*(6), 337–340.

Robinson, K., Sportsman, S., Eschiti, V. S., Bradshaw, P., & Bol, T. (2006). Preparing faculty and students for an international nursing education experience. *Journal of Continuing Education in Nursing, 37*(1), 21–29.

Ross, M. E. T. (2012). Linking classroom learning to the community through service learning. *Journal of Community Health Nursing, 29,* 53–60.

Rowthorn, V. (2012). Teaching health law: Health law service-learning trip, a how-to guide. *Journal of Law, Medicine & Ethics, 40*(2), 401–408.

Schneider, C. G., & Humphreys, D. (2005). Putting liberal education on the radar screen. *Chronicle of Higher Education*. Retrieved from http://chronicle.com/article/Putting-Liberal-Education-on/26781

Schoener, L., & Hopkins, M. L. (2004). Service learning: A tuberculosis screening clinic in an adult residential care facility. *Nurse Educator, 29*(6), 242–245.

Scott, S. B., Harrison, A. D., Baker, T., & Wills, J. D. (2005). Interdisciplinary community partnership for health professional students: A service-learning approach. *Journal of Allied Health, 34*(1), 31–35.

Seifer, S. D. (1998). Service-learning: Community–campus partnerships for health professions education. *Academic Medicine, 73*(3), 273–277.

Seifer, S. D., & Vaughn, R. L. (2002). Partners in caring and community: Service-learning in nursing education. *Journal of Nursing Education, 41*(10), 437–439.

Shinnamon, A., Gelmon, S. B., & Holland, B. A. (1999). *Methods and strategies for assessing service-learning in the health professions*. San Francisco, CA: CCPH.

Tabi, M. M., & Mukherjee, S. (2003). Nursing in a global community: A study abroad program. *Journal of Transcultural Nursing, 14*(2), 134–138.

University of Vermont. (2013). *Community-university partnerships & service learning*. Retrieved from http://www.uvm.edu/partnerships/?Page=courses.php

University of Vermont, College of Medicine. (2013). *Office of Primary Care and Area Health Education Centers*. Retrieved from http://www.uvm.edu/medicine/ahec

Walsh, L. V., & DeJoseph, J. (2003). "I saw it in a different light": International learning experiences in baccalaureate nursing education. *Journal of Nursing Education, 42*(6), 266–272.

Warner, J. R. (2002). Cultural competence immersion experiences. Public health among the Navajo. *Nurse Educator, 27*(4), 187–190.

Worrell-Carlisle, P. (2005). Service-learning: A tool for developing cultural awareness. *Nurse Educator, 30*(5), 197–202.

CHAPTER 25

Engaging Students in Global Health Endeavors

Lori A. Spies

Now more than ever, global issues and interconnectedness have an impact on healthcare professionals, and students in the health disciplines are seeking relevant experiences (Memmott et al., 2010). Global experiences are offered at more than 85% of U.S. institutions (Whalen, 2015). In 2013–2014, more than 300,000 students from the United States took a study-abroad course (Open Doors, 2015). Students can be engaged globally through a range of activities. Study abroad, service learning, joining faculty in global capacity-building activities, or discipline-specific missions can all be a part of the healthcare student's learning experience.

The access to travel and number of people venturing to remote parts of the world bring motivation to seek knowledge in distant lands (Kulbok, Mitchell, Glick, & Greiner, 2012). Healthcare students seek new challenges and ways to learn and engage in the world, because today global health is local health. There is an increase in the movement of people transiently on vacations, for adventure travel, and for longer durations or permanently in migration and immigration; all of these factors require expanded health knowledge. There is an ever-increasing refugee population that requires specialized health care. Increasing students' knowledge of working cross-culturally, enhancing their awareness of global health, and expanding their view of themselves as global leaders and citizens of the world are potential outcomes of a well-crafted global student experience (Delpech, 2013).

The growing mobility of people all over the world impacts the delivery of health care in a myriad of ways. The diversity of society necessitates new skills. This chapter provides information on how to craft a global learning experience for healthcare students to prepare them for changing healthcare needs. The focus of this chapter is the types of global student experiences that can be developed. Elements such as student safety, costs, and housing are considered, among others, and informational resources and checklists are included.

■ Definition and Purposes

There is huge variation in types of global experience and terms used. The terms *global* and *international* are used interchangeably in the general press, but how they are defined is important to include when engaging students.

Originating from public health, the term *international health* is generally used when speaking of work in other countries, but the term *global health* is used in issues related to the provision of health care that crosses borders (Koplan et al., 2009). During an international health-related learning experience, global health skills that are locally applicable can be developed in students.

There are many reasons to provide students with an out-of-country opportunity. A global learning experience can foster cultural acumen to prepare students to address the increasingly diverse population in the United States (Ballestas & Roller, 2013). Working well cross-culturally is a skill that can enhance patient care and help improve outcomes. The myriad of cultures present in a typical healthcare setting calls for more than memorized rudimentary knowledge of a few cultures. A holistic approach includes acknowledging differences and interacting respectfully to accomplish mutually agreeable goals; this is ideally developed in the global experience. Cultural navigation skills can be developed and refined through student global experiences that incorporate intentional cross-cultural interaction (Carpenter & Garcia, 2012).

There is an increasing need for healthcare students to become—and remain— aware of conditions previously unseen or uncommon in the United States. The febrile patient from East Asia may have malaria; the musculoskeletal issue in the African may be related to childhood polio. There has been an increase in vector-borne diseases such as dengue and chikungunya, previously seen primarily in tropical regions but now found in the United States as well due to global climate change (World Health Organization, n.d.). The importance of understanding global health was tragically illustrated by the cases of Ebola in Dallas, Texas, in 2014. Guiding students in global experiences can help them be more cognizant of the interconnected nature of health on a small planet.

Students across all disciplines are seeking ways to have international experiences (National League for Nursing [NLN], 2011; Delpech, 2013; Sachau, Brasher, & Fee, 2010; Whalen, 2015)). Universities are expanding their global presence, exchange programs are increasing, international research is expanding, faculty development partnerships are emerging, and mission and service learning opportunities are readily available (Scarr et al., 2012). Exposure to people who have had global experiences and ready access to global information has piqued student interest in global engagement. However, turning awareness and interest into enriching learning global experiences is a multifaceted task.

■ Theoretical Rationale

Global endeavors, almost by definition, are rooted in experiential learning theory (ELT). The requirement to be able to comprehend and apply knowledge is a clear need in health care. A key construct of ELT is that learning is a process and results from the interaction of a person with his or her environment (Kolb, 1984; Passarelli & Kolb, 2012). Placing a student in an international setting manipulates the usual environment and orchestrates a relevant opportunity. The in-country experience can epitomize ELT's process of "experiencing, reflecting, thinking and acting" (Kolb & Kolb, 2012, p. 49). Learning through global endeavors reflects ELT in the processes of preparation, travel, being in country, and reflecting on the process as an unfolding experience that continues to provide insight after returning home. The consideration of that which is new and the challenges of being outside of one's comfort zone require resolution of conflict and are drivers of the learning process (Kolb & Kolb, 2012; Passarelli & Kolb, 2012). The health-related global experience can be strengthened by the inclusion of theory that considers culture and intentional incorporation of reflective practice.

Cultural humility theory involves active reflection and cultivation of sensitivity to those from other cultures (Tervalon & Murray-Garcia, 1998). It focuses on awareness of one's personal perspective on culture in relation to others rather than on the mastery of a list of cultural skills. Cultural humility stresses cultural parity and the acceptance of cultural differences, and is applicable across professional experiences. Placing personal culture in the context of "one of many" rather than regarding it as the superior or even the normal way characterizes cultural humility (Schuessler, Wilder, & Byrd, 2012; Tervalon & Murray-Garcia, 1998).

Although attaining true cultural competence is outside the scope of the vast majority of educational global experiences, the students preparing to travel internationally will need concrete details about the practices of the destination. More important, however, is the development of an appropriate approach to cross-cultural interactions. Global experiences can provide structured cultural interactions and planned reflections to raise awareness of cultural preconceived thoughts and expectation. Cultural skill acquisition can be linked to diverse theories, and program organizers should consider what would best mesh with the specific program or institution. To be culturally humble requires a reflective attitude about one's personal culture and belief in the cultural parity of all those with whom one interacts (Isaacson, 2014; Tervalon & Murray-Garcia, 1998). A good practice is to design the global experience following tenets of ELT and cultural humility. During each phase of planning, ELT and cultural humility can be incorporated to lead to a learning experience that enriches students after graduation and movement into their professions.

■ Crafting the Global Experience

Creating a student global experience is a multifaceted process with a plethora of variables. Leaders of global endeavors need to accept that although every detail is planned, and contingency strategies are outlined, inevitably there will be change. It is important to take exquisite care in the details, but equally important to be able to be flexible as the global experience unfolds.

Orchestrating a global endeavor from start to finish provides an opportunity for experiential learning for the faculty. Developing and leading any sort of global experience for students is labor intensive. A study-abroad course incorporates all of the usual required course preparation, as well as the additional international trip planning, student recruiting, and university approval seeking. During the time out of country, the faculty will need to be available to the student(s) around the clock. On a 2-week trip of 8-hour days, there will be 112 hours of direct student contact and 168 hours of being on call—far more than a course taught in a traditional 15-week format (Sachau et al., 2010). Faculty who lead global endeavors usually find the effort well rewarded, but the time and attention to detail required may be more than anticipated.

Determining the learning objectives for the experience is frequently the first step. The decision can then be made about what sort of global endeavor might facilitate meeting of the learning objectives. It is important to consider objectives in the context of the academic program and institution's learning environment (Delpech, 2013). Broad educational goals can enhance the development of knowledge and skills, cultivate cultural acumen, and enrich and expand worldviews (Sachau et al., 2010). Prioritizing student learning and adopting standards of good practice do not dictate the type of trip, but can guide the development of the experience (Whalen, 2015). Objectives can spring from the course and from the cultural experiences anticipated (Delpech, 2013). Learning priorities can be focused on clinical skill and knowledge acquisition in addition to the attainment of discipline-encouraged cultural competency (American Association of Colleges of Nursing [AACN], 2008, 2011). Pre-trip preparation and in-country experiences can subsequently be developed to facilitate achievement of the objectives.

Examples of global experience include mission, study abroad, and research. Each is likely to have varying institutional requirements and processes for approval. The destination should be selected to meet the learning objectives and to be consistent with the type of experience sought. With those two components in place, the details of student orientations, assignments, and outcomes can be delineated. It is recommended that the course faculty contact the appropriate office at the academic institution early in the process for guidance on all aspects of the course and travel. Travel arrangements and safety plans can be formulated quite early in the process. Appropriate "on the ground" contacts should be cultivated, and long-term engagement can be considered from the outset. This process ideally begins a year or more before the global experience is launched.

Types of Experiences for Global Learners

Common categories of student global experiences include study abroad, mission, and research- and project-directed initiatives. Each category has many permutations and specific details to be attended to. Consistent across innovative teaching modalities is the principle that the desired learning outcome must be well thought out and carefully outlined. Setting the learning, service, or research goals and determining the desired learning outcomes will help determine which type of activity will best meet the curricular needs. There are many ways to get students involved in learning experiences that include international involvement. Begin by becoming familiar with format options at the host and destination institutions to determine which type of global endeavor best meets your students' learning needs.

Study Abroad

Study abroad is a general term for learning that can be implemented in several ways. It can be universities exchanging students for a semester or year of study. The short- and long-term faculty-led models are frequently used, and required courses are often also designed with time allotted for regional travel and exploration (Sachau et al., 2010). A *study tour* is a variation of study abroad involving faculty-guided travel to multiple sites to expound on the course theme (Sachau et al., 2010). A study abroad can be embedded in a course that starts and ends at the home university but requires a mandatory trip mid-semester. Students can join in-country university students for lecture, work alongside local healthcare providers for a clinical course, or participate in an independent study involving the use of local resources to expand their knowledge on a specific topic using an independent study model. Study-abroad courses offer a way for students in health-related majors to develop relevant knowledge and skills, adding an enriching, albeit challenging, cross-cultural dimension.

Regardless of the type of course—didactic, clinical, or independent study—the course must be designed to work within the existing curriculum. Creating and having a study-abroad course adopted into a curriculum will necessitate a broad array of support by faculty and administration. A new course will require approval from multiple curriculum committees in the school or college and at the institutional level. Students should be encouraged to check with the financial aid officer to determine if scholarships or loans can be applied to study-abroad courses or expenses. Study-abroad cost must also factor in required faculty time and expenses. These costs are reflected in the tuition, trip fees, and travel expenses that each student typically pays.

Mission

Taking part in a global *mission* has many of the same components as study abroad. The student is expected to achieve specific goals, and objectives are clearly delineated. The mission has an added component of being consistent with an ideological perspective, often religious. Mission efforts do not include tuition, nor are faculty paid for leading students on missions. Approval for the effort involved in the mission experience may be reflected in the service portion of the annual faculty evaluation. Students may be able to count mission effort as volunteer hours. Faculty-led student missions are often scheduled during semester breaks.

Missions, like study abroad, often involve formal university procedures. The mission experience is often funded through donations. Raising support can be included as a learning objective and part of the pre-trip orientation. The language surrounding missions often emphasizes the team and working to accomplish the goal of the group or mutually recognized goals. *Discipline-specific mission* is a model that incorporates students being on mission and receiving course credit for the work accomplished (Kennedy, n.d.). This model has been successfully used in several healthcare disciplines to provide credit for an experience that focuses on expansion of ministry in a faith-based setting.

Scholarship

Scholarship can be embedded in both mission and study-abroad trips. It is also possible to focus a trip on developing scholarship in students and global collaborative partners, and finding opportunities for faculty research.

Research

International research is increasingly common across health disciplines. Planning for students to join faculty in research projects is a way to garner student interest and develop research, cross-cultural, and often interprofessional skills. Collaboratively building meaningful research capacity is a faculty and student cooperative undertaking. Conducting research with a faculty member is an ideal learning experience, paving the way to early involvement in scholarly activities while cultivating an expanded worldview and cultural humility. An important component of successful international research is the mutually beneficial nature of the endeavor. Faculty and students from both countries should be able to provide meaningful input as to how best to achieve shared scholarly goals (Spies, Garner, Prater, & Riley, 2015).

Student and Faculty Projects

Related to research but broader in reach is having the student experience be project focused. Students and faculty can collaborate with in-country partners to implement evidence-based projects. Students' understanding of the application of research is cultivated and enhanced through carefully selected projects. These projects should meet a need in country while expanding participants' skill sets. Engaging students and faculty from both countries provides an avenue for directed cultural interaction.

Service Learning

Service learning is another well-established way for students to be engaged globally. For more information on service learning and best practices, please refer to Chapter 24.

Country Selection

Selection of the type of experience should be concurrently explored with where the experience will take place. There are many facets to consider when choosing a destination, and being aware of your institution's policies and protocols will help in the process. Approval of the destination, like having a course approved, can involve communicating with multiple people within the institutions before final arrangements are established. Working with your institution's center for international education or global endeavors office early in the planning will help avoid putting time and effort into plans and preparations that may eventually not be approved.

Consider existing contacts of faculty and programs in other departments when trying to select a destination. A well-established education department relationship might be an ideal connection and easily built on for the creation of a healthcare-related endeavor. Where is work being done that is most relevant to the learning goals of the program? A faculty member with strong connections can make introductions and share contacts to begin to create a robust global experience.

Safety

Safety should be considered early when selecting a region of the world. The U.S. Department of State has a website for current travel warnings (Travel.State.Gov), and it is prudent to check this source early in the selection process. Few new programs in the United States will be approved if the U.S. government has placed limits on tourist and business interaction in the destination.

Language

Language factors into the selection of a location. Courses are often designed to develop language skills in healthcare students. Language may be perceived as a barrier, but interpreters are widely available—and learning to work with an interpreter is a skill that may be useful in a student's clinical practices after graduation. Interpreters frequently also function as cultural guides and provide helpful insight.

Timing

The amount of time that can be allotted to travel and stay at the destination is a big consideration. Thirty-six hours of travel to arrive at a remote location may not be practical for an eight-day endeavor. Linked to time is also the consideration of jet lag on the way to the experience and on the return home. A trip of equal length in the same time zone may provide significantly more productive time than traveling across multiple time zones. A traveler's rule of thumb is to allow one day for each hour of time difference on the return trip for full recovery. This is rarely an option for a global experience planned during the academic year. Keep the time change and jet lag adjustment in mind when examining what will be expected of students and faculty on their return; this is a part of choosing a location as well as the timing of the trip.

Cost

Aside from tuition, the next predictably largest expense is likely to be airfare. Trip budgets vary widely: Study abroad in Hong Kong will cost significantly more than a research trip to Mexico. Trip costs affect who elects to participate and often the viability of the entire endeavor. A quick conversation with a travel agent or exploration of costs on travel websites may rule out some potential destinations. Students and faculty will need the estimated cost to be as accurate as possible. Faculty costs are usually subsumed in the students' trip fees (Sachau et al., 2010). It behooves the planner to estimate with a margin of error. Costs can rise unexpectedly; however, if actual costs are less than expected, a special team dinner or gift for the host can be arranged. Some global endeavors include all meals and every excursion, whereas other leaders arrange for optional excursions and certain meals to be separately funded. This is decided by the team leader, but the details and expectations must be clearly conveyed to all participants.

Housing

Housing selection is designed to promote team building, provide reflective time, and/or enhance cultural engagement. The cost of room and board varies significantly. Staying with host families makes a trip more affordable while enhancing the cultural immersion experience. Dormitory rooms at universities may be available inexpensively during the summer semester (Sachau et al., 2010). Considering alternatives to hotel rooms, such as renting a house or apartments, may also provide more flexibility in cost.

Global Learning Experiences

Assignments are incorporated to take advantage of the multifaceted opportunities present in the global setting. Learning objectives from both the course and the global experience should be considered in crafting each assignment. Guest lectures from local university professors, community workers, and health professionals will augment information provided by course faculty (Sachau et al., 2010). Contacting hospitals, schools, and professional organizations can provide diverse in-country experts as speakers.

Teaching projects to deliver in country can be developed based on, and derived from, students' cultural preparation about the destination and the target audience (Delpech, 2013). Reading and communication with in-country contacts provides information on possible topics. For example, graduate nursing students are required to develop continuing education for clinicians. The students may be surprised to learn that the topics most needed might not be what they anticipated; desired topics could be something commonly known to healthcare providers in the United States, such diabetes or breast cancer. Assessing the in-country learning need helps students apprehend the knowledge of topics, such as the significant increase in chronic disease in developing countries, in an especially meaningful way. Preparing a workshop requires students to become familiar with the usual in-country care and available resources. Preparing and leading a culturally appropriate workshop increases comfort with the clinical topics, enriches cultural interaction, and deepens understanding of health disparities and the provision of health care in environments of scarcity.

Journaling is a particularly useful tool that faculty can adapt to encourage reflective practice and enhance learning (Delpech, 2013; Savicki & Price, 2015). The process of reflective practice and journaling can be in a paper notebook, a series of short writing assignments, or an electronic blog (Sachau et al., 2010). Reflective practice can allow students to track their cultural and clinical learning experiences (Delpech, 2013; Passarelli & Kolb, 2012; Schuessler et al., 2012). Carefully designed critical reflection can target deeper exploration of key objectives and solidify experiential learning (Ash & Clayton, 2009).

Assigning students a topical paper focusing on a clinical or cultural issue provides a rich learning opportunity. A case study assignment, with the review of the literature completed prior to departure, enhances baseline knowledge. Scholarship is cultivated by requiring students to work with faculty and prepare a manuscript to be submitted for publication.

Clinical visits can be an important part of global experiential learning. Touring hospitals and clinics can provide insight into the usual standard of care and cultural norms. The use of traditional medicine in a modern hospital in Asia can provide the healthcare student with an expanded world-view. The philosophical and cultural differences of health care are brought to life when seeing acupuncture and herbal treatments being used one floor away from a Western-style intensive care unit.

Clinical participation may be arranged through local contacts (Delpech, 2013). Arranging for students to shadow a provider for a portion of the day brings insight into the local professional standards and practice. Seeking permission and obtaining local approval for students' clinical experience is best navigated by an in-country contact. Faculty and students should make themselves aware of licensure and practice rules before travel. Students and faculty must often submit copies of licensure, degrees, and transcripts before entry into clinical sites is permitted. An important standard is that students' activity must remain within their skill set and scope of practice. Ethically, students should not be allowed to take on tasks that they are not prepared for, or use clinical skills they could not perform in the United States and for which they have not obtained competency through their nursing education program.

Introducing students from both countries via social media before the trip is one way to enhance the experience and cultural exchange (Sachau et al., 2010). By building on those contacts, student interactions may be planned to increase students' personal cultural interactions, and local activities may be safely explored. Increasing cultural interaction in daily activities, in addition to excursions to healthcare facilities and historical sites, enhances the development of cultural humility (Delpech, 2013; Sachau et al., 2010).

■ Learners: Recruiting and Cultivating Interest

Students have multiple demands on their time. Developing interest and participation in study-abroad or mission trips can be challenging, especially if it is a new endeavor. Plan to get the details in front of those students who are most likely to be interested. It is a good idea to have students exposed to information about the global opportunities on several occasions. Encourage students early in their programs to think about where they can best include a global activity in their degree plan. If multiple options are available, provide snapshot information in a single brochure with contact e-mails of the point person(s). The information should include approximate cost and when the experience is held. Students will want to know if the experience is for credit and what the course expectations are.

Highlighting the main activities of a trip is a useful tool in cultivating interest. Studying traditional Chinese medicine in Hong Kong or working to provide physical therapy in an orphanage will draw student attention. Student interest is piqued by the clinical or didactic focus of the course or trip, but also by the culture and environment in which it takes place. Drawing students' attention to the need in an area is also helpful. The shocking statistics about maternal infant morbidity may drive a student to want to be a part of a team going to India to teach about delayed cord clamping. As awareness of needs is raised, students can identify the gaps they wish to fill in their global endeavors (Houghton, 2014).

Student Selection

Student selection is typically a multistep process, with participation criteria set prior to recruitment. This can include the student's current GPA, travel experience, health status, and completion of certain prerequisite courses. Fragile health, pregnancy, or certain preexisting conditions will be cause for exclusion. During recruitment, students are given a specific application deadline. In addition to demographic information on the application, students will usually provide answers to essay questions generally geared to determine why they are interested in the trip. Each student should be interviewed by the team leader and at least one additional person. For a larger team, a committee will be helpful in selecting participants. The process of determining who joins the team can be difficult. Revisiting the demand of the course and making the importance of interpersonal interaction a priority in selection can enhance flexibility (Delpech, 2013). If a second team sponsor or faculty member is needed, sometimes recruiting can expand to alumni and graduate students who are further along in the program (Palmer, Wing, Miles, Heaston, & de la Cruz, 2013).

Pre-Trip

The pre-trip phase of the experience is largely focused on creating a cohesive group and sharing information. Frequent meetings will help to establish the team and provide a venue to share the large amount of information that must be transmitted. It would be difficult to overstate the importance of meeting regularly to prepare students for the experience (Behrnd & Porzelt, 2012; Delpech, 2013). Safety, expectations, country orientation, and travel and packing-related information can be provided to students. A folder or notebook can be provided to give the student a central location of information. A linked website or course module can also be used (Sachau et al., 2010). Guidelines to assist in developing a credit-based study-abroad course are found at the end of this chapter.

Orientation Topics

Safety

The faculty or team sponsor should work closely with institutional global endeavors and risk management departments. Safety includes considering political and weather conditions and food and travel safety. Travel and liability waivers will be needed, and travel insurance will be required. Universities typically have mechanisms in place to assure that travelers are safe, the trips are registered, contact information is available, and itinerary and emergency contact information has been shared.

Travel health information and resources should be provided. Required immunizations and routine food precautions should be reviewed. This information is readily available from the Centers for Disease Control and Prevention. Directions on how to handle money in public and rules for behavior should all be discussed in detail. The level of information and structure is determined by the level of risk. In some settings, it is prudent for the student never to leave the guest house unattended; in other locations, a courtesy text to the faculty may be required. The rules regarding student behavior must be clearly explained and the ramifications identified. An example: "If you leave the compound without permission from your instructor in person, you will be sent home on the next flight at your own expense." These matters are reviewed during orientation; the student is asked to sign an agreement and is provided a copy.

Students are required to provide their emergency contact with a detailed itinerary. Team leaders, and in some cases all participants, will be required to have a working phone. A phone tree can be prepared, but leaders would be prudent to clearly convey to students that emergency situations are not to be texted, tweeted, or posted until the team leader has made official contact.

Country

Students should be provided basic information about the country where the global experience will occur. Exposure to online resources allows independent exploration of country-specific information (Delpech, 2013). Providing a map increases students' geographical awareness, and the corresponding weather information is helpful in deciding what to pack. The student should be aware of defining historical events, key geographical features, and key facets of the economy. Information about government, economic, and healthcare systems increases student understanding of the complex and interconnected nature of global health care. The student must be aware of relevant health information, such as the leading causes of morbidity and mortality, and the usual population access to healthcare providers. The specific information shared will be determined by the destination and the objectives.

Culture

There are many ways to educate students about working cross-culturally, and many theoretical approaches to culture can be incorporated into the planning and implementation of the global experience. Pre-trip information about culture has the purpose of providing student information about both the destination culture and guidelines for cultural skill acquisition.

How the destination culture impacts daily work can be explored from several perspectives. Questions such as "What are the usual birth practices?" and "How does the culture view illness?" can be presented as homework and brought into discussions. Students may be made aware of cultural issues by lecture or assigned reading (Ballestas & Roller, 2013). The level of comfort that students have working cross-culturally and their experience in travel can be assessed and used as a guide (Johns & Thompson, 2010).

Packing

Students will almost certainly be limited as to the amount of luggage they can take. The airlines have specific and clear guidelines on their websites about weight and size limitations. It is also prudent to review what cannot go in the carry-on or checked bags. Checking the Transportation Security Administration website can clarify the items on the most current "no fly" list. This should be emphasized with all travelers. Students should also be made aware if it is an expectation that a portion of their allotment is for team supplies. For a clinical trip, a packing day for the entire team to sort donated supplies and weigh suitcases is helpful.

What to pack presents a challenge as well. Students will benefit from clear guidelines for what they will be expected to wear while touring, while in the clinical setting, while in the classroom, and during downtime. Consideration of the cultural norms of dress, depending on the destination, is crucial. The clinic may require a lab jacket; women may be expected to always wear long skirts; head coverings may be the norm. A faculty-determined uniform of a school collared shirt and khaki pants or skirts to wear on clinical tours may streamline packing. A schedule with clothing requirements and a packing checklist may be helpful. A travel checklist for the supervising faculty appears at the end of this chapter.

■ The In-Country Experience

Every global endeavor provides unique opportunities. Before arriving at the destination, the faculty leader has carefully developed the course and itinerary. Students are oriented to the course and to travel, and provided with information and resources about the country, culture, and course. The in-country global learning experience incorporates the global learning assignments and is augmented by what is available in the destination.

A typical day in a study-abroad course begins with a morning student and faculty meeting. Depending on the type of course, the morning may be used for a lecture from a partner university, or perhaps for a clinical experience in a dental clinic, physical therapy department, or hospital inpatient area. Lunch with in-country students or professional colleagues provides an opportunity to develop relationships and explore cultural norms. The afternoon might include a cultural excursion related to course content or a community outreach activity. Activities are selected to augment learning. Opportunities such as participating in local feeding programs, providing community education on dental health, and working with physical therapists in an orphanage can enhance student learning in-country. Students can attend professional meetings, tour local facilities, and shadow providers as they make in-home follow-up visits. The list of options is endless.

Students will gain insight into the local culture by interacting away from the clinical settings as well. Being a guest in someone's home for tea, eating in a local market, shopping in the grocery store, visiting a temple, and simply walking in the community will raise cultural awareness.

Communication

While in the country, faculty and students should meet face to face frequently and at regularly scheduled times. Twice-daily meetings circumvent issues on short trips. A morning meeting during or after breakfast provides an opportunity to review the day's schedule and answer questions. Students should be reminded about appropriate attire and required equipment. This is also a good time to verify that students have identification, the address of the hotel, and a working phone with them, and to reinforce other safety concerns. An evening meeting is an opportunity to hear about the successes of the day, address any concerns, and make adjustments as needed. Student input is helpful, but limiting the number of choices the students make for the group will help eliminate grumbling and discord (Sachau et al., 2010). Allow time each evening for reflective journaling; for this activity, supplying topic prompts is helpful (Ash & Clayton, 2009; Ballestas & Roller, 2013). The journaling then becomes a natural segue into relaxed free time.

Frequent meetings also provide an avenue to revisit pre-trip teaching. It is often necessary to reinforce warnings about avoiding tap water and uncooked foods. Encouraging students to rest and stay hydrated is a good idea. Charging students with caring for one another, watching out for safety issues, or even synchronizing taking anti-malarial medication helps the team work together.

Rules about taking photographs and posting information to social media must be clear before the trip and emphasized during the experience. A typical rule is that no photographs are to be taken without consent and no photographs taken in the clinical setting may be posted to any social media site. Designating a daily student photographer and incorporating photo sharing into the evening debriefing eliminates multiple duplicate photos. A blog without public access provides a place to post updates and share photographs. Establishing a person to update the blog, either for the trip or daily, helps with information sharing. The faculty should make a habit of reviewing the blog each day.

Post-Trip Debriefing and Follow-Up

Debriefing is an important component of many experiential learning experiences. It provides an opportunity for students and faculty to examine and evaluate the global experience. Structured debriefing can be used to enhance students' global learning experiences and assist them in relating their experience in other countries to their profession at home (Bender & Walker, 2013). The debriefing can include informal sharing of pictures and memories and/or a guided consideration of experiences. This can refer to and reinforce issues evoked by the reflective journaling, helping to bring closure or to provide resources for additional contemplation.

Setting the date for debriefing prior to departure can overcome the distracted business and activity that inevitably follows a return from a trip. Opportunities for the returning students to share information with students, staff, faculty, and the community can be scheduled separately from the debriefing, but can be used as a time to share pictures and key thoughts and begin recruiting for the next trip.

■ Resources
Travel

Transportation Security Administration: https://www.tsa.gov
U.S. passports and international travel: http://travel.state.gov/content/travel/en.html
The World Factbook: https://www.cia.gov/library/publications/the-world-factbook

Health

Centers for Disease Control and Prevention: http://www.cdc.gov
World Health Organization International Travel and Health: http://www.who.int/ith/en

Global Learning

National League for Nursing (NLN) Faculty Preparation for Global Experiences tool kit: http://www.nln.org/docs/default-source/default-document-library/toolkit_facprepglobexp5a3fb25c78366c709642ff00005f0421.pdf

Cultural Competence

American Association of Colleges of Nursing (AACN). Tool kit of resources for cultural competent education for baccalaureate nurses: http://www.aacn.nche.edu/education-resources/toolkit.pdf

American Association of Colleges of Nursing (AACN). Tool kit for graduate cultural competence: http://www.aacn.nche.edu/education-resources/Cultural_Competency_Toolkit_Grad.pdf

Guidelines for Developing a For-Credit, Elective Study-Abroad Program for Student Nurses

The use of recommendations based on the collective wisdom of experienced nursing faculty who have participated in experiential learning can provide a rubric for successful study-abroad courses. Whether the program is in the beginning stages of development or has been functioning for many years, working with diverse and international populations presents challenges for faculty and student learning. The following guidelines may provide a rubric for structure, evaluation, and outcomes.

1. Create a proposal with the following:
   a. Goals and objectives of proposed program
   b. Location—distance, safety, costs, local interest and support for program, easy accessibility; collaborate with study-abroad office
   c. Experiences for students and faculty—clinical experiences, participation in cultural activities, local language lessons
   d. Safety plan—political safety and stability, environmental safety (climate, local disease threats), health insurance and local health care available for participants, emergency evacuation plan
   e. Student prerequisites—nursing skills, language background, grade point average, orientation, disciplinary rules
   f. Number of faculty needed
   g. Number of students expected (interest survey given to students may yield a more precise idea)
   h. Transportation—round trip to destination, as well as local transportation
   i. Estimated costs
2. Obtain support from the university's president, provost, dean, department chairs, and whoever else who may have to approve the endeavor. Obtain seed money to investigate the feasibility of the program and provide transportation, housing, and other costs needed to explore an area to make initial preparations for the proposed program. Gifts may also be required in some cultures to facilitate appointments for key people in the local proposed site.
3. Make a preparation visit to the proposed location.
   a. If possible, arrange all transportation and housing as you would expect to with students. Stay in a hotel or with a local family as you would expect students to, to see how the experience would be for students. Always ask permission to take pictures to show the university administrators as well as prospective students.
   b. Keep a detailed record book of all costs encountered. This will help in designing a course with an accurate price to reflect real costs.

c. Find a person who has experience and is willing to coordinate housing for students. This person will require a placement fee per student. Often the local university has such a person, or a secretary may be able to handle this. See if the university already has someone who assists foreign students with housing. Visit several homes or hotels for proposed housing and get specifics with prices.

d. Obtain local language lessons. Find a local university or language school that is willing to give lessons to students at a reasonable price for 1 hour per day. This will help students to enhance their language and cultural background while they are at the proposed location.

e. Meet with the minister of health (or equivalent person of high rank in the community) to discuss the students' participation in caring for local patients within a healthcare setting (hospitals or clinics). Specifically discuss student roles, supervision by faculty, dress codes, hours of work, and length of stay, among other issues. If it is culturally appropriate, get a written contract. Ask which types of supplies or equipment are needed for the purpose of donations in the future. After the meeting, send flowers and a thank-you note to the person for giving his or her time and attention. Note: Students working within a different culture and language should not be giving medications because of safety issues, which could be further threatened by a language barrier.

4. Meet with a tourist travel agency or find a specific person in the community who will agree to provide transportation and help with an agenda for visiting sites of interest. Take advantage of all local tourist attractions, emphasizing anything reflecting health care if available.

5. Recruit students.

a. Prior to recruitment, make all decisions about transportation, tuition, housing, food, cultural sites, donations, health insurance, availability of scholarships, and other factors, and prepare a formal budget. Decide how much it will cost per student for the entire package.

b. Create a brochure for the course/trip with detailed specifics of costs, inclusions, dates, course credits, prerequisites, and other information, and print flyers for a recruitment session. Several recruitment sessions may be necessary to contact all available students who may be interested in the program. Arrange a date, time, and location for the recruitments, and order food. If possible, bring photos or present a PowerPoint slide show of pictures of the area. Obtain a list of interested students with names and e-mail contacts, and provide a way for students to sign up for the course. If the university already has other study-abroad programs in place, they may be extremely helpful in planning your program.

c. Collect all fees prior to departure. Assemble supplies or equipment donations. Pack donations and send boxes with students to avoid mailing costs and possible theft of items.

    d. Create a mandatory orientation program prior to departure. Make sure that all students have all necessary passports, visas, and vaccinations. Supply food and invite all family or friends who are interested in the trip details. Review and give written handouts relating a typical day, dress and behavior codes, and health guidance (including what to eat and which medications to bring). Include a list of what to pack, identifying the weight and number limitations for luggage. State where to meet at the airport and at what time. Emphasize the safety and health plan. Review rules and regulations. Pass out the course syllabus and review pre-trip readings available. A survey of student perceptions of the trip prior to leaving would make an interesting point of comparison to impressions after having had the experience. Encourage students to bring small gifts for their host family and nurse mentors at their location.

    e. Have students review and sign a code of behavior while studying in the location. Include the following:

       i. No alcohol or drug use is permitted.

      ii. Dress codes and rules for expected behavior with family, faculty, and all members of local community are to be written and enforced.

     iii. No leaving of the city, under any circumstances, without permission of faculty.

     iv. All students will stay all night with their host family, with no exceptions.

      v. Students will always follow the faculty's instructions and are subject to being sent home, incurring their own extra expenses, if they do not behave.

     vi. Students will fail the course if they do not behave as instructed by faculty.

6. Plan and document the experience while at the location.

    a. Plan an orientation with local health administration for tours and work assignments, to give donations of supplies, and offer to pay for snacks served. Bring a gift for key health administrator contacts.

    b. Keep a daily journal of visits, contacts, phone numbers, and e-mail addresses; costs; problems to be solved; and daily agenda.

    c. Make student assignments with local agency administrators. Give students preferences when possible according to their previous experiences and language abilities.

    d. Make local community contacts on your own time. Meet the directors of all hospitals, clinics, housing, group excursions, and language centers. Bring small gifts or take them for coffee and pastries when meeting with them. Emphasize how much you appreciate the help that they are giving to you.

    e. Make friends in the local community with merchants, taxi drivers, restaurant owners, and other service providers, and if relationships are successful, bring students to them. Often you will receive a group discount on tickets, transportation, food, and other items with these relationships.

f. Participate in all student activities. Take local language classes with students and assist with supervision in hospitals, in clinics, and on all cultural excursions. Find out about other activities in the community that may interest students.

Checklist for Supervising Faculty

1. Code of behavior signed by all participants.
2. Review health precautions, arrange travel health insurance that will cover emergency evacuation.
3. Review safety precautions for money (under-the-clothing money bags for traveling) and locking up valuables such as passports, money, credit cards, and cameras.
4. Review food- and hygiene-related safety.
5. Frequent reminders on health and safety topics for students.
6. Always watch luggage and carry-ons at airports. Things may disappear very quickly, especially in developing countries, if they are valuable and unattended. Use a team sticker or ribbon to identify luggage of all group members easily.
7. Be prepared to deal with culture shock. Language, customs, and in some locations tremendous, never-before-seen poverty can overwhelm faculty and students. Many poor people, including those begging in the streets, can be overwhelming. Developing a way to give to the community will begin to address the overwhelming feelings of frustration.
8. Have students always travel in groups and always carry information with them regarding where they are staying and contact information for reaching faculty 24/7.
9. Always be available to students 24/7. This is not like the responsibility of a classroom on campus.

■ Conclusion

Many students preparing to be healthcare professionals are interested in and can benefit from a global experience. Faculty efforts to incorporate an international experience into the curriculum can be well rewarded in student learning. Time taken to identify desired learning outcomes and incorporate experiential learning and activities to facilitate growth is usually very well spent. Activities can be crafted to develop skills, knowledge, and confidence in providing health care. Students can benefit from being part of an international partnership that contributes sustainably to global health care. International experiences provide opportunities for students to work with interpreters; teach clinical topics; learn about new countries, diseases, and ways of providing health care; and gain personal insight that enhances cross-cultural acumen. Careful planning and appropriate follow-up can create life-changing experiences for both faculty and students.

Discussion Questions

1. What might hinder student acquisition of cultural skills on a global experience?
2. What type of global endeavor would programmatically be a good fit for your academic program?
3. What institutional barriers to creating a global endeavor might be anticipated?

References

American Association of Colleges of Nursing (AACN). (2008). *Tool kit of resources for cultural competent education for baccalaureate nurses.* Retrieved from http://www.aacn.nche.edu/education-resources/toolkit.pdf

American Association of Colleges of Nursing (AACN). (2011). *Tool kit for cultural competence in master's and doctoral nursing education.* Retrieved from http://www.aacn.nche.edu/education-resources/Cultural_Competency_Toolkit_Grad.pdf

Ash, S. L., & Clayton, P. H. (2009). Generating, deepening, and documenting learning: The power of critical reflection in applied learning. *Journal of Applied Learning in Higher Education, 1,* 25–48. Retrieved from http://webii.eckerd.edu/qep/faculty/files/Ash_Clayton_Generating_Deepening_and_Documenting_Learning.pdf

Ballestas, H. C., & Roller, M. C. (2013). The effectiveness of a study abroad program for increasing students' cultural competence. *Journal of Nursing Education and Practice, 3*(6), 125.

Behrnd, V., & Porzelt, S. (2012). Intercultural competence and training outcomes of students with experiences abroad. *International Journal of Intercultural Relations, 36*(2), 213–223.

Bender, A., & Walker, P. (2013). The obligation of debriefing in global health education. *Medical Teacher, 35*(3), e1027–e1034.

Carpenter, L. J., & Garcia, A. A. (2012). Assessing outcomes of a study abroad course for nursing students. *Nursing Education Perspectives, 33*(2), 85–89.

Delpech, P. A. (2013). Developing a short-term international study-abroad program: From beginning to end. *PRISM: A Journal of Regional Engagement, 2*(2), 5.

Houghton, S. A. (2014). Exploring manifestations of curiosity in study abroad as part of intercultural communicative competence. *System, 42,* 368–382.

Isaacson, M. (2014). Clarifying concepts: Cultural humility or competency. *Journal of Professional Nursing, 30*(3), 251–258.

Johns, A., & Thompson, C. W. (2010). Developing cultural sensitivity through study abroad. *Home Health Care Management & Practice, 22*(5), 344–348.

Kennedy, R. (n.d.). *Baylor University Missions.* Retrieved from http://www.baylor.edu/missions/index.php?id=867914

Kolb, A. Y., & Kolb, D. A. (2012). Experiential learning theory. In N. Seel (Ed.), *Encyclopedia of the sciences of learning* (pp. 1215–1219). New York, NY: Springer.

Kolb, D. A. (1984). *Experiential learning: Experience as the source of learning and development.* Englewood Cliffs, NJ: Prentice-Hall.

Koplan, J. P., Bond, T. C., Merson, M. H., Reddy, K. S., Rodriguez, M. H., Sewankambo, N. K., . . . Consortium of Universities for Global Health Executive Board. (2009). Towards a common definition of global health. *Lancet, 373*(9679), 1993–1995.

Kulbok, P. A., Mitchell, E. M., Glick, D. F., & Greiner, D. (2012). International experiences in nursing education: A review of the literature. *International Journal of Nursing Education Scholarship, 9*(1), 1–21. doi:10.1515/1548-923X.2365

Memmott, R. J., Coverston, C. R., Heise, B. A., Williams, M., Maughan, E. D., Kohl, J., & Palmer, S. (2010). Practical considerations in establishing sustainable international nursing experiences. *Nursing Education Perspectives, 31*(5), 298–302.

National League for Nursing (NLN). (2012). Faculty preparation for global experiences tool kit. http://www.nln.org/docs/default-source/default-document-library/toolkit_facprepglobexp5a3fb25c78366c709642ff00005f0421.pdf

Open Doors. (2015). Fast facts. *Institute of International Education.* Retrieved from http://www.iie.org /Research-and-Publications/Open-Doors

Palmer, S., Wing, D., Miles, L., Heaston, S., & de la Cruz, K. (2013). Study abroad programs: Using alumni and graduate students as affiliate faculty. *Nurse Educator, 38*(5), 198–201. doi:10.1097 /NNE.0b013e3182a0e587

Passarelli, A., & Kolb, D. A. (2012). Using experiential learning theory to promote student learning and development in programs of education abroad. In M. V. Berg, R. M. Paige, & K. H. Lou (Eds.), *Student learning abroad: What our students are learning, what they're not, and what we can do about it* (pp. 137–162). Sterling, VA: Stylus.

Sachau, D., Brasher, N., & Fee, S. (2010). Three models for short-term study abroad. *Journal of Management Education, 34*(5), 645–670.

Savicki, V., & Price, M. V. (2015). Student reflective writing: Cognition and affect before, during, and after study abroad. *Journal of College Student Development, 56*(6), 587–601.

Scarr, E. M., Pulcini, J., Makonnen, J., Turk, K. A., Wheeler, K., Eissler, L. A., . . . Krauskopf, P. B. (2012). International nursing partnerships. *The Nurse Practitioner, 37*(6), 11–12. doi:10.1097/01 .NPR.0000414598.24648.00

Schuessler, J. B., Wilder, B., & Byrd, L. W. (2012). Reflective journaling and development of cultural humility in students. *Nursing Education Perspectives, 33*(2), 96–99.

Spies, L. A., Garner, S. L., Prater, L., & Riley, C. (2015). Building global nurse capacity through relationships, education, and collaboration. *Nurse Education Today, 35*(5), 653–656. doi:10.1016/j .nedt.2015.01.014

Tervalon, M., & Murray-Garcia, J. (1998). Cultural humility versus cultural competence: A critical distinction in defining physician training outcomes in multicultural education. *Journal of Health Care for the Poor and Underserved, 9*(2), 117–125.

Whalen, B. (2015). The management and funding of US study abroad. *International Higher Education,* (50), 15–16.

World Health Organization (WHO). (n.d.). *All about climate change and vectorborne diseases.* Retrieved from http://www.wpro.who.int/mvp/climate_change/about/en

Evaluation

The final section of this text presents components of a key aspect of any educational program: evaluation. Although evaluation is often overlooked, it is an essential part of the teaching–learning process. Educators predominantly think of evaluation either in the form of testing and grading or in the form of clinical evaluation. These are microlevel forms of measurement linked directly to course, program, and school evaluation. Successful school and program appraisals reflect the quality of the programs and are essential for accreditation or endorsement by related professional organizations. Chapters in this section describe innovative approaches to evaluation that educators use. Program evaluation also is presented, to assist educators in updating and improving current programs and developing new ones.

CHAPTER 26

Concept Mapping: A Meaningful Learning Tool to Promote Conceptual Understanding and Clinical Reasoning

Gregory G. Passmore

Instruction can be described as existing on a continuum from teacher-centered/ content-oriented to student-centered/learner-oriented actions (Ertmer & Newby, 1993; Passmore, Owen, & Prabakaran, 2011). Various models of this continuum exist in health professions instruction, eliciting reactive to proactive student behavior and participation and passive to active involvement of the instructor in learning. Traditionally, curricula for health professions instruction have been developed to meet the behavioral learning outcomes desired by national accrediting and credentialing bodies. These traditional curricula are often content centered to meet these desired outcomes. However, the current healthcare environment is demanding graduates who can think critically and problem solve in a variety of clinical practice areas (Daley & Torre, 2010; Edmondson, 1994; Novak & Cañas, 2008; Passmore et al., 2011; Pinto & Zeitz, 1997; Regan-Smith et al., 1994; Rendas, Fonseca, & Rosado-Pinto, 2006; Wheeler & Collins, 2003). Critical thinking, problem solving, and clinical reasoning are poorly served by most content-centered instruction. Educational theorists such as Novak and Gowin (1984) believe that the key to successful critical thinking and problem solving is methods of instruction centered in cognitivist/constructivist meaningful learning, to promote active processing of concepts leading to problem-solving skills.

The key to meaningful learning is that learning is an individual, cognitive process, in which each learner must construct his or her own understanding of concepts, relationships, and procedures. For a student to accomplish this style of learning, a learner would have to mentally integrate the new information acquired during learning activities into what the learner already knows or differentiate what the learner knows to accommodate the new information (Ausubel, 1968; Ausubel, Novak, & Hanesian, 1978; Heinze-Fry & Novak, 1990; Novak, 1990, 2003; Novak & Cañas, 2008; Novak & Gowin, 1984; Passmore, 1995; West, Park, Pomeroy, & Sandoval, 2002).

Meaningful learning, then, is how the student organizes, saves, and retrieves information or knowledge in a relational fashion. Meaningful learning is based on the premise that knowledge is bundled in packets called *concepts* (defined as recognized regularities in events or objects) and recalled from memory based on how the concepts are attached to one another. New information is nonarbitrarily attached to concepts already familiar to the learner through linkages that the learner identifies as meaningful. In contrast to rote learning, the outcome of meaningful learning is that the new information is transferred into long-term memory through a meaningful linkage, thus enabling the retrieval needed for critical thinking and problem solving (Novak, 1990; Novak & Cañas, 2008; Pinto & Zeitz, 1997).

The purpose of instruction is for the student to develop a knowledge base within the discipline, but also to be able to acquire new knowledge as the discipline changes with advancements in technology and practice. Students who are taught how to learn meaningfully by the nonarbitrary assimilation of new concepts and procedures into their knowledge structure, or by accommodating their knowledge structures to accept the new information, should be able to meet the discipline's needs today and tomorrow. One learning intervention that helps identify an individual's unique knowledge structure of a topic or process is a graphic organizer of topical concepts commonly known as a *concept map*. Concept maps provide both teacher and student a guide on which to base further learning (Ausubel, 1968; Novak, 1990; Novak & Gowin, 1984; Passmore, 1996; Pinto & Zeitz, 1997).

■ Definition and Purposes

A *concept map* is a concise, two-dimensional, schematic representation of the collection of concepts and linking relationships in a student's knowledge set of a topic or process. Two or more concepts and their linking relationships become meaningful statements about some object or event one is trying to define, classify, or purpose. It is the identification of the linking relationship between concepts in a concept map that makes this graphic organizer unique and separates the concept map from other less communicative organizing techniques, such as outlines, nursing process care plans, or flow charts. Concept maps can be used by individual students and groups as tools for learning, by teachers and students for remediation, and by teachers for assessment (Adler, Wilson, & Coulter, 2008; Dansereau & Cross, 1990; Edmondson, 1994; Hsu & Hsieh, 2005; Novak, 1990; Novak & Gowin, 1984; Novak & Wandersee, 1990; Passmore, 1995, 1996; West et al., 2002).

Concept maps have been used as a learning intervention for individuals and groups in traditional didactic and distance courses, in laboratories, in clinical courses, and in critical thinking and problem-solving courses, with the emphasis in the healthcare literature on clinic, critical thinking, and problem solving (Daley & Torre, 2010; Pinto & Zeitz, 1997). By creating concept maps, students learn that the conceptual understanding they gain in their didactic coursework has a procedural counterpart in their laboratory and/or clinical application courses and clerkships (Hunter-Revell, 2012; Passmore, 1996, 1998). In essence, using concept maps as a meaningful learning intervention helps students to develop a more complete and meaningful understanding of the theoretical knowledge they gain didactically and to bridge the gap between the theoretical knowledge and the procedural knowledge they gain in the laboratory and the clinic (Hicks-Moore, 2005; Novak & Gowin, 1984; Passmore, 1998). Further, the concept map's visual interpretation of an individual's knowledge structure can simplify discussion and lead to enhanced understanding between individuals, either in groups or by providing an opportunity between teacher and student for misconception remediation (Dansereau & Cross, 1990; Novak & Cañas, 2008; Novak & Gowin, 1984; Passmore, 1995, 1996, 1998). Additionally, the concept map lends itself to quantitative and qualitative assessment using rubrics such as the one developed by Novak and Gowin (1984), allowing a teacher and the student to measure the extent of the knowledge represented by the concept map.

■ Theoretical Rationale

The continuum of learning theories begins with the behaviorist theory, where learning is confirmed by specific behavioral responses to specific stimuli; passes through the cognitivist theory, where learning is confirmed by the behavioral and mental solutions to specific stimuli; and ends with the constructivist theory, where learning is individualized and based on the stimuli as they are presented. More simply, this continuum might be described as moving from rote learning or memorization through meaningful learning and problem solving to autonomous learning and invention (Novak & Cañas, 2008; Passmore et al., 2011).

The shortcomings of behaviorist learning theory applied to students in the health professions can be seen in the example of the student who correctly performs a healthcare protocol in clinical practice, but who fails when he or she is exposed to variations in the protocol or patients. If the student has been conditioned to respond to certain stimuli in the protocol, when the learning stimuli are different, the learner may not be able to respond appropriately until he or she has memorized all possible variations of the protocol.

Further, the student taught using cognitivist learning theories and given the same set of variations in clinical protocols as previously mentioned understands the need for or existence of the variations. This student does not see the required variations as an impediment to accomplishing the task, since he or she has developed a mental schema that allows for processing of critical thinking and problem-solving strategies that come with meaningful learning.

Students taught in the constructivist learning environment may or may not be able to accomplish a health professions–associated task. Constructivist learning theory supports creativity in problem solving because it asks the student to approach the problem from different perspectives where knowledge of previous protocols may be advantageous, but not necessary. However, by its definition, a protocol establishes a set of procedures used to carry out a task. Reinventing that set of procedures every time the task is required would be inefficient and time consuming, and it is a weakness with constructivist learning in situations where conformity is essential and divergent thinking may cause problems.

The cognitive psychologist David Ausubel (1968) summed up the purpose of learning interventions as actions designed to "ascertain this [what the student already knows] and teach him accordingly" (p. vi). The fundamental idea in Ausubel's cognitive psychology is that learning takes place either by the assimilation of new concepts into existing conceptual or cognitive structures held by the learner or by accommodation of the learner's cognitive structure to the new concept (also see Chapter 1). Thus, personal knowledge is typically constructed like a house or a car, and not usually discovered like oil or a new planet (Novak & Gowin, 1984).

The learning theory that is utilized in instruction is the one that best meets the outcomes of the learning objectives, the type of learning task, and the student's level of competence. In the health professions, this leads to instruction that both meets the predicated curricular objectives of accrediting agencies and promotes meaningful learning to best meet the needs of the student. Instruction is provided for the student to develop a knowledge base within the discipline. However, the student has to be able to learn new knowledge as the discipline changes with advancements in technology and practice. Rote learning will provide most students with a body of facts, such as lab values, anatomy and physiology, and even some clinical protocols. However, students who are taught how to learn meaningfully by the nonarbitrary assimilation of new information or new concepts and procedures into their knowledge structure have been shown to be better critical thinkers/problem solvers, and thus should be able to more completely meet their discipline's needs and challenges (Daley & Torre, 2010; Edmondson, 1994; Ertmer & Newby, 1993; Passmore et al., 2011; Wheeler & Collins, 2003).

How the student organizes and recalls knowledge is the key to meaningful learning. Meaningful learning is based on the premise that knowledge is bundled in concept packets and recalled from memory based on how the concepts are attached or linked to one another when stored in long-term memory. Concept maps are two-dimensional graphic representations or organizers of multiple concepts designed to help students recall and structure their knowledge in relational maps. It is this process of identifying or naming the linking relationships between concepts in the map that makes this graphic organizer an effective learning intervention (Novak & Cañas, 2008; Passmore, 1995).

Well-developed concept maps also display cross-links. These are linking relationships between concepts in different levels or conceptual clusters of the concept map and are an important characteristic of concept maps. Cross-links help us see how a concept or process in one domain of knowledge represented on the map is related to a concept in another domain shown on the map, indicating a deeper level of understanding (Angelo & Cross, 1993; Dansereau & Cross, 1990; Novak, 1990; Novak & Cañas, 2008; Novak & Gowin, 1984; Passmore, 1995, 1996, 1998).

Meaningful learning requires the learner to become an active participant in the learning process. The process of creating a concept map, by identifying relevant concepts and the relationships between them, is an active learning process. Meaningful learning strategies, such as concept mapping, allow learners to actively organize their knowledge structures into powerful, integrated patterns. A concept map becomes a concise, visual interpretation of an individual's knowledge structure (Angelo & Cross, 1993; Dansereau & Cross, 1990; Heinze-Fry & Novak, 1990; Novak, 1990; Novak & Cañas, 2008; Novak & Gowin, 1984; Passmore, 1995, 1996, 1998). Whereas rote memorization is typically static, concept mapping supports the growth of the individual's knowledge structure. **Figure 26-1** represents a student concept map depicting understanding of fundamental radiation safety concepts before (a) and after (b) multiple teacher–student remediation activities. Note that a relational linking term exists between concepts, and the postremediations map has several levels of hierarchies and clusters of understanding. This pair of maps shows how a student's understanding can grow following instruction, laboratory, or remediation.

■ Conditions

Concept maps have been used as guides to instruction, meaningful learning organizers, misconception remediation facilitators, and assessment tools across all levels of education. Construction of concept maps requires reflection on the part of the individual constructing the map, whether student or teacher (Novak & Gowin, 1984). Individuals with a penchant for rote learning activities and assessments should be given the opportunity to familiarize themselves with the processes of map construction. Teachers and students who focus more on memorization rather than deep understanding have expressed state anxiety in using mapping activities. This is exemplified in Roth and Roychoudhury's 1993 study of elementary education majors taking a physical science course for their specialty certification. These researchers found that the concept mapping activity was attitudinally accepted by 81% of the student teachers in the program, leaving 19% to declare themselves attitudinally resistant as they were being moved from rote learning to meaningful learning practices. Similarly, Passmore (1996) found some attitudinal resistance in his longitudinal study of radiologic science students; however, these feelings of resistance seem to be abated with long-term

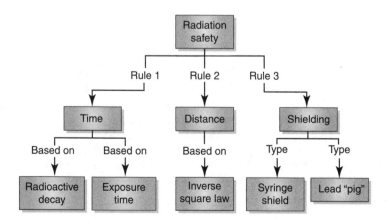

■ **Figure 26-1a**   Student concept map depicting understanding of fundamental radiation safety concepts prior to remediation.

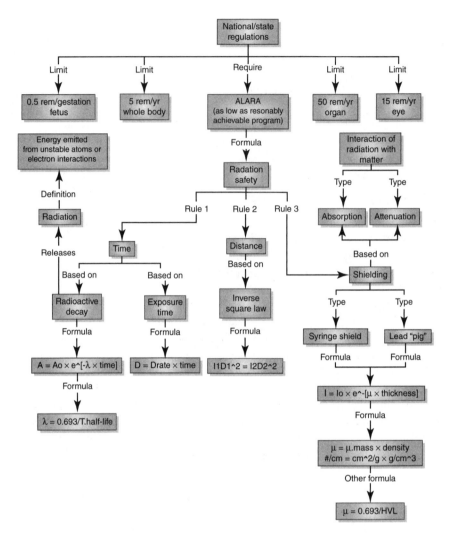

■ **Figure 26-1b** After remediation: Student concept map depicting understanding of fundamental radiation safety concepts.

Terminology Key: rem = unit of dose equivalent (J/kg); HVL = half-value layer measure of attenuation in linear dimension units (e.g., mm); D = dose or amount of energy deposited in matter (J/kg); Drate = rate of energy deposited in matter (J/kg/unit time); μ = linear attenuation coefficient derived from the ratio of the ln2/HVL; T = half-life, the time required for a radioactive sample to decay to one-half the sample's original activity; λ = radioactive decay constant derived from the ratio of the ln2/T; inverse square law = I = radiation intensity, D = distance from source from which radiation intensity was measured or for which it is to be calculated.

use (Feldsine, 1987; Passmore, 1998). Concept maps have been used successfully in the academic environment, the business environment, and the military environment (Novak & Cañas, 2008).

Implementation

Concept mapping has to be taught to students, researchers, or clinicians when the method is intended to be utilized in the classroom, laboratory, or clinic (Adler et al., 2008; Novak & Cañas, 2008; Novak & Gowin, 1984; Passmore, 2008; Pinto & Zeitz, 1997). This is a process activity, and it should be treated just like any other process, with stepwise instruction and practice (Gagne, 1985). Passmore (2008) uses a 2- to 4-hour workshop to introduce the mapping process to health professions students and teachers. Because the audience for this workshop is discipline diverse, the workshop is initiated by having participants identify concepts and relationships from a general list of biologic and sociology concepts and relationships (Dansereau & Cross, 1990). The workshop concludes with participants (in small-group units) developing a concept map from a two-paragraph description of the information-processing model of memory using long-term and short-term memory, using a skeleton map as a starting point. In this instructional process, it is important to begin with a limited domain of knowledge that is familiar to the student. This creates a context that will help determine the structure of the concept map. Although experienced map makers may employ topical, broad-scope maps, novice map makers should be provided with a clear, specific domain, root concepts or skeleton map, and/or focus question around which they can develop their maps (Cañas, Novak, & Reiska, 2012; Novak & Cañas, 2008; Passmore, 2008).

The next step is for the map maker to list the key concepts in the domain. From this list, the map is developed with the most general concepts at the top and the most specific concepts at the bottom. One technique for identifying subordinate concepts from the superordinate, general concept is to ask descriptive questions about the general concept (Dansereau & Cross, 1990), such as questions of types, characteristics, and parts that pertain to the general concept; or questions of process, such as what leads to the general concept or what follows.

Once this list is generated, map construction can begin, typically with a preliminary map. In the preliminary map, the concepts can be positioned in a fashion that is unique to the map maker. Lines are drawn between concepts and labeled with a few relational words that describe the relationship between the concepts. As this map develops, the maker usually sees that the most organized fashion for the map is with the most general, superordinate concept at the top with the subordinate concepts clustered beneath. However, whereas these hierarchical maps seem intuitive in science-based fields, this may not be the case in all disciplines. Many maps start with the most general concept as a central node, and the subordinate concepts radiate out and beneath the central concept (Dansereau & Cross, 1990; Passmore, 2004). Dynamic or cyclic maps can also be generated as the discipline requires to indicate temporal distributions in the conceptual structures, such as the assessment, evaluation, and follow-up process involved in many patient care activities (Dansereau & Cross, 1990; Safayeni, Derbentseva, & Cañas, 2005).

One notable aspect of concept maps that makes the intervention such a powerful, meaningful learning tool is that cross-links between subordinate concepts or clusters of concepts should be sought and labeled, as these indicate a deeper understanding of the relationships in any domain. Another feature that may be added to concept maps is specific examples of events or objects that help to clarify the meaning of a given concept. These early drafts are followed by subsequent drafts until the final draft is reached, which the map maker feels explains his or her understanding of the response to the initial question or domain. Revisions using pencil and paper can be somewhat cumbersome and time consuming. There are software packages available that allow for frequent revisions, but these may be a little restrictive compared to pencil-and-paper mapping activities (Novak & Cañas, 2008). The revisions also provide an orderly sequence of iterations between working memory and long-term memory, using the map as the scaffold or template to build knowledge frameworks (Novak, 1990). The concept maps can now be used as an individual study guide, as a collaborative group discussion format, as a basis from which misconceptions can be identified and remediated prior to testing (Figure 26-1), and as a form of assessment (**Figure 26-2**) (Abel & Freeze, 2006; Adler et al., 2008; All & Huycke, 2007; Daley & Torre, 2010; Gonzalez, Palencia, Umana, Galindo, & Villafrade, 2008; Hinck et al., 2006; Hsu & Hsieh, 2005; Mahler, Hoz, Fischl, Tov-Ly, & Lernau, 1991; Novak & Gowin, 1984; Passmore, 1996; Passmore et al., 2011; West et al., 2002; West, Pomeroy, Park, Gerstenberger, & Sandoval, 2000).

◼ Types of Learners

The physical construction of concept maps as a learning intervention has been shown to facilitate meaningful learning by enabling students from elementary school through college and graduate school to actively seek and develop conceptual relationships. Researchers have shown the utility of concept mapping as a learning and evaluation tool in multiple educational environments, including expository lecture, laboratory, critical thinking, problem solving, cooperative group learning, clinical, case study analysis, patient care planning, and distance learning (Daley & Torre, 2010; Novak & Cañas, 2008; Passmore, 1996; Passmore et al., 2011; Preszler, 2004).

Research into multiple intelligences (Gardner, 1983) and learning styles (Felder, 1993; Kolb & Kolb, 2005) has been well accepted and draws attention to the wide range of differences in student abilities for various types of learning and performances. Concept mapping, being a form of graphic organizer, would seem to fit well with those individuals who rely on visual/spatial techniques for learning. Other forms of learning preferences, such as verbal/auditory and tactile, can also benefit from generating concept maps. If learning style preferences are long-term learner adaptations to facilitate learning, then activities that enhance meaningful learning should be adapted to just as readily, given time and practice, irrespective of the learning style (Laight, 2004; Novak & Cañas, 2008).

◼ Using the Method

Concept maps can be used for a variety of educational processes from the perspective of the teacher and the student, in the form of knowledge acquisition/structuring template, critical-thinking/problem-solving intervention, misconception remediation

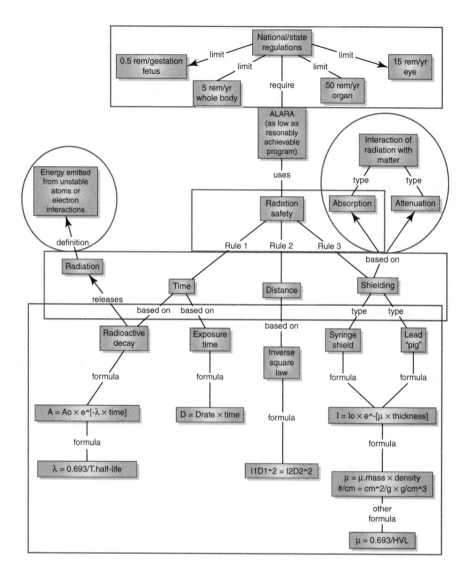

■ **Figure 26-2**   The scoring process applied to Figure 26-1b. Note that a relational linking term exists between concepts, and the postremediation map has several levels of hierarchies and clusters of understanding. Each map was scored based on the rubric described here. This map shows how a student's increased understanding following instruction, laboratory, or remediation can be quantified in place of other formal or summative assessments.

Score: 28 conceptual links × 1 point each; 1 definition × 1 point; 4 levels of hierarchy × 10 points each; 1 supporting cluster × 10 points; = 79 points

Terminology Key: rem = unit of dose equivalent (J/kg); HVL = half-value layer measure of attenuation in linear dimension units (e.g., mm); D = dose or amount of energy deposited in matter (J/kg); Drate = rate of energy deposited in matter (J/kg/unit time); μ-linear attenuation coefficient derived from the ratio of the ln2/HVL; T = half-life, the time required for a radioactive sample to decay to one-half the sample's original activity; λ-radioactive decay constant derived from the ratio of the ln2/T; inverse square law = I = radiation intensity, D = distance from source from which radiation intensity was measured or for which it is to be calculated.

guide, meaningful-learning/authentic-assessment template, research/project-planning guide, and curriculum-planning guide. These tasks are applied in several different curriculum models to include lecture/laboratory, critical thinking/problem solving, cooperative learning, clinical processes, case study analysis, case/care planning, distance learning environments, and postprofessional continuing education (Cañas et al., 2003; Daley & Torre, 2010).

Student Uses of Concept Maps

Meaningful Learning from Lecture/Laboratory Curriculum

Concept maps can be used as meaningful learning tools within a lecture-based course. Students can map lectures and textbook passages to gain a meaningful understanding of the material presented. Students can use concept mapping to organize and integrate multiple concepts and as a template for growing their conceptual understanding. As a meaningful learning activity, students can document their existing knowledge, gain new understandings, and then relate the new information to what they already know. In addition, students can detect areas where there are misconceptions, expressed as dissatisfaction with their own cognitive structures in trying to connect concepts in a meaningful and organized way. Whether self-determined or discovered through study group or teacher–student interaction, misconceptions provide an opportunity for remediation, a process in which student misconceptions are replaced with more scientifically valid concepts and relationships, which is discussed more fully in the "Teacher Uses of Concept Maps" section later in this chapter (Daley & Torre, 2010; Novak & Cañas, 2008; Novak & Gowin, 1984; Passmore, 1995, 1996, 1998; Pinto & Zeitz, 1997; Roth & Roychoudhury, 1993).

Concept maps also can be used in other study methods, such as distance learning and laboratory. Distance learning demands communication between students and teachers, as well as between students. Concept maps make excellent vehicles for long-distance discussion between individuals, to include misconception remediation activities (Coffey & Cañas, 2000; Novak & Cañas, 2008; Passmore et al., 2011; Pinto & Zeitz, 1997).

Additionally, concept maps used in laboratory will help students understand the relationships between the concepts that are driving the procedures the students are following. Many laboratory study guides provide the conceptual understanding required for purposeful learning in a laboratory protocol. However, unless the student is acting on the information in a meaningful fashion, the student may miss the understanding and simply follow the procedure. Having students construct a relational concept map can help them identify how the laboratory procedures are derived from the theoretical and conceptual basis. Concept maps used this way will tend to have a descriptive component as well as a dynamic, procedural component, thus giving students access to the "Why is the procedure done this way?" instead of "It is done this way" encountered so often in laboratory and clinical practice (Dansereau & Cross, 1990; Hicks-Moore, 2005; Novak & Gowin, 1984; Passmore, 1998; Safayeni et al., 2005).

One goal of radiologic science physics teaching has traditionally been to help students become proficient problem solvers. Several studies point out that traditional methods of applying formulas to sets of problems at the end of a chapter fail to encourage concept development; thus, the student has no knowledge base (appropriate memory) from which to draw the needed information and procedures to develop a solution set (Champagne & Klopfer, 1984; Glynn, Yeany, & Britton, 1991; Novak, Gowin, & Johansen, 1983; Passmore, 1998; Prankratius, 1990; Roth & Roychoudhury, 1993). Prankratius (1990) compared concept mapping groups to nonconcept mapping groups in physics instruction and concluded that the groups that often performed concept mapping scored significantly higher on a problem-solving assessment than traditionally instructed groups that relied on practice alone.

Meaningful Learning from Critical Thinking/Problem-Based Learning Curriculum

Students in a problem-based learning (PBL) program use their concept maps to identify the student-generated informational learning opportunities that emerge during case study. Additionally, each PBL group can create a concept map of a model specific to the case study. A case-specific concept map would have the students incorporate basic science concepts, clinical science concepts, procedural concepts, and student-generated hypotheses into a case-specific model of the case study that would potentially include multiple cross-linkages and layers (Dansereau & Cross, 1990; Pinto & Zeitz, 1997). Giddens (2006) based a curriculum development activity for graduate student nurses on using concept maps as a guide to critical thinking and deeper understanding. Attitudinal outcomes were positive, as participants felt that the mapping activity led to discussions of content and theory. These were possible after organizing, analyzing, and communicating interrelationships among concepts identified in the mapping process. Hicks-Moore and Pastirik (2006) quantified critical thinking in a study to assess the level of critical thinking with concept maps. Their results indicate that critical thinking was enhanced by developing concept maps. (See Chapter 12 for more on problem-based learning.)

Meaningful Learning from Clinical Curriculum

Students in clinical courses, to include community health care, preventive medicine, allied health sciences, and healthcare delivery, can use concept mapping when learning important concepts and procedures that are the basis for their clinical rotations or clerkships. As described previously in the "Meaningful Learning from Lecture/Laboratory Curriculum" section, the concept map processes used for meaningful learning of basic science knowledge also can be used for meaningful learning of clinical procedures, ensuring that students understand the science behind the procedures they are learning and enhancing students understanding in both the declarative or conceptual and the procedural knowledge bases.

One example of this process applied clinically is in clinical care plans that incorporate concept maps as part of the critical thinking and problem-solving process. Concept mapping encourages a patient-centered focus in a comprehensive care environment (Abel & Freeze, 2006; Atay & Karabacak, 2012; Hinck et al., 2006; Novak & Gowin, 1984; Passmore, 1998; Pinto & Zeitz, 1997; Wheeler & Collins, 2003; Weiss & Levison, 2000). **Figure 26-3** is an example of a nuclear medicine technology

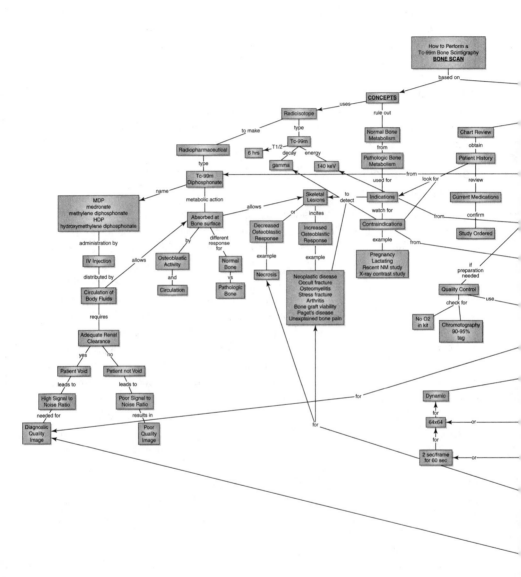

■ **Figure 26-3** Postremediation student concept map depicting both conceptual and procedural knowledge structures used to perform a Tc-99m bone scan in the nuclear medicine clinic. Relationships between the two domains indicate interplay required to understand processes.

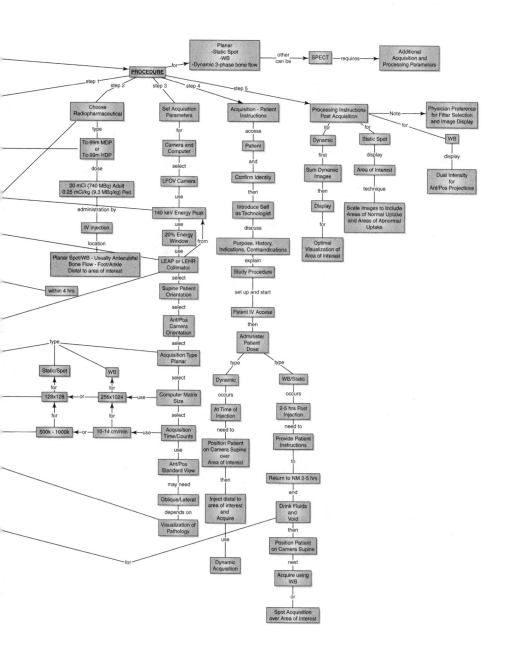

student's clinical protocol concept map for Tc-99m Bone Scintigraphy—Bone Scan developed after remediation sessions involving both the teacher and the student (see the following subsection on "Teacher Uses of Concept Maps: Concept Maps as Misconception Remediation Tools"). Significant to this clinical protocol map is the organization of both the conceptual knowledge required for the bone scan as well as the procedural knowledge required for completing the study. This particular organization is a variation of Gowin's vee diagram (Afamasaga-Fuata'i, 2004; Novak & Gowin, 1984; Passmore, 1998; Roth & Roychoudhury, 1993), a meaningful learning tool designed to help the learner "see" the relationship between the conceptual knowledge he or she possesses going into the laboratory and the procedural knowledge produced during the laboratory experience, used here to represent clinical activity. Note in Figure 26-3 how the conceptual nature of the bone scan study aligns to the left side of the figure, and the dynamic procedural nature of the bone scan study aligns to the right side of the figure. The cross-links between the right and left sides indicate relationships where protocol actions are relationally explained through the conceptual knowledge base. The interplay between concepts and procedures may be categorized differently depending on discipline needs. For example, Baugh and Mellott (1998), as well as Abel and Freeze (2006), describe the use of clinical concept maps by nursing students with relational concept maps indicating the interplay between pathophysiological and psychosocial characteristics as part of a nursing care plan.

Some teachers prefer to use hub-and-spoke, radially oriented maps for protocol representation, as in the manner of Dansereau and Cross (1990). Schuster (2000) describes transforming a traditional four-column patient care plan into a radial map with the pathology at the center and the nursing care plan with patient response to treatments radiating away from the center. This version of a clinical care concept map also was used by Hill (2006) as a platform for teacher-student conferences when planning nursing interventions and assessments. Derbentseva, Safayeni, and Cañas (2007) compared dynamic thinking with cyclic map relationships versus traditional hierarchical maps that use dynamic quantifiers in the concept in an undergraduate science course environment. Although there were no statistical differences between the cyclic and hierarchical maps in number of dynamic relationships, students found the cyclic concept map more interesting.

Adema-Hannes and Parzen (2005) report using student-generated clinical concept maps as misconception remediation/assessment tools with the additional benefit of replacing tedious care plan paperwork. Students rated their clinical reasoning as improved, versus no change, due to their newfound ability to organize their thoughts to link lab values, medications, pathophysiology, and plan to address patient care issues.

Meaningful Learning from Medical Residency Curriculum

Medical school programs consist of medical program education followed by a long period of residency training. A longitudinal use of concept maps is seen in medical residents' use of maps made during early clinical experiences as a basis for meaningful learning of new concepts encountered during residency training. These individually unique concept maps can serve as a means for integrating the new knowledge acquired during residency training with the knowledge achieved and meaningfully learned during medical school (Mahler et al., 1991; Pinto & Zeitz, 1997; West et al., 2002; West et al., 2000).

Meaningful Learning from Postprofessional Curriculum

For healthcare professionals, learning does not stop upon completion of professional training. New knowledge emerges with increasing frequency, a fact not lost on the certification/registry boards that require either recertification every few years or continuous education every year. Thus, healthcare professionals are obligated to gain a meaningful understanding of the new science and care concepts developed in their discipline, and to integrate these new concepts with prior concepts retained in long-term memory. Concept mapping can be used as a meaningful learning strategy for knowledge identification in this lifelong, often self-directed, postprofessional learning environment (Cañas et al., 2003; Pinto & Zeitz, 1997).

Teacher Uses of Concept Maps

Concept Maps as Planning Tools

Teachers can make a concept map to use as a teaching guide to help organize a lecture. This helps the teacher identify what he or she feels is important for students to understand. Also, this strategy promotes a conceptual flow in the lecture. Programmatic curriculum and lesson planning through the use of concept mapping have been suggested by Novak and Gowin (1984) and documented by Starr and Krajcik (1990), who studied the development of a curriculum by elementary teachers using the concept map technique. These group concept maps were analyzed for levels of hierarchical structure, topical differentiation, and integrative reconciliation. As each curriculum map revision took place, the curricular concepts to be learned and the relationships between them were clarified until a conceptually cohesive, integrated, and hierarchically arranged curriculum guide was produced. This process can also enhance authentication of teacher evaluation. Teachers who use concept maps to guide their lectures and curricula will be in a better position to evaluate their teaching performance when they consider how well their knowledge set describes the hierarchical relationships and complexity of the material to be taught (Dansereau & Cross, 1990; Glynn et al., 1991; Trowbride & Wandersee, 1994).

Giddens (2006) used concept mapping in a group activity to promote critical thinking about curriculum design. Graduate student nurses were asked to develop nursing curricula while working in groups. The activity generated much discussion and problem solving within the groups, and positive affective outcomes were noted. Additionally, participants claimed that the concept mapping activity provided a guide that led to group discussions concerning related reading assignments. A deeper understanding was the most cited outcome of these discussions.

Daley and Torre (2010) report on a research effort in which teacher-generated concept maps were used to augment didactic learning materials. However, caution suggests that complete teacher maps should not be shared with students. Recall that concept maps are individually unique; expert maps have been shown to either be so complex that the learning objectives and concepts are difficult for the viewer to identify, or too simplistic, because much of what the expert knows is subsumed in more general concepts, which are not elaborated upon in the expert's map (Bogden, 1977). Also, the action of a teacher handing out a teacher-prepared concept map sets up the condition for students to memorize the map by rote, which does little in helping them to cognitively understand or integrate the material (Cañas et al., 2012; Novak, personal communication, September 3, 2012). However, it has been shown that a skeleton map of a few main concepts and initial relationships may be given as a guide to help students see the organization and integration of the important concepts, allowing students to build or expand on these maps, which will negate rote memorization and encourage meaningful learning (Novak & Cañas, 2008).

Concept Maps as Assessment Tools

Concept maps are a tool for teachers wanting a more authentic or meaningful evaluation than standardized achievement tests. Meaningful learning activities such as concept mapping should be followed by meaningful evaluation, and using the student-generated concept map as the evaluation tool is one method for achieving this goal. Scoring concept maps for the validity or completeness of conceptual or procedural relationships, for what the teacher or discipline determines to be correct conceptions, for multiple levels of hierarchical structure, and for complexity described by concept differentiation and integration yields a more authentic assessment than end-of-course achievement tests, which are often oriented to rote memorization (Abel & Freeze, 2006; Daley & Torre, 2010; Markham, Mintzes, & Jones, 1984; Novak & Gowin, 1984; Novak, 1990; Passmore, 1995, 1996, 1998; Roth & Roychoudhury, 1993; West et al., 2002).

To use the concept map as an assessment tool, the teacher must construct a domain-specific expert concept map, and compare each student's map to the "expert" map. A scoring scheme based on Novak and Gowin's (1984) suggestion follows:

1. 1 point for each correct conceptual relationship and concept example or definition,
2. 5 points for cross-linking relationships, and
3. 10 points for conceptual clusters and hierarchical structure.

This process can be used as a pre- and/or postlesson formative or summative assessment, or to assist in the remediation process discussed earlier, as the change in quantitative values attached to a student's concept map can serve as extrinsic motivators to reinforce the learning process (Abel & Freeze, 2006; Daley & Torre, 2010; Novak & Gowin, 1984; Passmore, 1995, 1996, 1998; West et al., 2002). Figure 26-2 shows a score associated with a student's concept map following several remediation efforts. A change in map complexity before and after instruction activity or remediation activity reflects the increase in the student's learning and can be quantified by scoring the pre/post activity concept maps.

Assessing concept maps through manual quantification algorithms, as described earlier, requires teacher time commitments similar to those of other manual grading techniques of student authentic assessment tools. There have been some attempts at reducing teacher assessment effort by giving the student a central or core concept, then only scoring the significant concepts and neighboring relationships extending from the core concept (Correia & Cicuto, 2014), as these core concepts/significant concept relationships are thought to represent the significant learning from the instructional activity. Alternatively, using computer-aided data mining or pattern analysis techniques similar to those used by algorithms examining customer transactions has shown some utility (Chiu & Lin, 2012). However, irrespective of the variations in the concept map grading algorithms, all seem to compare an "expert" conceptual knowledge structure with its inherent conceptual relationships to a "novice" conceptual knowledge structure and relationships to assess student meaningful learning.

The teacher should be aware that assessment of concept maps may well indicate differences in success for students who typically score well on standardized assessments. Novak et al's (1983) analysis suggested that students who best understood the science concepts were not necessarily the students who received the best grades on standardized tests. Additionally, Passmore's (1995) study outcomes using concept map assessment showed that concept mapping altered the predictive ability of SAT scores. West et al. (2000) compared pre/post instruction concept map scores, noting improvement. However, the improvement in map scores did not correlate with course outcomes or standardized test scores. These observations support the differences in assessment, and achievement, between rote and meaningful learning.

Concept Maps as Misconception Remediation Tools

Having students concept-map a lecture can give the teacher feedback information on student misconceptions, thus prompting mentoring and/or misconception remediation. Misconceptions that have occurred as a result of the interaction of the student and the instruction from lecture, laboratory, or clinic must be successfully identified and remediated (Griffiths, Thomey, Cooke, & Normore, 1988; Renner, Abraham, Grzybowski, & Marek, 1990; Roth, 1990; Wandersee et al., 1994). Misconceptions are identified in concept maps as a linkage between two concepts that is false or as a linkage that fails to address the main idea relating the two or more concepts (Novak & Gowin, 1984). One method of examining the student's concepts and relationships is through a preinstruction and postinstruction interview. Because concept maps are a concise representation of the concepts and relationships in a learner's knowledge set, they allow teachers to quickly recognize invalid or underdeveloped knowledge claims, which would suggest a need for remediation (Novak, 1990; Novak & Gowin, 1984; Roth, 1990; Wandersee et al., 1994).

Passmore (1995, 1996) used concept maps as a postinstruction format for misconception remediation prior to formal assessment with radiologic science students (Figure 26-1), finding concept maps to be both an efficient and effective form of communication between student and teacher. Learning gains were evident in the concept mapping group, as evidenced by the ability of the concept mapping intervention to alter the predictive ability of SAT scores in the concept mapping group. Student attitudes toward having remediation before the assessment instead of traditionally after the assessment were positive. Wallace and Mintzes (1990) used concept maps to document conceptual change in biology for elementary education majors. These authors note that a teacher can observe how the student's individual cognitive structures grow and mature by comparing successive student concept maps as the student gains mastery of the domain.

Correcting long-held misconceptions of basic science or social science phenomena requires conceptual change. Students' dissatisfaction with their own cognitive structures in trying to connect concepts in a meaningful and organized way is a requirement in cognitive/constructivist philosophy as a first step in conceptual change, a process in which student misconceptions are replaced with more scientifically valid concepts and relationships, ideally through meaningful learning activities (Roth & Roychoudhury, 1993).

■ Conclusion

Meaningful learning for health professions students and practitioners is an important, individual cognitive skill that can be enhanced through the use of concept mapping. Concept maps can be used by teachers, students, and postgraduate professionals to enable meaningful learning for themselves, their students, and their colleagues. Educationally oriented research using these two-dimensional graphic organizers has shown that students can benefit from drawing how they are integrating new knowledge, as well as identifying misconceptions, and from using them as a guide for discussion and understanding in group work, critical thinking/problem solving, and relation of conceptual knowledge to the procedural knowledge needed for clinical reasoning and performance. Teachers can use concept maps as meaningful assessments, as enablers for misconception remediation, as guides in group work, and as devices that allow for a complete lesson and/or curriculum-planning process. Professionals, too, can gain from the process of concept mapping by integrating new concepts required for current practice with previously learned concepts in a format that allows information to be recalled in a usable manner. The multiplicity of researched uses of this graphic organizer show the extent of the utility of this meaningful learning tool in helping students and professionals shift from rote learners to meaningful learners.

Discussion Questions

1. What is an advantage of using concept mapping techniques compared to an outline when designing teaching for the healthcare environment?
2. How can a teacher use the concept map as part of the assessment of student understanding of a laboratory activity?
3. When using concept maps as clinical protocol guides or care plans, the student can capture both conceptual and procedural knowledge. How does this type of mapping activity compare to and/or contrast with a purely textual protocol description or care plan?

References

Abel, W., & Freeze, M. (2006). Evaluation of concept mapping in an associate degree nursing program. *Journal of Nursing Education, 45*(9), 356–364.

Adema-Hannes, R., & Parzen, M. (2005). Concept mapping: Does it promote meaningful learning in the clinical setting? *College Quarterly, 8*(3). Retrieved from http://www.senecac.on.ca/quarterly/2005-vol08 -num03-summer/adema-hannes_parzen.html

Adler, S. R., Wilson, E., & Coulter, Y. Z. (2008). Assessing students' socio-cultural knowledge frameworks through concept mapping. *Medical Education, 42,* 1125.

Afamasaga-Fuata'i, K. (2004). Students' conceptual understanding and critical thinking: A case for concept maps and vee-diagrams in mathematics problem solving. In J. Anderson, M. Coupland, & T. Spencer (Eds.), *Making mathematics vital (Proceedings of the Twentieth Biennial Conference of The Australian Association of Mathematics Teachers Inc.)*. Adelaide: Australia. (EJ802692).

All, A. C., & Huycke, L. I. (2007). Serial concept maps: Tools for concept analysis. *Journal of Nursing Education, 46*(5), 217–224.

Angelo, T. A., & Cross, K. P. (1993). *Classroom assessment techniques: A handbook for college teachers* (2nd ed.). San Francisco, CA: Jossey-Bass.

Atay, S., & Karabacak, U. (2012). Care plans using concept maps and their effects on the critical thinking dispositions of nursing students. *International Journal of Nursing Practice, 18,* 233–239.

Ausubel, D. P. (1968). *Educational psychology: A cognitive view*. New York, NY: Holt, Rinehart, & Winston.

Ausubel, D. P., Novak, J. D., & Hanesian, H. (1978). *Educational psychology: A cognitive view*. New York, NY: Holt, Rinehart, & Winston.

Baugh, N. G., & Mellott, K. G. (1998). Clinical concept mapping as preparation for student nurses' clinical experiences. *Journal of Nursing Education, 37*(6), 253–256.

Bogden, C. A. (1977). *The use of concept mapping as a possible strategy for instructional design and evaluation in college genetics*. Master's thesis, Cornell University, Ithaca, NY.

Cañas, A. J., Coffey, J. W., Carnot, M. J., Feltovich, P., Hoffman, R. R., & Novak, J. D. (2003). *A summary of literature pertaining to the use of concept mapping techniques and technologies for education and performance support*. Prepared for the Chief of Naval Education and Training, Pensacola, FL. Pensacola, FL: *Institute for Human and Machine Cognition*. Retrieved from http://www.ihmc.us/users/acanas /publications/conceptmaplitreview/ihmc%20literature%20review%20on%20concept%20mapping.pdf

Cañas, A. J., Novak, J. D., & Reiska, P. (2012). Freedom vs. restriction of content and structure during concept mapping: Possibilities and limitations for construction and assessment. In A. J. Cañas, J. D. Novak, & J. Vanhear (Eds.), *Concept maps: Theory, methodology, technology (Proceedings of the Fifth International Conference on Concept Mapping* (Vol. 2, pp. 247–257). Valletta, Malta: Institute for Human and Machine Cognition, University of Malta. Retrieved from http://cmc.ihmc.us/cmc2012Proceedings /cmc2012%20-%20Vol%202.pdf

Champagne, A. B., & Klopfer, L. E. (1984). Research in science education: The cognitive psychology perspective. In D. Holdzkom & P. Lutz (Eds.), *Research within reach: Science education* (pp. 171–189). Washington, DC: National Science Teachers Association.

Chiu, C. H., & Lin, C. L. (2012). Sequential pattern analysis: Method and application in exploring how students develop concept maps. *Turkish Online Journal of Educational Technology, 11*(1), 145–153.

Coffey, J. W., & Cañas, A. J. (2000). A learning environment organizer for asynchronous distance learning systems. In *Proceedings of the Twelfth IASTED International Conference on Parallel and Distributed Computing and Systems*, Las Vegas, NV. Retrieved from www.ihmc.us

Correia, P. R. M., & Cicuto, C. A. T. (2014). Neighbourhood analysis to foster meaningful learning using concept mapping in science education. *Science Education International, 24*(3), 259–282.

Daley, B. J., & Torre, D. M. (2010). Concept maps in medical education: An analytical literature review. *Medical Education, 44*(5), 440–448.

Dansereau, D. F., & Cross, D. R. (1990). *Knowledge mapping: Cognitive software for thinking, learning, and communicating*. Ft. Worth, TX: Department of Psychology, Texas Christian University.

Derbentseva, N., Safayeni, F., & Cañas, A. J. (2007). Concept maps: Experiments on dynamic thinking. *Journal of Research in Science Teaching, 44*(3), 448–465.

Edmondson, K. M. (1994). *Concept mapping for the development of medical curricula*. Paper presented at the Annual Conference of the American Educational Research Association, Atlanta, GA. Retrieved from ERIC database (ED 360 322).

Ertmer, P. A., & Newby, T. J. (1993). Behaviorism, cognitivism, constructivism: Comparing critical features from an instructional design perspective. *Performance Improvement Quarterly, 6*(4), 50–72.

Felder, R. M. (1993). Reaching the second tier: Learning and teaching styles in college science education. *Journal of College Science Teaching, 23,* 286–290.

Feldsine, J. E. (1987). *The construction of concept maps facilitates the learning of general college chemistry: A case study.* PhD dissertation, Cornell University. Ann Arbor, MI: Dissertation Information Service.

Gagne, R. (1985). *The conditions of learning and theory of instruction* (4th ed.). New York, NY: Holt, Rinehart, & Winston.

Gardner, H. (1983). *Frames of mind: The theory of multiple intelligences.* New York, NY: Basic Books.

Giddens, J. (2006). Concept mapping as a group learning activity in graduate nursing education. *Journal of Nursing Education, 45*(1), 45–46.

Glynn, S. M., Yeany, R. H., & Britton, B. K. (1991). A constructive view of learning science. In S. M. Glynn, R. H. Yeany, & B. K. Britton (Eds.), *The psychology of learning science* (pp. 3–20). Hillsdale, NJ: Lawrence Erlbaum.

Gonzalez, H. L., Palencia, A. P., Umana, L. A., Galindo, L., & Villafrade, M. L. A. (2008). Mediated learning experience and concept maps: A pedagogical tool for achieving meaningful learning in medical physiology students. *Advances in Physiology and Education, 32*(4), 312–316.

Griffiths, A. K., Thomey, K., Cooke, B., & Normore, G. (1988). Remediation of student-specific misconceptions relating to three science concepts. *Journal of Research in Science Teaching, 25*(9), 709–719.

Heinze-Fry, J. A., & Novak, J. D. (1990). Concept mapping brings long-term movement toward meaningful learning. *Science Education, 74*(4), 461–472.

Hicks-Moore, S. L. (2005). Clinical concept maps in nursing education: An effective way to link theory and practice. *Nurse Education Practice, 5,* 348–352.

Hicks-Moore, S. L., & Pastirik, P. J. (2006). Evaluating critical thinking in clinical concept maps: A pilot study. *International Journal of Nursing Education Scholarship, 3,* Article 27.

Hill, C. M. (2006). Integrating clinical experiences into the concept mapping process. *Nurse Educator, 31*(1), 36–39.

Hinck, S. M., Webb, P., Sims-Giddens, S., Helton, C., Hope, K. L., Utley, R., & Yarbrough, S. (2006). Student learning with concept mapping of care plans in community-based education. *Journal of Professional Nursing, 22*(1), 23–29.

Hsu, L., & Hsieh, S. I. (2005). Concept maps as an assessment tool in a nursing course. *Journal of Professional Nursing, 21*(3), 141–149.

Hunter-Revell, S. M. (2012). Concept maps and nursing theory: A pedagogical approach. *Nurse Educator, 37*(3), 131–135.

Kolb, A. Y., & Kolb, D. A. (2005). Learning styles and learning spaces: Enhancing experiential learning in higher education. *Academy of Management Learning & Education, 4*(2), 193–212.

Laight, D. W. (2004). Attitudes to concept maps as a teaching/learning activity in undergraduate health professional education: Influence of preferred learning style. *Medical Teacher, 26*(3), 229–233.

Mahler, S., Hoz, R., Fischl, D., Tov-Ly, E., & Lernau, O. Z. (1991). Didactic use of concept mapping in higher education: Applications in medical education. *International Sciences, 20,* 25–47.

Markham, K. M., Mintzes, J. J., & Jones, M. G. (1994). The concept map as a research and evaluation tool: Further evidence of validity. *Journal of Research in Science Teaching, 31*(1), 91–101.

Novak, J. D. (1990). Concept mapping: A useful tool for science education. *Journal of Research in Science Teaching, 27,* 937–949.

Novak, J. D. (2003, Summer). The promise of new ideas and new technology for improving teaching and learning. *Cell Biology Education, 2,* 122–132.

Novak, J. D., & Cañas, A. J. (2008). *The theory underlying concept maps and how to construct them* (Technical report; IHMC CmapTools 2008-01). Florida Institute for Human and Machine Cognition. Retrieved from https://www.uibk.ac.at/tuxtrans/docs/TheoryUnderlyingConceptMaps-1.pdf

Novak, J. D., & Gowin, D. B. (1984). *Learning how to learn.* New York, NY: Cambridge University Press.

Novak, J. D., Gowin, D. B., & Johansen, G. T. (1983). The use of concept mapping and knowledge vee mapping with junior high school science students. *Science Education, 67*(5), 625–645.

Novak, J. D., & Wandersee, J. H. (1990). Perspectives on concept mapping. *Journal of Research in Science Teaching, 27*(10), 921–1075.

Passmore, G. G. (1995). Constructing concept maps facilitates learning in radiologic technologies education. *Radiologic Science and Education, 2*(2), 50–59.

Passmore, G. G. (1996). *The effects of Gowin's vee heuristic diagramming and concept mapping on meaningful learning in the radiation science classroom and laboratory.* Doctoral dissertation, University of Missouri, Columbia, MO.

Passmore, G. G. (1998). Using vee diagrams to facilitate meaningful learning and misconception remediation in radiologic technologies laboratory education. *Radiologic Science and Education, 4*(1), 11–28.

Passmore, G. G. (2004). Extending the power of the concept map. *Alberta Journal of Educational Research, 50*(4), 370–390.

Passmore, G. G. (2008). *Concept mapping construction: Meaningful learning activity and assessment tool. A report on the empirical evidence.* Multimedia Educational Resource for Learning and Online Teaching—MERLOT Tegrity presentation, learning materials category. Retrieved from http://www.merlot.org/merlot/viewMaterial.htm?id=317905

Passmore, G. G., Owen, M. A., & Prabakaran, K. (2011). Empirical evidence of the effectiveness of concept mapping as a learning intervention for nuclear medicine technology students in a distance learning radiation protection and biology course. *Journal of Nuclear Medicine Technology, 39,* 284–289.

Pinto, A. J., & Zeitz, H. J. (1997). Concept mapping: A strategy for promoting meaningful learning in medical education. *Medical Teacher, 19*(2), 114–122.

Prankratius, W. J. (1990). Building an organized knowledge base: Concept mapping and achievement in secondary school physics. *Journal of Research in Science Teaching, 27*(4), 315–333.

Preszler, R. W. (2004). Cooperative concept mapping improves performance in biology. *Journal of College Science Teaching, 33,* 30–35.

Regan-Smith, M. G., Obenshain, S. S., Woodward, C., Richards, B., Zeitz, H. J., & Small, P. A., Jr. (1994). Rote learning in medical school. *Journal of the American Medical Association, 272,* 1380–1381.

Rendas, A. B., Fonseca, M., & Rosado-Pinto, P. (2006). Toward meaningful learning in undergraduate medical education using concept maps in a PBL pathophysiology course. *Advances in Physiology Education, 30,* 23–29.

Renner, J. W., Abraham, M. R., Grzybowski, E. B., & Marek, E. A. (1990). Understandings and misunderstandings of eighth graders of four physics concepts found in textbooks. *Journal of Research in Science Teaching, 27*(1), 35–54.

Roth, W. M. (1990). Map your way to a better lab. *Science Teacher, 57*(4), 31–34.

Roth, W. M., & Roychoudhury, A. (1993). Using vee and concept maps in collaborative settings: Elementary education majors construct meaning in physical science courses. *School Science and Mathematics, 93*(5), 237–244.

Safayeni, F., Derbentseva, N., & Cañas, A. J. (2005). A theoretical note on concepts and the need for cyclic concept maps. *Journal of Research in Science Teaching, 42*(7), 741–766.

Schuster, P. M. (2000). Concept mapping: Reducing clinical careplan paperwork and increasing learning. *Nurse Educator, 25*(2),76-81.

Starr, M. L., & Krajcik, J. S. (1990). Concept maps as a heuristic for science curriculum development: Toward improvement in process and product. *Journal of Research in Science Teaching, 27*(10), 987–1000.

Trowbride, J. E., & Wandersee, J. H. (1994). Identifying critical junctures in learning: A college course on evolution. *Journal of Research in Science Teaching, 31*(5), 459–473.

Wallace, J. D., & Mintzes, J. J. (1990). The concept map as a research tool: Exploring conceptual change in biology. *Journal of Research in Science Teaching, 27*(10), 1033–1052.

Wandersee, J. H., Mintzes, J. J., & Novak, J. D. (1994). Research on alternative conceptions in science. In D. Gabel (Ed.), *Handbook of research on science teaching and learning* (pp. 177–203). Washington, DC: National Science Teachers Association.

Weiss, L. B., & Levison, S. P. (2000). Tools for integrating women's health into medical education: Clinical cases and concept mapping. *Academic Medicine, 75*(1), 1081–1086.

West, D. C., Park, J. K., Pomeroy, J. R., & Sandoval, J. (2002). Concept mapping assessment in medical education: A comparison of two scoring systems. *Medical Education, 36,* 820–826.

West, D. C., Pomeroy, J. R., Park, J. K., Gerstenberger, E. A., & Sandoval, J. (2000). Critical thinking in graduate medical education: A role for concept mapping assessment? *Journal of the American Medical Association, 284,* 1105–1110.

Wheeler, L. A., & Collins, S. K. R. (2003). The influence of concept mapping on critical thinking in baccalaureate nursing students. *Journal of Professional Nursing, 19*(6), 339–346.

CHAPTER 27

The Clinical Pathway: A Tool to Evaluate Clinical Learning

Martha J. Bradshaw

■ Introduction

The clinical pathway is a strategy that uses specific, essential evaluation criteria in unique clinical learning settings.

■ Definition and Purpose

The clinical pathway is an abbreviated form of clinical evaluation that provides a means for the instructor to evaluate student progress using specified criteria. Clinical pathways can be used to evaluate applied practice and clinical learning that occur in time-limited, less traditional care settings. Learning activities are directed toward the same clinical outcomes as would be expected in traditionally structured patient care settings. The emphasis is on application of principles in a new setting, versus gaining experience via repeated opportunities in a familiar setting. As students apply principles, they recognize the development of individual practice-based judgment and decision making, and they begin to visualize themselves as professional healthcare providers. Faculty can determine how well the student uses guided thinking and clinical reasoning in unfamiliar settings, yet at the same time provides familiar and appropriate interventions.

■ Theoretical Foundations

Clinical pathways, also called *critical pathways*, are being used by nurses and other members of the healthcare team as a directed approach to goal-based outcomes; they are especially beneficial in quality improvement for cost-effectiveness (Broughton, 2011). Most nursing literature describes pathways for use in complex patient care situations, and use of pathways can have a positive influence on patient mortality (Panella, 2009). Consequently, if one thinks of clinical failure by a student as "mortality," then a pathway can be a valuable tool to avert student loss.

Pathways also are used for orientation of new nursing staff, quality improvement, evaluation and improvement of patient care interventions, and student-precepted experiences (Hunter & Segrott, 2010; Kersbergen & Hrbosky, 1996; Kinsman & James, 2001). One of the advantages of a pathway is that it is a cost-effective means, in both time and money, by which the individual is directed to the goal(s) and progress is measured (Renholm, Leino-Kilpi, & Suominen, 2002). Pathways also enable all individuals involved to know exactly what the goals are, thus clarifying expectations and making energy expenditure more efficient (Kersbergen & Hrbosky, 1996). Clinical faculty are able to collaborate on student evaluations by examining how well the student meets outcome criteria from more than one perspective. This principle is similar to how integrated-care pathways are used in interdisciplinary clinical situations, in that student progress and achievement of outcomes are the focus (Atwal & Caldwell, 2002).

■ Conditions

In selected situations, student clinical learning activities are one-time experiences and may deviate from the more structured patient care experiences. In addition, many clinical experiences are short term because of decreases in hospitalization length and emphasis on wellness programs. Examples of these clinical experiences in nursing are community health fairs, outpatient surgery, and pediatric health screenings in day-care settings. Whereas these unique clinical opportunities provide expanded observations and open up new areas of practice, one-time experiences do not always lend themselves to achievement of established clinical learning outcomes. If the learning outcomes are not readily identified, then the clinical instructor cannot easily evaluate clinical progress based on the experience. Therefore, instructors traditionally create one-time experiences as observation-only activities, or as task-focused activities that may not represent a professional nursing approach. In doing so, many valuable learning opportunities may be lost to the students. Instructors also lose the opportunity to determine the extent to which students are able to adapt to unique settings, apply principles, and enact new roles. For these reasons, a clinical pathway should be developed for virtual learning experiences, such as with high-fidelity patient simulators. These behaviors, as part of clinical reasoning (see Chapter 5), are essential in evaluating patient safety. Tanicala, Sheffer, and Roberts (2011) address the need to effectively evaluate behaviors in students that have a bearing on patient safety and could make the difference between a passing and failing student.

Use of a clinical pathway for student experiences enables continued learning by students and maximizes the benefits of the one-time clinical opportunities. Just as the critical pathway is an abbreviated version of a patient's plan of care, the student clinical pathway is an abbreviated version of the clinical evaluation tool. A major advantage of the pathway for both the student and course faculty is that it reduces the inconsistency or inadequacy of evaluation of one-time or isolated clinical learning opportunities. Variations in expectations and evaluation lead to variations in outcomes among students (Holaday & Buckley, 2008; Tanicala et al., 2011), and the pathway is a means to correct this problem.

At the time of the clinical experience, the student uses the pathway as a guide for fulfilling selected roles and completing specific responsibilities. Simultaneously, the student is aware of the criteria by which evaluation will take place. Therefore, use of clinical time and experience is maximized. The clinical pathway makes unique clinical experiences more purposeful, thus improving student clinical learning outcomes (Kinsman, 2004). Student clinical pathways are based on the same purposes as are patient- or staff-oriented pathways: they are goal directed, designed to be efficient, and effective in terms of time and energy. The components of the clinical pathway are derived directly from the clinical evaluation tool used by faculty in student evaluation.

■ Types of Learners

Whereas the clinical pathway could be used with learners of all levels, it is best used with undergraduate students who are engaged in directed clinical learning experiences. The clinical pathway offers specific learning outcomes and can include recommended or structured activities that enable the student to meet these outcomes. Students in undergraduate clinical settings generally have more faculty supervision, which creates opportunity for direct observation and evaluation. The clinical pathway is designed for intended learning, even though students often acquire additional personal growth during the clinical experience.

The pathway also is quite suitable for students of all levels in brief clinical learning settings with a preceptor, such as a one-day event. The preceptor should not be expected to conduct an in-depth evaluation of the student, but preceptor feedback is exceedingly helpful in compiling comprehensive information on a student. Therefore, a succinct and purposeful tool such as a clinical pathway can be easily completed and provide needed information. Preceptors also feel more empowered in their ability to make decisions about students and promote accountability for care (Kersbergen & Hrbosky, 1996).

■ Resources

The basis for a clinical pathway is the learning outcomes for the course. These outcomes are based upon professional competencies (Oermann & Gaberson, 2006). Evaluation tools used by all clinical instructors are directed toward course outcomes and ultimately professional standards for practice. Instructors supervising students in selected experiences identify outcomes and expected behaviors from the evaluation tool. Based on anticipated clinical learning opportunities, the instructor develops a clinical pathway that guides the student in what will be accomplished during the experience and the activities or behaviors the instructor expects to observe in each learner.

■ Using the Method

Implementation of an education-focused clinical pathway enables the faculty to develop student learning experiences that are directly related to the outcomes for the total clinical course. Two examples demonstrate how pathways are derived from the clinical evaluation tool and how components of the tool can be applied to more than one setting. Hearing and vision screening with school-age children can be conducted with nursing students at any level in the educational program. Such screenings have a place in a fundamentals course, a course on nursing care of children, or in a community nursing course. A more sophisticated version of the screening (to include patient referral) can be developed for nurse practitioner students.

When students are assigned to a unique, one-time clinical experience, they may have some apprehension about being responsible for patient care in a new setting. Knowing that they have only one opportunity to demonstrate competence, students benefit from the direction that a pathway provides. In fact, many students like the opportunity to test themselves in the new setting. Time and opportunity do not permit students to meet all criteria on the standard, comprehensive course evaluation tool. To maximize the learning experience, a sample pathway (see **Box 27-1**) was developed based on the following items from the course clinical evaluation tool:

- Demonstrates preparation for assignment
- Performs nursing skills correctly
- Maintains professionalism
- Demonstrates professional inquiry activities

As can be seen by the example in Box 27-1, other expectations are specified under the broad clinical outcomes. The pathway expectations are derived from the clinical evaluation tool and applied to the situation, such as communications with

---

Box 27-1   Course Outcomes Applied to Clinical Pathways

Learning Outcomes of Clinical Pathways

1. Demonstrates professional behaviors and inquiry activities.
2. Demonstrates preparation and use of principles in screening techniques.
3. Assesses behaviors of patient and family/support in ambulatory surgery and provides appropriate nursing interventions.
4. Provides nursing interventions for a patient in the ambulatory surgery/operative unit.

Clinical Learning Outcomes of Course

1. Demonstrates professional behavior and accountability.
2. Demonstrates preparedness for assignment.
3. Provides a safe environment.
4. Complies with the regulations of the school of nursing and clinical agency.
5. Performs nursing skills or interventions appropriate to the patient's health.
6. Demonstrates safe administration of medications.
7. Establishes rapport and demonstrates good communication skills.
8. Demonstrates collaboration with other care disciplines.
9. Demonstrates patient and family teaching.
10. Demonstrates appropriate documentation.
11. Maintains confidentiality and respect for others.
12. Completes assignments on time.
13. Seeks assistance/guidance appropriately.
14. Adapts to changing or stressful situations.
15. Uses critical thinking skills.
16. Demonstrates professional inquiry activities.

children or use of critical thinking. The expectations also indicate specific behaviors related to the clinical activity that must be demonstrated by the student, such as ability to complete vision screening.

Additional information that leaves no room for guesswork regarding preparation and professional behaviors is provided in the pathway for the student. Also, the standard for acceptable behavior (pass) is indicated as part of the directions, so that in the event a student demonstrates unacceptable behaviors, he or she has a clear understanding of how the final evaluation was determined (see **Box 27-2**).

In developing the pathway, the focus is on outcomes (student learning), not process (tasks or activities). Therefore, the instructor may designate specified activities or behaviors that direct the student to the outcomes; not all behaviors must be seen in order to attain the goal. Furthermore, other, unanticipated activities related

---

Box 27-2   Clinical Pathway: Hearing and Vision Screening

The clinical pathway identifies the specific nursing activities that will enable the student to meet the objectives for this one-time clinical experience. The student will be evaluated based on completion of items on this pathway. A student who fails this clinical pathway (i.e., fails to pass at least 7 of the 12 items on the clinical pathway) has failed the clinical day.

Objectives and Student Nursing Activities:

1. Demonstrates preparation and use of principles in screening techniques:
   - Attends clinical experience promptly, appropriately attired, and with own supplies.
   - Establishes a positive working relationship with patient(s).
   - Initiates and completes screening in timely manner.
   - Correctly follows sequence of steps in screening assessment(s).
   - Shows familiarity with equipment, screening criteria, and documentation.
   - Individualizes assessments as needed based on unique attributes of each patient.
2. Demonstrates professional behaviors and inquiry activities:
   - Uses principles of therapeutic and professional communications when interacting with patient(s).
   - Shows appropriate level of independence and self-direction.
   - Demonstrates critical thinking and problem-solving skills regarding screenings or patient interactions.
   - Documents or reports results of screening exam.
   - Seeks guidance or advice from instructor as needed.
   - Discusses screening results and/or patient responses with instructor and fellow students.

Student Preparation

- Complete check-off on hearing and vision screening equipment in the skills lab. If needed, practice again before clinical experience.
- You are permitted to bring your Hearing and Vision (H&V) booklet or some guidelines written on a card. This does not take the place of preparation and familiarity with the procedure. If you make too many references to the guidelines, your instructor will consider you unprepared. Bring these pathway sheets to give to your instructor.

to the patient situation that enable the student to meet the outcomes may present themselves.

An evaluation sheet provides feedback to the student regarding the experience and serves as the evaluation measure and anecdotal record for the instructor. Information regarding clinical activities and evaluation is found in the clinical section of the course syllabus. In that section is the detailed information indicating that the one-time activity is a clinical day of equal importance to a day caring for a hospitalized patient. Clinical instructors use the information from the pathway when formulating a final clinical evaluation report on each student.

Box 27-3 is a clinical pathway developed for use with nursing students in an ambulatory surgery unit. In addition to typical nursing activities related to an operative experience, an emphasis of this experience includes patient and caregiver interaction, alleviation of anxiety, provision of information about the procedure, and presentation of postoperative teaching prior to discharge. The ambulatory surgery pathway

---

Box 27-3 Clinical Pathway: Ambulatory Surgery Experience

For this one-time clinical experience, the clinical pathway identifies the specific nursing care activities on which the student will be evaluated. Items on this pathway will enable the student to meet the objectives for the ambulatory surgery experience for NUR 3102 (listed below). A student who fails the ambulatory surgery experience (i.e., receives a failing evaluation on two of the three sections of the clinical pathway) has failed a clinical day.

Objectives and Student Nursing Activities:

1. Assesses behaviors of patient and family/support in ambulatory surgery and provides appropriate nursing interventions:
   - Introduces self to patient and family/support person; establishes a working relationship.
   - Identifies behaviors related to hospitalization and surgery; discusses conclusions regarding behaviors with instructor, giving specific examples.
   - Indicates how patient behaviors influence preoperative, surgical, and postoperative periods.
   - Gives specific examples of family/support coping abilities.
   - Makes conclusions and interventions that are correctly based on patient's developmental level.
2. Provides nursing interventions for a patient in the ambulatory surgery/operative unit:
   - Demonstrates preparedness regarding knowledge of surgical procedure; discusses procedure and pertinent information with instructor.
   - Reviews patient's health history, lab, and other data as available on unit.
   - Teams with staff RN to provide care for patient.
   - Conducts assessments, including vital signs, in a timely manner, using correct technique.
   - Recognizes comfort and safety needs, specific for operative patients.
   - Provides interventions promptly.
   - Administers medications, based on the "five rights" and according to school of nursing guidelines.
   - Practices professional therapeutic communication skills in the areas of teaching, reassurance, and collaboration.

3. Demonstrates professional behaviors and inquiry activities:
   - Selects appropriate priorities for patient and family/support.
   - Conducts self in dignified, professional manner, including conversation and general appearance.
   - Shows organization and good use of time.
   - Demonstrates initiative to be involved in patient care and to further own learning.
   - Evaluates outcomes of patient's surgical experience; discusses patient responses and readiness for discharge/transfer with instructor.

Ambulatory Surgery Experience Clinical Pathway: Evaluation

Note: The student must receive a passing evaluation for at least two of the objectives in order to receive a passing grade for this clinical day.

1. Assess behaviors of patient and family/support in ambulatory surgery and provide appropriate nursing interventions.

   Pass/Fail   Comments:

2. Provide nursing interventions for a patient in the ambulatory surgery/operative unit.

   Pass/Fail   Comments:

3. Demonstrate professional behaviors and inquiry activities.

   Pass/Fail   Comments:

_____   _____

   Instructor   Date

also is constructed to indicate to the students what the expectations are for patient care. Prior to use of the pathway, students may be unsure of what they are permitted to do, and thus miss many learning opportunities.

Because the ambulatory surgery pathway is broader in scope, it uses both basic care items (same as in Box 27-1) and specific items:

- Provides a safe environment
- Establishes good rapport and maintains good communication
- Recognizes skill and knowledge limitations and seeks assistance appropriately
- Demonstrates safe administration of medications
- Uses critical thinking in decision making and applying various problem-solving methods

For this clinical experience, the student may be evaluated either by a different instructor or by a staff preceptor. Evaluation information is shared with the clinical instructor, added to other evaluation data, and used as part of the final course evaluation. One benefit of using the pathway in total course evaluation is that it provides the instructor with a glimpse of behavior patterns in a student, regardless of setting. In the event that the pathway does not provide beneficial evaluative feedback, the faculty must determine if the clinical experience and learning opportunities cannot be measured the way the pathway was constructed, or if the course evaluation tool should be revised to better reflect student learning outcomes (Kinsman, 2004).

■ Potential Problems

Any difficulties encountered in using the clinical pathway are related to the nature of this evaluation measure. It is intended to evaluate the student in a one-time experience, based on selected criteria. Potential problems with this method include:

- Inability of the instructor to observe and evaluate all behaviors. The type of clinical activity and spontaneous events govern the student's participation in care and types of care provided.
- The new environment may have a negative effect on students' behavior. Some students adapt more quickly than others to working in new settings. This is especially true of more experienced students and field-independent students who are able to sort out and select relevant information about the clinical setting. Students who are less able to adapt are therefore hampered in their performance and may appear to be weak in clinical judgment or nursing skills.
- It is easy to "rubber-stamp" evaluation remarks. For the instructor who has 40 or 50 students progressing through the one-time experience, the evaluation remarks become repetitive and tiresome. Instructors must endeavor to make individual comments that are an accurate description of the student. Remarks that reflect abilities in other clinical settings will validate the student's total clinical evaluation.
- To some instructors, the clinical pathway may be seen as too behavioral. In some cases, this is the intent of the pathway: to evaluate psychomotor skills. An immunization pathway is an example of psychomotor evaluation. The clinical pathway can be constructed in such a way as to provide opportunities for the student to use critical thinking and problem-solving abilities in ways that the instructor can readily observe and evaluate. An example is priority setting and decision making related to immediate patient care needs. This is an advantage of the pathway in that it facilitates evaluation in spontaneous situations.

■ Conclusion

Clinical pathways are a means by which an instructor can objectively and effectively evaluate student learning and progress toward clinical outcomes. An advantage to use of pathways in one-time experiences is that the pathway serves as a criterion-based frame of reference for both the student and the instructor, because the criteria are the same as for other clinical experiences in that course. The faculty member thus has an objective measure of student learning and performance, and the student always knows the measure on which he or she will be evaluated.

Clinical pathways are limited to brief experiences and are not designed to show professional growth and progress in learning over time. However, a pathway could be designed to appraise critical thinking and professional behaviors associated with spontaneous incidents, such as a problem patient. Nurse educators can use pathways as a creative means to address student performance in a variety of situations.

Discussion Questions

1. Discuss the strategy of having a student develop his or her personalized learning objectives to add to a clinical pathway.
2. When using a clinical pathway, is there too much emphasis on psychomotor skills?
3. If a student receives a weak/failing evaluation for a one-time experience, to what extent should that factor into the full clinical evaluation course grade?

References

Atwal, A., & Caldwell, K. (2002). Do multidisciplinary integrated care pathways improve interprofessional collaboration? *Scandinavian Journal of Caring Sciences, 16*, 360–367.

Broughton, E. I. (2011). The "how" and "why" of cost-effectiveness analysis for care pathways. *International Journal of Care Pathways, 15*, 76–81.

Holaday, S. D., & Buckley, K. M. (2008). A standardized clinical evaluation tool-kit: Improving nursing education and practice. *Annual Review of Nursing Education, 6*(ch.7), 123–149.

Hunter, B., & Segrott, J. (2010). Using a clinical pathway to support normal birth: Impact on practitioner roles and working practices. *Birth: Issues in Perinatal Care, 37*, 227–236.

Kersbergen, A. L., & Hrbosky, P. E. (1996). Use of clinical map guides in precepted clinical experiences. *Nurse Educator, 21*(6), 19–22.

Kinsman, L. (2004). Clinical pathway compliance and quality improvement. *Nursing Standard, 18*, 33–35.

Kinsman, L., & James, E. L. (2001). Evidence-based practice needs evidence-based implementation. *Lippincott's Case Management, 5*, 208–219.

Oermann, M. H., & Gaberson, K. (2006). *Evaluation and testing in nursing education* (2nd ed.). New York, NY: Springer.

Panella, M. (2009). The impact of pathways: A significant decrease in mortality. *International Journal of Care Pathways, 13*, 57–61.

Renholm, M., Leino-Kilpi, H., & Suominen, T. (2002). Critical pathways: A systematic review. *Journal of Nursing Administration, 32*, 196–202.

Tanicala, M. L., Scheffer, B. K., & Roberts, M. S. (2011). Defining pass/fail. Nursing student clinical behaviors phase I: Moving toward a culture of safety. *Nursing Education Perspectives, 32*, 155–161. doi:10.5480/1536-5026-32.3.155

CHAPTER 28

Truth or Consequences: The Significance of Giving and Receiving Evaluation Feedback

Lyn S. Prater
Stephanie S. Allen

. . . women and men as beings who cannot be truly human apart from communication, for they are essentially communicative creatures. To impede communication is to reduce people to the status of "things."

—*Paulo Freire (1970)*
International Educator, Community Activist

■ Introduction

Feedback is an essential component of the practice of health professionals and is a significant attribute in both professional education and practice settings. As valuable as feedback is, many educators struggle with giving and receiving feedback and thus do not benefit from its intended purposes. This chapter addresses the use of feedback in both practice and academic settings. Purposes of feedback are explained, types of relationships seen with feedback are explored, and the characteristics of effective feedback are delineated. Recommendations for the giving and receiving of feedback are presented, with the goal being growth of the healthcare professional.

■ Definition and Purpose

Feedback has many purposes and benefits. In didactic settings, feedback to students is typically given on exams, quizzes, papers, and projects. The feedback often is in a numerical form, is objective, and is compiled into a course grade. In applied practice settings, feedback is derived from information or behaviors that have taken place in the past and is used for advisory purposes and ongoing development. A primary aim of feedback is to explain the differences between expected and actual behaviors.

Feedback is also used for evaluative purposes tied to advancement. This could be for job retention, promotion, or advancement in the academic setting. Novices to the profession need to understand that evaluative feedback will be an ongoing component of their professional careers. Feedback that is student centered is used to bring awareness of commendable behavior as well as areas for correction. In Scott's (2014) study, finding out what students understood about feedback was an important step in increasing student satisfaction with the feedback provided. Scott points out that "there is no widely agreed scholarly definition of 'feedback'" (p. 49). Implicit in the word *feedback* is an exchange of information that has occurred or will occur between two parties. One party has recognized behavior that is worthy of comment and wishes to give or "feed" this information to the other party. The intended goal of feedback is for the receiver of feedback to be able to improve performance (Maynard, 2012). Feedback that is clear, descriptive, balanced, and well-timed can provide beneficial insights to the recipient, thus allowing for self-reflection and contributing to potential changes in behavior.

Recipients can learn from effective feedback. It is important that students take in and accept feedback and thus take responsibility for their behaviors (Fitzgerald, Gibson, & Gunn, 2010). Giles, Gilbert, and McNeill (2014) found that nursing students wished to be engaged with the feedback process, and have indicated that helpful written feedback enhances their learning. Nursing students also reported that absent or inadequate feedback hindered their learning. In a qualitative study by Nottingham and Henning (2014), athletic training students reported a strong association between correct and incorrect behavior from the feedback they received. The benefits of feedback for the giver include enriched interpersonal communication, while the process allows the giver to formally capture the state of an individual at one point in time and use that as a basis for ongoing evaluation and guiding future decisions.

The individual who is the recipient of feedback often perceives the process as critical, derogatory, or judgmental. These feelings likely are genuine, as a result of an encounter with one or more persons who do not know how to provide feedback appropriately. The feedback process and the mindset it creates must be addressed, because feedback should have numerous positive outcomes for the receiver. These may include increasing motivation, improving interpersonal relationships, and validating competence. By incorporating feedback into daily practice, direct care providers can enhance the quality of care delivered to patients. By applying best practices in the giving and receiving of feedback, leaders can better guide and support others. Effective feedback enhances self-esteem and self-confidence, which in turn strengthen assertiveness and promote action. Thus, feedback can be very empowering.

■ Theoretical Foundations

To understand how feedback shapes and supports learning outcomes, classic learning theories must be considered. Behavioral scientists describe feedback as a way of reinforcing or modifying behavior. Cognitive theorists focus on how information is acquired, processed, and stored, while humanists view learning as self-actualization with a focus on personal goals and stress the importance of engaging the individual as a partner in the encounter (see Chapter 1). Constructivists and social theorists believe learning is a function of experiences and social interactions. Therefore, various perspectives should be considered throughout the feedback process.

Feedback is most effective when the theoretical foundations are employed in combination with strategies and approaches tailored to an individualized context. Contextual strategies and individualized approaches begin with respectful consideration for the dignity of the recipient, while at the same time adhering to the professional standard(s) and context of the necessary feedback. In some instances, the delicate nature of the content creates reluctance and procrastination on the part of the giver, which inhibits the feedback process. It is a moral imperative for the giver of feedback to assume the professional responsibility and provide feedback based upon the principles described by Duffy (2013; see "Using the Method" section). Ultimately, it should encourage the giver to remember that initiating this type of feedback is geared toward benefiting the recipient.

In some instances, assertiveness is required on the part of the giver to initiate needed feedback. Simultaneously, the giver must keep in mind the delicate balance of maintaining the recipient's self-esteem while upholding best practice. Assertiveness is an interpersonal behavior that contributes to more effective ongoing feedback. The research of Unal (2012) pointed out that there is a positive relationship between assertiveness and self-esteem. The more opportunities one has for strengthening personal self-esteem, the more assertive one becomes. The giver of feedback must utilize the appropriate communication techniques, being assertive and not aggressive, angry, or demeaning. By showing a respectful and supportive attitude, along with providing specific and detailed information, the feedback is received positively and usually increases self-awareness in the recipient. This self-awareness allows the learner to experience growth in the areas of interpersonal communication, safe patient care delivery, and the development of successful relationships with patients, families, and colleagues.

In addition to the theory base on feedback as associated with clinical evaluation, the report from the Institute of Medicine (IOM, 2010) redirected the emphasis of student clinical evaluation to better meet industry standards. The report called for health education programs to better integrate patient safety core competencies in the measurement of student performance. The goal of these recommendations for students, instructors, and programs is the delivery of high-quality care (IOM, 2010). The IOM report focused on nursing, because it is the largest work-force group in the health professions, but the recommendations apply to all health professions programs.

Relationships

When considering the individuals involved, the nature of the feedback that is given and received depends upon the relationship of the individuals. The three most common relationships where feedback occurs are authoritarian, developmental, and lateral. When giving feedback, it is an essential component of the relationship to acknowledge the human capital of an individual. Royal (2012) explains that an individual's human capital is comprised of his or her specific values, knowledge, ideas, education, expertise, and skills. These traits influence how the individual relates with and to others. This is key when both giving and integrating feedback, and when initiating a process of personal change. An understanding of human capital is important during the process of giving feedback. Consideration of the perspectives of others facilitates the intended goals of the feedback session while upholding the self-esteem of both parties.

Authoritarian

The first encounter a health professions student may have with professional feedback is as an entry-level student. Professional disciplines utilize feedback for instructional and role development purposes. The roles of faculty member or instructor and student automatically create this authoritarian relationship where the power differential places the student in a position of vulnerability and perceived helplessness. The faculty member collects the data that comprise the evaluative feedback. The student must listen and receive the feedback given and recognize that it is more than part of receiving a grade: it is part of the professional growth process. The faculty member has the obligation to give specific and timely feedback, which affords the student the opportunity to learn and grow in the professional role (Aston & Hallam, 2011). This also is an opportunity for the faculty member to role model open and clear dialogue as a component of feedback related to safe professional practice. Because she or he is the established professional in the relationship, it is imperative that the faculty member promote a culture of trust and respect. If the foundation for feedback has been well established, the student is more likely to see feedback as a constructive component of her or his professional development during transition into professional practice.

Developmental

A prototype of a developmental relationship is that of a mentor and protégé or preceptor and preceptee. In a relationship of this nature, an individual with experience and insight shepherds and oversees the novice in the selected role. This relationship is different from one of authority in that there is a vested interest in outcome versus reward. The goal of the relationship is that the protégé or preceptee will become a part of the team as the preceptor's colleague; thus, the focus of the relationship is on the development of the preceptee into the designated role (Morgan, Mattison, Stephens, & Medows, 2012). In the mentor-protégé relationship, the mentor should focus on the cultivation of self-reflection or critically reflective work behavior (CRWB), as defined by de Groot and colleagues. These are internal tools that promote the development of an individual's cognitive processes. De Groot et al. (2012) point out that, "Social aspects of CRWB include asking others for feedback, sharing critical opinions, challenging group-think, and being open with others about mistakes" (p. 49). Engaging in these behaviors invites lateral feedback, promoting critically reflective behavior.

Preceptors often use the technique of peer coaching, an adult learning approach for skill proficiency and patient safety. "Peer-to-peer coaching is not about telling, criticizing, or instructing peers; it is about observing, giving effective feedback, and motivating" (Maynard, 2012, p. 203). Staff engaged in the formal process of precepting students in a capstone clinical internship are invaluable in student professional development. The quality of the feedback that preceptors provide to both students and the faculty instructors is critical to the final summative evaluation.

A unique feature of the association of preceptor–preceptee is the reciprocity of the relationship, where the responsibility is shared by both parties. According to Maynard (2012), effective feedback on the part of the preceptor is nonevaluative in nature, but must be descriptive and specific. The preceptee has the obligation to give feedback about the types and quality of the developmental experiences while progressing through the orientation. As the preceptee achieves independence in the role, she or he gains a greater sense of empowerment, which results in a sense of personal satisfaction in both the preceptor and the preceptee (Giles et al., 2014). The preceptor–preceptee relationship and the quality and timeliness of feedback serve as a bridge for the new graduate's transition into practice.

Lateral

In a lateral relationship, peers have the responsibility to provide feedback for the purpose of supportive or corrective action, in order to promote or sustain the integrity of a healthy work environment. This feedback is purposeful in nature, may be formal or informal, and often occurs only when the situation requires. For example, in the practice setting, one nurse or student may observe another breaking sterile technique and recognize that action and feedback are needed. In the academic setting, a faculty member may realize that a colleague needs advice and feedback on test construction. In both examples, one person is aware that he or she needs to give feedback to another and must do so utilizing the key principles of effective feedback. Depending upon the nature of the problem and the outcome of the feedback, the two individuals may find benefit in entering into a mentor–protégé relationship. In this relationship the components of human capital can be supported.

Many evaluative situations call for input from more than one peer. This can be problematic when the peers have not gathered periodic or thorough evidence. At times, the peers or preceptors are reluctant to give the constructive feedback that is important for growth but may be perceived as negative or critical. This commonly occurs in the preceptor–student relationship because the preceptor does not want to discourage the emerging professional (Hicks & McCracken, 2011).

Regardless of the type of relationship, key points to remember when giving and receiving feedback are that it is social in nature and is best accomplished face to face. Creating a positive, open atmosphere for feedback generates trust and collegiality. The desired outcome of giving and receiving effective feedback is personal and professional growth.

■ Types of Learners

Whereas feedback is useful in a myriad of work and academic settings, the focus of this chapter is on feedback as it relates to students and learning achievement. Because all students are the recipients of feedback, it is incumbent upon instructors to acknowledge that not all learners are the same: each will respond differently to the feedback process. Students arrive in the clinical setting from many backgrounds. Some students are of traditional age, and others may be second-career adult learners; therefore, maturity levels will vary greatly. Feedback should be given in clinical courses on both the undergraduate and graduate levels. Consequently, the graduate student is not a novice in receiving feedback and may have different expectations regarding the timing, depth, amount of feedback given, and the opportunity to respond.

Academically strong students often have high expectations of themselves and are comfortable with eliciting feedback in order to improve their work. In some cases, their expectations are not congruent with their performance, so the feedback process can be challenging for both instructor and student. Many programs typically have a cadre of students who fall into the statistically "average" academic category. It is easy for these students to blend in with the large group and, often due to age and level of academic achievement, they may not elicit feedback. For these reasons, the instructor must be careful not to overlook providing individualized attention and feedback to help each student reach her or his full potential.

Academically challenged students present complex issues related to feedback and evaluation. For example, students previously undiagnosed with learning disorders may discover during their first clinical rotation that they may not be suited to an applied practice profession. It may be that such a student lacks particular mental capabilities, such as executive functions, to be successful. In the healthcare professions, essential executive functions are the ability to plan patient care, set personal or patient goals, be flexible, and take in and monitor feedback in self and others (Bradshaw & Salzer, 2003). A student with a spatial recognition problem will have great difficulty with psychomotor skills, and faculty need to be sensitive to this because this may be a neurocognitive problem and not just awkwardness. Feedback regarding poor performance based upon newly discovered deficits can be very disheartening to a student who wishes to be part of a health profession.

More often, academically weak students are those who lack the background and are unable to acquire and/or transfer the learning from theory to practice. Some students lack the prerequisite foundation before entering the health professions program. Other students have personal issues that interfere with their ability to meet the requirements of the academic program. In these circumstances, the feedback session may call for a discussion regarding a change in personal strategies, such as adjusting priorities, time management, or altering the program progression plan.

Adult learners, many of whom are second-degree students, enter a health professions program with career and personal goals and have high expectations of themselves and the program they have chosen (McNiesh, 2011; Payne, 2013). Frequently these students approach clinical learning experiences in a planned and purposeful manner, similar to their previous work or domestic situations. Whereas many students are strongly competent in their abilities, some are anxious due to their self-imposed pressure to succeed. In some situations, adult learners in a new learning environment appear overconfident, and may be resistant to constructive feedback in their desire to appear successful. Conducting a feedback session for these students calls for a special consideration of the perspectives of adult learners and may require additional preparation.

Self-directed learners are individuals who know what they want to learn or accomplish and how to achieve it. Unfortunately, this process that they have used effectively in the past can become a liability in the healthcare setting. More frequent monitoring and immediate feedback are called for by the instructor. This will guide learners in comprehending and adhering to the boundaries of their student role. Regardless of the type or personal characteristics of the student, the principles and processes of providing feedback are universally applied. When feedback is given well, students are apt to recognize it as such, respond positively, and act upon the feedback.

■ Conditions for Giving Feedback (Where, When, and Why)

When giving feedback, the context is just as important as the content. The *context* is the circumstance upon which feedback is required. The context for feedback includes the setting (environmental) and skill in delivery (personal).

Environmental

In the practice setting, it may be in the best interest of patient safety for the preceptor or instructor to intervene immediately, withdrawing from the situation in order to provide critical feedback. To preserve the receiver's privacy, one should make every effort to find a location where the conversation cannot be overheard. This may have to be a less-than-ideal location, such as a supply closet, but it will do as long as it is private. A planned feedback session is typically held in a prearranged location such as a conference room or private office. In both situations, whenever possible, every effort should be made to reduce or eliminate extraneous noise and control as many distractions as possible. Good lighting, ambient room temperature, and ample personal body space must be taken into consideration. Regarding the seating arrangement, efforts should be made to minimize authoritarian or intimidating barriers. For example, whereas chairs placed opposite each other across a large desk may inhibit engagement, two chairs placed at the corner of a conference table may be more conducive for engagement.

Personal

Even though the giver of feedback may intend to communicate a positive, supportive, and developmental message, it may not be viewed as such by the receiver. In an effort to maximize the intended benefit of the message, the giver must consider body language, verbal and nonverbal characteristics. A landmark study by Mehrabian and Ferris (1967) pointed out that only 7% of a message's meaning is actually conveyed by the words that are used; 93% of the meaning of any communication is relayed by the speaker's tone of voice and body language. Therefore, the giver of feedback must engage the conversation by making eye contact, speaking in a neutral or welcoming tone of voice, and assessing for behaviors that validate engagement has occurred. This research also supports the importance of giving feedback face to face, rather than through e-mail or even a telephone call. Electronic communications are not linear, and the intent can be interpreted differently by all parties involved. Thus, the perceived meaning can be altered based on the receiver's interpretation (Littlejohn, 2002).

Appropriate body language includes staying focused on the recipient. This means you do not answer a cell phone, e-mail messages, or text during the feedback session. Be aware of restless motions such as finger tapping, leg moving, or rocking. Subtle body language such as the raising of eyebrows or turning of the head may communicate doubt or dissatisfaction to the receiver. Demonstrating active listening helps recipients feel supported and conveys that what they have to say is important. In addition, the giver of the feedback should be aware of subtle body-language signs coming from the recipient. An individual who has lost eye contact, begins to appear restless, is distracted, or falls silent indicates diminished engagement. The art of reading these signs will help the giver redirect or validate the message being conveyed. This is a skill that develops with practice over time.

For someone who is new to giving feedback, there are several ways to attain constructive feedback skills. Suggestions are seeking opportunities to shadow a more experienced role model, practicing giving feedback with colleagues, and taking a course or attending a conference on providing feedback or dealing with difficult conversations (Duffy, 2013).

■ Using the Method

Prompt Feedback versus Bad Practice

The impetus for a feedback session begins with a decision to provide information based upon observed behaviors. Whether giving negative or positive feedback, an effective feedback session should be conducted in a planned and purposeful manner. Contained in this section are general recommendations to be followed when giving feedback, keeping in mind the goal of benefiting the recipient while maintaining that person's dignity and self-esteem. It is important to note that each session is highly individualized and can be unpredictable. Reluctance to initiate feedback may stem from previous experiences that did not reach the intended outcome. These negative results could be based upon lack of preparation on the part of the giver or lack of readiness on the part of the recipient to hear and accept feedback. Therefore, a well-planned and well-conducted feedback session provides a higher likelihood of attaining the intended outcome. Duffy (2013) has defined five principles for providing constructive feedback: Gather and compile information, set realistic goals, gauge expectations of feedback, act on information gathered, and be specific.

Preparing

When an instructor determines that a feedback session is warranted, that individual is obligated to initiate a conference with the intended recipient. The conference may

---

Box 28-1   Sample Statements for Initiating Feedback

- The reason I want to meet with you today is because . . . .
- I think now that some time has passed, let's debrief on how things have gone and what you could differently next time
- I think you know we are meeting for . . . .
- You may not be aware that . . . .
- It has come to my attention that . . . .
- Let's step outside for just a moment . . . .
- Let's go in here; I'd like to give you some feedback about . . . .

---

occur either spontaneously or as a planned session. By providing feedback in a timely manner, one capitalizes on the "teachable moment" in which the context and behaviors are still fresh. Because this is an isolated incident, this type of feedback calls for minimal planning and information gathering. Spontaneous feedback often occurs in lateral relationships, and is seen with the preceptor–preceptee relationship as well as in clinical instruction with students. (See **Box 28-1** for an example of how to initiate this type of conversation.)

Whether spontaneous conversation or planned conference, the what, where, when, and how must be considered. This supports the value of maintaining the recipient's privacy and self-esteem. The giver of feedback should always remember: "praise in public; coach in private." Based upon the information gathered, the goals and outcomes for the session can be predetermined. Planning includes considering strategies that will most effectively meet these goals and outcomes. For example, using a reflective discussion strategy may encourage the recipient of feedback to reflect upon the context and behaviors in a meaningful way (Price, 2012). To bring this about, planning should include thoughtful consideration about the needed amount of time and the pace of the conversation. The giver must take into account that periods of quiet reflection and response by the recipient will be needed. As an outcome of the session, the giver also needs to prepare recommendations for the next steps.

The giver of feedback notifies the recipient of the need for a conference and seeks a mutually agreed-upon time and location. In the event the recipient demands an immediate meeting, best practice calls for the person initiating the feedback session to consider the nature of the request. The person giving feedback must maintain control of the situation. Giving feedback as close to the actual event will have the greatest effect (Royal College of Nursing, 2007).

Presenting the Matter Under Discussion

There is an art to presenting the information related to the matter at hand. The feedback session begins with an explanation of the purpose for the session, with an emphasis on the session being an opportunity for growth. The information must be clear, current, factual, and presented in an objective manner. The giver must remember to guard body language, maintain a level tone of voice, and be genuine in delivery.

The giver of feedback reviews roles and responsibilities for both parties and ties them to the purpose of the current meeting. As an example, a preceptor may say, "I have a professional obligation to give you feedback . . .," or a faculty member may say, "Part of my teaching role is to provide specific feedback about your documentation . . . ." The giver of feedback can help the recipient view the session as collegial and beneficial by conveying a positive intent.

Many disciplines endorse use of the "sandwich approach" for giving feedback: Begin with positive comments, address problematic areas, and end with positive or encouraging remarks (Clynes & Raftery, 2008; Walsh, 2010). Elcigil and Sari (2008) discovered that motivational aspects of feedback were important and encouraged students to take more initiative for their own learning. Once all of the information has been presented, the giver should seek validation on the information given. This verification provides the foundation for discussion on the recipient's perspective. Doing so allows an opportunity for the recipient to assume ownership of the topic and express additional concerns, both of which can be very empowering for the individual. At the same time, the giver may glean additional insights from what the receiver shares. More detailed discussion then can ensue regarding future plans. This may include a specific new behavior, outlining corrective action, or providing the resources necessary to accomplish the desired targets.

Planning for Improvement, Growth, Autonomy, and Independence

The endpoint of the discussion must allow time for planning steps/actions for improvement. This often is addressed in a discussion encompassing, "What can be done differently next time?" The plan should include mutually agreed-upon goals with a delineation of role responsibilities. A defined time frame, follow-up, and review of achievements should occur before alternate plans are developed. It is crucial that summaries of the feedback session and plan be documented (Duffy, 2013).

Often the written plan includes signatures of both parties. The need to obtain the signatures varies depending upon the relationship of the parties in the feedback session. In a developmental relationship (preceptor–preceptee), the feedback session may have been conducted with no printed documentation. If so, the preceptor should inform the preceptee that she or he will summarize their discussion, make contact with the preceptee for the purpose of communication, and present the plan in writing. Two copies should be available so that each party can retain the information. The benefit for the preceptee is that she or he can have the printed plan available for reference. The benefit for the preceptor is in having a reference source for follow-up and evaluation.

In an authoritarian relationship, the formal evaluation may be on a preprinted document and the developmental plan added during discussion. Consequently, the documented information can be signed at the conclusion of the meeting. Typically these signed documents are owned and housed by the institution, yet are available for review by either party at any time. In both situations, the giver of feedback, who is obtaining the signatures, must inform the feedback recipient signee that the signature indicates only that the recipient has read the document, and does not imply agreement with the content of the document.

■ Potential Problems
Matching the Learner and the Learning Experience

At times, the instructor may discover that the student and the clinical placement and/or preceptor are not a good match. Debriefing and addressing the issues first with the student and then with the preceptor is a priority for resolution of the issue. Or, change in patient status may create a challenging learning environment. In both situations, the important cycle of feedback exists; the instructor must obtain feedback from the appropriate sources and process the information before giving feedback to the student.

Conversely, a situation may be discovered in which a student has been placed in a clinical setting that is not challenging enough, or a preceptor does not give beneficial evaluative feedback. Based on feedback and observation, it may be necessary to adjust the student assignment to create a more challenging learning experience. This can be done by adding another patient to the present assignment, if feasible, or by giving the student a more challenging patient assignment in the future.

As mentioned previously, the quality of feedback from the preceptor to the instructor is essential to the final summative evaluation. Consequently, not receiving the desired type of feedback can have a negative effect. Often preceptors are reluctant to provide negative feedback, for fear of damaging the preceptor–student relationship and discouraging students in their academic progress. Furthermore, if the potential exists for the student as a new graduate, negative feedback comments could impair the formation of a future peer relationship. A proactive approach for avoiding a problematic feedback experience is to provide either formal or informal education to the preceptor about the evaluation.

Trust, Triangulation, and Transparency

Essential to the outcome is a trusting relationship between the giver and the receiver of feedback. The giver trusts that the recipient will hear the feedback in the spirit in which it is intended, within the framework of the professional discipline, and will take appropriate actions as a result. The recipient trusts the giver to provide honest, objective, and timely feedback that is supported by evidence. Both parties trust that the conversation will be kept confidential and nonjudgmental and will have mutual benefits. Therefore, both parties are accountable for the integrity of the process and the results.

Triangulation occurs when the recipient of feedback vents disappointments, frustrations, and other emotions to a third party. Sometimes this triangulation is an effort to obtain support or validation, and sometimes this triangulation is a strategy intended to weaken or demean the giver of feedback. Another form of triangulation occurs when feedback is not given directly to the person who could best benefit from it, but is shared with a third party instead. When any triangulation occurs, it destroys the intended purposes of feedback: open, honest, and direct communication, with discussion and plans for growth. Triangulation also contributes to a culture of mistrust that is counterproductive to professional relationships and communication. Trust must be maintained; a no-tolerance policy against triangulation must be adopted, and transparency must be a cornerstone of open communication in the feedback process.

Feedback as Part of a Clinical Grade

Every program uses a different system for grading the clinical student. One of the purposes of feedback is to assign a clinical course grade, so programs must have a standard tool and grading system used consistently in all courses. There is debate about the advantages and disadvantages of the pass-fail system versus the numeric grading system. Any clinical evaluation tool must contain expected clinical behaviors that are tied to course objectives and program outcomes. The pass-fail grading system is a very black-and-white system, even though it measures whether students are safe in the clinical arena, whether students can apply knowledge to practice, and whether students understand their professional roles and responsibilities. For the instructor, the decision is easy to make: it is yes or no. Historically, the pass-fail system lacked quality indicators; however, efforts are under way to apply the IOM's culture of safety to student pass-fail behaviors (Tanicala, Schaeffer, & Roberts, 2011). Consequently, the pass-fail system may be best suited for introductory courses such as the skills lab.

A benefit of the numeric or letter grading system for the instructor is that the tool provides performance categories to indicate the level or quality of student achievement. (See Chapter 21.) Based upon accumulated anecdotal information, it is recommended that the instructor develop a method to provide feedback based upon each clinical experience. This ongoing feedback may prevent the problem of a contentious final evaluation session. The biggest disadvantage to a graded evaluation method is the subjectivity among instructors regarding their interpretation of the performance indicators. Many instructors struggle with whether student performance is B level or C level. Some instructors operating under "wishful thinking" may assign an introductory student a low grade in hopes that the student will improve, rather than actually failing the student (Amicucci, 2012).

Regardless of which system of grading is utilized, it is imperative that the instructor maintain ongoing anecdotal documentation of student performance. The more descriptive the instructor can be with these anecdotal notes, the more helpful it is for student growth. In addition, well-documented student behaviors provide helpful, supportive evidence in the event of a grade appeal.

What to Do When a Feedback Session Does Not Go Well

If a student begins to argue during the feedback session, the instructor must stay objective, focusing on the expected behaviors and performance standards. A repeated review of the anecdotal notes may be needed. In some instances, students who are receiving a less-than-desired grade may be silent throughout the feedback session or cry. After reflecting on the feedback session, the student may contact the instructor at a later time and request a meeting for grade reconsideration. This is when the due process begins. Every school or program will have a designated method through which to handle appeals, but regardless of the system, peer faculty support is essential. Although no one wishes to engage in a grade appeal, this due process allows all parties to be heard fairly and the evidence at hand to be given careful consideration.

Additional Challenges

There are instances in which a member of the workforce is compelled to give feedback to a senior leader in the organization. Such feedback may be prompted by safety concerns, lack of adherence to policies or procedures, personnel issues, or lack of academic integrity. This encounter can be most effective when utilizing the steps of the feedback process, accompanied by an expression of unbiased concern. Recognizing that the senior leader is a busy administrator, the giver of feedback must make the message succinct and to the point. Part of this message may be that there is a barrier to meeting organizational goals. This will stimulate the leader's attention and open the door for the presentation of evidence. It is the leader's decision on whom to include in the resolution of the problem. *Leaders beware*: The compelling nature of the evidence obligates you to act upon it. To close this feedback loop with the member of the workforce, the leader must communicate the decisions made or actions taken.

■ Conclusion

Professionals utilize the feedback process in many ways, often with the goal of promoting growth in the profession. The role one plays as a giver or receiver of feedback is affected by one's relationship or professional status. The approach should be highly individualized and coupled with best practices to accomplish the intended outcomes. Despite best intentions and efforts on the part of the giver of feedback, the human element cannot be overlooked; therefore, unintended outcomes and consequences may occur. These consequences can be either positive or negative. Validation or confirmation that the message was heard by the receiver is a key step for the sender throughout the feedback process. Feedback contributes to professional insight and development. Therefore, feedback should occur in an atmosphere of diplomacy, honesty, and compassion.

Discussion Questions

1. What three common relationships must be taken into consideration when individuals are involved with the giving and receiving of feedback? How should the feedback process be adjusted based on these three common relationships?
2. What is the unique feature that affects effective feedback in the preceptor–preceptee relationship? How is this different from the mentor–protégé relationship?
3. What is a leader's role when receiving feedback regarding safety, lack of adherence to policies, or academic honesty?

References

Amicucci, B. (2012). What nurse faculty have to say about clinical grading. *Teaching and Learning in Nursing, 7,* 51–55.

Aston, L., & Hallam, P. (2011). *Successful mentoring in nursing.* Exeter, England: Learning Matters.

Bradshaw, M. J., & Salzer, J. S. (2003). The nursing student with attention deficit hyperactivity disorder. *Nurse Educator, 28*(4), 161–165.

Clynes, M. P., & Raftery, S. E. (2008). Feedback: An essential element of student learning in clinical practice. *Nurse Education in Practice, 8,* 405–411.

de Groot, E., Jaarsma, D., Endedijk, M., Mainhard, T., Lam, E., Simons, R.-J., & van Beukelen, P. (2012). Critically reflective work behavior of health care professionals. *Journal of Continuing Education in the Health Professions, 32*(1), 48–57.

Duffy, K. (2013). Providing constructive feedback to students during mentoring. *Nursing Standard, 27*(31), 50–56.

Elcigil, A., & Sari, H. Y. (2008). Students' opinions about and expectations of effective nursing clinical mentors. *Journal of Nursing Education, 47*(3), 120–123.

Fitzgerald, M., Gibson, F., & Gunn, K. (2010). Contemporary issues relating to assessment of pre-registration nursing students in practice. *Nurse Education in Practice, 10,* 158–163.

Freire, P. (1970). *Pedagogy of the oppressed.* New York, NY: Continuum.

Giles, T. M., Gilbert, S., & McNeill, L. (2014). Nursing students' perceptions regarding the amount and type of written feedback required to enhance their learning. *Journal of Nursing Education, 53,* 23–30. doi:10.3928/01484834-20131209-02

Hicks, R., & McCracken, J. (2011, May–June). How to give difficult feedback. *Physician Executive Journal,* 84–87.

Institute of Medicine (IOM). (2010). *The future of nursing: Leading change, advancing health. Report brief.* Washington, DC: Author.

Littlejohn, S. (2002). *Theories of human communication (7th ed.).* Belmont, CA: Wadsworth.

Maynard, L. (2012). Using clinical peer coaching for patient safety. *Association of periOperative Registered Nurses Journal, 96,* 203–205. doi:doi.org/10.1016/j.aorn.2012.05.002

McNiesh, S. (2011). The lived experience of students in an accelerated nursing program: Intersecting factors that influence experiential learning. *Journal of Nursing Education, 50*(4), 197–203.

Mehrabian, A., & Ferris, S. R. (1967). Inference of attitudes from nonverbal communication in two channels. *Journal of Consulting Psychology, 31,* 248–252. doi:10.1037/h0024648

Morgan, A., Mattison, J., Stephens, M., & Medows, S. (2012). Implementing structured preceptorship in an acute hospital. *Nursing Standard, 26*(28), 35–39.

Nottingham, S., & Henning, J. (2014). Feedback in clinical education, part II: Approved clinical instructor and student perceptions and influences on feedback. *Journal of Athletic Training, 49*(1), 58–67.

Payne, L. (2013). Comparison of students' perceptions of educational environment in traditional vs. accelerated second degree BSN programs. *Nurse Education Today, 33*(11), 1388–1392.

Price, B. (2012). Key principles in assessing students' practice-based learning. *Nursing Standard, 26*(49), 49–55.

Royal, J. (2012). Evaluating human, social and cultural capital in nurse education. *Nurse Education Today, 32,* e19–e22.

Royal College of Nursing. (2007). *Guidance for mentors of nursing students and midwives: An RCN toolkit.* London, United Kingdom: Author.

Scott, S. (2014). Practising what we preach: Towards a student-centered definition of feedback. *Teaching in Higher Education, 19*(1), 49–57.

Tanicala, M., Scheffer, B., & Roberts, M. (2011). Defining PASS/FAIL nursing student clinical behaviors phase I: Moving toward a culture of safety. *Nursing Education Perspectives, 32*(3), 155–161.

Unal, S. (2012). Evaluating the effect of self-awareness and communication techniques on nurses' assertiveness and self-esteem. *Contemporary Nurse, 43*(1), 90–98.

Walsh, D. (2010). *The nurse mentor's handbook: Supporting students in clinical practice.* Maidenhead, England: Open University Press.

CHAPTER 29

Evaluating a Program's Teaching Resources

Shanti Freundlich

The evaluation of teaching resources—the resources that exist to support an academic program—must be part of a holistic, systematic, and ongoing evaluation. In this context, *program evaluation* is defined as "a systematic operation of varying complexity involving data collection, observations and analyses, and culminating in a value judgement with regard to quality" (Mizikaci, 2006, p. 40). To holistically evaluate the resources available to support teaching and teachers in a professional health sciences program, the context must always be examined. According to the National League for Nursing Accreditation Commission (2012), teaching resources include fiscal, physical, and learning resources. At a more granular level, they include:

- the physical—buildings, classrooms, lab space
- the technology—the learning management platform, the library's electronic databases and other information resources
- simulation lab spaces
- the staff available to support all of these resources
- teaching and learning centers—curriculum and professional development resources for the faculty, opportunities for professional growth and interprofessional opportunities
- the fiscal resources to support them all

As with any form of evaluation, the program should choose highly regarded and relevant standards as a measure against which to compare itself, and this self-reported perspective should be incorporated into future changes to the program. Quite simply, if the results of an evaluation are not going be used as part of an ongoing evidence-based decision-making process, there is little value in evaluating a program's resources. The accreditation standards for health education programs all have unique requirements, but there are enough commonalities among the resources needed that the context, resources, models, and future challenges discussed here will speak to a wide variety of programs.

■ Context

Nursing and other professional health sciences programs exist within larger health and higher education contexts that continue to change dramatically, and these contexts affect the goals and essential resources of nursing and other professional health sciences programs. There are recent and significant pieces of legislation affecting the work environment that newly graduated students enter: namely, the Patient Protection and Affordable Care Act (ACA) and the Health Information Technology for Economic and Clinical Health Act (HITECH). These are affecting the professional environment in which students have their clinical placements and where they will be working after graduation. The changes mandated by these laws are also affecting faculty members, who are adopting new systems and technologies in their places of work and into their teaching as they prepare students to enter this changed professional world.

The ACA affects nursing education in multiple ways: addressing faculty shortages through raising funding caps; instituting faculty and student loans programs, including an emphasis on diversity; updating the Nurse Education, Practice and Retention grant program; and expanding the National Health Services Corps, among other grants and programs (Wakefield, 2010). It also affects educational programs indirectly; students need to be prepared for an increased number of patients as health care becomes more accessible and care models in hospitals and community health settings change.

Meanwhile, HITECH calls for the implementation of electronic health records (EHRs) and the achievement of meaningful use—the use of EHRs to achieve health and efficiency goals (National Coordinator for Health Information Technology, 2013). In order for students to be part of these health information technology standards, programs must train them to be proficient EHR users, to be comfortable integrating technology into practice, and to understand meaningful use standards so that they can help achieve them and improve quality of care.

Simultaneously, professional health education programs also exist within the context of academia: strategic plans; institutional mission and vision statements; accreditation standards; tenure concerns; faculty shortages; teaching versus research mentalities; high-stakes conversations about online education, including blended courses, fully online programs, and massive open online courses (MOOCs); as well as changing student demographics, dynamics, and expectations. Program evaluation must also examine how and if multiple learning styles are addressed, how they are reflected in student learning outcomes, and how faculty members' professional development around teaching techniques is being supported.

Any one of the ACA, HITECH, or academia-related factors would have significant impact on the shape of a program and require fiscal, physical, and learning resources. However, programs are affected by all of them and so must allocate resources to address all of them—and an evaluation is a chance to examine current levels of support and identify future goals in resource management.

■ Teaching Resources

To determine what resources are needed to support a curriculum, Schug (2012) recommends asking the following: "What resources (e.g. library, information technology) contribute to the curricular implementation? What features of the physical facilities

---

Box 29-1   Resource Categorization

Resources can be categorized more specifically as:

- Physical resources—including the buildings, classrooms, lab spaces, and the geographic location.
- Simulation/clinical resources—necessary for students to gain hands-on experience and learn how to work with real patients, clinicians, and doctors under pressure.
- Technology resources—the electronic and print resources (via the library), learning management platforms, electronic health records, and the support to offer training and ensure functionality.
- Online learning resources—the specialized software and support necessary to ensure that students enrolled in blended or fully online courses receive the same level of attention and interaction as those enrolled in in-person courses.
- Curriculum/teaching resources—the materials and personnel usually found in co-curricular support centers that offer opportunities to refine teaching techniques, explore innovative teaching methods, and encourage the incorporation of new learning theories and styles.

---

were conductive to learning? What presented barriers/challenges?" (p. 303). These fiscal, physical, and learning resources (National League for Nursing *Accreditation* Commission, 2012) that support faculty in their teaching are just one aspect of an academic program. Evaluating the resources that faculty use to create an environment that facilitates learning is separate from evaluating teaching (i.e., faculty output) or learning (i.e., what students take in). See **Box 29-1**.

Before it can be evaluated, a program must define and articulate its resources, map them to course and curricular goals, and describe at what level they currently exist.

■ Theoretical Framework

At the program level, strategic mission statements and learning outcomes set the standards that a program aspires to meet. Based on these, resources can be evaluated to determine if they meet these standards. Once the program being evaluated has clear strategic goals, a theoretic framework on which to base the evaluation process can be chosen. Not every aspect of a program's resources should or can be evaluated at once, but Gard, Flannigan, and Cluskey (2004, p. 176) recommend that any evaluation process start with the following four clear, practical questions:

- What do we want to know?
- Why do we want to know it?
- What should we measure?
- How should we measure it?

Once these questions have been answered, a more in-depth theoretical model can be chosen as a framework, or aspects of multiple frameworks can be combined into a customized model to best evaluate the program's resources. The literature is full of potential frameworks, and one should be chosen based on what aspect of the program is being evaluated; some focus on simulations (Jeffries, 2005), and others focus on online or distance education curricula (Avery, Cohen, & Walker, 2008), whereas many take a systematic approach (Gard et al., 2004; Hamner & Bentley, 2003; Kalb, 2009; Matthiesen & Wilhelm, 2006). When developing or adopting a framework, consider the aspirational goals of the program as well. For example, if a school is planning to start a new online program, the teaching resources can be evaluated with an eye toward the soon-to-be-developed online program.

Matthiesen and Wilhelm (2006) use a case study approach to argue that evaluation should not limit its scope solely to the curriculum, but rather should be an ongoing and systematic view of the program and the core components required by multiple accreditation bodies and licensure and certification boards. Schug (2012) chooses to focus on just the curricular aspects of a program; however, she also acknowledges that these are components of a larger evaluation process. Her schema for curricular evaluation can be used to inventory and evaluate resources at a micro (i.e., course) level by asking what resources are available to support each aspect of a course, and whether there is any room to improve said resource. Instead of simply asking if the following aspects are present in a course, Schug (2012) recommends evaluating what resources are available to faculty and students to best facilitate the creation, maintenance, use, or understanding of:

- Course objectives
- Curricular threads
- Course content
- Schedule
- Teaching and learning strategies
- Evaluation of student performance
- Textbooks/library holdings
- Student evaluations of the course
- Accrediting standards
- Liberal arts requirements

Evaluation is an evidence-based judgment process, and a theoretical framework serves as a scaffold for evaluation as a program articulates to itself what it wants to know and why, and what it wants to measure and how (Gard et al., 2004). As a program evaluates itself systematically, the findings of an in-depth examination of resources can help project its potential future directions.

■ Evaluation Process

One method to help jump-start the evaluation process is to consider the program through the eyes of a new faculty member or student. Determine the resources that are immediately available to them, those that are lacking, and what additional support for teaching/learning would ideally be present. This exercise can offer an outsider's perspective on the familiar and prompt a deep examination of program resources. This is a method that usability experts often use, including to experience a library's physical space from a student's perspective.

Much of the literature on program evaluation agrees that accreditation visits are often the catalyst for ongoing program evaluation (Gard et al., 2004; Hamner & Bentley, 2003; Jeffries, 2005; Suhayda & Miller, 2006), and a programmatic evaluation will often be led by a committee of invested faculty and administrators. This helps ensure that the process garners support and buy-in from the larger department, and that the self-report and evaluation plan work with the academic calendar and accreditation schedules, rather than attempting to work independently from them. A comprehensive evaluation plan can combine theoretical elements from the systematic approach of Hamner and Bentley (2003) and the ongoing schedule of Gard and colleagues (2004). Hamner and Bentley's (2003) matrix includes space for the resource being evaluated, supporting documentation, the person responsible, the evaluation method, the evaluation standard, the committee findings, and the committee's recommendations for action. Gard and colleagues' (2004) schedule recommends planning the process in August, reviewing the existing documentation during the fall semester, focusing on the resources in the latter half of it, and collecting course evaluation data at the end. The fall semester can be used to focus on external accreditation; meanwhile, the spring semester can be used to write recommendations, and alumni feedback is collected throughout the year.

As a program initiates an evaluation process, it is essential to connect to the departmental, school, and institutional strategic planning processes so that the evaluation has a clear purpose and it is simpler to connect the work of a single program to the mission, vision, and strategic plan of the larger institution. Hamner and Bentley (2003) also recommend clearly defining the program resources and elements that are being evaluated from the outset, so that it is a more manageable process. Once a framework has been articulated, a committee formed, and a schedule agreed upon, the information being gathered must be shared between committee members so that work is not duplicated. It will also benefit the evaluation committee to draw on documents the program has already created in response to other nationally recognized accreditation standards. To encourage faculty to participate in a program evaluation, it must be clear that the data collected are completely separate from individual faculty evaluations, so that the committee can work from comprehensive data. These steps—gathering complete and comprehensive data, sharing information, and drawing on previous work—will make it more straightforward to reuse the findings and recommendations for other reports.

■ Evaluating Resources, Not Learning

The evaluation of student learning is core to all academic programs, and this discussion of teaching resources examines the context in which that learning occurs. Assessing how and what students are learning is an integral part of teaching, and assessment can be built into the essential aspects of each lesson, as well as the midterm and final exams that serve as comprehensive assessment measures.

Similar to evaluating resources, learning is more effectively measured if clear learning outcomes are set ahead of time, as outlined by Wiggins and McTighe's (2005) backwards approach to curricular design. In their approach, course design starts with course outcomes, which learning outcomes connect back to, and which are tied directly to the program's mission, vision, and goals. Having a strategic scaffold in place means that faculty are under less pressure to develop all of those outcomes from scratch every time they teach, and if faculty lead the development of the program's learning outcomes as part of an ongoing process, no faculty member will feel too far removed from these goals in his or her own teaching.

Without a doubt, evaluating student learning is part of program evaluation, but when taking a holistic approach to evaluation, the measure of a program does not rest solely on students, but rather on all the elements that come together to create an environment that facilitates and encourages learning—one that is supported by teaching resources.

■ Future Challenges

A program that teaches evidence-based practice must also draw on the same principles to inform its own teaching practices. Evaluating teaching resources is an integral part of a larger systematic program evaluation, and both the elements and process will benefit from being clearly defined from the outset. Although evaluation examines the past and present, the findings and recommendations can inform future opportunities, even as events outside a program continue to evolve and shape expectations.

Nursing and professional health sciences programs are exploring interprofessional learning opportunities—in classrooms, clinical training settings, and community settings. As these interprofessional plans solidify, all the academic programs involved must ensure that they are held to the same evaluation standards as all of the other program elements. Interprofessional learning opportunities may also require different or additional teaching resources, so, as these opportunities grow, faculty will need to look closely at their programs to ensure that the resources are still meeting the program's needs.

As programs consider moving more teaching to blended or fully online formats, they must continue to evaluate resources, outcomes, and students at the same standard as in-person programs. They will also have to determine what additional teaching resources must be provided to ensure that faculty members are able to deliver the same high-quality teaching in a completely different format, which will offer new challenges as well as benefits.

■ Conclusion

Once program evaluation becomes an ongoing process, the findings and recommendations for changes to teaching resources may seem overwhelming and challenging to implement. Rather than attempting to enact every recommendation simultaneously and at full scale, programs may consider running pilot projects and implementing incremental change. Scaling of efforts also acknowledges that faculty and staff have limited amounts of time in which to participate in evaluation efforts and program reviews on top of existing teaching, service, and clinical responsibilities. An organization that is serious about creating an environment that uses the results of an evaluation for program improvement will encourage the implementation of the recommendations, even if it just starts at a small scale.

Evidence-based decisions are a driving force in health care and healthcare education today. Ensuring that the same evidence-based mindset is also applied to the teaching resources that are being using to prepare the next generation of healthcare providers is a natural and essential step of the process.

Discussion Questions

1. How have past self-reports and accreditation patterns shaped changes to your program? Are these evaluation activities considered to be constructive activities for your program, or are they outside exercises?
2. What teaching resources exist on your campus—are faculty members encouraged to work with teaching and learning centers? Do faculty members collaborate with each other to offer classroom teaching observations? What could you do to encourage a culture that offers this kind of collaborative teaching support?

References

Avery, M. D., Cohen, B. A., & Walker, J. (2008). Evaluation of an online graduate nursing curriculum: Examining standards of quality. *International Journal of Nursing Education Scholarship, 5*(1), 1–17.

Gard, C. L., Flannigan, P. N., & Cluskey, M. (2004). Program evaluation: An ongoing systematic process. *Nursing Education Perspectives, 25*(4), 176–179.

Hamner, J. B., & Bentley, R. W. (2003). A systematic evaluation plan that works. *Nurse Educator, 28*(4), 179–184.

Jeffries, P. R. (2005). A framework for designing, implementing, and evaluating simulations used as teaching strategies in nursing. *Nursing Education Perspectives, 26*(2), 96–103.

Kalb, K. A. (2009). The Three Cs Model: The context, content, and conduct of nursing education. *Nursing Education Perspectives, 30*(3), 176–180.

Matthiesen, V., & Wilhelm, C. (2006). Quality outcomes and program evaluation in nursing education: An overview of the journey. *Quality Management in Healthcare, 15*(4), 279–284.

Mizikaci, F. (2006). A systems approach to program evaluation model for quality in higher education. *Quality Assurance in Education, 14*(1), 37–53.

National Coordinator for Health Information Technology. (2013). *HealthIT: The official site for Health IT information*. Retrieved from http://www.healthit.gov

National League for Nursing Accrediting Commission, Inc. (2012). *NLNAC Accreditation Manual: Including the 2008 Standards and Criteria*. Atlanta, GA: Author.

Schug, V. (2012). Curriculum evaluation using National League for Nursing accrediting commission standards and criteria. *Nursing Education Perspectives, 33*(5), 302–305.

Suhayda, R., & Miller, J. M. (2006). Optimizing evaluation of nursing education programs. *Nurse Educator, 31*(5), 200–206.

Wakefield, M. K. (2010). Nurses and the Affordable Care Act. *The American Journal of Nursing, 110*(9), 11.

Wiggins, G., & McTighe, J. (2005). *Understanding by design* (2nd ed.). Alexandria, VA: Association for Supervision and Curriculum Development.

CHAPTER 30

Program Evaluation

Shelley F. Conroy

Academic institutions and healthcare facilities are required to be accountable to their stakeholders and can no longer only be judged by reputation and resources. The public wants academic institutions and healthcare facilities to demonstrate measurable outcomes of their work. Educators are accountable to their students to provide a quality education. For example, in health professions, licensure and certification pass rates are frequently used to assess the quality and outcome of a program, assure the competency of its graduates, and ensure students the ability to be employed (Parker, Burrows, Nash, & Rosenblum, 2011; Stufflebeam & Shinkfield, 2007). Likewise, the public has access to hospital mortality and morbidity rates and can make decisions whether to use those facilities with undesirable rates. Program evaluation can assure the public that academic institutions and healthcare facilities provide quality instruction and quality health care. This chapter defines program evaluation, details the benefits of evaluation, discusses the importance of evaluations to accreditation, and provides examples of evaluation research.

■ Evolving Significance

As early as the 1940s, Ralph Tyler described a behavioral objective model examining whether educational learning experiences produced the desired educational outcomes (Tyler, 1949). This was a summative evaluation model. In the 1980s, Stufflebeam (1983) advocated for also including the use of formative evaluation by assessing the process of program implementation. In the 1980s, in response to requirements by the U.S. Department of Education, accrediting bodies began mandating outcomes assessment for programs in order to ensure a continuous process of quality improvement and demonstrate accountability (Haleem et al., 2010; Sauter, Gillespie, & Knepp, 2012). Each accrediting body (and often state regulatory bodies as well) specifies required outcome indicators that should be included in the programmatic assessment. These are often included in a written program evaluation plan, as is required by the three nursing accreditors: the Commission on Collegiate Nursing Accreditation (CCNE), Accreditation Commission for Education in Nursing (ACEN), and Commission for Nursing Education Accreditation (CNEA).

The author wishes to thank Astrid H. Wilson for her review and contributions to this chapter.

This process of systematically assessing and reviewing data to make decisions and improvements in the program is detailed in the program evaluation plan. The plan is like the blueprint to guide the ongoing systematic assessment of the components of the program, as well as to examine the relationships and contexts of how and why processes are or are not working (Haji, Morin, & Parker, 2013). The program identifies goals or targets to achieve, and the systematic evaluation plan describes evaluation approaches to collect relevant data to analyze and interpret to make decisions toward the attainment of these goals (Ellis & Hallstead, 2012).

This information is used for decision making and program improvement. Unless a program examines outcomes, it is easy to continue with the same practices and processes without knowing whether or not they are effective (Lewallen, 2015). In addition, building the outcome indicators required by state, programmatic, regional, and national accrediting or regulatory bodies into the evaluation plan helps to ensure maintenance of compliance (Sauter et al., 2012). Often, a program evaluation committee composed of representatives from various groups associated with the program is responsible for implementing the plan, collecting the data, and reporting to the faculty for decision making. Evaluation should be a collaborative process that involves active and ongoing engagement among stakeholders (O'Sullivan, 2012). Program changes are generally accepted more readily if they are based on data that support the recommendations. Used regularly and systematically, program evaluation allows a program to maximize its strengths and make needed improvements (Lewallen, 2015).

■ Definition

There are numerous definitions of *program evaluation* in the literature (Chen, 2005; Davidson, 2005; Fink, 2005; McNamara, 2006; Mertz, 2007). The common theme in the definitions is that of program evaluation being a process of collecting data to determine the effectiveness of a selected program and to make decisions, using sound methodology, in order to improve the effectiveness of the program. The evaluator chooses from a range of appropriate, sound approaches, based on the component being evaluated. There is also an emphasis on systematic methods in collecting data to include process and outcome evaluations (Parker et al., 2011).

■ Purpose

Program evaluation may be comprehensive or directed at specific aspects of a program. There are many different types of evaluations and reasons to conduct program evaluation, such as effectiveness, accreditation, outcomes, impact, cost/benefit analysis, needs assessment, and research to provide empirical support (Haji et al., 2013). In addition, program evaluation can be used to demonstrate program effectiveness if the program has been funded and may be used to request additional funding. It is a valuable way to record the program's accomplishments. Most importantly, it is an opportunity to honestly consider ways to improve the implementation (process) and the effectiveness (outcome) of the program.

Data can be collected from an educational program to determine a program's worth and the success of its graduates (Bell, Pestka, & Forsyth, 2007). Chen (2005) stresses the role of evaluation in fostering program improvement via three steps: (1) systematic identification of stakeholder needs, (2) selection of evaluation options suited to those needs, and (3) putting the selected approach(es) into action. Inexpensive methods to collect information for a program evaluation include questionnaires, surveys, and checklists, which can be anonymous and provide a large amount of data. Interviews can elicit more information than questionnaires, surveys, and checklists and allow the interviewer to validate statements, but they take more time and are more costly due to the personnel needed. Focus groups, usually audiotaped, can yield rich narratives from groups of 4 to 12 participants; however, a skilled moderator is needed to lead each group. Transcribing and analyzing the tapes may be cost-prohibitive. Case studies fully depicting participants' experiences can be used to showcase the program, but are time consuming to develop. Qualitative methods to capture formative and summative evaluation data include portfolios and capstone assessments.

■ Benefits

There are many benefits to conducting program evaluation—both to the members of the program and to outside stakeholders such as administrators, accreditation boards, and grant funders. The members of the program benefit by gaining self-understanding and self-accountability and having a way to show the accomplishments of the program. Also, knowledge gained shows program strengths and identifies ineffective practices, which can be helpful to program faculty and staff. In academic health-related programs and other programs, administrators such as deans, provosts, and presidents are keenly interested in the success of the university's programs, as this success leads to credibility and visibility. The primary purpose of evaluation is to provide stakeholders with data for decision making regarding program improvement and measurement of outcomes. We view this process as an appraisal of the program's quality. The data collected in a program evaluation can also be used for strategic planning and can substantiate requests for increased resources by demonstrating need and/or providing evidence of effectiveness. Educational researchers also hope to gain information for curricular design to inform the work of others as to best practices (Haji et al., 2013).

■ Conceptual Models

Organizational Model

Using an organizational model helps ensure that the evaluation plan is comprehensive and provides an organizing framework (Suhayda & Miller, 2006). The Context, Inputs, Process and Product (CIPP) Model (Stufflebeam, 1983) is an effective and widely used model for organizing the program evaluation process. The CIPP Model emphasizes both evaluation for program improvement (formative) and evaluation to assess program quality (summative). Formative evaluation is conducted while the program is operating and the student is progressing through the curriculum. It examines program processes, policies, and the curriculum. Evaluators look at periodic reports and make decisions. Summative evaluation takes place after the student has completed the program. It asks questions such as: Did the student achieve the expected competencies? How well were the outcomes achieved? (Lewallen, 2015; Story et al., 2010).

With the CIPP Model, data can be triangulated through multiple methodologies of data collection. It easily incorporates various criteria and outcomes required by accreditation bodies. For example, the "Context" component allows one to look at relevant mission and appropriate stakeholders. The "Input" component evaluates human, fiscal, and physical resources. "Process" examines the curriculum and policies, while "Product" evaluates the outcomes such as licensure and certification pass rates, job placement, achievement of professional competencies expected of graduates, and accomplishments of the faculty (Singh, 2004). The program evaluation plan should identify each component to be evaluated using the CIPP Model, ask relevant questions to be investigated, identify sources of data and methods to collect the information to be analyzed, assign responsibility to specific persons to carry out the assessment, and set the frequency for collection and review. Once the data are analyzed and reviewed over time, the faculty can make evidence-based decisions to improve the quality of the program.

Accreditation Model

Accreditation for healthcare programs is usually developed through a nongovernmental accrediting agency set up through the board of directors of a specific national professional organization within a specialty profession such as medicine, nursing, physical therapy, dietetics, or other healthcare specialty. Each healthcare profession should have an accreditation process for educational programs that develop practitioners in its specialty. These educational programs are usually located within an institution of higher learning, although some healthcare agencies may provide programs in a specific profession, such as diploma nursing or radiography schools. There is a financial cost to the programs for the accreditation process and survey site visit.

The accreditation agency for the profession will develop standards, guidelines, and requirements that the program will have to meet to achieve accreditation for undergraduate and graduate programs in a specific profession. Accreditation may be granted for a specific number of years (up to 10 years), depending on the accrediting agency's standards and policies. New programs receiving accreditation for the first time may have a shorter accreditation time frame; or, if a program does not fully meet the criteria, the agency may require an earlier review.

An example of a comprehensive program evaluation in nursing is an accreditation review and site visit by peer evaluators. One such accrediting agency is the Commission on Collegiate Nursing Education (CCNE). The CCNE was developed by the American Association of Colleges of Nursing (AACN) to improve the existing accreditation process for baccalaureate and graduate nursing programs. The AACN developed a task force to explore the issue of developing an accrediting agency, and the CCNE program was developed and approved by the AACN membership in 1997 (CCNE, 2008). The CCNE was established as an autonomous agency contributing to the improvement of the public's health and does not report to the AACN, so conflict of interest is not an issue. The program was developed to ensure the quality and integrity of baccalaureate, graduate, and residency programs in nursing and serves the public interest by assessing and identifying programs that engage in effective educational practices. The CCNE accreditation is a nongovernmental peer review process that operates in accordance with nationally recognized standards established for the practice of accreditation in the United States (CCNE, 2008, 2013).

An educational organization applies to the CCNE for initial accreditation of existing and new programs. Nursing programs with continuing accreditation are notified of the dates of an on-site visit and the process for reaccreditation about a year before the accreditation is due to expire. The accreditation process and site visit provide a nursing program the opportunity to conduct its own program evaluation using the CCNE's four standards and key elements of each standard. Standards I–III relate to program quality of the mission and governance, institutional commitment and resources, and curriculum and teaching–learning practices; Standard IV is focused on program effectiveness with aggregate student and faculty outcomes (CCNE, 2013).

The nursing program must develop a system to collect data related to the standards and prepare an analytical self-study report. Program faculty should be actively involved in collecting data and developing the report. The university administration also is involved in collecting administrative and financial data relating to the program. Documentation is a critical part of the program evaluation process. Faculty meeting minutes are helpful to document discussion of data and resultant decisions for program improvement that were made. This is an ongoing documentation of the process over time (Lewallen, 2015).

CCNE peer evaluators read the program's self-study report and visit the campus to validate what is contained in the report. During the visit to the institution, the site visitors meet with university and program administrators, faculty, students, and community agencies that employ graduates. At the end of the visit, they hold an open forum to discuss their preliminary findings of standards that appear to be met, as well as noting areas that may require some improvement. The evaluators do not make recommendations about accreditation, but rather prepare a report describing the results of their visit and send it to the CCNE, which in turn forwards the final report to the chief nurse administrator of the program. The chief nurse administrator has an opportunity to respond to the report in writing. This response may include additional data that were not available at the time of the site visit and what was done to respond to suggestions for improvement. The program's self-study report, the evaluators' report and response, and third-party comments are forwarded to the CCNE Accreditation Review Committee. That group reviews all materials and makes a confidential recommendation to the CCNE board of commissioners regarding accreditation. It is the board of commissioners that makes the final accreditation decisions.

Many aspects of a quality nursing program are addressed in the CCNE accreditation review process, such as mission, goals, student and faculty expectations and outcomes, student and faculty governance, institution support and resources, curriculum and teaching–learning practices, and program effectiveness based on aggregate data. Ongoing evaluation of these components of an educational program assists in program improvement and effectiveness. For example, ongoing review of teaching–learning practices gives the program the opportunity to self-reflect on its teaching strategies and student learning in the classroom, clinical setting, and online instruction. Research studies to develop evidence for effective teaching strategies and student learning can enhance program effectiveness. Any empirical data developed by a program provide strong evidence for accreditation review. Additionally, programs are required by CCNE to submit evidence to support the ongoing comprehensive program review process via a "Continuous Improvement Progress Report" at the midpoint of the 10-year accreditation cycle (Ellis & Hallstead, 2012).

■ Evaluation Research

Evaluation research provides empirical findings that can strengthen the value of selected programs and determine how they are working. It can provide stakeholders with knowledge about a program's intended outcomes, as well as the educational processes employed (Parker et al., 2011). Evaluation research can focus on the entire program or specific aspects of a program. More than one part of the program may be evaluated, such as the process or implementation, outcome, impact, or cost analysis (Polit & Beck, 2012). Currently, evaluating program outcomes is a major emphasis expected of educational programs by accrediting bodies. Different quantitative and qualitative research methodologies can be used when assessing program outcomes, such as surveys, pretest-posttest designs, and qualitative methods, such as 1:1 exit interviews, focus groups, capstone projects, external evaluation, and portfolios. Examples of the use of different methodologies in diverse program evaluations are provided here.

Survey

Survey research is a method commonly used in social science research to collect data. Surveys have been used in evaluation research for many years. The advantages of surveys include their flexibility, broad scope, and ability to focus on diverse topics (Polit & Beck, 2012). Surveys can be used to obtain data through personal interviews, questionnaires, and telephone interviews. They are frequently used when one needs to reach a large audience. Web-based surveys have become increasingly popular in today's landscape due to the relative convenience of distribution and ease of use. Pen-and-paper surveys are becoming increasingly inefficient due to being viewed as outdated by today's graduates, resulting in a poor response rate. One educational program found that moving to online alumni surveys increased the response rate from near zero to 52% (Story et al., 2010).

A program evaluation was conducted using questionnaires to determine nursing school instruction and students' perceived competence to empathetically communicate with patients (McMillan & Shannon, 2011). Six hundred nursing students from 14 nursing programs completed this *Nursing Student Empathic Communication Questionnaire,* using a five-point Likert scale. As the questionnaire was used for the first time, there was no prior reliability coefficients report; however, in this population, the Cronbach's alpha for subscales ranged from 0.63 to 0.83. The results drove changes in the program, including practical steps to enhance classroom and clinical pedagogy, such as providing situations that foster empathetic communication development, improving teaching methods, and providing evidence-based studies showing the relationship between empathetic communications in improving patient outcomes.

Story et al. (2010) used survey research with a Likert scale to have external evaluators (preceptors) assess student achievement of the CCNE *BSN Essentials* as a basis for program evaluation. Morris and Hancock (2013) used the Institute of Medicine's 2003 core competencies to evaluate a program's curriculum by both students and faculty.

Another program evaluation study—focusing on a transplantation specialty pharmacy (TSP) program—utilized surveys to determine the impact on patients' and healthcare providers' satisfaction, identified outcomes, and cost margin (Hlubocky, Stuckey, Schuman, & Stevenson, 2012). In addition, data were collected related to medication adherence and hospital readmission within 90 days of the surgery. There was an almost 35% response rate ($n = 290$) from the surveys. The results were favorable for patients' and healthcare providers' satisfaction, continuity of care, and a substantial cost margin. These empirical findings supported the use of the TSP program at this institution.

Pretest-Posttest Design

The pretest-posttest design involves the collection of data prior to an intervention and then again after the intervention. With this design, researchers can determine which changes occurred and see if any statistical significance was found in a quantitative study (Polit & Beck, 2012).

An evaluation study was conducted in a bachelor of nursing program in Australia to determine whether a structured learning program influenced student anxiety and efficacy (Watt, Murphy, Pascoe, Scanlon, & Gan, 2011). A pretest-posttest design was used to study three cohorts of students ($n = 118$), who completed questionnaires before and after participating in a structured learning program. There were statistically significant results in the scores on the posttest, with anxiety being decreased and efficacy being increased. This study supported the implementation of a structured learning program at this school.

Focus Groups

Focus groups are held to obtain perceptions about an area of interest. Their size may vary from 4 to 12 depending on the sensitivity of the discussion and the number of participants available. This method enables a researcher to take advantage of the participants' discussion to collect more in-depth data (Doody, Slevin, & Taggart, 2013). Evaluators then engage in a methodic process to determine recurring themes emerging from the interviews. This information is then summarized and reported.

An evaluation study of a mentoring program designed to increase the diversity of the nursing workforce was conducted using focus groups. The purpose was to determine the effectiveness of a formal mentoring program entitled "Preparing the

Next Generation of Nurses Mentoring Program" (Wilson, Sanner, & McAllister, 2010). The program paired at-risk nursing students (mentees) with a faculty mentor. Focus groups were conducted annually over a 3-year period separately among mentors and mentees. Themes flowing from the discussions described faculty and student perceptions of the overall program and both groups' perceptions of a good mentor and mentee. The findings were helpful and in part refined the role of a faculty mentor and showed how to overcome some of the challenges, including scheduling conflicts.

Both surveys and focus groups were used in evaluating teams of interdisciplinary staff in an interprofessional education program (Bajnok, Puddester, MacDonald, Archibald, & Kuhl, 2012). The purpose was to determine whether interprofessional team development made a difference in team functioning, satisfaction, and improved patient well-being. The overall goals of the education project were met, including a positive reaction to the learning experience, an increased awareness of the roles and responsibilities of other healthcare providers, participants' ability to transfer their learning to the workplace, and greater collaboration in care decision making.

Case Studies

Case studies are in-depth descriptions of selected phenomena including an individual, group, or social unit. Data collection may relate to a present state or other factors related to the subject of interest (Polit & Beck, 2012).

Researchers used a qualitative, cross-case analysis to describe evaluation systems related to comprehensive developmental school counseling (CDSC) programs in two states, Missouri and Utah (Martin & Carey, 2012). Results of the study provided in-depth descriptions of the evaluation programs and the differences in each state's approach. Lessons learned included the importance of building the capacity of school counselors to evaluate their own programs with state leadership. The authors suggest that one advantage for state leaders is that a systematic state evaluation program can be used to advocate for the necessity of school counseling in the educational system.

Portfolios

Portfolios can be used for both formative and summative evaluation. They usually contain a collection of student work across the curriculum intended to demonstrate achievement of competencies. They are individual snapshots that reflect the breadth and depth of student attainment of program outcomes (Haverkamp & Vogt, 2015). In Haverkamp and Vogt's (2015) study, Doctor of Nursing Practice (DNP) students developed and submitted e-portfolios with at least one assignment per course to demonstrate growth and development of the core competencies reflected in the *Essentials of Doctoral Education for Advanced Nursing Practice* (AACN, 2006). The faculty used the portfolios to organize and categorize outcomes related to these program outcomes. They found that the e-portfolios demonstrated this growth and reflected each student's learning journey through the curriculum.

One-on-One Interviews

One-on-one or face-to-face interviews are a qualitative summative assessment technique to help the program's faculty understand why the program is or is not working. Parker et al. (2011) conducted face-to-face interviews with all graduates and noncompleters as they left the program. The interview data were summarized and analyzed for recurring themes. They also involved employers and their advisory committee in examining the data and interpreting the implications. As O'Sullivan (2012) points out, collaborative evaluation should involve stakeholders to help interpret the data. This information is then shared with faculty for informed programmatic improvement decision making.

■ Conclusion

This chapter addressed program evaluation and its importance for improving and maintaining high-quality nursing and other healthcare programs. The purposes and benefits of program evaluation were discussed and the term defined. The CIPP Model was described as a common organizing framework employed for continuous monitoring. The role of accreditation in identifying effective nursing programs was discussed using the standards and key elements of the CCNE. Examples of program evaluation research studies were presented, including the effect of a nursing school instructional program on students' perceived competence to empathetically communicate with patients, a structured nursing program to reduce student anxiety and increase efficacy, a nursing mentoring program for at-risk nursing students, and the assessment of DNP students' attainment of the CCNE *Essentials of Doctoral Education for Advanced Nursing Practice*. Additional studies presented were from other disciplines: an evaluation of a transplantation specialty pharmacy program, the effectiveness of interprofessional teams in the practice setting, and the evaluation of capacity with state-level school counseling programs. Examples of qualitative research methods for formative and summative evaluation were also presented. Using data from program evaluation can be useful in better understanding a program, and it can provide insights into necessary changes for improvement. Also, research evaluations provide empirical data to support needed changes in specified programs.

Discussion Questions

1. How can your program's terminal student objectives/competencies be translated into measureable outcomes that can be assessed as part of program evaluation?
2. Using the CIPP Model, identify one major evaluation question that is relevant to your educational program evaluation that can be asked for each of the four main components of the model. What indicators and corresponding data would you select to measure for each?
3. Describe examples of formative and summative evaluation research methods that would be a good match for each of the components you identified in question 2.

References

American Association of Colleges of Nursing (AACN). (2006). *Essentials of doctoral education for advanced practice nursing.* Washington, DC: Author.

Bajnok, I., Puddester, D., MacDonald, C. J., Archibald, D., & Kuhl, D. (2012). Building positive relationships in healthcare: Evaluation of the teams of interprofessional staff interprofessional education program. *Contemporary Nurse, 42*(1), 77–89.

Bell, D. F., Pestka, E., & Forsyth, D. (2007). Outcome evaluation: Does continuing education make a difference? *Journal of Continuing Education, 38*(4), 186–190.

Chen, H. (2005). *Practical program evaluation: Assessing and improving planning, implementation, and effectiveness.* London, UK: Sage.

Commission on Collegiate Nursing Education (CCNE). (2008). *Achieving excellence in accreditation.* Washington, DC: Author. Retrieved from http://www.aacn.nche.edu/ccne-accreditation/about /mission-values-history

Commission on Collegiate Nursing Education (CCNE). (2013). *Standards for accreditation of baccalaureate and graduate nursing programs.* Washington, DC: Author.

Davidson, E. J. (2005). *Evaluation methodology basics: The nuts and bolts of sound evaluation.* Thousand Oaks, CA: Sage.

Doody, O., Slevin, E., & Taggart, L. (2013). Focus group interviews in nursing research: Part 1. *British Journal of Nursing, 22*(1), 16–19.

Ellis, P., & Hallstead, J. (2012). Understanding the Commission on Collegiate Nursing Education accreditation process and the role of the continuous improvement progress report. *Journal of Professional Nursing, 28*(1), 18–26.

Fink, A. (2005). *Evaluation fundamentals: Insights into the outcomes, effectiveness, and quality of health programs.* London, UK: Sage.

Haji, F., Morin, M., & Parker, K. (2013). Rethinking programme evaluation in health professions education: Beyond "did it work?" *Medical Education, 47*(4), 342–351.

Haleem, D. M., Evanina, K., Gallagher, R., Golden, M. A., Healy-Karabell, K., & Manetti, W. (2010). Program evaluation: How faculty addressed concerns about the nursing program. *Nurse Educator, 35*(3), 118–121.

Haverkamp, J., & Vogt, M. (2015). Beyond academic evidence: Innovative uses of technology within e-portfolios in a doctor of nursing practice program. *Journal of Professional Nursing, 31*(4), 284–289.

Hlubocky, J. M., Stuckey, L. J., Schuman, A. D., & Stevenson, J. G. (2012). Evaluation of a transplantation specialty pharmacy program. *American Journal of Health-System Pharmacy, 69*, 340–347. doi:10.2146 /ajhp110350

Lewallen, L. P. (2015). Practical strategies for nursing education program evaluation. *Journal of Professional Nursing, 31*(2), 133–140.

Martin, J., & Carey, J. C. (2012). Evaluation capacity within state-level school counseling programs: A cross-case analysis. *Professional School Counseling, 15*(3), 132–143.

McMillan, L. R., & Shannon, D. (2011). Program evaluation of nursing school instruction in measuring students' perceived competence to empathetically communicate with patients. *Nursing Education Perspectives, 32*(3), 150–154.

McNamara, C. (2006). *Field guide to nonprofit program design, marketing and evaluation.* Minneapolis, MN: Authenticity Consulting.

Mertz, A. J. (2007). *Why conduct a program evaluation? Five reasons why evaluation can help an out-of-school time program* (Publication #2007-31). Washington, DC: Child Trends.

Morris, T. L., & Hancock, D. R. (2013). Institute of Medicine core competencies as a foundation for nursing program evaluation. *Nursing Education Perspectives, 34*(1), 29–33.

O'Sullivan, R. G. (2012). Collaborative evaluation within a framework of stakeholder-oriented evaluation approaches. *Evaluation and Program Planning, 35*(4), 518–522.

Parker, K. P., Burrows, G., Nash, H., & Rosenblum, N. D. (2011). Going beyond Kirkpatrick in evaluating a clinician scientist program: It's not "if it works" but "how it works." *Academic Medicine, 86*(11), 1389–1396.

Polit, D. F., & Beck, C. T. (2012). *Nursing research: Generating and assessing evidence for nursing practice* (9th ed.). Philadelphia, PA: Wolters Kluwer/Lippincott Williams & Wilkins.

Sauter, M. K., Gillespie, N. N., & Knepp, A. (2012). Educational program evaluation. In D. M. Billings & J. A. Hallstead (Eds.), *Teaching in nursing: A guide for faculty* (pp. 503–549). St. Louis, MO: Elsevier.

Singh, M. D. (2004). Evaluation framework for nursing education programs: Application of the CIPP model. *International Journal of Nursing Education Scholarship, 1*(1), Article 13. doi:10.2202/1548-923X.1023

Story, L., Butts, J. B., Bishop, S. B., Green, L., Johnson, K., & Mattison, H. (2010). Innovative strategies for nursing education program evaluation. *Journal of Nursing Education, 49*(6), 351–354. doi:10-3928/01484834-20100217-07

Stufflebeam, D. L. (1983). The CIPP model for program evaluation. In G. Madaus, M. Scriven, & D. Stufflebeam (Eds.), *Evaluation models: Viewpoints on educational and human services evaluation* (pp. 117–141). Boston, MA: Kluwer-Nijoff.

Stufflebeam, D. L., & Shinkfield, A. J. (2007). *Evaluation theory, models, and applications*. San Francisco, CA: Jossey-Bass.

Suhayda, R., & Miller, J. M. (2006). Optimizing evaluation of nursing education programs. *Nurse Educator, 31*(5), 200–206.

Tyler, R. W. (1949). *Basic principles of curriculum and instruction*. Chicago, IL: University of Chicago Press.

Watt, E., Murphy, M., Pascoe, E., Scanlon, A., & Gan, S. (2011). An evaluation of a structured learning programme as a component of the clinical practicum in final year bachelor of nursing programme: A pre-post-test analysis. *Journal of Clinical Nursing, 20*, 2286–2293. doi:10.1111/j.1365-2702.2010.0362

Wilson, A. H., Sanner, S., & McAllister, L. E. (2010). An evaluation study of a mentoring program to increase the diversity of the nursing workforce. *Journal of Cultural Diversity, 17*(4), 144–150.

Index

Note: Page numbers followed by *b*, *f*, or *t* indicate material in boxes, figures, or tables, respectively.